Medications and Mothers' Milk

A Manual of Lactational Pharmacology

Medications and Mothers' Milk

Eleventh Edition

Thomas W. Hale, R.Ph., Ph.D.
Professor of Pediatrics
Texas Tech University
School of Medicine
Amarillo, Texas 79106-1708

Pharmasoft Publishing

Medications and Mothers' Milk

Eleventh Edition

© Copyright 1992-2004

Pharmasoft Publishing L.P.

1712 North Forest

Amarillo, TX 79106-7017

(806)-376-9900

(800)-378-1317

DISCLAIMER

ISBN 0-9636219-8-X
RJ216 .H25 1995
96-143153

Ordering Information

Pharmasoft Publishing L.P.

1712 N. Forest

Amarillo, Texas, USA 79106

8:00 AM to 5:00 PM CST

Call......   806-376-9900

Sales.....   800-378-1317

FAX......   806-376-9901

http://www.iBreastfeeding.com

Common Abbreviations

ACEi	Angiotensin converting enzyme inhibitor
AUC	Area under the Curve
BID	Twice daily
Cmax	Plasma or milk concentration at peak
MAOI	Monoamine oxidase inhibitors
μCi	Microcurie of Radioactivity
μg/L	Microgram per liter
μmol	Micromole of weight
mg/L	Milligram per liter
mL	Milliliter. One cc
mmol	Millimole of weight
M/P	Milk/Plasma Ratio
MW	Molecular Weight
ng/L	Nanogram per liter
NSAIDs	Non-steroidal anti-inflammatory
Oral=	Oral bioavailability (adult)
PB=	Percent of protein binding in maternal circulation
PHL=	Pediatric elimination half-life
pKa	pH
PRN	As needed
q	Every
QD	Daily
QID	Four times daily
RID	Relative Infant Dose
T½=	Adult elimination half-life
TID	Three times daily
Tmax	Time to peak plasma level (PK)
Vd	Volume of Distribution
X	Times

Preface

New data continues to be published almost monthly which supports that human milk is the finest source of nutrition for human infants. During the first week postnatally, human milk is filled with immunoglobulins (IgG, IgA, and IgM), interferons, and other antibacterial substances which results in colonization of the GI tract of the newborn with benign bacterial flora. The presence of numerous growth factors(IgF-1), cytokines, and gastric hormones enhance development of protective barriers in the GI tract and stimulate elimination of meconium present during gestation. Other key benefits to the infant include perfect nutrition, enhanced neurocognitive development, stronger immune function, and at least a three fold reduction in infectious disease such as upper respiratory infections, otitis media, and necrotizing enterocolitis.

Although recent studies have suggested that the number of women who choose to breastfeed their infant is presently 72% and rising in the USA, the number of women who discontinue breastfeeding in order to take a medication is still significant. Surveys in many countries indicate that 90-99% of women who breastfeed will receive at least some medication during the first week postpartum. Other studies suggest that the use of medications is one of the major reasons women discontinue breastfeeding prematurely. The most frequently used drugs include analgesics, hypnotics, and methylergometrine.

Because so many women ingest medications during the early neonatal period, it is not surprising that one of the most common questions encountered in pediatrics is concerning the use of various drugs during lactation. Unfortunately, most physicians simply review the package insert, or advise the mother to not breastfeed without having done a thorough study of the literature to find the true answer. Discontinuing breastfeeding is often the wrong decision and most mothers could easily continue to breastfeed their infants and take the medication without risk to the infant.

In the past 20 years, a large number of studies have been published providing a better understanding of the kinetics of drug entry into human milk. Most of the physiocochemical properties that facilitate transfer (molecular weight, pKa, lipophilicity) are well known but ultimately the degree of transfer of the medication must be determined in humans. Rodent studies are virtually worthless as the albumin content in rodent milk is many times higher than in humans. This may account for the fact that most of the rodent studies show milk levels that are many times too high and simply do not correlate with human studies.

Benefits to breastfeeding women are significant and include a major reduction in bone loss in later life, and a reduction in the incidence of breast and ovarian cancer. Other benefits include enhanced weight loss, reduced blood loss postpartum, and a more desirable inter-pregnancy interval.

The publication several years ago by the American Academy of Pediatrics recommending at least one year of breastfeeding was a major step in acceptance by a major medical body that breastfeeding is immunologically and nutritionally the best way to feed infants. The Academy, provided with evidence by numerous publications that breastfed infants are not only healthier but may also gain in developmental skills as well, finally felt that the evidence was overwhelming and justified a stronger stance by this large body of pediatricians. Due to enormous support for breastfeeding in the medical community, many mothers are now resistant to discontinuing breastfeeding just to take a medication, particularly if the interruption is based solely on the recommendation of their physician. Although interrupting breastfeeding may appear safest to the physician, it is simply not necessary in most cases as the amount of drug transferred to milk is normally quite small.

We all know that most medications penetrate milk to some degree. However, the amount transferred into human milk is generally low. With only a few exceptions, the dose of the medication transferred to the infant via milk is generally far subclinical. It is ultimately the clinician's responsibility to review the documentation available before coming to a decision as to breastfeeding. There are almost always other medications that could be substituted that are safe for both mother and infant.

> *The pharmaceutical manufacturer's resistance to using medications in breastfeeding mothers is almost always based on legal reasons not clinical reasons.*

Because the PDR basically lists only the pharmaceutical's package insert, the standard recommendation is to not take the medication while breastfeeding. The PDR is the poorest source for obtaining accurate breastfeeding information.

The amount of drug excreted into milk depends on the following factors:

> **Drugs transfer into human milk if they :**
>
> - Are highly lipid soluble.
> - Attain high concentrations in maternal plasma.
> - Are low in molecular weight (< 500).
> - Are low in protein binding.
> - Pass into the brain easily.

However, once medications are transferred into human milk then other kinetic factors are involved. One of the most important is the oral bioavailability of the medication to the infant. Numerous medications are either destroyed in the infant's gut, fail to be absorbed through the gut wall, or are rapidly picked up by the liver. Once in the liver, they are either metabolized or stored.

Drugs enter milk primarily by diffusion driven by equilibrium forces between the maternal plasma compartment and the maternal milk compartment. They pass from the maternal plasma through capillary walls into the alveolar cell lining the alveolus. Medications must generally pass through both lipid membranes of the alveolar cell to penetrate milk; although, early on they may pass between the alveolar cells (first 72 hours postpartum). During the first three days of life, large gaps between alveolar cells exist. These gaps permit enhanced access for most drugs, many immunoglobulins, maternal living cells (lymphocytes, leukocytes, macrophages), and other maternal proteins to the milk. By the end of the first week, the alveolar cells swell under the influence of prolactin; subsequently closing the intracellular spaces and reducing the intracellular entry of most maternal drugs, proteins, and other substances to the milk compartment. It is generally agreed that medications penetrate into milk more during the colostral period than in mature milk. However, the absolute dose transferred during the colostral period is still low as the total volume of milk is generally less than 30-100 mL total volume/day.

In most instances, the most important determinant of drug penetration into milk is the mother's plasma level. Almost without exception, as the level of the medication in the mother's plasma rises, the concentration in milk increases as well. Drugs enter milk and exit milk as a function of the mother's plasma level. As soon as the maternal plasma level of a medication begins to fall, equilibrium forces drive the medication out of the milk compartment back into the maternal plasma for elimination. In some instances, drugs are trapped in milk (ion trapped). This means that due to the lower pH of human milk (7.0-7.2) the ionic state of the drug changes and prevents its exit back into the maternal circulation. This is important in weakly basic drugs such as the barbiturates. With the iodides, such as ^{131}I or any ionic form of iodine, the drug may concentrate in milk due to a pumping system on the alveolar cell wall. Thus iodides, particularly radioactive ones, should be avoided as their milk concentrations are exceedingly high.

Two other physicochemical factors are important in evaluating drugs in breastfeeding mothers. These are the degree of protein binding and lipid solubility. Drugs that are very lipid soluble penetrate into milk in higher concentrations almost without exception. Of particular interest are the drugs that are active in the central nervous system (CNS). CNS-active drugs invariably have the unique characteristic requisite to enter milk. Therefore, if a drug is active in the central nervous system, higher levels in milk can be expected; although, they still are often subclinical. Many of the neuroactive drugs produce Relative Infant Doses of >5%. Protein binding also plays an important role. Drugs circulate in the maternal plasma either bound to albumin or freely soluble in the plasma. It is the free component (unbound) that transfers into milk while the bound fraction stays in the maternal circulation. Therefore, drugs that have high maternal protein binding (warfarin) have reduced milk levels simply because they are excluded from the milk compartment.

First Four Days Postpartum

Maternal Capillary

After 14 Days Postpartum

Once a drug has entered the mother's milk and has been ingested by the infant, it must traverse through the infant's GI tract prior to absorption. Some drugs are poorly stable in this environment due to the proteolytic enzymes and acids. In general, the infant's stomach is quite acidic and the acidity can denature many drugs. This includes the aminoglycoside family, Omeprazole, and large peptide drugs such as Heparin or Insulin. Other drugs are simply poorly absorbed by the gastrointestinal tract, and are poorly absorbed into the infant's blood stream. Oral bioavailability is a useful tool to estimate just how much of the drug will be absorbed by the infant. In addition, many drugs are sequestered in the liver (first pass) and may never actually reach the plasma compartment where they are active. Such absorption characteristics tend ultimately to reduce the overall effect of many drugs. There are certainly exceptions to this rule and one must always be aware that the action of a drug in the GI tract can also be profound producing diarrhea, constipation, and occasionally syndromes such as pseudomembranous colitis.

One of the more popular methods for estimating risk is to determine the Relative Infant Dose (RID). The RID is calculated by dividing the infant's dose via milk (mg/kg/day) by the mothers dose in mg/kg/day. The RID gives the clinician a feeling for just how much medication the infant is exposed to on a weight-normalized basis. However, many authors calculate the infant dose without normalizing for maternal and infant weight so be cautious.

Key Points About Breastfeeding and Medications

- Avoid using medications where possible. Herbal drugs, high dose vitamins, unusual supplements, etc. are simply not necessary; recommend avoiding the risk.
- If the Relative Infant Dose is less than 10%, most medications are quite safe to use. The RID of the vast majority of drugs is < 1%.
- Choose drugs for which we have published data rather than those recently introduced.
- Evaluate the infant for risks. Be slightly more cautious with premature infants or neonates. Be less concerned about older infants.
- Observe breastfeeding mothers for depression as the incidence is high.
- Recommend antidepressants in depressed breastfeeding mothers. The risks of a depressed mother to the infant are simply too high.
- Most drugs are quite safe in breastfeeding mothers while the risks of not breastfeeding and of using infant formulas are much higher for the infant.
- Discontinuing breastfeeding for some hours/days may be required particularly with radioactive compounds.
- Choose drugs with short half-lives, high protein binding, low oral bioavailability, or high molecular weight.

Adapted from Hale TW, Ilett KF. Drug Therapy and Breastfeeding: From Theory to Clinical Practice, First Edition ed. London: Parthenon Publishing; 2002.

Lastly, it is extremely important to always evaluate the infant's ability to handle small amounts of medications. Some infants, such as premature or ill infants, may not be suitable candidates for certain medications. But remember that early postpartum the amount of milk produced is so low that the clinical dose of drug transferred is often low. So even in premature neonates, the dose is still probably low because of the limited amount of milk used in these infants.

Evaluation of the Infant

- **Inquire about the infant** - Always inquire as to the infant's age, size, and stability. It's an important criteria before using medications in breastfeeding mothers.
- **Infant age** - premature and newborn infants are at somewhat greater risk.
- **Infant stability** - unstable infants with poor GI stability may increase the risk of using medications.
- **Pediatric Approved Drugs** - generally are less hazardous if long-term history of safety is recognized.
- **Dose** - in a premature infant various doses may be more risky than in a 1 year old healthy infant.
- **Drugs that alter milk production** - may be much more risky during the neonatal period than after the milk supply is well established.

General Suggestions for the Clinician

1.   Determine if the drug is absorbed from the GI tract. Many drugs such as the aminoglycosides, vancomycin, cephalosporin antibiotics (third generation), morphine, magnesium salts, and large protein drugs (heparin) are so poorly absorbed that it is unlikely the infant will absorb significant quantities. At the same time, observe for GI side effects from the medication trapped in the GI compartment of the infant (e.g. diarrhea).

2.   Review the monograph provided herein on the drug. Review the theoretical infant dose and the relative infant dose (RID) and compare that to the pediatric dose if known. Remember, most of the Theoretic Infant Doses were derived from the C_{max} (highest milk concentration of the drug) that is published. Unfortunately, the milk/plasma ratio is virtually worthless information unless you know the maternal plasma level. It does not provide the user with information as to the absolute amount of drug transferred to the infant via milk. Even if the drug has a high

milk/plasma ratio, if the maternal plasma level of the medication is very small (such as with propranolol), then the absolute amount (dose) of a drug entering milk will still be quite small and often subclinical.

3.   Try to choose shorter half-life drugs as they generally peak rapidly and then are eliminated from the maternal plasma thus exposing the milk compartment (and the infant) to reduced levels of medication. Urge the mother not to breastfeed while the drug is at it's peak level in the maternal plasma. Determine the time-to-peak interval as this will indicate how long the mother must wait before feeding. However, you must first determine the dosage form administered. If the tablet formulation is a prolonged release form, then all prior assumptions about half-life are pointless and you must assume that the drug has a long half-life (12-24 hours). Unfortunately, avoiding peaks early postpartum is simply not very practical and drugs with low milk levels should be chosen.

4.   Be cautious of drugs (or their active metabolites) that have long pediatric half-lives as they can continually build up in the infant's plasma over time. The barbiturates, benzodiazepines, meperidine, and fluoxetine are classic examples where higher levels in the infant can and do occasionally occur.

5.   If you are provided a choice, choose drugs that have higher protein binding because they are more often sequestered in the maternal circulation and do not transfer as readily to the milk or the infant. Remember, it's the free drug that transfers into the milk compartment. Without doubt, the most important parameter that determines drug penetration into milk is plasma protein binding. Choose drugs with high protein binding.

6.   Although not always true, I have generally found neuroleptic drugs frequently penetrate milk in higher levels simply due to their physicochemistry. If the drug in question produces sedation, depression, or other neuroleptic effects in the mother, it is likely to penetrate the milk and may produce similar effects in the infant. Sedative drugs (particularly phenothiazines) may contribute to an elevated risk of SIDS; although, this is poorly documented.

7.   Be cautious of herbal drugs as many contain chemical substances that may be dangerous to the infant. Numerous poisonings have been reported. Prior to using, advise the mother to contact a lactation consultant or herbalist who is knowledgeable about their use in breastfeeding mothers. Do not exceed standard recommended doses. Try to use pure forms not large mixtures of unknown herbals. Do not overdose. Use only minimal amounts.

8.   With radioactive compounds, check the NRC table in the index of this volume. The NRC recommendations are quite good. They can be

copied and provided to your radiologist. They are available from the Nuclear Regulatory Commission's web page address in the appendix. Also, I've included a number of new tables in the appendix on radioisotopes and radioactive procedures.

9.   Use the **Theoretic Infant Dose** to estimate the maximum dose the infant would receive per kilogram per day. This data is derived from the literature and is a close estimate of the peak amount an infant would receive. Another very useful evaluation of the dose is to determine the **Relative Infant Dose.** The box below shows the calculation. In general, a Relative infant dose of < 10% is considered safe and its use is becoming increasingly popular by numerous investigators. But you will still find many useful drugs may approach 20% RID (metronidazole, fluconazole, etc.). Because they are incredibly safe medications, they are still quite useful in breastfeeding mothers. Remember the RID is only a guideline; certain safer medications simply don't fall within this rule.

$$ RID = \frac{Dose.infant\left(\dfrac{mg/kg}{d}\right)}{Dose.mother\left(\dfrac{mg/kg}{d}\right)} $$

Dose.infant   = dose in infant
Dose.mother = dose in mother

10.   Hence, it is important that the clinician evaluate all the risks of the drug in relationship to the absolute dose received by the infant and the ability of the infant to handle even that dose. It is no longer acceptable for the clinician to interrupt lactation merely because of heightened anxiety on their part. The risks of formula feeding are significant and should not be trivialized. There are few drugs that have well documented and significant toxicity in infants as a result of breastfeeding and we know most of these. At the same time, no medication should be used lightly in a breastfeeding mother.

The following review of drugs is a compilation of what has been published concerning the use of various medications in breastfeeding women. It is unfortunate that manufacturers are not required by law to provide breastfeeding data on all their products. This would make evaluation of using new products in breastfeeding women much easier.

THE AUTHOR MAKES NO RECOMMENDATIONS AS TO THE SAFETY OF THESE MEDICATIONS DURING LACTATION, BUT ONLY REVIEWS WHAT IS CURRENTLY PUBLISHED IN THE SCIENTIFIC LITERATURE. INDIVIDUAL USE OF MEDICATIONS MUST BE LEFT UP TO THE JUDGEMENT OF THE PHYSICIAN, THE PATIENT, AND OTHER HEALTHCARE CONSULTANTS.

Thomas W. Hale

How to Use this Book

This section of the book is designed to aid the reader in determining risk to an infant from maternal medications and in using the pharmacokinetic parameters throughout this reference.

Drug Name and Generic Name
Each monograph begins with the generic name (capitalized in index)of the drug. Several of the most common USA trade names are provided under the *Trade* section.

Can/Aus/UK:
Most, but not all, of the most common trade names used in Canada, Australia, and the United Kingdom are provided.

Uses:
This lists the general use of the medication such as penicillin antibiotic, or antiemetic, or analgesic, etc. Remember, many drugs have multiple uses in many syndromes. I have only listed the most common use.

AAP:
This entry lists the new recommendations provided by the American Academy of Pediatrics as published in their document, *The transfer of drugs and other chemicals into human milk* (Pediatrics. 2001 Sep;108(3):776-89.). Drugs are listed in tables according to the following recommendations: Cytotoxic drugs that may interfere with cellular metabolism of the nursing infant; Drugs of abuse for which adverse effects on the infant during breastfeeding have been reported; Radioactive compounds that require temporary cessation of breastfeeding; Drugs for which the effect on nursing infants is unknown but may be of concern; Drugs that have been associated with significant effects on some nursing infants and should be given to nursing mothers with caution; Maternal medication usually compatible with breastfeeding. In this book, the AAP recommendations have been paraphrased to reflect these recommendations. Because the AAP recommendations do not cover all drugs, "Not Reviewed" simply implies that the drug has not yet been reviewed by this committee. The author recommends that each user review these recommendations for further detail.

Drug Monograph
The drug monograph lists what we currently understand about the drug, its ability to enter milk, the concentration in milk at set time intervals, and other parameters that are important to a clinical consultant. I have reported only what the references have documented.

Pregnancy Risk Category:
Pregnancy risk categories have been assigned to almost all medications by their manufacturers and are based on the level of risk the drug poses to the fetus during gestation. They are not useful in assigning risk via breastfeeding. The FDA has provided these five categories to indicate the risk associated with the induction of birth defects. Unfortunately, they do not indicate the importance of when during gestation the medication is used since some drugs are more dangerous during certain trimesters of pregnancy. The definitions provided below are, however, a useful tool in determining the possible risks associated with using the medication during pregnancy. Some newer medications may not yet have pregnancy classifications and are therefore not provided herein.

Category A:
Controlled studies in women fail to demonstrate a risk to the fetus in the first trimester (and there is no evidence of a risk in later trimesters) and the possibility of fetal harm appears remote.

Category B:
Either animal-reproduction studies have not demonstrated a fetal risk but there are no controlled studies in pregnant women or animal-reproduction studies have shown an adverse effect (other than a decrease in fertility) that was not confirmed in controlled studies in women in the first trimester (and there is no evidence of a risk in later trimesters).

Category C:
Either studies in animals have revealed adverse effects on the fetus (teratogenic or embryocidal, or other) and there are no controlled studies in women, or studies in women and animals are not available. Drugs should be given only if the potential benefit justifies the potential risk to the fetus.

Category D:
There is positive evidence of human fetal risk but the benefits from use in pregnant women may be acceptable despite the risk (e.g., if the drug is needed in a life-threatening situation or for a serious disease for which safer drugs cannot be used or are ineffective).

Category X:
Studies in animals or human beings have demonstrated fetal abnormalities or there is evidence of fetal risk based on human experience, or both, and the risk of the use of the drug in pregnant women clearly outweighs any

possible benefit. The drug is contraindicated in women who are or may become pregnant.

Lactation Risk Category:

L1   SAFEST:
Drug which has been taken by a large number of breastfeeding mothers without any observed increase in adverse effects in the infant. Controlled studies in breastfeeding women fail to demonstrate a risk to the infant and the possibility of harm to the breastfeeding infant is remote or the product is not orally bioavailable in an infant.

L2   SAFER:
Drug which has been studied in a limited number of breastfeeding women without an increase in adverse effects in the infant. And/or the evidence of a demonstrated risk which is likely to follow use of this medication in a breastfeeding woman is remote.

L3   MODERATELY SAFE:
There are no controlled studies in breastfeeding women; however, the risk of untoward effects to a breastfed infant is possible or controlled studies show only minimal non-threatening adverse effects. Drugs should be given only if the potential benefit justifies the potential risk to the infant.

L4   POSSIBLY HAZARDOUS:
There is positive evidence of risk to a breastfed infant or to breastmilk production but the benefits from use in breastfeeding mothers may be acceptable despite the risk to the infant (e.g., if the drug is needed in a life-threatening situation or for a serious disease for which safer drugs cannot be used or are ineffective).

L5   CONTRAINDICATED:
Studies in breastfeeding mothers have demonstrated that there is significant and documented risk to the infant based on human experience or it is a medication that has a high risk of causing significant damage to an infant. The risk of using the drug in breastfeeding women clearly outweighs any possible benefit from breastfeeding. The drug is contraindicated in women who are breastfeeding an infant.

Theoretic Infant Dose:
This is an estimate (hence the term "Theoretic") of the maximum likely dose per kilogram per day that an infant would ingest via milk. Because the literature is highly variable, I used several methods to calculate this estimate. First, if the authors provided milk AUC information or clear estimates of the average amount in milk during the day, I used this data to estimate the dose to the infant as it is much more accurate. But more commonly, the only data provided was the peak milk level also called C_{max}. In these cases, I used this data to derive the theoretic infant dose. For

determining dose, I used the standard milk intake of 150 mL/kg/day multiplied times the concentration of medication in milk (C_{max}/Liter X 0.150 mL/kg/day= TID). Please remember, this is generally the **maximum** concentration that would be transferred. Most often, the actual dose to the infant would be much lower. If you know the maternal dose, calculate the **Relative Infant Dose** using the formula below. It may prove very useful.

Relative Infant Dose: The relative infant dose (RID) is calculated by dividing the infants dose via milk (Theoretic Infant Dose) in "mg/kg/day" by the maternal dose in " mg/kg/day" (see box above). This weight-normalizing method gives one a feeling for just how much of the "maternal dose" the infant is receiving. Many authors now use this preferred method because it gives the reader a better idea of the relative dose transferred to the infant. These same authors also suggest that anything less than 10% of the maternal dose is probably safe. This is usually correct. However; some drugs (metronidazole, fluconazole) actually have much higher relative infant doses but because they are quite non-toxic they do not often bother an infant. To calculate this dose, I chose the data I felt was best and this often included larger studies with AUC calculations of mean concentrations in milk. I also chose an average body weight of 70 kg for an adult. Thus the RIDs herein are calculated assuming a maternal average weight of 70 kg and a daily intake of 150 mL/kg/day in the infant. Please note, many authors fail to normalize their data for weight. Others provide a RID for 'each' feeding not a daily average. Therefore, my values may vary slightly from others due simply to differences in the method of calculation.

Adult Concerns:
This section lists the most prevalent undesired or bothersome side effects listed for adults. As with most medications, the occurrence of these is often quite rare, generally less than 1-10% of the time. Side effects vary from one patient to another and should not be overemphasized since most patients do not experience untoward effects.

Pediatric Concerns:
This section lists the side effects noted in the published literature as associated with medications transferred **via human milk**. Pediatric concerns are those effects that were noted by investigators as being associated with drug transfer via milk. They are not the effects that would result from direct administration to the infant. In some sections, I have added comments that may not have been reported in the literature, but are well known attributes of this medication and are useful information to provide the mother so that she can better care for her infant ("Observe for weakness, apnea").

Drug Interactions:
Drug interactions generally indicate which medications when taken

together may produce higher or lower plasma levels of other medications or they may decrease or increase the effect of another medication. These effects may vary widely from minimal to dangerous. Because some medications have hundreds of interactions and because I had limited room to provide this information, I have listed only those that may be highly significant. Therefore, please be advised that this section may not be complete. In several references, I have suggested that due to the large number of interactions the reader consult a more complete drug interaction reference. Please remember that the drugs administered to a mother could interact with those being administered concurrently to an infant. Example: Maternal fluconazole and pediatric cisapride.

Alternatives:
Drugs listed in this section may be suitable alternate choices for the medication listed above. In many instances, if the patient cannot take the medication or it is a poor choice due to high milk concentrations, these alternates may be suitable candidates. **WARNING**: The alternates listed are only suggestions and may not be at all proper for the syndrome in question. Only the clinician can make this judgment. For instance, nifedipine is a calcium channel blocker with good antihypertensive qualities but poor antiarrhythmic qualities. In this case, verapamil would be a better choice.

Adult Dosage:
This is the usual adult oral dose provided in the package insert. While these are highly variable, I chose the dose for the most common use of the medication.

T½ =
This lists the most commonly recorded adult half-life of the medication. It is very important to remember that short half-life drugs are preferred. Use this parameter to determine if the mother can successfully breastfeed around the medication by nursing the infant—then taking the medication. If the half-life is short enough (1-3 hours), then the drug level in the maternal plasma will be declining when the infant feeds again. This is ideal. If the half-life is significantly long (12-24 hours), then find a similar medication with a shorter half-life (compare ibuprofen with Naproxen).

PHL=
This lists the most commonly recorded pediatric half-life of the medication. Medications with extremely long half-lives (>12 hours) in pediatric patients may accumulate to high levels in the infant's plasma. Pediatric half-lives are difficult to find due to the paucity of studies.

M/P=
This lists the Milk/plasma ratio. This is the ratio of the concentration of drug in the mother's *milk* divided by the concentration in the mother's *plasma*. If high (> 1 to 5), it is useful as an indicator of drugs that may

sequester in milk in high levels. If low (< 1), it is a good indicator that only minimal levels of the drug are transferred into milk (this is preferred). While it is best to try to choose drugs with LOW milk/plasma ratios, the amount of drug which transfers into human milk is largely determined by the level of drug in the mother's plasma compartment. Even with high M/P ratios and LOW maternal plasma levels, the amount of drug that transfers is still low. Therefore, the higher M/P ratios often provide an erroneous impression that large amounts of drug are going to transfer into milk. This simply may not be true.

T_{max} (formerly PK)

This lists the time interval from administration of the drug until it reaches the highest level in the mother's plasma (C_{max}) which we call the peak or "time to max" hence T_{max}. The peak is when you do not want the mother to breastfeed her infant; rather, wait until the peak is subsiding or has at least dropped significantly. Remember, drugs enter breastmilk as a function of the maternal plasma concentration. The higher the mother's plasma level; the greater the entry of the drug into her milk. If possible, choose drugs that have short peak intervals and suggest mom not breastfeed when it is at C_{max}.

PB=

This lists the percentage of maternal protein binding. Most drugs circulate in the blood bound to plasma albumin. If a drug is highly protein bound, it cannot exit the plasma compartment as well. The higher the percentage of binding the less likely the drug is to enter the maternal milk. Try to choose drugs that have high protein binding in order to reduce the infant's exposure to the medication. Good protein binding is typically greater than 90%.

Oral=

Oral bioavailability refers to the ability of a drug to reach the systemic circulation after oral administration. It is generally a good indication of the amount of medication that is absorbed into the blood stream of the patient. Drugs with low oral bioavailability are generally either poorly absorbed in the gastrointestinal tract or they are sequestered by the liver prior to entering the plasma compartment. The oral bioavailability listed in this text is the adult value; almost none have been published for children or neonates. Recognizing this, these values are still useful in estimating if a mother or perhaps an infant will actually absorb enough drug to provide clinically significant levels in the plasma compartment of the individual. The value listed estimates the percent of an oral dose that would be found in the plasma compartment of the individual after oral administration. In many cases, the oral bioavailability of some medications is not listed by manufacturers, but instead terms such as "Complete", "Nil", or "Poor" are used. For lack of better data, I have included these terms when no data is available on the exact amount (percentage) absorbed.

Vd=
The volume of distribution is a useful kinetic term that describes how widely the medication is distributed in the body. Drugs with high volumes of distribution (Vd) are distributed in higher concentrations in remote compartments of the body, and may not stay in the blood. For instance, digoxin enters the blood compartment and then rapidly leaves to enter the heart and skeletal muscle. Most of the drug is sequestered in these remote compartments (100 fold). Therefore, drugs with high volumes of distribution (1-20 liter/kg) generally require much longer to clear from the body than drugs with smaller volumes (0.1 liter/kg). For instance, whereas it may only require a few hours to totally clear gentamycin (Vd=0.28 l/kg), it may require weeks to clear amitriptyline (Vd=10 l/kg) which has a huge volume of distribution. In addition, some drugs may have one half-life for the plasma compartment, but may have a totally different half-life for the peripheral compartment as half-life is a function of volume of distribution. For a complete description of Vd, please consult a good pharmacology reference. In this text, the units of measure for Vd are liters/kg.

pKa=
The pKa of a drug is the pH at which the drug is equally ionic and nonionic. The more ionic a drug is the less capable it is of transferring from the milk compartment to the maternal plasma compartment. Hence, they become trapped in milk (ion-trapping). This term is useful because drugs that have a pKa higher than 7.2 may be sequestered to a slightly higher degree than one with a lower pKa. Drugs with higher pKa generally have higher milk/plasma ratios. Hence, choose drugs with a lower pKa.

MW=
The molecular weight of a medication is a significant determinant as to the entry of that medication into human milk. Medications with small molecular weights (< 200) can easily pass into milk by traversing small pores in the cell walls of the mammary epithelium (see ethanol). Drugs with higher molecular weights must traverse the membrane by dissolving in the lipid bilayer which may significantly reduce milk levels. As such, the smaller the molecular weight the higher the relative transfer of that drug into milk. Protein medications (e.g. Heparin, Insulin) which have enormous molecular weights transfer at much lower concentrations, and are virtually excluded from human breastmilk. Therefore, when possible, choose drugs with higher molecular weights to reduce their entry into milk.

5-HYDROXYTRYPTOPHAN
Trade: Powersleep, Oxitriptan
Can/Aus/UK:
Uses: Precursor of serotonin
LRC: L3
AAP: Not reviewed

5-Hydroxytryptophan(5-HTP) is a natural aromatic amino acid which is the immediate precursor of the neurotransmitter serotonin. L-Tryptophan is another amino acid formerly used to treat depression.

L-Tryptophan:
L-tryptophan (LTP), once absorbed, is rapidly transported to the liver where some of it is incorporated into proteins, and some passes unchanged into the general circulation. It is a precursor of serotonin. One of the major problems with the use of LTP is that when used at higher doses, metabolism to kynurenine is highly induced, and the majority of LTP is subsequently metabolized rather than converted into serotonin. Even under the best of circumstances, less than 3% of the LTP is likely to be converted to serotonin in the brain. L-Tryptophan crosses the blood-brain barrier only poorly. As the doses increase, the creation of the metabolite kynurenine tends to block entry of LTP into the brain. As the doses of LTP used are extraordinarily high 2000-6000 mg/d cost and adverse effects are significant.[1] Older formulations created with contaminates were responsible for the eosinophilia-myalgia syndrome.

5-HTTP:
5-HTP is rapidly absorbed, and approximately 70% of the dose is bioavailable. The remaining 30% is converted to serotonin by intestinal cells which may lead to some nausea. 5-HTP readily crosses the blood-brain barrier (24% in CSF) and is one step closer to serotonin production. The dose of 5-HTP is much lower, averaging 100-300 mg/d, and some studies have found it equivalent to tricyclic antidepressants[2] and fluvoxamine (an SSRI) in treating depression.[3] Although several cases of eosinophilia-myalgia syndrome have been reported with the use of 5-HTP[4,5] both of these patients had defective metabolic mechanisms for converting 5-HTP.

Unfortunately, there are no data on the transfer of exogenously supplied LTP or 5-HTP into human milk. For instance, it is not apparently known if high maternal plasma levels would produce high milk levels. While it is true human milk contains higher levels of LTP, presumably to stimulate serotonin levels in the infant's CNS, it is not known if high maternal doses would likewise produce high milk levels. Because the infant's neurologic development is incredibly sensitive to serotonin levels, and because we do not know if supplementation with LTP or 5-HTP could produce high milk levels leading to overdose in the infant, this author does not recommend the use of L-tryptophan or 5-HTP supplementation in breastfeeding mothers until we know corresponding milk levels.

Pregnancy Risk Category:

Lactation Risk Category: L3

Adult Concerns: Adverse anorexia, diarrhea, nausea, and vomiting have been reported.

Pediatric Concerns: None reported via milk.

Drug Interactions: Carbidopa may increase absorption of 5-HT. Use with MAOi is potentially dangerous. 5-HT may potentiate the serotonergic effect of selective serotonin reuptake inhibitors (SSRIs).

Theoretic Infant Dose:

Relative Infant Dose:

Adult Dose:

Alternatives:

T½ =	4.3hours	M/P =	
PHL =		PB =	19%
T$_{max}$ =	3-6 hours	Oral =	< 70%
MW =	393	pKa =	6.96
Vd =	0.6		

References:

1. Murray MT, Pizzorno JE. 5-Hydroxytryptophan. In: Murray MT, Pizzorno JE, editors. Textbook of Natural Medicine. Churchill Livingstone, 1999: 783-796.
2. van Praag HM. Management of depression with serotonin precursors. Biol Psychiatry 1981; 16(3):291-310.
3. Poldinger W, Calanchini B, Schwarz W. A functional-dimensional approach to depression: serotonin deficiency as a target syndrome in a comparison of 5-hydroxytryptophan and fluvoxamine. Psychopathology 1991; 24(2):53-81.
4. Sternberg EM, Van Woert MH, Young SN, Magnussen I, Baker H, Gauthier S, Osterland CK. Development of a scleroderma-like illness during therapy with L-5-hydroxytryptophan and carbidopa. N Engl J Med 1980; 303(14):782-787.
5. Michelson D, Page SW, Casey R, Trucksess MW, Love LA, Milstien S, Wilson C, Massaquoi SG, Crofford LJ, Hallett M, . An eosinophilia-myalgia syndrome related disorder associated with exposure to L-5-hydroxytryptophan. J Rheumatol 1994; 21(12):2261-2265.

ACARBOSE

Trade: Precose, Prandase
Can/Aus/UK: Prandase, Glucobay
Uses: Delays carbohydrate absorption
LRC: L3
AAP: Not reviewed

Acarbose is an oral alpha-glucosidase inhibitor used to reduce the absorption of carbohydrates in the management of Type II (NIDDM) diabetics.[1]   The reduction of carbohydrate absorption reduces the rapid rise in glucose following a meal; hence, glycosylated hemoglobin (Hemoglobin A1c) levels are reduced.   Acarbose is less than 2% bioavailable as an intact molecule.[2] No data are available on the transfer of acarbose into human milk, but with a bioavailability of less than 2%, it is very unlikely any would reach the milk compartment or be orally absorbed by the infant.

Pregnancy Risk Category: B

Lactation Risk Category: L3

Adult Concerns: Adverse effects include flatulence, abdominal pain and distention, diarrhea, and borborygmi. Isolated cases of elevated liver enzymes have been reported.   Elevate liver enzymes occurred in approximately 15% of acarbose-treated patients and is apparently dose related with doses > 300 mg daily.

Pediatric Concerns: None reported via milk.

Drug Interactions: May increase hypoglycemia when used with other antidiabetic medications such as the sulfonylureas.

Theoretic Infant Dose:

Relative Infant Dose:

Adult Dose: 50-100 mg TID

Alternatives:

T½ =	< 2 hours	M/P =	
PHL =		PB =	
T$_{max}$ =		Oral =	0.7- 2%
MW =	645	pKa =	
Vd =	0.32		

References:
1.   Pharmaceutical Manufacturer Prescribing Information. 1999.
2.   Balfour JA, McTavish D. Acarbose. An update of its pharmacology and therapeutic use in diabetes mellitus. Drugs 1993; 46(6):1025-1054.

ACEBUTOLOL

Trade: Sectral
Can/Aus/UK: Monitan, Sectral
Uses: Antihypertensive, beta blocker
LRC: L3
AAP: Maternal Medication Usually Compatible with Breastfeeding

Acebutolol is predominately a beta-1 blocker but can block beta-2 receptors at high doses. It is low in lipid solubility and contains some intrinsic sympathetic activity (partial beta agonist activity). It increases cold sensitivity. Studies indicate that on a weight basis, acebutolol is approximately 10-30% as effective as propranolol. It is 35-50% bioavailable orally.[1]

After relatively high doses in animal studies, acebutolol does not appear to be overly teratogenic or harm the fetus. Acebutolol is well tolerated by pregnant hypertensive women.

In a study of seven women receiving 200-1200 mg/day acebutolol, the highest milk concentration occurred in the women receiving 1200 mg/day and was 4123 µg/L.[2] In women receiving 200, 400, or 600 mg/day of acebutolol, milk levels were 286 µg/L, 666 µg/L and 539 µg/L respectively. Acebutolol and diacetolol (its major metabolite) appear in breastmilk with a milk/plasma ratio of 1.9 to 9.2 (acebutolol) and 2.3 to 24.7 for the metabolite (diacetolol).

These levels are considered relatively high and occurred following maternal doses of 400-1200 mg/day. When the metabolite is added, the dose may approach 10% of maternal dose. Neonates appear much more sensitive to acebutolol.

Pregnancy Risk Category: B

Lactation Risk Category: L3

Adult Concerns: Hypotension, bradycardia, and transient tachypnea have been reported. Drowsiness has been reported.

Pediatric Concerns: Hypotension, bradycardia, and transient tachypnea have been reported. Drowsiness has been reported.

Drug Interactions: Decreased effect when used with aluminum salts, barbiturates, calcium salts, cholestyramine, NSAIDs, ampicillin, rifampin, and salicylates. Beta blockers may reduce the effect of oral sulfonylureas (hypoglycemic agents). Increased toxicity/effect when used with other antihypertensives, contraceptives, MAO inhibitors, cimetidine, and numerous other products. See drug interaction reference for complete listing.

Theoretic Infant Dose: 618 µg/kg/day

Relative Infant Dose: 3.6%

Adult Dose: 200-400 mg BID

Alternatives: Propranolol, Metoprolol

T½ =	3-4 hours	M/P =	7.1-12.2
PHL =		PB =	26%
T$_{max}$ =	1-4 hours	Oral =	35-50%
MW =	336	pKa =	
Vd =	1.35		

References:
1. Drug Facts and Comparisons 1995 ed. ed. St. Louis: 1995.
2. Boutroy MJ, Bianchetti G, Dubruc C, Vert P, Morselli PL. To nurse when receiving acebutolol: is it dangerous for the neonate? Eur J Clin Pharmacol 1986; 30(6):737-739.

ACETAMINOPHEN
Trade: Tempra, Tylenol, Paracetamol
Can/Aus/UK: Apo-Acetaminophen, Tempra, Tylenol, Paracetamol, Panadol, Dymadon, Calpol
Uses: Analgesic
LRC: L1
AAP: Maternal Medication Usually Compatible with Breastfeeding

Only small amounts are secreted into breastmilk and are considered too small to be hazardous. In a study of 11 mothers who received 650 mg of acetaminophen orally, the highest milk levels reported were from 10-15 mg/L.[1] The milk/plasma ratio was 1.08. In another study of three patients who received a single 500 mg oral dose, the reported milk and plasma concentrations of acetaminophen was 4.2 mg/L and 5.6 mg/L respectively.[2] The milk/plasma ratio was 0.76. The maximum observed concentration in milk was 4.4 mg/L. In another study of women who ingested 1000 mg acetaminophen, milk levels averaged 6.1 mg/L and provided an average dose of 0.92 mg/kg/d according to the authors.[3] There seems to be wide variation in the milk concentrations in these studies, but the relative infant dose is probably less than 6.4% of the maternal dose. This is significantly less than the pediatric therapeutic dose. Acetaminophen is probably safe for breastfeeding mothers.

Pregnancy Risk Category: B

Lactation Risk Category: L1

Adult Concerns: Few when taken in normal doses. Diarrhea, gastric upset sweating in overdose. Note: numerous cases of liver toxicity have been reported following 'chronic' abuse of acetaminophen at > 200 mg/kg/day.

Pediatric Concerns: None reported via milk. Probably safe.

Drug Interactions: Rifampin can interact to reduce the analgesic effect of acetaminophen. Increased acetaminophen hepatotoxicity when used with barbiturates, carbamazepine, hydantoins, sulfinpyrazone, and chronic alcohol abuse.

Theoretic Infant Dose: 0.91 µg/kg/day

Relative Infant Dose: 6.4%

Adult Dose: 325-650 mg q 4-6 hours PRN

Alternatives:

T½ =	2 hours	M/P =	0.91-1.42
PHL =	1-3 hours	PB =	25%
T$_{max}$ =	0.5-2 hours	Oral =	> 85%
MW =	151	pKa =	9.5
Vd =	0.8-1.0		

References:
1. Berlin CM, Jr., Yaffe SJ, Ragni M. Disposition of acetaminophen in milk, saliva, and plasma of lactating women. Pediatr Pharmacol (New York) 1980; 1(2):135-141.
2. Bitzen PO, Gustafsson B, Jostell KG, Melander A, Wahlin-Boll E. Excretion of paracetamol in human breastmilk. Eur J Clin Pharmacol 1981; 20(2):123-125.
3. Notarianni LJ, Oldham HG, Bennett PN. Passage of paracetamol into breastmilk and its subsequent metabolism by the neonate. Br J Clin Pharmacol 1987; 24(1):63-67.

ACETAZOLAMIDE
Trade: Dazamide, Diamox
Can/Aus/UK: Acetazolam, Apo-Acetazolamide, Diamox
Uses: Diuretic
LRC: L2
AAP: Maternal Medication Usually Compatible with Breastfeeding

Acetazolamide is a carbonic anhydrase inhibitor dissimilar to other thiazide diuretics. In general, diuretics may decrease the volume of breastmilk although this is rare. In a patient receiving 500 mg of acetazolamide twice daily, acetazolamide concentrations in milk were 1.3 to 2.1 mg/L while the maternal plasma levels ranged from 5.2-6.4 mg/L.[1] Plasma concentrations in exposed infants were 0.2 to 0.6 µg/mL 2 to 12 hours after breastfeeding. These amounts are unlikely to cause adverse effects in the infant.

Pregnancy Risk Category: C

Lactation Risk Category: L2

Adult Concerns: Anorexia, diarrhea, metallic taste, polyuria, muscular weakness, potassium loss. Malaise, fatigue, depression, renal failure have been reported.

Pediatric Concerns: None reported via milk.

Drug Interactions: Increases lithium excretion, reducing plasma levels. May increase toxicity of cyclosporine. Digitalis toxicity may occur if hypokalemia results from acetazolamide therapy.

Theoretic Infant Dose: 0.31 mg/kg/day

Relative Infant Dose: 2.21%

Adult Dose: 500 mg BID

Alternatives:

T½ =	2.4-5.8 hours	M/P =	0.25
PHL =		PB =	70-95%
T$_{max}$ =	1-3 hours	Oral =	Complete
MW =	222	pKa =	7.4
Vd =	0.2		

References:
1. Soderman P, Hartvig P, Fagerlund C. Acetazolamide excretion into human breastmilk. Br J Clin Pharmacol 1984; 17(5):599-600.

ACETOHEXAMIDE

Trade: Dimelor
Can/Aus/UK: Dimelor, Diamox
Uses: Hypoglycemic agent
LRC: L3
AAP: Not reviewed

Acetohexamide is an intermediate-acting hypoglycemic sulfonylurea antidiabetic agent.[1] Its structure is similar to tolbutamide, chlorpropamide, and tolazamide. No data are available on its transfer to human milk, but other sulfonylureas transfer to milk in minimal levels (see tolbutamide). The use of sulfonylureas in breastfeeding mothers is somewhat controversial due to limited studies but has not been noted in the literature to produce any problems. Observe infant closely for hypoglycemia if used.

Pregnancy Risk Category: C

Lactation Risk Category: L3

Adult Concerns: The most common adverse effects include hypoglycemia, nausea, epigastric fullness, heartburn, and rashes.

Pediatric Concerns: None reported via milk.

Drug Interactions: Numerous drugs interact with sulfonylureas; please consult further references. Increased hypoglycemic effects occur when used with salicylates, beta blockers, MAO inhibitors, oral anticoagulants, NSAIDs, sulfonamides, insulin, etc. Reduced hypoglycemic effects may occur when used with cholestyramine, diazoxide, hydantoins, rifampin, and thiazides.

Theoretic Infant Dose:

Relative Infant Dose:

Adult Dose: 250-1000 mg daily

Alternatives: Metformin

$T^{1/2}$ =	1.3-6 (metabolite) hours	M/P =	
PHL =		PB =	65-90%
T_{max} =	3 hours	Oral =	Good
MW =	324	pKa =	
Vd =	0.2		

References:
1. Pharmaceutical Manufacturer Prescribing Information. 1999.

ACYCLOVIR

Trade: Zovirax
Can/Aus/UK: Zovirax, Aviraz, Apo-Acyclovir, Acyclo-V, Zyclir, Aciclover
Uses: Antiviral, for herpes simplex
LRC: L2
AAP: Maternal Medication Usually Compatible with Breastfeeding

Acyclovir is converted by herpes simplex and varicella zoster virus to acyclovir triphosphate which interferes with viral HSV DNA polymerase. It is currently cleared for use in HSV infections, Varicella-Zoster, cytomegalo virus and Epstein-Barr infections. There is virtually no percutaneous absorption following topical application and plasma levels are undetectable. The pharmacokinetics in children are similar to adults. In neonates, the half-life is 3.8-4.1 hours, and in children one year and older it is 1.9-3.6 hours.

Acyclovir levels in breastmilk are reported to be 0.6 to 4.1 times the maternal plasma levels.[1] Maximum ingested dose was calculated to be 1500 µg/day assuming 750 mL milk intake. This level produced no overt side effects in one infant. In a study by Meyer,[2] a patient receiving 200 mg five times daily produced breastmilk concentrations averaging 1.06 mg/L. Using this data an infant would ingest less than 1 mg acyclovir daily. In another study, doses of 800 mg five times daily produced milk levels that ranged from 4.16 to 5.81 mg/L (total estimated infant ingestion per day = 0.73 mg/kg/day).[3]

Topical therapy on lesions other than nipple is probably safe. If applied to nipples, any residual acyclovir cream should be removed prior to feeding. Toxicities associated with acyclovir are few and usually minor. Acyclovir therapy in neonatal units is common and produces few toxicities. Calculated intake by infant would be less than 0.87 mg/kg/d.

Pregnancy Risk Category: C

Lactation Risk Category: L2

Adult Concerns: Nausea, vomiting, diarrhea, sore throat, edema, and skin rashes

Pediatric Concerns: None reported via milk in several studies.

Drug Interactions: Increased CNS side effects when used with zidovudine and probenecid.

Theoretic Infant Dose: 0.87 mg/kg/day

Relative Infant Dose: 1.5%

Adult Dose: 200-800 mg q 4-6 hours

Alternatives:

$T\frac{1}{2}$ =	2.4 hours	M/P =	0.6-4.1
PHL =	3.2 hours (neonates)	PB =	9-33%
T_{max} =	1.5 - 2 hours	Oral =	15-30%
MW =	225	pKa =	
Vd =			

References:

1. Lau RJ, Emery MG, Galinsky RE. Unexpected accumulation of acyclovir in breastmilk with estimation of infant exposure. Obstet Gynecol 1987; 69(3 Pt 2):468-471.
2. Meyer LJ, de Miranda P, Sheth N, Spruance S. Acyclovir in human breastmilk. Am J Obstet Gynecol 1988; 158(3 Pt 1):586-588.
3. Taddio A, Klein J, Koren G. Acyclovir excretion in human breastmilk. Ann Pharmacother 1994; 28(5):585-587.

ADALIMUMAB

Trade: Humira
Can/Aus/UK:
Uses: Anti-rheumatic, anti-tumor necrosis antibody
LRC: L3
AAP: Not reviewed

Adalimumab is a recombinant human IgG1 monoclonal antibody specific for human tumor necrosis factor (TNF). TNF is implicated in the pain and destructive component of arthritis and other autoimmune syndromes. This product would be similar to others such as etanercept (Enbrel) and infliximab(Remicade). IgG transfer into human milk is significant the first 4 days postpartum, then is minimal afterwards. The primary immunoglobulin in mature human milk is IgA. Immunoglobulins are transferred into human milk by a very specific carrier protein. It is not known if these unusual immunoglobulins are transferred, but it is unlikely. Specific data from my laboratories suggests that no infliximab transfers into human milk in mothers receiving IV doses.[1] It is not likely that adalimumab would transfer in clinically relevant amounts after the first week postpartum but no data are available at this time.

Pregnancy Risk Category: B

Lactation Risk Category: L3

Adult Concerns: May induce tuberculosis reactivations. May induce immunosuppression and reduce host defences against infections. Serious infections, neurologic events, and malignancies have been reported.

Pediatric Concerns: None reported via milk. Unlikely to enter milk.

Drug Interactions: None reported.

Theoretic Infant Dose:

Relative Infant Dose:

Adult Dose: 40 mg every other week subcutaneously.

Alternatives: Infliximab

$T^{1/2}$ =	2 weeks	M/P =	
PHL =		PB =	Nil
T_{max} =	131 hours	Oral =	Low
MW =	148,000	pKa =	
Vd =	4.7		

References:
1. Hale TW, Fasanmade A. Unpublished data. 2002.

ADAPALENE
Trade: Differin
Can/Aus/UK: Differin
Uses: Topical acne remedy
LRC: L3
AAP: Not reviewed

Adapalene is a retinoid-like compound (similar to Tretinoin) used topically for treatment of acne. No data are available on its transfer into human milk. However, adapalene is virtually unabsorbed when applied topically to the skin.[1] Plasma levels are almost undetectable (< 0.25 ng/mL plasma), so milk levels would be infinitesimally low and probably undetectable.[2]

Pregnancy Risk Category: C

Lactation Risk Category: L3

Adult Concerns: Exacerbation of sunburn, irritation of skin, erythema, dryness, scaling, burning, itching

Pediatric Concerns: None reported via milk. Very unlikely due to minimal maternal absorption.

Drug Interactions:

Theoretic Infant Dose:

Relative Infant Dose:

Adult Dose: Apply topical daily.

Alternatives: Tretinoin

References:
1. Pharmaceutical Manufacturer Prescribing Information. 1999.
2. Drug Facts and Comparisons 1999 ed. ed. St. Louis: 1999.

ALBUTEROL
Trade: Proventil, Ventolin
Can/Aus/UK: Novo-Salmol, Ventolin, Asmavent, Respax, Respolin, Asmol, Salbulin, Salbuvent, Salamol
Uses: Bronchodilator for asthma
LRC: L1
AAP: Not reviewed

Albuterol is a very popular beta-2 adrenergic agonist that is typically used to dilate constricted bronchi in asthmatics[1]. It is active orally but is most commonly used via inhalation. When used orally, significant plasma levels are attained and transfer to breastmilk is possible. When used via inhalation, less than 10% is absorbed into maternal plasma. Small amounts are probably secreted into milk although no reports exist. It is very unlikely that pharmacologic doses will be transferred to the infant via milk following inhaler use. However, when used orally, breastmilk levels could be sufficient to produce tremors and agitation in infants. Commonly used via inhalation in treating pediatric asthma. This product is safe to use in breastfeeding mothers.

Pregnancy Risk Category: C

Lactation Risk Category: L1

Adult Concerns: Observe infant for tremors and excitement.

Pediatric Concerns: None reported via milk

Drug Interactions: Albuterol effects are reduced when used with beta blockers. Cardiovascular effects are potentiated when used with MAO inhibitors, tricyclic antidepressants, amphetamines, and inhaled anesthetics (enflurane).

Theoretic Infant Dose:

Relative Infant Dose:

Adult Dose: 2-4 mg TID or QID

Alternatives:

$T\frac{1}{2}$ =	3.8 hours	M/P =	
PHL =		PB =	
T_{max} =	5-30 minutes (inhaled)	Oral =	100%
MW =	239	pKa =	10.3
Vd =	2.2		

References:
1.   Pharmaceutical Manufacturer Prescribing Information. 1997.

ALBUTEROL AND IPRATROPIUM BROMIDE

Trade: Duoneb
Can/Aus/UK:
Uses: Bronchodilators
LRC:
AAP: Not reviewed

Duo Neb is a combination product containing 0.103 mg albuterol and 0.018 mg of ipratropium bromide per metered-dose inhalation. See the individual monographs on this product.

ALEMTUZUMAB

Trade: Campath
Can/Aus/UK:
Uses: Anti-leukemic agent
LRC: L3
        L4 during first week postpartum.
AAP: Not reviewed

Alemtuzumab is a recombinant DNA-derived humanized monoclonal antibody that is directed against specific cell receptors on leukemic cells.[1] It is a large IgG1 antibody. No data are available on its transfer to human milk, but it is very unlikely to enter milk due to its large size. However, the first 72 hours postpartum, IgG levels in milk are higher and this should be considered with this agent. While some IgG is still transferred into human milk, it is done so by a very specialized transporter. It is unlikely this transporter would transport this unusual monoclonal antibody.

Pregnancy Risk Category: C

Lactation Risk Category: L3
                          L4 during first week postpartum

Adult Concerns: Adverse events include rigors post-infusion, fever, nausea, vomiting, hypotension, rash, fatigue, urticaria, dyspnea, pruritus, headache, and diarrhea. An elevated risk of infections is reported.

Pediatric Concerns: None reported via milk. Unlikely to penetrate milk after first week postpartum.

Drug Interactions:

Theoretic Infant Dose:

Relative Infant Dose:

Adult Dose: Maintenance dose is 30 mg/day three times weekly on alternate days.

Alternatives:

T½ =	12 days	M/P =	
PHL =		PB =	Nil
T$_{max}$ =		Oral =	Nil
MW =	150,000	pKa =	
Vd =			

References:
1. Pharmaceutical Manufacturers prescribing information, 2003.

ALENDRONATE SODIUM

Trade: Fosamax
Can/Aus/UK: Fosamax
Uses: Inhibits bone resorption
LRC: L3
AAP: Not reviewed

Alendronate is a specific inhibitor of osteoclast-mediated bone resorption, thus reducing bone loss and bone turnover.[1] While incorporated in bone matrix, it is not pharmacologically active. Because concentrations in plasma are too low to be detected (< 5 ng/mL), it is very unlikely that it would be secreted into human milk in clinically relevant concentrations. Concentrations in human milk have not been reported. Because this product has exceedingly poor oral bioavailability, particularly when ingested with milk, it is very unlikely that alendronate would be orally absorbed by a breastfeeding infant.

Pregnancy Risk Category: C

Lactation Risk Category: L3

Adult Concerns: Abdominal pain, nausea, dyspepsia, constipation, muscle cramps, headache, taste perversion. There are a number of case reports of esophagitis and esophageal ulceration in patients taking Fosamax.

Pediatric Concerns: None reported via milk.

Drug Interactions: Ranitidine will double the absorption of alendronate. Calcium, milk, and other multivalent cation containing foods reduce the bioavailability of alendronate.

Theoretic Infant Dose:

Relative Infant Dose:

Adult Dose: 10 mg daily

Alternatives:

$T\frac{1}{2}$ =	< 3 hours(plasma)	M/P =		
PHL =		PB =	78%	
T_{max} =		Oral =	< 0.7%	
MW =	325	pKa =		
Vd =	0.4			

References:
1. Pharmaceutical Manufacturer Prescribing Information. 1997.

ALFENTANIL
Trade: Alfenta
Can/Aus/UK: Alfenta, Rapifen
Uses: Narcotic analgesic
LRC: L2
AAP: Not reviewed

Alfentanil is secreted into breastmilk. Following a dose of 50 μg/kg IV (plus several additional 10 μg/kg doses), the mean levels of alfentanil in colostrum at 4 hours varied from 0.21 to 1.56 μg/L of colostrum, levels probably too small to produce overt toxicity in breastfeeding infants.[1] Mean levels 28 hours post-alfentanil were 0.05 μg/L.

Pregnancy Risk Category: C

Lactation Risk Category: L2

Adult Concerns: Observe for bradycardia, shivering, constipation, and sedation.   In neonates observe for severe hypotension.

Pediatric Concerns: None reported via milk.

Drug Interactions: Phenothiazines may antagonize the analgesic effects of opiates.   Dextromethorphan may increase the analgesia of opiate agonists.   Other CNS depressants such as benzodiazepines, barbiturates, tricyclic antidepressants, erythromycin, reserpine, and beta blockers may increase the toxicity of this opiate.

Theoretic Infant Dose: 0.23 μg/kg/day

Relative Infant Dose: 0.5%

Adult Dose: 8-40 μg/kg

Alternatives: Remifentanil

T½ =	1-2 hours	M/P =	
PHL =	5-6 hours (neonates)	PB =	92%
T$_{max}$ =	immediate	Oral =	
MW =	417	pKa =	6.5
Vd =	0.3-1.0		

References:
1. Giesecke A, Rice L, Lipton J. Alfentaril in colostrum. Anesthesiology 63:A284 1985.
2. Spigset O. Anaesthetic agents and excretion in breastmilk. Acta Anaesthesiol Scand 1994; 38(2):94-103.

ALLERGY INJECTIONS
Trade:
Can/Aus/UK:
Uses: Desensitizing injections
LRC: L1
AAP: Not reviewed

Allergy injections consist of protein and carbohydrate substances from plants, animals, and other species. There are no reported untoward effects. They are unlikely to enter milk.

Pregnancy Risk Category:

Lactation Risk Category: **L1**

Adult Concerns: Allergic pruritus, anaphylaxis, other immune reactions

Pediatric Concerns: None reported in breastfeeding mothers.

ALLOPURINOL
Trade: Zyloprim, Lopurin
Can/Aus/UK: Alloprin, Apo-Allopurinol, Novo-Purol, Zyloprim, Allorin, Capurate, Zygout, Aluline, Caplenal, Cosuric, Hamarin, Zyloric
Uses: Reduces uric acid levels
LRC: L2
AAP: Maternal Medication Usually Compatible with Breastfeeding

Allopurinol is a potent antagonist of xanthine oxidase, an enzyme involved in the production of uric acid. It is used to reduce uric acid levels in gouty individuals. In a nursing mother receiving 300mg/d allopurinol, the breastmilk concentration at 2 and 4 hours was 0.9 and 1.4 µg/mL respectively.[1] The concentration of the metabolite, oxypurinol, was 53.7 and 48.0 µg/mL at 2 and 4 hours respectively. The milk/plasma ratio ranged from 0.9 to 1.4 for allopurinol and 3.9 for its metabolite, oxypurinol. The average daily dose that an infant would receive from milk would be approximately 0.14-0.20 mg/kg of allopurinol and 7.2-8.0 mg/kg of oxypurinol. No adverse effects were noted in the infant after 6 weeks of therapy. Pediatric dosages for ages 6 and under is generally 10 mg/kg/24 hours.

Pregnancy Risk Category: **C**

Lactation Risk Category: **L2**

Adult Concerns: Itching skin rash, fever, chills, nausea and vomiting, diarrhea, gastritis

Pediatric Concerns: No adverse effects were noted in one infant after 6 weeks of therapy.

Drug Interactions: Alcohol decreases allopurinol efficacy. Inhibits metabolism of azathioprine and mercaptopurine. Increased incidence of skin rash when used with amoxicillin and ampicillin. Increased risk of kidney stones when used with high doses of vitamin C. Allopurinol prolongs half-life of oral anticoagulants, theophylline, and chlorpropamide.

Theoretic Infant Dose: 0.21 μg/kg/day

Relative Infant Dose: 4.9%

Adult Dose: 100-400 mg BID

Alternatives:

T½ =	1-3 hours (allopurinol)	M/P =	0.9-1.4
PHL =		PB =	0%
T$_{max}$ =	2-6 hours	Oral =	90%
MW =	136	pKa =	
Vd =	1.6		

References:
1. Kamilli I, Gresser U. Allopurinol and oxypurinol in human breastmilk. Clin Investig 1993; 71(2):161-164.

ALMOTRIPTAN

Trade: Axert
Can/Aus/UK: Almogran
Uses: Acute migraine treatment
LRC: L3
AAP: Not reviewed

Almotriptan is a selective serotonin receptor antagonist similar to sumatriptan although it is slightly more bioavailable orally. No data are available on its transfer to human milk. Clinically, it is not much better than oral sumatriptan[1], which has been well studied in breastfeeding women. See sumatriptan for alternative.

Pregnancy Risk Category: C

Lactation Risk Category: L3

Adult Concerns: Nausea, somnolence, headache, dry mouth, tachycardia, myocardial ischemia

Pediatric Concerns: None reported.

Drug Interactions: Higher plasma level of almotriptan could result from use with ketoconazole, amiodarone, cimetidine, clarithromycin, erythromycin, nefazodone, and other inhibitors of CYP3A4. Do not use with ergot alkaloids, MAO inhibitors, verapamil, SSRIs such as fluoxetine, sertraline, etc.

Theoretic Infant Dose:

Relative Infant Dose:

Adult Dose: 6.25-12.5 mg

Alternatives: Sumatriptan

T½ =	3-4 hours	M/P =	
PHL =		PB =	35%
Tmax =	2-4 hours	Oral =	80%
MW =		pKa =	
Vd =	2.85		

References:
1. Spierings EL, Gomez-Mancilla B, Grosz DE, Rowland CR, Whaley FS, Jirgens KJ. Oral almotriptan vs. oral sumatriptan in the abortive treatment of migraine: a double-blind, randomized, parallel-group, optimum-dose comparison. Arch Neurol 2001; 58(6):944-950.

ALOE VERA
Trade: Aloe Vera, Cape, Zanzibar, Socotrine
Can/Aus/UK:
Uses: Extract from A. Vera
LRC: L3
AAP: Not reviewed

There are over 500 species of aloes. The aloe plant yields two important products: Aloe latex derived from the outer skin and Aloe gel, a clear, gelatinous material derived from the inner tissue of the leaf. The aloe gel is the most commonly used product in cosmetic and health food products. The gel contains a polysaccharide glucomannan, similar to guar gum, which is responsible for its emollient effect. Aloe also contains tannins, polysaccharides, organic acids, enzymes, and other products. Bradykininase, a protease inhibitor, is believed to relieve pain and decrease swelling and pruritus. Other components such as an anti-prostaglandin compound is believed to reduce inflammation.[1]

Aloe latex, a bitter yellow product derived from the outer skin, is a drastic cathartic and produces a strong purgative effect on the large intestine due to its anthraquinone barbaloin content. Do not use the latex orally in children.[1] The most common use of the aloe gel is in burn therapy for minor burns and skin irritation. Thus far, well controlled studies do not provide evidence of a clear advantage over aggressive wound care. Two FDA advisory panels failed to find sufficient evidence to show Aloe Vera is useful in treatment of minor burns, cuts, or vaginal irritation.

Recent evidence suggests that A.vera may accelerate wound healing such as in frostbite and in patients undergoing dermabrasion although another study suggests a delay in healing.[2,3] Numerous studies have suggested accelerated wound healing, reduction in arthritic inflammation, and other inflammatory diseases although these are, in many cases, poorly controlled.

The toxicity of A.vera gel when applied topically is minimal. Oral use of the latex derived from the outer skin of A. vera is strongly discouraged as they are drastic cathartics. Aloe emodin and other anthraquinones present in A. vera latex may cause severe gastric cramping and should never be used in pregnant women and children. Aloe has been suggested to inhibit infection and promote healing of minor burns and wounds.[4]

Pregnancy Risk Category:

Lactation Risk Category: L3

Adult Concerns: Severe gastric irritation, strong purgative effect and diarrhea when gel used orally.

Pediatric Concerns: No reports of untoward effects following maternal use or via milk ingestion.

Drug Interactions:

Theoretic Infant Dose:

Relative Infant Dose:

Adult Dose: N/A

Alternatives:

References:
1. Review of Natural Products Ed: Facts and Comparisons 1997.
2. Leung AY. Encyclopedia of Common Natural Ingredients used in Food, Drugs and Cosmetics. J Wiley and Sons, 1980.
3. Fulton JE, Jr. The stimulation of postdermabrasion wound healing with stabilized aloe vera gel-polyethylene oxide dressing. J Dermatol Surg Oncol 1990; 16(5):460-467.
4. Schmidt JM, Greenspoon JS. Aloe vera dermal wound gel is associated with a delay in wound healing. Obstet Gynecol 1991; 78(1):115-117.

ALOSETRON

Trade: Lotronex
Can/Aus/UK:
Uses: Treatment of Irritable Bowel Syndrome
LRC: L3
AAP: Not reviewed

Alosetron (Lotronex) is a new 5-HT3 receptor antagonist which is used to control the symptoms of irritable bowel syndrome. No data are available on the transfer of this medication into human milk. While the manufacturer suggests it is present in animal milk, no data are provided.[1] The peak plasma levels (in young women) of this product are quite small, only averaging 9 nanogram/mL following a 1 mg dose. Although the half-life of the parent alosetron is short (1.5 hours), its metabolites have much longer half-lives although their importance is unknown. Bioavailability is lessened (< 25%) when admixed with food. With this data it is unlikely milk levels will be extraordinarily high or that the levels transferred to the infant will be clinically relevant to the infant. However, its use in breastfeeding patients should be approached with caution until we have more clinical experience with this new product.

Pregnancy Risk Category: B

Lactation Risk Category: L3

Adult Concerns: Constipation is very common, hypertension, nausea less so

Pediatric Concerns: None reported via milk, but no studies exist.

Drug Interactions: It is unlikely alosetron will inhibit the metabolism of drugs metabolized by the major CYP 450 enzymes.

Theoretic Infant Dose:

Relative Infant Dose:

Adult Dose: 1 mg twice daily

Alternatives:

$T\frac{1}{2}$ =	1.5 hours	M/P =		
PHL =		PB =	82%	
T_{max} =	1 hour	Oral =	50-60%	
MW =		pKa =		
Vd =	1.36			

References:
1. Manufacturers package insert Glaxo-Wellcome 2000.

ALPRAZOLAM

Trade: Xanax
Can/Aus/UK: Apo-Alpraz, Novo-Alprazol, Xanax, Kalma, Ralozam
Uses: Benzodiazepine antianxiety agent
LRC: L3
AAP: Drugs whose effect on nursing infants is unknown but may be of concern

Alprazolam is a prototypical benzodiazepine drug similar to Valium but is now preferred in many instances because of its shorter half-life. In a study of 8 women who received a single oral dose of 0.5 mg, the peak alprazolam level in milk was 3.7 µg/L which occurred at 1.1 hours; the observed milk/serum ratio (using AUC method) was 0.36.[1] The neonatal dose of alprazolam in breastmilk is low. The author estimates the average between 0.3 to 5 µg/kg per day. While the infants in this study did not breastfeed, these doses would probably be too low to induce a clinical effect.

In a brief letter, Anderson reports that the manufacturer is aware of withdrawal symptoms in infants following exposure in utero and via breastmilk.[2] In a mother who received 0.5 mg 2-3 times daily (PO) during pregnancy, a neonatal withdrawal syndrome was evident in the breastfed infant the first week postpartum. This data suggests that the amount of alprazolam in breastmilk is insufficient to prevent a withdrawal syndrome following prenatal exposure. In another case of infant exposure solely via breastmilk, the mother took alprazolam (dosage unspecified) for nine months while breastfeeding and withdrew herself from the medication over a 3 week period. The mother reported withdrawal symptoms in the infant including irritability, crying, and sleep disturbances.

The benzodiazepine family, as a rule, are not ideal for breastfeeding mothers due to relatively long half-lives and the development of dependence. However, it is apparent that the shorter-acting benzodiazepines are safest during lactation provided their use is short-term or intermittent, low dose, and after the first week of life.[3]

Pregnancy Risk Category: D

Lactation Risk Category: L3

Adult Concerns: Drowsiness, fatigue, insomnia, confusion, dry mouth, constipation, nausea, vomiting

Pediatric Concerns: Rarely, withdrawal syndrome reported in one breastfed infant. Observe for sedation, poor feeding, irritability, crying, insomnia on withdrawal. Use on an acute or short term basis is not contraindicated.

Drug Interactions: Decreased therapeutic effect when used with carbamazepine, disulfiram. Increased toxicity when used with oral contraceptives, CNS depressants, cimetidine and lithium.

Theoretic Infant Dose: 0.55 µg/kg/day

Relative Infant Dose: 7.8%

Adult Dose: 0.5-1 mg TID

Alternatives: Lorazepam

T½ =	12-15 hours	M/P =	0.36
PHL =		PB =	80%
T$_{max}$ =	1-2 hours	Oral =	Complete
MW =	309	pKa =	
Vd =	0.9-1.3		

References:
1. Oo CY, Kuhn RJ, Desai N, Wright CE, McNamara PJ. Pharmacokinetics in lactating women: prediction of alprazolam transfer into milk. Br J Clin Pharmacol 1995; 40(3):231-236.
2. Anderson PO, McGuire GG. Neonatal alprazolam withdrawal--possible effects of breast feeding. DICP 1989; 23(7-8):614.
3. Maitra R, Menkes DB. Psychotropic drugs and lactation. N Z Med J 1996; 109(1024):217-218.

ALTEPLASE

Trade: Activase
Can/Aus/UK: Actilyse
Uses: Thrombolytic agent
LRC: L3
AAP: Not reviewed

Alteplase is a thrombolytic agent commonly known as tissue-type plasminogen activator (tPA). Alteplase is a large protein with 527 amino acids and with a large molecular weight. It binds to fibrin in a thrombus and converts the plasminogen to plasmin which subsequently leads to a breakdown of the clot. Alteplase is rapidly cleared from the plasma, with an initial half-life of 5 minutes following rapid IV therapy and a somewhat longer half-life of 26-46 minutes following prolonged infusion.[1,2] Its transfer into mature milk would be negligible, but it could potentially pass in small amounts in colostrum. Whether it would be bioavailable in the gut of a newborn infant is questionable, but it would almost certainly not be bioavailable in an older infant. It is very unlikely it would produce adverse effects in breastfed infants.

Pregnancy Risk Category: C

Lactation Risk Category: L3

Adult Concerns: Hemorrhage, reperfusion arrhythmias, bradycardia and possibly seizures

Pediatric Concerns: None reported.

Drug Interactions: May potentiate hemorrhage when used with other anticoagulants such as dicoumarol, warfarin, anisindione, acenocoumarol, phenindione, heparin and etc.   Nitroglycerin may increase clearance of TPA.

Theoretic Infant Dose:

Relative Infant Dose:

Adult Dose: 100 mg

Alternatives:

T½ =	26-46 minutes	M/P =	
PHL =		PB =	
T$_{max}$ =	20-40 minutes	Oral =	Nil
MW =	Large	pKa =	
Vd =	8.1		

References:
1.   Pharmaceutical Manufacturer Prescribing Information.
2.   Verstraete M, Su CA, Tanswell P, Feuerer W, Collen D. Pharmacokinetics and effects on fibrinolytic and coagulation parameters of two doses of recombinant tissue-type plasminogen activator in healthy volunteers. Thromb Haemost 1986; 56(1):1-5.

AMANTADINE

Trade: Symmetrel, Symadine
Can/Aus/UK: Symmetrel, Endantanine, Gen-Amantadine, Mantadine
Uses: Anti-viral
LRC: L3
AAP: Not reviewed

Amantadine is a unique compound that has both antiviral activity against influenza A and is effective in treating Parkinsonian symptoms.[1] Pediatric indications for prevention of influenza for ages 1-10 are available.   Only trace amounts are believed to be secreted in milk although no reports are found. Adult plasma levels following doses of 200 mg daily are 400-900 nanograms/mL.[2]   Even assuming a theoretical milk/plasma ratio of 1.0, the average daily dose to a breastfeeding infant would be far less than 0.9 mg, a dose that would be clinically irrelevant compared to the 4-8 mg/kg dose used in 1 year old infants.

However, amantadine is known to suppress prolactin production and should not be used in breastfeeding mothers or at least used with caution while observing for milk suppression.[3,4]

Pregnancy Risk Category: **C**

Lactation Risk Category: **L3**

Adult Concerns: Urinary retention, vomiting, skin rash in infants. Insomnia, depression, confusion, disorientation, nausea, anorexia, constipation, vomiting

Pediatric Concerns: None reported via milk but a major reduction in prolactin levels has been reported. Avoid.

Drug Interactions: May increase anticholinergic effects when used with anticholinergic or CNS active drugs. Increased toxicity and plasma levels when used with hydrochlorothiazide plus triamterene, or amiloride.

Theoretic Infant Dose:

Relative Infant Dose:

Adult Dose: 100 mg BID

Alternatives:

$T\frac{1}{2}$ =	1-28 hours	M/P =	
PHL =		PB =	67%
T_{max} =	1-4 hours	Oral =	86-94%
MW =	151	pKa =	10.1
Vd =	4.4		

References:
1. Pharmaceutical Manufacturer Prescribing Information. 1997.
2. Cedarbaum JM. Clinical pharmacokinetics of anti-parkinsonian drugs. Clin Pharmacokinet 1987; 13(3):141-178.
3. Correa N, Opler LA, Kay SR, Birmaher B. Amantadine in the treatment of neuroendocrine side effects of neuroleptics. J Clin Psychopharmacol 1987; 7(2):91-95.
4. Siever LJ. The effect of amantadine on prolactin levels and galactorrhea on neuroleptic-treated patients. J Clin Psychopharmacol 1981; 1(1):2-7.

AMIKACIN
Trade: Amikin
Can/Aus/UK: Amikin
Uses: Aminoglycoside antibiotic
LRC: L2
AAP: Not reviewed

Amikacin is a typical aminoglycoside antibiotic used for gram negative infections. Other aminoglycoside antibiotics are poorly absorbed from

GI tract in infants although they could produce changes in GI flora. Only very small amounts are secreted into breastmilk. Following 100 and 200 mg IM doses, only trace amounts have been found in breastmilk and then in only 2 of 4 patients studied.[1] In another study of 2-3 patients who received 100 mg I.M., none to trace amounts were found in milk.[2]

Pregnancy Risk Category: C

Lactation Risk Category: L2

Adult Concerns: Diarrhea, changes in GI flora

Pediatric Concerns: None reported via milk. Commonly used in neonates.

Drug Interactions: Increased aminoglycoside toxicity when used with indomethacin, amphotericin, loop diuretics, vancomycin, enflurane, methoxyflurane, depolarizing neuromuscular blocking agents.

Theoretic Infant Dose:

Relative Infant Dose:

Adult Dose: 5-7.5 mg/kg/dose TID

Alternatives:

$T\frac{1}{2}$ =	2.3 hours	M/P =	
PHL =	4-5 hours	PB =	4%
T_{max} =	0.75-2.0 hours	Oral =	Poor
MW =	586	pKa =	
Vd =	0.28		

References:
1. Matsuda C. A study of amikacin in the obstetrics field. Jpn J Antibiot 1974; 27:633-636.
2. Matsuda S. Transfer of antibiotics into maternal milk. Biol Res Pregnancy Perinatol 1984; 5(2):57-60.

AMINOSALICYLIC ACID (PARA)
Trade: Paser, PAS
Can/Aus/UK: Tubasal, Nemasol
Uses: Antitubercular
LRC: L3
AAP: Drugs associated with significant side effects and should be given with caution

PARA inhibits folic acid synthesis and is selective only for tuberculosis bacteria. Following a maternal dose of 4.0 gm/day, the peak maternal plasma level was 70.1 mg/L and occurred at 2 hours. The breastmilk concentration of 5-ASA at 3 hours was 1.1 mg/L.[1] In another study, the concentration in milk ranged from 0.13 to 0.53 μmol/liter.[2] In a 29 year old mother who received 3 gm/day of 5-ASA for ulcerative colitis, the estimated intake for an infant receiving 120-200 mL of milk was 0.02 to 0.012 mg of 5-ASA.[3] The concentrations of 5-ASA and its metabolite Acetyl-5-ASA present in milk appear too low to produce overt toxicity in most infants. Only one report of slight diarrhea in one infant has been reported.

Pregnancy Risk Category: C

Lactation Risk Category: L3

Adult Concerns: Nausea, vomiting, diarrhea

Pediatric Concerns: Only one report of slight diarrhea in one infant has been reported.

Drug Interactions: Reduces levels of digoxin and vitamin B-12.

Theoretic Infant Dose: 0.16 mg/kg/day

Relative Infant Dose: 0.29%

Adult Dose: 150 mg/kg/day BID or TID

Alternatives:

T½ =	1 hour	M/P =	0.09-0.17
PHL =		PB =	50-73%
T_{max} =	2 hours	Oral =	> 90%
MW =	153	pKa =	
Vd =			

References:

1. Holdiness MR. Antituberculosis drugs and breast-feeding. Arch Intern Med 1984; 144(9):1888.
2. Christensen LA, Rasmussen SN, Hansen SH. Disposition of 5-aminosalicylic acid and N-acetyl-5-aminosalicylic acid in fetal and maternal body fluids during treatment with different 5-aminosalicylic acid preparations. Acta Obstet Gynecol Scand 1994; 73(5):399-402.
3. Klotz U, Harings-Kaim A. Negligible excretion of 5-aminosalicylic acid in breastmilk. Lancet 1993; 342(8871):618-619.

AMIODARONE

Trade: Cordarone

Can/Aus/UK: Cordarone, Aratac

Uses: Strong antiarrhythmic agent

LRC: L5

AAP: Drugs whose effect on nursing infants is unknown but may be of concern

Amiodarone is a potent and sometimes dangerous antiarrhythmic drug and requires close supervision by clinicians. Although poorly absorbed by the mother (<50%), maximum serum levels are attained after 3-7 hours. This drug has a very large volume of distribution, resulting in accumulation in adipose, liver, spleen, and lungs and has a high rate of fetal toxicity (10-17%). It should not be given to pregnant mothers unless critically required.

Significant amounts are secreted into breastmilk at levels higher than the plasma level. Breastmilk samples obtained at birth and at 2 and 3 weeks post-partum in 2 patients contained levels of amiodarone and desethylamiodarone varying from 1.7 to 3.0 mg/L (mean =2.3 mg/L) and 0.8 to 1.8 mg/L (mean =1.1 mg/L), respectively.[1] Despite the concentrations of amiodarone in milk, the amounts were apparently not high enough to produce plasma levels of both drugs higher than about 0.1 µg/mL, which are minimal compared to the maternal plasma levels of 1.2 µg/mL or higher.

McKenna reported amiodarone milk levels in a mother treated with 400 mg daily.[2] In this study, at 6 weeks postpartum, breastmilk levels of amiodarone and desethylamiodarone varied during the day from 2.8-16.4 mg/L and 1.1-6.5 mg/L respectively. Reported infant plasma levels of amiodarone and desethylamiodarone were 0.4 and 0.25 respectively. The dose ingested by the infant was approximately 1.5 µg/kg/day. The authors suggest that the amount of amiodarone ingested was moderate and could expose the developing infant to a significant dose of the drug and should be avoided. Because amiodarone inhibits extrathyroidal deiodinases, conversion of T4 to T3 is reduced. One reported case of hypothyroidism has been reported in an infant following therapy in the mother. Because of the long half-life and high concentrations in various organs, amiodarone could continuously build up to higher levels in the infant although it was not reported in the above studies. This product should be used only under the most extraordinary conditions, and the infant should be closely monitored for cardiovascular and thyroid function.

Pregnancy Risk Category: C

Lactation Risk Category: L5

Adult Concerns: Hypothyroidism, myocardial arrhythmias, pulmonary toxicity, serious liver injury, congestive heart failure

Pediatric Concerns: Hypothyroidism has been reported. Extreme caution is urged.

Drug Interactions: Amiodarone interferes with the metabolism of a number of drugs including: oral anticoagulants, beta blockers, calcium channel blockers, digoxin, flecainide, phenytoin, procainamide, quinidine. Plasma levels of these drugs tend to be increased to hazardous levels.

Theoretic Infant Dose: 2.46 mg/kg/day

Relative Infant Dose: 43.05%

Adult Dose: 200-800 mg BID

Alternatives: Disopyramide, Mexiletine

$T\frac{1}{2}$ =	26-107 days	M/P =	4.6-13
PHL =		PB =	99.98%
T_{max} =	3-7 hours	Oral =	22-86%
MW =	643	pKa =	6.6
Vd =	18-148		

References:
1. Plomp TA, Vulsma T, de Vijlder JJ. Use of amiodarone during pregnancy. Eur J Obstet Gynecol Reprod Biol 1992; 43(3):201-207.
2. McKenna WJ, Harris L, Rowland E, Whitelaw A, Storey G, Holt D. Amiodarone therapy during pregnancy. Am J Cardiol 1983; 51(7):1231-1233.

AMITRIPTYLINE

Trade: Elavil, Endep
Can/Aus/UK: Apo-Amitriptyline, Elavil, Novo-Tryptin, Amitrol, Endep, Mutabon D, Tryptanol, Domical, Lentizol
Uses: Tricyclic antidepressant
LRC: L2
AAP: Drugs whose effect on nursing infants is unknown but may be of concern

Amitriptyline and its active metabolite, nortriptyline, are secreted into breastmilk in small amounts. In one report of a mother taking 100 mg/day of amitriptyline, milk levels of amitriptyline and nortriptyline (active metabolite) averaged 143 μg/L and 55.5 μg/L respectively; maternal serum levels averaged 112 μg/L and 72.5 μg/L respectively.[1] No drug was detected in the infants serum. From this data, an infant would consume approximately 21.5 μg/kg/day, a dose that is unlikely to be clinically relevant.

In another study following a maternal dose of 25 mg/day, the amitriptyline and nortriptyline(active metabolite) levels in milk were 30 μg/L and < 30 μg/L respectively.[2] In the same study when the dosage was 75 mg/day, milk levels of amitriptyline and nortriptyline averaged 88 μg/L and 69 μg/L respectively. Both drugs were essentially undetectable in the infant's serum. Therefore, the authors estimated that a nursing infant would receive less than 0.1 mg/day.

Pregnancy Risk Category: D

Lactation Risk Category: L2

Adult Concerns: Anticholinergic side effects, such as drying of secretions, dilated pupil, sedation

Pediatric Concerns: No untoward effects have been noted in several studies.

Drug Interactions: Phenobarbital may reduce effect of amitriptyline. Amitriptyline blocks the hypotensive effect of guanethidine. May increase toxicity of amitriptyline when used with clonidine. Dangerous when used with MAO inhibitors, other CNS depressants. May increase anticoagulant effect of coumadin, warfarin. SSRIs (Prozac, Zoloft,etc) should not be used with or soon after amitriptyline or other TCAs due to serotonergic crisis.

Theoretic Infant Dose: 21.4 μg/kg/day

Relative Infant Dose: 1.5%

Adult Dose: 15-150 mg BID

Alternatives: Amoxapine, Imipramine

T½ =	31-46 hours	M/P =	1.0
PHL =		PB =	94.8%
T$_{max}$ =	2-4 hours	Oral =	Complete
MW =	277	pKa =	9.4
Vd =	6-10		

References:
1. Bader TF, Newman K. Amitriptyline in human breastmilk and the nursing infant's serum. Am J Psychiatry 1980; 137(7):855-856.
2. Brixen-Rasmussen L, Halgrener J, Jorgensen A. Amitriptyline and nortriptyline excretion in human breastmilk. Psychopharmacology (Berl) 1982; 76(1):94-95.
3. Matheson I, Skjaeraasen J. Milk concentrations of flupenthixol, nortriptyline and zuclopenthixol and between-breast differences in two patients. Eur J Clin Pharmacol 1988; 35(2):217-220.

AMLODIPINE BESYLATE

Trade: Norvasc
Can/Aus/UK: Norvasc, Istin
Uses: Antihypertensive, calcium channel blocker
LRC: L3
AAP: Not reviewed

Amlodipine is a typical calcium channel blocker, antihypertensive agent which has greater bioavailability and a longer duration of action.[1] No data are currently available on transfer of amlodipine into breastmilk. Because most calcium channel blockers (CCB) readily transfer into milk, we should assume the same for this drug. Use caution if administering to lactating women.

Pregnancy Risk Category: C

Lactation Risk Category: **L3**

Adult Concerns: Hypotension, bradycardia, edema, headache, or nausea

Pediatric Concerns: None reported but observe for bradycardia, hypotension upon prolonged use.

Drug Interactions: Cyclosporine levels may be increased when used with calcium channel blockers. Use with azole antifungals (fluconazole, itraconazole, ketoconazole, etc) may lead to enhanced amlodipine levels. Use with rifampin may significantly reduce plasma levels of calcium channel blockers.

Theoretic Infant Dose:

Relative Infant Dose:

Adult Dose: 5-10 mg daily

Alternatives: Nifedipine, Nimodipine

$T^{1/2}$ =	30-50 hours	M/P =	
PHL =		PB =	93%
T_{max} =	6-9 hours	Oral =	64-65%
MW =	408	pKa =	
Vd =	21		

References:
1. Pharmaceutical Manufacturer Prescribing Information. 2002

AMOXAPINE
Trade: Asendin
Can/Aus/UK: Asendin, Asendis
Uses: Tricyclic antidepressant
LRC: L2
AAP: Drugs whose effect on nursing infants is unknown but may be of concern

Amoxapine and its metabolite are both secreted into breastmilk at relatively low levels. Following a dose of 250 mg/day, milk levels of amoxapine were less than 20 µg/L and 113 µg/L of the active metabolite.[1] Milk levels of active metabolite varied from 113 to 168 µg/L in two other milk samples. Maternal serum levels of amoxapine and metabolite at steady state were 97 µg/L and 375 µg/L respectively.

Pregnancy Risk Category: **C**

Lactation Risk Category: **L2**

Adult Concerns: Dry mouth, constipation, urine retention, drowsiness or sedation, anxiety, emotional disturbances, parkinsonism, tardive dyskinesia, seizures

Pediatric Concerns: None reported via milk.

Drug Interactions: Decreased effect of clonidine, guanethidine. Amoxapine may increase effect of CNS depressants, adrenergic agents, anticholinergic agents. Increased toxicity with MAO inhibitors.

Theoretic Infant Dose: 16.9 µg/kg/day

Relative Infant Dose: 0.5%

Adult Dose: 25 mg BID or TID

Alternatives:

T½ =	8 hours(parent)	M/P =	0.21
PHL =		PB =	15-25%
Tmax =	2 hours	Oral =	18-54%
MW =	314	pKa =	
Vd =	65.7		

References:
1.   Gelenberg AJ. Single case study. Amoxapine, a new antidepressant, appears in human milk. J Nerv Ment Dis 1979; 167(10):635-636.

AMOXICILLIN
Trade: Larotid, Amoxil
Can/Aus/UK: Amoxil, Apo-Amoxi, Novamoxin, Alphamox, Moxacin, Cilamox, Betamox
Uses: Penicillin antibiotic
LRC: L1
AAP: Maternal Medication Usually Compatible with Breastfeeding

Amoxicillin is a popular oral penicillin used for otitis media and many other pediatric/adult infections. In one group of 6 mothers who received 1 gm oral doses, the concentration of amoxicillin in breastmilk ranged from 0.68 to 1.3 mg/L of milk (average = 0.9 mg/L).[1]   Peak levels occurred at 4-5 hours. Milk/plasma ratios at 1,2, and 3 hours were 0.014, 0.013, and 0.043.   Less than 0.95% of the maternal dose is secreted into milk. No harmful effects have been reported.

Pregnancy Risk Category: B

Lactation Risk Category: L1

Adult Concerns: Diarrhea,   rashes, and changes in GI flora. Pancytopenia, rarely pseudomembranous colitis

Pediatric Concerns: None reported. Commonly used in neonates and children.

Drug Interactions: Efficacy of oral contraceptives may be reduced. Disulfiram and probenecid may increase plasma levels of amoxicillin. Allopurinol may increase the risk of amoxicillin skin rash.

Theoretic Infant Dose: 0.13 mg/kg/day

Relative Infant Dose: 0.95%

Adult Dose: 500-875 mg BID

Alternatives:

$T\frac{1}{2}$ =	1.7 hours	M/P =	0.014-0.043
PHL =	4 hours (neonate)	PB =	18%
T_{max} =	1.5 hours	Oral =	89%
MW =	365	pKa =	
Vd =	0.3		

References:

1. Kafetzis DA, Siafas CA, Georgakopoulos PA, Papadatos CJ. Passage of cephalosporins and amoxicillin into the breastmilk. Acta Paediatr Scand 1981; 70(3):285-288.

AMOXICILLIN + CLAVULANATE

Trade: Augmentin

Can/Aus/UK: Clavulin, Augmentin

Uses: Penicillin antibiotic, extended spectrum

LRC: L1

AAP: Not reviewed

Addition of clavulanate extends spectrum of amoxicillin by inhibiting beta lactamase enzymes. Small amounts of amoxicillin (0.9 mg/L milk) are secreted in breastmilk. No harmful effects have been reported[1]. See amoxicillin. Although clavulanic acid is well absorbed and widely distributed, no reports of secretion into human milk exist, but it should be expected ($T\frac{1}{2}$= 1 hour). May cause changes in GI flora and possibly fungal (candida) overgrowth.

Pregnancy Risk Category: B

Lactation Risk Category: L1

Adult Concerns: Diarrhea, rash, thrush, or diarrhea

Pediatric Concerns: None reported but observe for diarrhea, rash.

Drug Interactions: Efficacy of oral contraceptives may be reduced. Disulfiram and probenecid may increase plasma levels of amoxicillin. Allopurinol may increase the risk of amoxicillin skin rash.

Theoretic Infant Dose: 0.135 mg/kg/day

Relative Infant Dose: 0.95%

Adult Dose: 875 mg BID

Alternatives:

T½ =	1.7 hours	M/P =	0.014-0.043
PHL =	4 hours (neonate)	PB =	18%
T$_{max}$ =	1.5 hours	Oral =	89%
MW =	365	pKa =	
Vd =	0.3		

References:
1. Kafetzis DA, Siafas CA, Georgakopoulos PA, Papadatos CJ. Passage of cephalosporins and amoxicillin into the breastmilk. Acta Paediatr Scand 1981; 70(3):285-288.

AMPHETAMINES, HALLUCINOGENIC
Trade: Ecstasy, Adam, Eve, Harmony, Love
Can/Aus/UK:
Uses: Amphetamines
LRC: L5
AAP: Contraindicated by the American Academy of Pediatrics in Breastfeeding Mothers

Hallucinogenic amphetamines are a group of illegal amphetamines synthesized specifically for inducing hallucinogenic stimulation. While their use in breastfeeding mothers is certainly contraindicated, their illicit use is increasing. There is a widely held belief among users that it is safe. In the last several years there have been a number of reports of the drug producing severe acute toxicity and death and there are concerns that it may produce long-term damage to the serotonin nerve terminals.[1] MDMA, MDEA, and MDA are three of the most prevalent of this group. Their "street names" are: MDMA=Adam, Ecstasy, MDM=XTC, Essence; MDEA= Eve; MDA=Harmony, Love, Love Drug, Speed for Lovers. All of these agents are amphetamine derivatives with extreme hallucinogenic and stimulant activity. As with most amphetamines, their half-lives are rather brief (less than 8 hours). Urinary excretion of these agents is generally complete within 24 hours but this depends on dose and individual.[2] Their duration of action varies with dose and individual but is 4-6 hours with doses of 75-150 mg. Because their structures are similar to methamphetamine, it is likely that significant amounts can transfer into human milk. Hallucinations, extreme agitation and seizures would be likely if an infant were exposed early in the administration of these agents. It is not known when it would be safe to reinitiate breastfeeding, but 24-48 hours should be sufficient to reduce risks to the infant. Again this depends on the dose administered.

Pregnancy Risk Category:

Lactation Risk Category: L5

Adult Concerns: Hallucinations, agitation, seizures, acute paranoid psychosis, extreme hypertension, hyperthermia, tachyarrhythmias may occur. Effects largely depend on the dose.

Pediatric Concerns: None reported via milk but breastfeeding should be interrupted for at least 24 hours following last administration.

Drug Interactions:

Theoretic Infant Dose:

Relative Infant Dose:

Adult Dose:

Alternatives:

T½ =	< 8 hours	M/P =	
PHL =		PB =	
T$_{max}$ =	1-5 hours	Oral =	Complete
MW =		pKa =	
Vd =			

References:
1. Green AR, Cross AJ, Goodwin GM. Review of the pharmacology and clinical pharmacology of 3,4-methylenedioxymethamphetamine (MDMA or "Ecstasy"). Psychopharmacology (Berl) 1995; 119(3):247-260.
2. Verebey K, Alrazi J, Jaffe JH. The complications of 'ecstasy' (MDMA). JAMA 1988; 259(11):1649-1650.

AMPHOTERICIN B

Trade: Fungizone, Amphotec
Can/Aus/UK: Ambisome, Resteclin, Abelcet, Fungilin, Amphocel
Uses: Antifungal
LRC: L3
AAP: Not reviewed

Amphotericin B is an intravenous antifungal effective for the treatment of Cryptococcus neoformans, Candida albicans, Histoplasma capsulatum, Coccidioides immitis, and Aspergillus infections.[1] Amphotericin is significantly toxic and is reserved for life-threatening infections. No data are available on its transfer to human milk. However, it is virtually unabsorbed orally (< 9%) and is commonly used in pediatrics. It is quite unlikely the amount in milk would be clinically relevant to a breastfeeding infant.

Pregnancy Risk Category: B

Lactation Risk Category: L3

Adult Concerns: Adverse effects include anemia, thrombocytopenia, congestive heart failure, thrombophlebitis, paresthesias, hypokalemia, hyperthermia, nephrotoxicity, hepatotoxicity, pulmonary toxicity, erythematous reactions, and anaphylaxis.

Pediatric Concerns: None reported. Unlikely to be absorbed orally.

Drug Interactions: Antagonism with azole antifungals. Enhanced renal toxicity with cyclosporin. Enhanced digitalis toxicity due to hypokalemia.

Theoretic Infant Dose:

Relative Infant Dose:

Adult Dose: 0.25 to 1.0 milligram/kilogram (mg/kg) daily IV

Alternatives:

$T\frac{1}{2}$ =	15 days	M/P =		
PHL =		PB =	> 90%	
T_{max} =	< 1 hour	Oral =	< 9%	
MW =	924	pKa =		
Vd =	4			

References:
1.   Pharmaceutical Manufacturer Prescribing Information. 2002

AMPICILLIN
Trade: Polycillin, Omnipen
Can/Aus/UK: Apo-Ampi, Novo-Ampicillin, NuAmpi, Penbriton, Ampicyn, Austrapen, Amfipen, Britcin, Vidopen
Uses: Penicillin antibiotic
LRC: L1
AAP: Not reviewed

Low milk/plasma ratios of 0.2 have been reported.[1] In a study by Matsuda of 2-3 breastfeeding patients who received 500 mg of ampicillin orally,   levels in milk peaked at 6 hours and averaged only 0.14 mg/L of milk.[2] The milk/plasma ratio was reported to be 0.03 at 2 hours.   In a group of 9 breastfeeding women sampled at various times and who received doses of 350 mg TID orally, milk concentrations ranged from 0.06 to 0.17 mg/L with peak milk levels at 3-4 hours after the dose.[3] Milk/plasma ratios varied between 0.01 and 0.58. The highest reported milk level (1.02 mg/L) was in a patient receiving 700 mg TID. Ampicillin was not detected in the plasma of any infant.

Ampicillin is one of the most commonly used prophylactic antibiotics in pediatric neonatal nurseries. Neonatal half-life is 2.8 to 4 hours. Possible rash, sensitization, diarrhea, or candidiasis could occur, but unlikely. May alter GI flora.

Pregnancy Risk Category: B

Lactation Risk Category: L1

Adult Concerns: Diarrhea, rash, fungal overgrowth, agranulocytosis, pseudomembranous colitis, anaphylaxis

Pediatric Concerns: None reported but observe for diarrhea.

Drug Interactions: Efficacy of oral contraceptives may be reduced. Disulfiram and probenecid may increase plasma levels of ampicillin. Allopurinol may increase the risk of ampicillin skin rash.

Theoretic Infant Dose: 0.15 mg/kg/day

Relative Infant Dose: 1.5%

Adult Dose: 250-500 mg QID

Alternatives: Amoxicillin

T½ =	1.3 hours	M/P =	0.58
PHL =	1.7 hours (neonate)	PB =	8-20
T$_{max}$ =	1-2 hours	Oral =	50%
MW =	349	pKa =	
Vd =	0.38		

References:
1. Kafetzis DA, Siafas CA, Georgakopoulos PA, Papadatos CJ. Passage of cephalosporins and amoxicillin into the breastmilk. Acta Paediatr Scand 1981; 70(3):285-288.
2. Matsuda S. Transfer of antibiotics into maternal milk. Biol Res Pregnancy Perinatol 1984; 5(2):57-60.
3. Branebjerg PE, Heisterberg L. Blood and milk concentrations of ampicillin in mothers treated with pivampicillin and in their infants. J Perinat Med 1987; 15(6):555-558.

AMPICILLIN + SULBACTAM

Trade: Unasyn
Can/Aus/UK: Dicapen
Uses: Penicillin antibiotic with extended spectrum.
LRC: L1
AAP: Not reviewed

Small amounts of ampicillin may transfer (1 mg/L).[1] Possible rash, sensitization, diarrhea, or candidiasis could occur but are unlikely. May alter GI flora. There are no reports of sulbactam secretion into human milk, but it is probably low and largely without side effects (AHL= 1 hour PB= 38%).

Pregnancy Risk Category: B

Lactation Risk Category: L1

Adult Concerns: Diarrhea, rash, fungal overgrowth, agranulocytosis, pseudomembranous colitis, anaphylaxis

Pediatric Concerns: None reported but observe for diarrhea.

Drug Interactions: Efficacy of oral contraceptives may be reduced. Disulfiram and probenecid may increase plasma levels of amoxicillin. Allopurinol may increase the risk of amoxicillin skin rash.

Theoretic Infant Dose: 0.15 mg/kg/day

Relative Infant Dose: 1.5%

Adult Dose: 1.5-3 gm QID

Alternatives:

$T\frac{1}{2}$ =	1.3 hours	M/P =	0.01-0.5
PHL =	1.7 hours (15-30 days old)	PB =	28%
T_{max} =	1-2 hours	Oral =	60%
MW =	349	pKa =	
Vd =	0.38		

References:
1. Kafetzis DA, Siafas CA, Georgakopoulos PA, Papadatos CJ. Passage of cephalosporins and amoxicillin into the breastmilk. Acta Paediatr Scand 1981; 70(3):285-288.

ANAKINRA
Trade: Kineret
Can/Aus/UK: Kineret
Uses: Anti-rheumatic
LRC: L3
AAP: Not reviewed

Anakinra is a recombinant form of the human interleukin-1 receptor antagonist (IL-1RA) and is used to reduce the inflammatory stimuli that mediate various inflammatory and immunological responses common in rheumatoid arthritis. It is a large molecular weight protein (17,300 daltons) administered subcutaneously. Due to its size, it is very unlikely to enter milk after the first week postpartum. In addition it is not likely to be orally bioavailable in an infant. However, we do not have data on its transfer to human milk and if used the infant should be observed for increased risk of GI infections.

Pregnancy Risk Category: B

Lactation Risk Category: L3

Adult Concerns: Adverse events include a high risk of serious infections(2%), URI, headache, nausea, and diarrhea

Pediatric Concerns: None reported via milk. This agent is too large to enter milk effectively after the first week postpartum.

Drug Interactions: None

Theoretic Infant Dose:

Relative Infant Dose:

Adult Dose: 100 mg SC daily

Alternatives:

T½ =	4-6 hours	M/P =	
PHL =		PB =	Nil
T$_{max}$ =		Oral =	Nil
MW =	17,300	pKa =	
Vd =			

References:
1. Pharmaceutical Manufacturers prescribing information, 2003.

ANTHRALIN
Trade: Anthra-Derm, Drithocreme, Dritho-Scalp, Micanol
Can/Aus/UK: Anthraforte, Anthranol, Anthrascalp, Dithranol, Alphodith
Uses: Anti-psoriatic
LRC: L3
AAP: Not reviewed

Anthralin is a synthetic tar derivative used topically for suppression of psoriasis. Anthralin, when applied topically, induces burning and inflammation of the skin but is one of the most effective treatments for psoriasis. Purple-brown staining of skin and permanent staining of clothing and porcelain bathroom fixtures is frequent. Anthralin when applied topically is absorbed into the surface layers of the skin and only minimal amounts enter the systemic circulation. That absorbed is rapidly excreted via the kidneys almost instantly; plasma levels are very low to undetectable.[1] No data are available on its transfer into human milk. Most anthralin is eliminated by washing off and desquamation of insolubles.[2] For this reason, when placed directly on lesions on the areola or nipple, breastfeeding should be discouraged. Another similar anthraquinone is Senna (laxative), which even in high doses does not enter milk. While undergoing initial intense treatment, it would perhaps be advisable to interrupt breastfeeding temporarily, but this may be overly conservative. Observe the infant for diarrhea. It has been used in children over 2 years of age for psoriasis.

Pregnancy Risk Category: C

Lactation Risk Category: L3

Adult Concerns: Pruritus, skin irritation, and inflammation. Purple-brown staining of skin and permanent staining of clothing and porcelain bathroom fixtures is frequent. Anthralin may have carcinogenic properties following high doses in mice. This may have no relevance to humans at all.

Pediatric Concerns: Diarrhea, nausea, vomiting via milk, but no reports have been published.

Drug Interactions:

Theoretic Infant Dose:

Relative Infant Dose:

Adult Dose: Apply topical BID

Alternatives:

T½ =	Brief	M/P =	
PHL =		PB =	
T$_{max}$ =		Oral =	Complete
MW =	226	pKa =	
Vd =			

References:
1. Goodfield MJ, Hull SM, Cunliffe WJ. The systemic effect of dithranol treatment in psoriasis. Acta Derm Venereol 1994; 74(4):295-297.
2. Shroot B. Mode of action of dithranol, pharmacokinetics/dynamics. Acta Derm Venereol Suppl (Stockh) 1992; 172:10-12.

ANTHRAX (BACILLUS ANTHRACIS)
Trade: Anthrax Infection, Bacillus Anthracis
Can/Aus/UK:
Uses: Anthrax infection
LRC: L5 if infected
AAP: Maternal Medication Usually Compatible with Breastfeeding

Anthrax is caused by the gram-positive, spore-forming bacterium bacillus anthracis. The spore may persist in nature for many years and infect grazing animals such as sheep, goats, and cattle. The most common forms of the disease are inhaled, oral, and cutaneous. The Center for Disease Control has recently published guidelines for treating or prophylaxing exposed breastfeeding mothers. The following web site contains several treatment options.[1]

Thus far, all of the anthrax strains released by bioterrorists have been sensitive to ciprofloxacin, doxycycline, and the penicillin family. In breastfeeding women, amoxicillin (80 mg/kg/d in 3 divided doses) is an option for antimicrobial prophylaxis when B. anthracis is known to be penicillin-susceptible and no contraindication to maternal amoxicillin use is indicated. The American Academy of Pediatrics also considers ciprofloxacin and tetracyclines (which include doxycycline) to be usually compatible with breastfeeding because the amount of either drug absorbed by infants is small, but little is known about the safety of long-term use.

Until culture sensitivity tests have been completed, the breastfeeding mother should be treated with ciprofloxacin (see ofloxacin or levofloxacin as alternates) or doxycycline. Once cultures show that the anthrax strain is sensitive to penicillins, then the mother can switch to amoxicillin for long term use up to 60 days or more. Due to possible dental staining following prolonged exposure, this author would not suggest long-term use(60 days) of doxycycline in a breastfeeding mother. The CDC offers several alternative antibiotics such as rifampin, vancomycin, imipenem, clindamycin, and clarithromycin in those patients will allergic conditions.[2] Check the CDC web sites for the most current recommendations.[3]

Pregnancy Risk Category:

Lactation Risk Category: L5 if infected

References:

1.   http://www.cdc.gov/mmwr/preview/mmwrhtml/mm504a5.htm. 2004.
2.   Update: Investigation of bioterrorism-related anthrax and interim guidelines for exposure management and antimicrobial therapy, October 2001 MMWR Morb Mortal Wkly Rep 2001; 50(42):909-919.
3.   Center for Disease Control Web site: http://www.bt.cdc.gov/. 2004.

ANTHRAX VACCINE

Trade: Anthrax Vaccine
Can/Aus/UK:
Uses: Vaccination
LRC: L3
AAP: Not reviewed

The anthrax vaccine for humans, licensed for use in the United States, is a cell-free filtrate vaccine, which means it uses dead bacteria as opposed to live bacteria. The vaccine is reported to be 93% effective in protecting against cutaneous anthrax.[1] The vaccine should only be administered to healthy men and women from 18 to 65 years of age since investigations to date have been conducted exclusively in that population. Because it is not known whether the anthrax vaccine can cause fetal harm, pregnant women should not be vaccinated. There are no data or indications relative to its use in breastfeeding mothers. While it consists primarily of protein fragments of anthrax bacteria, it is very unlikely any would transfer into milk nor even be bioavailable in the infant. The CDC states that " No data suggest increased risk for side effects or temporally related adverse events associated with receipt of anthrax vaccine by breast-feeding women or breast-fed children."

Administration of nonliving vaccines (e.g., anthrax vaccine) during breast-feeding is not medically contraindicated."

Pregnancy Risk Category: C

Lactation Risk Category: L3

Adult Concerns: Mild local reactions occur in 30% of recipients and consist of slight tenderness and redness at the injection site. A moderate local reaction can occur if the vaccine is given to anyone with a past history of anthrax infection. Severe local reactions are very infrequent and consist of extensive swelling of the forearm in addition to the local reaction. Systemic reactions occur in fewer than 0.2% of recipients and are characterized by flu-like symptoms.

Pediatric Concerns: None reported via milk.

Drug Interactions:

Theoretic Infant Dose:

Relative Infant Dose:

Adult Dose: 2-30 mg per day

Alternatives:

References:
1. Center for Disease Control Web site: http://www.bt.cdc.gov/. 2004.

ANTIPYRINE
Trade: Antipyrine
Can/Aus/UK:
Uses: Analgesic, antipyretic
LRC: L5
AAP: Not reviewed

Insignificant secretion into breastmilk.[1] This product is no longer used in the USA due to high incidence of fatal bone marrow toxicity. Contraindicated.

Pregnancy Risk Category:

Lactation Risk Category: L5

Adult Concerns: Severe bone marrow toxicity

Pediatric Concerns: None reported but due to better medications, this product should never be used.

Drug Interactions:

Theoretic Infant Dose:

Relative Infant Dose:

Adult Dose:

Alternatives: Ibuprofen, acetaminophen

T½ =		M/P =	1.0
PHL =		PB =	< 1%
T$_{max}$ =	1-2 hours	Oral =	
MW =	188	pKa =	1.4
Vd =	0.56		

References:
1. Berlin CM, Jr., Vesell ES. Antipyrine disposition in milk and saliva of lactating women. Clin Pharmacol Ther 1982; 31(1):38-44.

ARGATROBAN
Trade: Argatroban
Can/Aus/UK:
Uses: Synthetic direct thrombin inhibitor: anticoagulant
LRC: L4
AAP: Not reviewed

Argatroban is a synthetic inhibitor of thrombin and is derived from L-arginine. It reversibly binds to the thrombin active site and exerts an anticoagulant effect by inhibiting thrombin-catalyzed reactions. It is primarily indicated as an anticoagulant for treatment of thrombosis in patients with heparin-induced thrombocytopenia. It is primarily in the extracellular fluid as evidenced by its low volume of distribution. No data are available on its transfer to human milk but it is reported present in rodent milk. It is not reported if this product is orally bioavailable. The presence of this product in milk could potentially induce GI hemorrhage in weak or susceptible infants including newborns, premature infants, infants with NEC, and other infants. Extreme caution is recommended until we know levels present in milk and more about its GI stability and absorption.

Pregnancy Risk Category: B

Lactation Risk Category: L4

Adult Concerns: Hemorrhage

Pediatric Concerns: None reported via milk.

Drug Interactions: Prolongation of prothrombin times when co-administered with heparin, warfarin and potentially aspirin. Angelica, Bilberry, Arnica, Astragalus, and Anise may increase the risk of bleeding.

Theoretic Infant Dose:

Relative Infant Dose:

Adult Dose: Initial: 25 μg/kg/minutes. Highly variable.

Alternatives:

T½ =	39-51 minutes	M/P =	
PHL =		PB =	54%
T$_{max}$ =	1-3 hours	Oral =	Unknown
MW =	526	pKa =	
Vd =	0.174		

References:
1. Pharmaceutical Manufacturers Prescribing Information, 2003.

ARGININE
Trade: L-Arginine, Arginine
Can/Aus/UK:
Uses: Amino Acid; test for Growth Hormone release
LRC: L3
AAP: Not reviewed

L-Arginine is a naturally-occurring basic amino acid. It is classified as a semi essential amino acid and is a potent stimulant of pituitary growth hormone and insuline release. Found in most foods, it can also easily be synthesized by the human. L-Arginine participates in many biochemical reactions but is most well known for its ability to stimulate "endothelium-derived relaxing factor" now known as nitric oxide (NO). NO plays critical roles in may diverse physiological processes including neurotransmission, vasorelaxation, and immune responses. There are "unconfirmed" reports that L-arginine may promote tumor growth in patients with malignancies and who receive supplements. Numerous other studies do not show this effect at all.

L-Arginine is not overly toxic. Doses as high as 30 g/day have been generally well tolerated in adults with the most common adverse effects of nausea and diarrhea being reported. No reports of its transfer into human milk are available. Most importantly, we do not know if high doses of L-Arginine subsequently increase Arginine levels in milk, although it would seem likely. As this product has limited usefulness in most patients, its use at high doses in breastfeeding mothers should be avoided until milk levels are reported.

Pregnancy Risk Category: B

Lactation Risk Category: L3

Adult Concerns: Allergic reactions have been reported to the administration of L-Arginine. When infused intravenous, local irritation, nausea and vomiting are reported. Hyperkalemia has occurred. Use cautiously in patients with liver and/or renal disease.

Pediatric Concerns: None reported via milk.

Drug Interactions: Potentially fatal hyperkalemia when used with spironolactone.

Theoretic Infant Dose:

Relative Infant Dose:

Adult Dose: 1-2 gm/day but highly variable. Doses as high as 30 gm/d have been used short-term.

Alternatives:

$T\frac{1}{2}$ =	< 2 hours	M/P =	
PHL =		PB =	
T_{max} =	1.5 hours	Oral =	70%
MW =	174	pKa =	2.18 & 9.0
Vd =			

References:

ARIPIPRAZOLE

Trade: Abilify
Can/Aus/UK:
Uses: Psychotropic drug for schizophrenia
LRC: L3
AAP: Not reviewed

Aripiprazole is an atypical antipsychotic agent that is indicated for the treatment of schizophrenia and schizoaffective disorder. It is apparently better tolerated than haloperidol. It should be comparatively similar to risperidone, olanzapine. But at this time, risperidone and olanzapine should be preferred due to published data in breastfeeding mothers.

Pregnancy Risk Category: C

Lactation Risk Category: L3

Adult Concerns: Orthostatic hypotension has been reported. Seizures, cognitive motor impairment, disruption of body temperature, esophageal dysmotility and aspiration have been reported. Elevated levels of prolactin, extrapyramidal symptoms, changes in weight, and somnolence have been reported.

Pediatric Concerns: None via milk but caution recommended until we have data.

Drug Interactions: Carbamazepine may stimulate metabolism and increase plasma clearance of aripiprazole. Inhibitors of CYP3A4 (ketoconazole) could increase plasma levels of aripiprazole.

Theoretic Infant Dose:

Relative Infant Dose:

Adult Dose: 10-15 mg/day

Alternatives: Risperidone, olanzapine

$T\frac{1}{2}$ =	75 hours(parent)	M/P =	
PHL =		PB =	99%
T_{max} =	3-5 hours	Oral =	87%
MW =	448	pKa =	
Vd =	4.9		

References:
1. Pharmaceutical Manufacturers prescribing information, 2003.

ASCORBIC ACID
Trade: Ascorbica, Cecon, Cevi-Bid, Ce-Vi-Sol, Vitamin C
Can/Aus/UK:
Uses: Vitamin C
LRC: L1
AAP: Not reviewed

Ascorbic acid is an essential vitamin. Without supplementation, 75 mg/day is excreted in the urine of the average individual due to overabundance. Renal control of vitamin C is significant and maintains plasma levels at 0.4 to 1.5 mg/dL regardless of dose. Ascorbic acid is secreted into human milk in well controlled sequence and mature milk contains 5 mg/100 mL.[1] Excessive Vitamin C intake in the mother does not alter (or increase) the controlled secretion into breastmilk. The RDA for mother is 100 mg/day. Maternal supplementation is only required in undernourished mothers.

Pregnant women should not use excessive ascorbic acid due to metabolic induction in the fetal liver, followed by a metabolic rebound scurvy early postpartum in the neonate. Ascorbic acid should not routinely be administered to breastfed infants unless to treat clinical scurvy.

Pregnancy Risk Category: A during 1st and 2nd trimester
C during 3rd trimester

Lactation Risk Category: L1

Adult Concerns: Renal calculi with large doses. Faintness, flushing, dizziness, nausea, vomiting, gastritis.

Pediatric Concerns: None reported via breastmilk, but excessive use prepartum is strongly discouraged.

Drug Interactions: Ascorbic acid decreases propranolol peak concentrations. Aspirin decreases ascorbate levels and increases aspirin levels. Reduced effect of warfarin when used with ascorbic acid. Urinary acidification results in decreased retention of many basic drugs, including tricyclic antidepressants, amoxapine, amphetamines. Do not use with aluminum antacids. Ascorbic acid reduces renal elimination of aluminum leading to encephalopathy, seizures, coma.

Theoretic Infant Dose:

Relative Infant Dose:

Adult Dose: 45-60 mg daily

Alternatives:

T½ =		M/P =	
PHL =		PB =	
Tmax =	2-3 hours	Oral =	Complete
MW =	176	pKa =	
Vd =			

References:
1. Sneed SM, Zane C, Thomas MR. The effects of ascorbic acid, vitamin B6, vitamin B12, and folic acid supplementation on the breastmilk and maternal nutritional status of low socioeconomic lactating women. Am J Clin Nutr 1981; 34(7):1338-1346.

ASPARTAME

Trade: Nutrasweet
Can/Aus/UK:
Uses: Artificial sweetener
LRC: L1
         L5 if used in infants with PKU
AAP: Not reviewed

Aspartame consists of two linked amino acids: aspartic acid and phenylalanine. Once in the GI tract, it is rapidly metabolized to phenylalanine and aspartic acid. Maternal ingestion of 50 mg/kg aspartame will approximately double (2.3 to 4.8 μmol/dL) aspartate milk levels. Phenylalanine milk levels similarly increased from 0.5 to 2.3 μmol/dL. This dose is 3-4 times the normal dose used, and these milk levels are too low to produce significant side effects in normal infants[1,2]. Contraindicated in infants with proven phenylketonuria.

Pregnancy Risk Category: B

Lactation Risk Category: L1
                              L5 if used in infants with PKU

Adult Concerns: Only contraindicated in infants with PKU.

Pediatric Concerns: None reported except contraindicated in infants with documented phenylketonuria.

Drug Interactions:

Theoretic Infant Dose:

Relative Infant Dose:

Adult Dose:

Alternatives:

T½ =		M/P =	
PHL =		PB =	
T$_{max}$ =		Oral =	Complete
MW =	294	pKa =	
Vd =			

References:
1. Levels of free amino acids in lactating women following ingestion of the sweetener aspartame Nutr Rev 1980; 38(5):183-184.
2. Stegink LD, Filer LJ, Jr., Baker GL. Plasma, erythrocyte and human milk levels of free amino acids in lactating women administered aspartame or lactose. J Nutr 1979; 109(12):2173-2181.

ASPIRIN

Trade: Anacin, Ecotrin, Aspergum, Empirin, Genprin, Arthritis Foundation Pain Reliever
Can/Aus/UK: Coryphen, Ecotrin, Novasen, Entrophen, Disprin, Aspro, Cartia
Uses: Salicylate analgesic
LRC: L3
AAP: Drugs associated with significant side effects and should be given with caution

Extremely small amounts secreted into breastmilk. Few harmful effects have been reported. Following single or multiple doses, peak levels occur at approximately 3 hours and vary from 1.12 to 1.69 mg/L.[1] In another study of a rheumatoid arthritis patient who received 4 gm/day, none was detectable in her milk (< 5mg/100cc).[2] Extremely high doses in mother could potentially produce slight bleeding in infant. Because aspirin is implicated in Reye's Syndrome in febrile-viral illnesses, it is a poor choice of analgesic to use in breastfeeding mothers. However, in rheumatic fever patients, it is still the anti-inflammatory drug of choice and a risk-vs-benefit assessment must be done in this case. See ibuprofen or acetaminophen as a better choice.

Pregnancy Risk Category: C during 1st and 2nd trimester
                                                    D during 3rd trimester

Lactation Risk Category: L3

Adult Concerns: GI ulceration, distress, esophagitis, nephropathy, hepatotoxicity, tinnitus, platelet dysfunction

Pediatric Concerns: None reported via milk, but aspirin use in pediatric patients may increase risk of Reye's syndrome in viral infections.

Drug Interactions: May decrease serum levels of other NSAIDs as well as GI distress. Aspirin may antagonize effect of probenecid. Aspirin may increase methotrexate serum levels, and increase free valproic acid plasma levels and valproate toxicity. May increase anticoagulant effect of warfarin.

Theoretic Infant Dose: 0.25 mg/kg/day

Relative Infant Dose: 0.04%

Adult Dose: 325-900 mg QID

Alternatives: Ibuprofen, Acetaminophen

T½ =	2.5-7 hours	M/P =	0.03-0.08
PHL =		PB =	88-93%
T$_{max}$ =	1-2 hours	Oral =	80-100%
MW =	180	pKa =	
Vd =	0.15		

References:
1. Findlay JW, DeAngelis RL, Kearney MF, Welch RM, Findlay JM. Analgesic drugs in breastmilk and plasma. Clin Pharmacol Ther 1981; 29(5):625-633.
2. Erickson SH, Oppenheim GL. Aspirin in breastmilk. J Fam Pract 1979; 8(1):189-190.

ATENOLOL

Trade: Tenoretic, Tenormin
Can/Aus/UK: Apo-Atenolol, Anselol, Noten, Tenlol, Tensig, Tenormin, Antipress
Uses: Antihypertensive beta blocker
LRC: L3
AAP: Drugs associated with significant side effects and should be given with caution

Atenolol is a potent cardio-selective beta blocker. Data conflict on the secretion of atenolol into breastmilk. One author reports an incident of significant bradycardia, cyanosis, low body temperature, and low blood pressure in breastfeeding infant of mother consuming 100 mg atenolol daily while a number of others have failed to detect plasma levels in the neonate or untoward side effects.[1]

Data seem to indicate that atenolol secretion into breastmilk is highly variable but may be as high as 10 times greater than for propranolol. In one study, women taking 50-100 mg/day were found to have M:P ratios of 1.5-6.8. However, even with high M:P ratios, the calculated intake per day (at peak levels) for a breastfeeding infant would only be 0.13 mg.[2]

In a study by White, breastmilk levels in one patient were 0.7, 1.2 and 1.8 mg/L of milk at doses of 25, 50 and 100 mg daily respectively.[3] In another study, the estimated daily intake for an infant receiving 500 mL milk per day would be 0.3 mg.[4] In these five patients who received 100 mg daily, the mean milk concentration of atenolol was 630 μg/L. In a study by Kulas, the amount of atenolol transferred into milk varied from 0.66 mg/L with a maternal dose of 25 mg, 1.2 mg/L with a maternal dose of 50 mg, and 1.7 mg/L with a maternal dose of 100 mg per day.[5] Although atenolol is approved by the AAP, some caution is recommended due to the milk/plasma ratios and the reported problem with one infant.

Pregnancy Risk Category: C

Lactation Risk Category: L3

Adult Concerns: Persistent bradycardia, hypotension, heart failure, dizziness, fatigue, insomnia, lethargy, confusion, impotence, dyspnea, wheezing in asthmatics

Pediatric Concerns: One report of bradycardia, cyanosis, low body temperature, and hypotension in a breastfeeding infant of mother consuming 100 mg atenolol daily, but other reports do not suggest clinical effects on breastfed infants.

Drug Interactions: Decreased effect when used with aluminum salts, barbiturates, calcium salts, cholestyramine, NSAIDs, ampicillin, rifampin, and salicylates. Beta blockers may reduce the effect of oral sulfonylureas (hypoglycemic agents). Increased toxicity/effect when used with other antihypertensives, contraceptives, MAO inhibitors, cimetidine, and numerous other products. See drug interaction reference for complete listing.

Theoretic Infant Dose: 94.5 μg/kg/day

Relative Infant Dose: 6.6%

Adult Dose: 50-100 mg daily

Alternatives: Propranolol, Metoprolol

T½ =	6.1 hours	M/P =	1.5-6.8
PHL =	6.4 hrs	PB =	5%
T_{max} =	2-4 hours	Oral =	50-60%
MW =	266	pKa =	9.6
Vd =	1.3		

References:
1. Schimmel MS, Eidelman AI, Wilschanski MA, Shaw D, Jr., Ogilvie RJ, Koren G, Schmimmel MS, Eidelman AJ. Toxic effects of atenolol consumed during breast feeding. J Pediatr 1989; 114(3):476-478.
2. Liedholm H, Melander A, Bitzen PO, Helm G, Lonnerholm G, Mattiasson I, Nilsson B, Wahlin-Boll E. Accumulation of atenolol and metoprolol in human breastmilk. Eur J Clin Pharmacol 1981; 20(3):229-231.
3. White WB, Andreoli JW, Wong SH, Cohn RD. Atenolol in human plasma and breastmilk. Obstet Gynecol 1984; 63(3 Suppl):42S-44S.
4. Thorley KJ, McAinsh J. Levels of the beta-blockers atenolol and propranolol in the breastmilk of women treated for hypertension in pregnancy. Biopharm Drug Dispos 1983; 4(3):299-301.
5. Kulas J, Lunell NO, Rosing U, Steen B, Rane A. Atenolol and metoprolol. A comparison of their excretion into human breastmilk. Acta Obstet Gynecol Scand Suppl 1984; 118:65-69.

ATOMOXETINE

Trade: Strattera
Can/Aus/UK:
Uses: Stimulant for treatment of ADHD
LRC: L4
AAP: Not reviewed

Atomoxetine is a selective norepinephrine reuptake inhibitor that is presently indicated for the treatment of Attention-Deficit/Hyperactivity Disorder (ADHD). Atomoxetine metabolism is highly variable. One group of poor metabolizers (7%) may have extended half-lives (22 hours) and higher plasma levels while another group of normal metabolizers has a half-life of about 5 hours. No data are available on the transfer of Atomoxetine into human milk. Because this is a lipophilic, neuroactive drug, there is some potential risk coincident with its use in a breastfeeding mother, and mothers should probably be cautioned about its use while breastfeeding.

Pregnancy Risk Category: C

Lactation Risk Category: L4

Adult Concerns: Adverse events include abdominal pain, dyspepsia, vomiting, decreased appetite, dizziness, headache, and cough

Pediatric Concerns: None reported via milk but no studies are available. If used, reduced weight gain, insomnia, and hyperactivity could occur.

Drug Interactions: Levels may be increased by inhibitors of CYP2D6 (paroxetine, fluoxetine, quinidine, etc). Albuterol may increase heart rate in patients treated with atomoxetine. Atomoxetine may increase plasma levels of midazolam. Do not use with or within two weeks of the use of a monoamine oxidase inhibitor (MAOi). Do not use in patients with narrow angle glaucoma.

Theoretic Infant Dose:

Relative Infant Dose:

Adult Dose: 0.5-1.2 mg/kg/day

Alternatives:

T½ =	5.2 hours	M/P =	
PHL =		PB =	98%
T_{max} =	1-2 hours	Oral =	63-94%
MW =	291	pKa =	
Vd =	0.85		

References:
1. Pharmaceutical Manufacturers prescribing information, 2003.

ATORVASTATIN CALCIUM
Trade: Lipitor
Can/Aus/UK: Lipitor
Uses: Cholesterol-lowering agent
LRC: L3
AAP: Not reviewed

Atorvastatin is a typical HMG Co-A reductase inhibitor for lowering plasma cholesterol levels. It is known to transfer into animal milk, but human studies are not available.[1] Due to its poor oral absorption and high protein binding, it is unlikely that clinically relevant amounts would transfer into human milk. Nevertheless, atherosclerosis is a chronic process and discontinuation of lipid-lowering drugs during pregnancy and lactation should have little to no impact on the outcome of long-term therapy of primary hypercholesterolemia. Cholesterol and other products of cholesterol biosynthesis are essential components for fetal and neonatal development, and the use of cholesterol-lowering drugs would not be advisable under any circumstances.

Pregnancy Risk Category: X

Lactation Risk Category: L3

Adult Concerns: Liver dysfunction, rhabdomyolysis with acute renal failure

Pediatric Concerns: None reported, but the use of these products in lactating women is not recommended.

Drug Interactions: Increased risk of myopathy when used with cyclosporin, fibric acid derivatives, niacin, erythromycin, and azole antifungals (Diflucan, etc). Decreased plasma levels of atorvastatin when used with antacids or colestipol.

Theoretic Infant Dose:

Relative Infant Dose:

Adult Dose: 10-80 mg daily

Alternatives:

T½ =	14 hours	M/P =	
PHL =		PB =	98%
T$_{max}$ =	1-2 hours	Oral =	12-30%
MW =	1209	pKa =	
Vd =	8		

References:
1. Pharmaceutical Manufacturer Prescribing Information. 1999.

ATOVAQUONE AND PROGUANIL
Trade: Malarone
Can/Aus/UK:
Uses: Antimalarials
LRC: L3
AAP: Not reviewed

Malarone is a fixed combination of atovaquone (250 mg) and proguanil (100 mg) (adult dose). The pediatric chewable tablet contains atovaquone (62.5) and proguanil (25 mg). Malarone is used both to prevent and treat malaria, particularly malaria resistant to certain other drugs. Both adult and pediatric formulations are available for treating pediatric patients down to 11 kg. There are no data available for transfer of these agents into human milk although the pharmaceutical company suggests that atovaquone concentrations in rodent milk were 30% of the concurrent concentrations in the maternal plasma. It is this author's experience that rodent levels are much higher than found in humans. Only trace quantities of proguanil were found in human milk. Further, while the pharmacokinetics of proguanil is similar in adults and pediatric patients, the elimination half-life of atovaquone is much shorter in pediatric patients (1-2 days) than in adult patients (2-3 days). Elimination half-life ranges from 32 to 84 hours for atovaquone and 12 to 21 hours for proguanil; the half-life of cycloguanil is approximately 14 hours.

For current information contact the CDC web site for information (www.cdc.gov). **According to the CDC, breastfeeding mothers with infants less than 11 kg should use mefloquine instead of malarone.**[2]

	Atovaquone	Progaunil
T½	32-84 h	12-21 h
Oral bioavailability	23%	Complete
Protein Binding	> 99%	75%

Pedi dose: One, two, or three MALARONE Pediatric Tablets (62.5 mg atovaquone and 25 mg proguanil hydrochloride) once a day depending on your child's body weight. For children over 40 kg (88 pounds) in weight, one MALARONE tablet (adult dose) once a day.

Pregnancy Risk Category: C

Lactation Risk Category: L3

Adult Concerns: Headache, fever, myalgia, abdominal pain, cough, diarrhea, dyspepsia, back pain, gastritis have been reported.

Pediatric Concerns: None reported via milk.

Drug Interactions: Major reductions in plasma levels of atovaquone have been reported following the use of tetracycline (40%), metoclopramide, rifampin (50%), or rifabutin (34%).

Theoretic Infant Dose:

Relative Infant Dose:

Adult Dose: Atovaquone (250 mg); Proguanil (100 mg) daily

Alternatives: Mefloquine

References:
1. Pharmaceutical Manufacturer Prescribing Information.
2. http://www.cdc.gov/ncidod/dpd/parasites/malaria/default.htm. 2004.

ATROPINE
Trade: Belladonna, Atropine
Can/Aus/UK: Atropine Minims, Atropisol, Isopto-Atropine, Atropt, Eyesule
Uses: Anticholinergic, drying agent
LRC: L3
AAP: Maternal Medication Usually Compatible with Breastfeeding

Atropine is a powerful anticholinergic that is well distributed throughout the body[1]. Only small amounts are believed secreted in milk[2]. Effects may be highly variable. Slight absorption together with enhanced neonatal sensitivity creates hazardous potential. Use caution. Avoid if possible but not definitely contraindicated.

Pregnancy Risk Category: C

Lactation Risk Category: L3

Adult Concerns: Dry, hot skin. Decreased flow of breastmilk.

Decreased bowel motility, drying of secretions, dilated pupil, and increased heart rate.

Pediatric Concerns: No reports are available, although caution is urged.

Drug Interactions: Phenothiazines, levodopa, antihistamines, may decrease anticholinergic effects of atropine. Increased toxicity when admixed with amantadine and thiazide diuretics.

Theoretic Infant Dose:

Relative Infant Dose:

Adult Dose: 0.6 mg every 6 hours

Alternatives:

T½ =	4.3 hours	M/P =	
PHL =		PB =	14-22%
T$_{max}$ =	1 hour	Oral =	90%
MW =	289	pKa =	9.8
Vd =	2.3-3.6		

References:
1. Drug Facts and Comparisons 1995 ed. ed. St. Louis: 1995.
2. Wilson J. Drugs in Breastmilk. New York: ADIS Press 1981.

AZAPROPAZONE
Trade:
Can/Aus/UK: Rheumox
Uses: Analgesic
LRC: L2
AAP: Maternal Medication Usually Compatible with Breastfeeding

Azapropazone a partial NSAID and anti-inflammatory. Unlike other NSAIDs its main effect is to stabilize the lysosomal membrane and only to a limited extent does it suppress prostaglandin synthetase. In a study of 4 patients each received 600 mg IV within 2 hours after giving birth, and thereafter, they received 600 mg twice daily.[1] Milk levels of azapropazone were measured on days 4 and 6 postpartum. The amount of azapropazone excreted in the breastmilk within 12 h ranged from 0.2 mg to 1.3 mg (mean 0.8 mg in 12 hours) or an average milk concentration of 2.43 μg/mL. The volume of milk produced during this 12 hour period averaged 329 mL. The relative infant dose over 24 hours would be 2.12% of the maternal dose. The authors did not report side effects in the infants.

Pregnancy Risk Category:

Lactation Risk Category: L2

Adult Concerns: Adverse effects include diarrhea, vomiting, nausea, GI distress, GI bleeding, headache, edema, GI ulceration, and other typical side effects of NSAID drugs.

Pediatric Concerns: None reported via milk in one study.

Drug Interactions: Increased azapropazone levels when mixed with cimetidine. Enhanced anticoagulant effect when mixed with coumarins, and other anticoagulants. Reduced excretion of lithium, and methotrexate when admixed with azapropazone. May block antihypertensive effects of beta-blockers, calcium channel blockers and other antihypertensives.

Theoretic Infant Dose: 0.36 mg/kg/day

Relative Infant Dose: 2.1%

Adult Dose: 600 mg twice daily

Alternatives: Celecoxib

$T\frac{1}{2}$ =	13-14 hours	M/P =	
PHL =		PB =	99%
T_{max} =	3-6 hours orally	Oral =	83%
MW =		pKa =	
Vd =	0.17		

References:
1. Bald R, Bernbeck-Betthauser EM, Spahn H, Mutschler E. Excretion of azapropazone in human breastmilk. Eur J Clin Pharmacol 1990; 39(3):271-273.

AZATHIOPRINE
Trade: Imuran
Can/Aus/UK: Imuran, Thioprine
Uses: Immunosuppressive agent
LRC: L3
AAP: Not reviewed

Azathioprine is a powerful immunosuppressive agent that is metabolized to 6-Mercaptopurine (6-MP). In two mothers receiving 75 mg azathioprine, the concentration of 6-Mercaptopurine in milk varied from 3.5-4.5 μg/L in one mother and 18 μg/L in the second mother[1]. Both levels were peak milk concentrations at 2 hours following the dose. The authors conclude that these levels would be too low to produce clinical effects in a breastfed infant. Using this data for 6-MP, an infant would absorb only 0.1 % of the weight-adjusted maternal dose, which is too low to likely produce adverse effects in a breastfeeding infant. Plasma levels in treated patients is maintained at 50 ng/mL or higher. One infant continued to breastfeed during therapy and displayed no immunosuppressive effects.

In another study of two infants who were breastfed by mothers receiving 75-100 mg/d azathioprine, milk levels of 6-MP were not measured. But both infants had normal blood counts, no increase in infections, and above-average growth rate[2]. Caution is recommended.

Pregnancy Risk Category: D

Lactation Risk Category: L3

Adult Concerns: Bone marrow suppression, megaloblastic anemia, infections, skin cancers, lymphoma, nausea, vomiting, hepatoxicity, pulmonary dysfunction, and pancreatitis

Pediatric Concerns: None reported, but caution is urged.

Drug Interactions: Increased toxicity when used with allopurinol. Reduce azathioprine dose to 1/3 to 1/4 of normal.   Use with ACE inhibitors has produced severe leukopenia.

Theoretic Infant Dose: 2.7 μg/kg/day

Relative Infant Dose: 0.25%

Adult Dose: 1-2.5 mg/kg/day

Alternatives:

T½ =	0.6 hour	M/P =	
PHL =		PB =	30%
Tmax =	1-2 hours	Oral =	41-44%
MW =	277	pKa =	
Vd =			

References:
1. Coulam CB, Moyer TP, Jiang NS, Zincke H. Breast-feeding after renal transplantation. Transplant Proc 1982; 14(3):605-609.
2. Grekas DM, Vasiliou SS, Lazarides AN. Immunosuppressive therapy and breast-feeding after renal transplantation. Nephron 1984; 37(1):68.

AZELAIC ACID
Trade: Azelex, Finevin
Can/Aus/UK: Skinoren
Uses: Topical treatment of acne
LRC: L3
AAP: Not reviewed

Azelaic is a dicarboxylic acid derivative normally found in whole grains and animal products. Azelaic acid, when applied as a cream, produces a significant reduction of P. acnes and an antikeratinizing effect as well. Small amounts of azelaic acid are normally present in human milk.[1] Azelaic acid is only modestly absorbed via skin (< 4%), and it is rapidly metabolized. The amount absorbed does not change the levels normally found in plasma nor milk. Due to its poor penetration into plasma and rapid half-life (45 min), it is not likely to penetrate milk or produce untoward effects in a breastfed infant.

Pregnancy Risk Category: B

Lactation Risk Category: L3

Adult Concerns: Pruritus, burning, stinging, erythema, dryness, peeling and skin irritation

Pediatric Concerns: None reported via milk. Normal constituent of milk.

Drug Interactions:

Theoretic Infant Dose:

Relative Infant Dose:

Adult Dose: Apply topical BID

Alternatives:

T½ =	45 minutes	M/P =	
PHL =		PB =	
T$_{max}$ =		Oral =	
MW =	188	pKa =	
Vd =			

References:
1. Pharmaceutical Manufacturer Prescribing Information. 1999.

AZELASTINE
Trade: Astelin, Optivar
Can/Aus/UK: Azep, Rhinolast, Optilast
Uses: Antihistamine
LRC: L3
AAP: Not reviewed

Azelastine (Astelin) is an antihistamine for oral, intranasal and ophthalmic administration. It is effective in treating seasonal and perennial rhinitis and nonallergic vasomotor rhinitis. Ophthalmically, it is effective for allergic conjunctivitis (itchy eyes). Oral bioavailability is 80%, and intranasal bioavailability is only 40%. No data are available on the transfer of azelastine into human milk. The doses used intranasally and ophthalmically are so low that it is extremely unlikely to produce clinically relevant levels in human milk. Oral administration could potentially lead to slightly higher levels, but azelastine is relatively devoid of serious side effects and it is doubtful that any would occur in a breastfed infant. However, this is an extremely bitter product. It is possible that even miniscule amounts in milk could alter the taste of milk leading to rejection by the infant.

Pregnancy Risk Category: C

Lactation Risk Category: L3

Adult Concerns: Intranasal: nasal burning and bitter taste, headache, somnolence.   Orally: drowsiness and bitter taste.   Ophthalmic: transient eye burning/stinging, headache, and bitter taste.

Pediatric Concerns: None reported via milk.   Levels in milk are unlikely to pose a problem.   May impart bitter taste to milk, infant may reject milk.

Drug Interactions: Avoid use in asthmatics.   Cimetidine significantly increases plasma levels of azelastine.

Theoretic Infant Dose:

Relative Infant Dose:

Adult Dose: Variable: 1-2 sprays(137 μg/spray) per nostrile BID.

Alternatives: Loratadine, cetirizine

$T\frac{1}{2}$ =	22 hour		M/P =	
PHL =			PB =	88%
T_{max} =	2-3 hours		Oral =	80%
MW =	418		pKa =	
Vd =	14.5			

References:
1. Pharmaceutical Manufacturers prescribing information, 2003.

AZITHROMYCIN

Trade: Zithromax
Can/Aus/UK: Zithromax
Uses: Erythromycin-like antibiotic
LRC: L2
AAP: Not reviewed

Azithromycin belongs to erythromycin family.   It has an extremely long half-life, particularly in tissues.[1]   Azithromycin is concentrated for long periods in phagocytes, which are known to be present in human milk. In one study of a patient who received 1 gm initially followed by two 500mg doses at 24 hr intervals, the concentration of azithromycin in breastmilk varied from 0.64 mg/L (initially) to 2.8 mg/L on day 3.[2]

The predicted dose of azithromycin received by the infant would be approximately 0.4 mg/kg/day.   This would suggest that the level of azithromycin ingested by a breastfeeding infant is not clinically significant. New pediatric formulations of azithromycin have been recently introduced. Pediatric dosing is 10 mg/kg STAT followed by 5 mg/kg per day for up to 5 days.

Pregnancy Risk Category: B

Lactation Risk Category: L2

Adult Concerns: Diarrhea, loose stools, abdominal pain, vomiting, nausea.

Pediatric Concerns: None reported via breastmilk. Pediatric formulations are available.

Drug Interactions: Aluminum and magnesium-containing antacids may slow but not reduce absorption of azithromycin. Increased effect/toxicity when used with tacrolimus, alfentanil, astemizole, terfenadine, loratadine, carbamazepine, cyclosporine, digoxin, disopyramide, triazolam.

Theoretic Infant Dose: 0.42 mg/kg/day

Relative Infant Dose: < 2.9%

Adult Dose: 250-500 mg daily
Alternatives:

$T\frac{1}{2}$ =	48-68 hours		M/P =	
PHL =			PB =	7-51%
T_{max} =	3-4 hours		Oral =	37%
MW =	749		pKa =	
Vd =	23-31			

References:
1. Pharmaceutical Manufacturer Prescribing Information. 1996.
2. Kelsey JJ, Moser LR, Jennings JC, Munger MA. Presence of azithromycin breastmilk concentrations: a case report. Am J Obstet Gynecol 1994; 170(5 Pt 1):1375-1376.

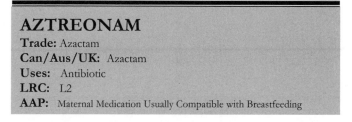

AZTREONAM
Trade: Azactam
Can/Aus/UK: Azactam
Uses: Antibiotic
LRC: L2
AAP: Maternal Medication Usually Compatible with Breastfeeding

Aztreonam is a monobactam antibiotic whose structure is similar but different than the penicillins and is used for documented gram-negative sepsis. Following a single 1 g IV dose, breastmilk level was 0.18 mg/L at 2 hours and 0.22 mg/L at 4 hours[1]. An infant would ingest approximately 33.0 µg/kg/day or < 0.03% of the maternal dose per day. The manufacturer reports that less than 1% of a maternal dose is transferred into milk.[2]   Due to poor oral absorption (< 1%), no untoward effects would be expected in nursing infants, aside from changes in GI flora.   Aztreonam is commonly used in pediatric units.

Pregnancy Risk Category: B

Lactation Risk Category: L2

Adult Concerns: Changes in GI flora, diarrhea, rash, elevations of hepatic function tests

Pediatric Concerns: None reported via milk.

Drug Interactions: Check hypersensitivity to penicillins and other beta-lactams. Requires dosage adjustment in renal failure.

Theoretic Infant Dose: 33 µg/kg/day

Relative Infant Dose: 0.23%

Adult Dose: 1-2 g BID or QID

Alternatives:

T½ =	1.7 hours	M/P =	0.005
PHL =	2.6 hours	PB =	60%
T$_{max}$ =	0.6-1.3 hours	Oral =	< 1%
MW =	435	pKa =	
Vd =	0.26-0.36		

References:
1.   Fleiss PM, Richwald GA, Gordon J, Stern M, Frantz M, Devlin RG. Aztreonam in human serum and breastmilk. Br J Clin Pharmacol 1985; 19(4):509-511.
2.   Pharmaceutical Manufacturer Prescribing Information. 1996.

BACLOFEN

Trade: Lioresal, Atrofen
Can/Aus/UK: Lioresal, Novo-Baclofen, Apo-Baclofen, Clofen
Uses: Skeletal muscle relaxant
LRC: L2
AAP: Maternal Medication Usually Compatible with Breastfeeding

Baclofen inhibits spinal reflexes and is used to reverse spasticity associated with multiple sclerosis or spinal cord lesions. Animal studies indicate baclofen inhibits prolactin release and may inhibit lactation. Small amounts of baclofen are secreted into milk. In one mother given a 20 mg dose, total consumption by infant over a 26 hr period is estimated to be 22 µg, about 0.1% of the maternal dose[1]. The milk half-life was 5.6 hours. It is quite unlikely that baclofen administered intrathecally would be secreted into milk in significant quantities.

Pregnancy Risk Category: C

Lactation Risk Category: **L2**

Adult Concerns: Drowsiness, excitement, dry mouth, urinary retention, tremor, rigidity, and wide pupils

Pediatric Concerns: None reported.

Drug Interactions: Decreased effect when used with lithium. Increased effect of opiate analgesics, CNS depressants, alcohol (sedation), tricyclic antidepressants, clindamycin (neuromuscular blockade), guanabenz, MAO inhibitors.

Theoretic Infant Dose:

Relative Infant Dose:

Adult Dose: 5-25 mg TID

Alternatives:

T½ =	3-4 hours	M/P =	
PHL =		PB =	30%
T$_{max}$ =	2-3 hours	Oral =	Complete
MW =	214	pKa =	
Vd =			

References:
1. Eriksson G, Swahn CG. Concentrations of baclofen in serum and breastmilk from a lactating woman. Scand J Clin Lab Invest 1981; 41(2):185-187.

BARIUM

Trade: Barium
Can/Aus/UK: ACB, Medebar, Medescan, Baritop
Uses: Radiopaque agent
LRC: L1
AAP: Not reviewed

Contrast agent used in radiology that is not absorbed orally. No reported harmful effects. Maternal absorption limited.

Pregnancy Risk Category:

Lactation Risk Category: **L1**

Adult Concerns: Nausea, vomiting, constipation

Pediatric Concerns: None reported, not absorbed.

Drug Interactions:

Theoretic Infant Dose:

Relative Infant Dose:

Adult Dose: N/A

Alternatives:

References:

BECLOMETHASONE

Trade: Vanceril, Beclovent, Beconase
Can/Aus/UK: Propaderm, Vanceril, Beconase, Becloforte, Aldecin, Beclovent, Becotide
Uses: Intranasal, intrapulmonary steroid
LRC: L2
AAP: Not reviewed

Beclomethasone is a potent steroid that is generally used via inhalation in asthma or via intranasal administration for allergic rhinitis. Due to its potency, only very small doses are generally used and ,therefore, minimal plasma levels are attained. Intranasal absorption is generally minimal.[1,2] Due to small doses administered, absorption into maternal plasma is extremely small. Therefore, it is unlikely that these doses would produce clinical significance in a breastfeeding infant. See corticosteroids.

Pregnancy Risk Category: C

Lactation Risk Category: L2

Adult Concerns: When administered intranasally or via inhalation, adrenal suppression is very unlikely. Complications include headaches, hoarseness, bronchial irritation, oral candidiasis, cough. When used orally, complications may include adrenal suppression.

Pediatric Concerns: None reported via milk and inhalation or intranasal use. Oral doses could suppress the adrenal cortex, and induce premature closure of the epiphysis, but would require high doses.

Drug Interactions: Corticosteroids have few drug interactions.

Theoretic Infant Dose:

Relative Infant Dose:

Adult Dose: 504-840 µg daily

Alternatives:

T½ =	15 hours	M/P =	
PHL =		PB =	87%
T$_{max}$ =		Oral =	90% (oral)
MW =	409	pKa =	
Vd =			

References:
1. Pharmaceutical Manufacturer Prescribing Information. 1996.
2. McEvoy GE. AFHS Drug Information. New York, NY: 1995.

BENAZEPRIL HCL

Trade: Lotensin, Lotrel
Can/Aus/UK: Lotensin
Uses: Antihypertensive, ACE inhibitor
LRC: L3
AAP: Not reviewed

Benazepril belongs to the ACE inhibitor family. Oral absorption is rather poor (37%). The active component (benazeprilat) reaches a peak at approximately 2 hours after ingestion. Generally, ACE inhibitors are seldom used during the early neonatal period due to profound neonatal hypotension. However, only minimal amounts are secreted into human milk. A newborn infant ingesting only breastmilk would receive less than 0.1% of the mg/kg maternal dose of benazepril and benazeprilat.

Lotrel is a combination product containing benazepril and amlodipine, a calcium channel blocker.

Pregnancy Risk Category: D

Lactation Risk Category: L3

Adult Concerns: Significant fetal and neonatal morbidity, hypotension

Pediatric Concerns: Neonatal morbidity, severe hypotension after in-utero exposure.

Drug Interactions: Decreased bioavailability with antacids. Reduced hypotensive effect with NSAIDS. Phenothiazines increase hypotensive effect. Allopurinol dramatically increase hypersensitivities (Steven-Johnson Syn.). ACE inhibitors dramatically increase digoxin levels. Lithium levels may be significantly increased with ACE use. Elevated potassium levels with oral potassium supplements.

Theoretic Infant Dose:

Relative Infant Dose:

Adult Dose: 20-40 mg daily

Alternatives: Enalapril, Captopril

T½ =	10-11 hours	M/P =	
PHL =		PB =	96.7%
T$_{max}$ =	0.5 - 1 hour	Oral =	37%
MW =		pKa =	
Vd =			

References:
1. Pharmaceutical Manufacturer Prescribing Information. 1996.

BENDROFLUMETHIAZIDE

Trade: Naturetin
Can/Aus/UK: Naturetin, Aprinox, Berkozide, Centyl, Urizid
Uses: Thiazide diuretic
LRC: L4
AAP: Maternal Medication Usually Compatible with Breastfeeding

Bendroflumethiazide is a thiazide diuretic sometimes used to suppress lactation. In one study, the clinician found this thiazide to effectively inhibit lactation[1]. Use with caution. Not generally recommended in breastfeeding mothers.

Pregnancy Risk Category: D

Lactation Risk Category: L4

Adult Concerns: Diuresis, fluid loss, leukopenia, hypotension, dizziness, headache, vertigo, reduced milk production

Pediatric Concerns: None reported, but may inhibit lactation.

Drug Interactions: Enhanced hyponatremia and hypotension when used with ACE inhibitors. May elevate lithium levels.

Theoretic Infant Dose:

Relative Infant Dose:

Adult Dose: 2.5-10 mg daily

Alternatives: Hydrochlorothiazide

$T\frac{1}{2}$ =	3-3.9 hours	M/P =	
PHL =		PB =	94%
T_{max} =	2-4 hours	Oral =	Complete
MW =	421	pKa =	
Vd =	1.48		

References:
1. Healy M. Suppressing lactation with oral diuretics. The Lancet 1961;1353-1354.

BENZONATATE

Trade: Tessalon Perles
Can/Aus/UK:
Uses: Antitussive
LRC: L3
AAP: Not reveiwed

Benzonatate is a nonnarcotic cough suppressant similar to the local anesthetic tetracaine. It anesthetizes stretch receptors in respiratory passages, dampening their activity and reducing the cough reflex.[1] There are little pharmacokinetic data on this product and no data on transfer into human milk. Because codeine is almost equally effective, and because we know that codeine only marginally transfers into human milk, it is probably a preferred antitussive in breastfeeding mothers.

Pregnancy Risk Category: C

Lactation Risk Category: L3

Adult Concerns: Sedation, headache, dizziness, constipation, nausea, pruritus have been reported.

Pediatric Concerns: None reported via milk.

Drug Interactions:

Theoretic Infant Dose:

Relative Infant Dose:

Adult Dose: 100 mg TID

Alternatives: Codeine

T½ =	< 8 hours	M/P =	
PHL =		PB =	
T$_{max}$ =	20 minutes	Oral =	Good
MW =		pKa =	
Vd =			

References:
1. Drug Facts and Comparisons 1998 ed. ed. St. Louis: 1998.

BEPRIDIL HCL

Trade: Vascor, Bepadin
Can/Aus/UK:
Uses: Antihypertensive, calcium channel blocker
LRC: L4
AAP: Not reviewed

Following therapy with bepridil, milk levels were reported to approach 1/3 of serum levels.[1,2] As with other calcium channel blockers, this family has been found to produce embryotoxic effects and should be used cautiously in pregnant women. Long half-life, enhanced oral absorption, and potency of this compound would increase the danger in nursing infant. Caution is recommended if used in nursing mother.

Pregnancy Risk Category: C

Lactation Risk Category: L4

Adult Concerns: Bradycardia, hypotension

Pediatric Concerns: None reported, but other calcium channel blockers may be preferred. See nifedipine.

Drug Interactions: H2 blockers may enhance oral absorption of bepridil. Beta blockers may enhance hypotensive effect. Bepridil may increase carbamazepine, cyclosporin, digitalis, quinidine, theophylline levels when used with these products.

Theoretic Infant Dose:

Relative Infant Dose:

Adult Dose: 300 mg daily

Alternatives: Nifedipine, Nimodipine

$T\frac{1}{2}$ =	42 hours	M/P =	0.33
PHL =		PB =	>99%
T_{max} =	2-3 hours	Oral =	60%
MW =	367	pKa =	
Vd =	8		

References:
1. Pharmaceutical Manufacturer Prescribing Information. 1996.
2. Drug Facts and Comparisons 1995 ed. ed. St. Louis: 1995.

BETAMETHASONE

Trade: Betameth, Celextone
Can/Aus/UK: Beben, Betadermetnesol, Celestone, Diprolene, Dipr, Betnovate, Betnelan, Diprosone
Uses: Synthetic corticosteroid
LRC: L3
AAP: Not reviewed

Betamethasone is a potent long-acting steroid. It generally produces less sodium and fluid retention than other steroids.[1] See prednisone.

Pregnancy Risk Category: C

Lactation Risk Category: L3

Adult Concerns: See prednisone.

Pediatric Concerns: None reported, used in pediatric patients.

Drug Interactions:

Theoretic Infant Dose:

Relative Infant Dose:

Adult Dose: 2.4-4.8 mg BID or TID

Alternatives:

$T\frac{1}{2}$ =	5.6 hours	M/P =	
PHL =		PB =	64%
T_{max} =	10-36 minutes	Oral =	Complete
MW =	392	pKa =	
Vd =			

References:
1.   Drug Facts and Comparisons 1995 ed. ed. St. Louis: 1995.

BETAXOLOL
Trade: Kerlone, Betoptic
Can/Aus/UK: Betoptic, Kerlone
Uses: Beta blocker antihypertensive
LRC: L3
AAP: Not reviewed

Betaxolol is a long-acting, cardioselective beta blocker primarily used for glaucoma but can be used orally for hypertension. No data are available on betaxolol except one report by manufacturer of side effects which occurred in one nursing infant[1]. Many in this family readily transfer into human milk (see atenolol, acebutolol). Manufacturer indicates that levels secreted in milk are sufficient to produce pharmacological effects in the infant. Caution is urged.

Pregnancy Risk Category: C

Lactation Risk Category: L3

Adult Concerns: Hypotension, bradycardia, fatigue

Pediatric Concerns: No data are available on betaxolol except one report by manufacturer of side effects which occurred in one nursing infant.

Drug Interactions: Decreased effect when used with aluminum salts, barbiturates, calcium salts, cholestyramine, NSAIDs, ampicillin, rifampin, and salicylates. Beta blockers may reduce the effect of oral sulfonylureas (hypoglycemic agents). Increased toxicity/effect when used with other antihypertensives, contraceptives, MAO inhibitors, cimetidine, and numerous other products. See drug interaction reference for complete listing.

Theoretic Infant Dose:

Relative Infant Dose:

Adult Dose: 10 mg daily

Alternatives: Propranolol, Metoprolol

T½ =	14-22 hours	M/P =	2.5-3.0
PHL =		PB =	50%
T$_{max}$ =	3 hours	Oral =	89%
MW =	307	pKa =	
Vd =	4.9		

References:
1. Pharmaceutical Manufacturer Prescribing Information. 1995.

BETHANECHOL CHLORIDE
Trade: Urabeth, Urecholine
Can/Aus/UK: Duvoid, Urecholine, Urocarb, Myotonine
Uses: Cholinergic stimulant
LRC: L4
AAP: Not reviewed

Bethanechol is a cholinergic stimulant useful for urinary retention. Although poorly absorbed from GI tract, no reports on entry into breastmilk are available. However, it could conceivably cause abdominal cramps, colicky pain , nausea, salivation, bronchial constriction, or diarrhea in infants. There are several reports of discomfort in nursing infants[1]. Use cautiously.

Pregnancy Risk Category: C

Lactation Risk Category: L4

Adult Concerns: Gastric distress such as colicky pain, cramping, nausea, salivation, breathing difficulties, diarrhea, hypotension, heart block, headache, urinary urgency

Pediatric Concerns: GI distress, discomfort, diarrhea.

Drug Interactions: Bethanechol when used with ganglionic blockers may lead to significant hypotension. Bethanechol effects may be antagonized by procainamide and quinidine.

Theoretic Infant Dose:

Relative Infant Dose:

Adult Dose: 10-50 mg BID-QID

Alternatives:

T½ =	1-2 hours	M/P =	
PHL =		PB =	
T$_{max}$ =	60-90 minutes (oral)	Oral =	Poor
MW =	197	pKa =	
Vd =			

References:
1. Shore MF. Drugs can be dangerous during pregnancy and lactation. Can Pharmaceut J 1970; 103:358.

BISACODYL

Trade: Bisacodyl, Dacodyl, Dulcolax
Can/Aus/UK: Bisacolax, Dulcolax, Laxit, Apo-Bisacodyl, Bisalax, Durolax, Paxolax
Uses: Laxative
LRC: L2
AAP: Not reviewed

Bisacodyl is a stimulant laxative that selectively stimulates colon contractions and defecation. It has only limited secretion into breastmilk due to poor gastric absorption and subsequently minimal systemic levels[1]. Little or no known harmful effects on infants.

Pregnancy Risk Category: C

Lactation Risk Category: L2

Adult Concerns: Diarrhea, GI cramping, rectal irritation

Pediatric Concerns: None reported via milk.

Drug Interactions: By speeding emptying of GI tract may reduce efficacy of warfarin and other products by reducing absorption.

Theoretic Infant Dose:

Relative Infant Dose:

Adult Dose: 10-15 mg daily

Alternatives:

T½ =		M/P =	
PHL =		PB =	
Tmax =		Oral =	< 5%
MW =	361	pKa =	
Vd =			

References:
1. Vorherr H. Drug excretion in breastmilk. Postgrad Med 1974; 56(4):97-104.

BISMUTH SUBSALICYLATE

Trade: Pepto-Bismol
Can/Aus/UK: Bismuth Liquid, Pepto-Bismol
Uses: Antisecretory, antimicrobial salt
LRC: L3
AAP: Drugs whose effect on nursing infants is unknown but may be of concern

Bismuth subsalicylate is present in many diarrhea mixtures. Although bismuth salts are poorly absorbed from the maternal GI tract, significant levels of salicylate could be absorbed from these products[1]. As such, these drugs should not be routinely used due to the association of salicylates in Reye's syndrome in children. Some forms (Parepectolin, Infantol Pink) may contain a tincture of opium (morphine).

Pregnancy Risk Category: C during 1st trimester
D during 2nd and 3rd trimester

Lactation Risk Category: L3

Adult Concerns: Constipation, salicylate poisoning (tinnitus). May enhance risk of Reyes syndrome in children.

Pediatric Concerns: Risk of Reyes syndrome in neonates, but has not been reported with this product in a breastfed infant.

Drug Interactions: May reduce effects of tetracyclines, and uricosurics. May increase toxicity of aspirin, warfarin, hypoglycemics.

Theoretic Infant Dose:

Relative Infant Dose:

Adult Dose: 524-2096 mg daily

Alternatives:

T½ =		M/P =	
PHL =		PB =	
Tmax =		Oral =	Poor
MW =	362	pKa =	
Vd =			

References:
1. Findlay JW, DeAngelis RL, Kearney MF, Welch RM, Findlay JM. Analgesic drugs in breastmilk and plasma. Clin Pharmacol Ther 1981; 29(5):625-633.

BISOPROLOL
Trade: Ziac, Zebeta
Can/Aus/UK: Amizide, Dichlotride, Emcor, Monocor
Uses: Beta-adrenergic antihypertensive
LRC: L3
AAP: Not reviewed

Bisoprolol is a typical beta blocker used to treat hypertension. The manufacturer states that small amounts (< 2%) are secreted into milk of animals[1]. Others in this family are known to produce problems in lactating infants (see atenolol, acebutolol). Ziac is a combination of bisoprolol and hydrochlorothiazide.

Pregnancy Risk Category: C

Lactation Risk Category: L3

Adult Concerns: Bradycardia, hypotension, fatigue, excessive fluid loss

Pediatric Concerns: None reported with this product, but other beta blockers have produced hypotension, hypoglycemia. See propranolol as alternative.

Drug Interactions: Decreased effect when used with aluminum salts, barbiturates, calcium salts, cholestyramine, NSAIDs, ampicillin, rifampin, and salicylates. Beta blockers may reduce the effect of oral sulfonylureas (hypoglycemic agents). Increased toxicity/effect when used with other antihypertensives, contraceptives, MAO inhibitors, cimetidine, and numerous other products. See drug interaction reference for complete listing.

Theoretic Infant Dose:

Relative Infant Dose:

Adult Dose: 5-10 mg daily

Alternatives: Propranolol, Metoprolol

T½ =	9-12 hours	M/P =	
PHL =		PB =	30%
Tmax =	2 - 3 hours	Oral =	80%
MW =	325	pKa =	
Vd =			

References:
1. Pharmaceutical Manufacturer Prescribing Information. 1995.

BLACK COHOSH
Trade: Baneberry, Black Snakeroot, Bugbane, Squawroot, Rattle Root
Can/Aus/UK:
Uses: Herbal estrogenic compound
LRC: L4
AAP: Not reviewed

The roots and rhizomes of this herb are used medicinally. Traditional uses include the treatment of dysmenorrhea, dyspepsia, rheumatisms, and as an antitussive. It has also been used as an insect repellant. The standardized extract, called Remifemin, has been used in Germany for menopausal management.[1] Black cohosh contains a number of alkaloids including N-methylcytosine, other tannins, and terpenoids. It is believed that the isoflavones or formononetic components may bind to estrogenic receptors.[2] Intraperitoneal injection of the extract selectively inhibits release of luteinizing hormone with no effect on the follicle-stimulating (FSH) hormone or prolactin.[3]   The data seems to suggest that this product interacts strongly at certain specific estrogen receptors and might be useful as estrogen replacement therapy in postmenopausal women although this has not been well studied. More studies are needed to address its usefulness in postmenopausal women and osteoporotic states.[1] Other effects of black cohosh include: hypotension, hypocholesterolemic activity, and peripheral vasodilation in vasospastic conditions (due to acetin content). Overdose may cause nausea, vomiting, dizziness, visual disturbances, bradycardia, and perspiration.   Large doses may induce miscarriage. This product should not be used in pregnant women.[4]   No data are available on the transfer of Black Cohosh into human milk, but due to its estrogenic activity, it could lower milk production although this is not known at this time. Caution is recommended in breastfeeding mothers. Use for more than 6 months is not recommended.[5]

Pregnancy Risk Category: X

Lactation Risk Category: L4

Adult Concerns: Large doses may induce miscarriage...this product should not be used in pregnant women. Other effects of black cohosh include: hypotension, hypocholesterolemic activity, and peripheral vasodilation in vasospastic conditions. Overdose may cause nausea, vomiting, dizziness, visual disturbances, bradycardia, and perspiration.

Pediatric Concerns: None reported via milk.

Drug Interactions:

Theoretic Infant Dose:

Relative Infant Dose:

Adult Dose:

Alternatives:

References:
1.   Murray M. Am.J.Nat.Med. 4(3): 3-5. 1997.
2.   Jarry H. et al Planta Medica 1885; 4:316-319.
3.   Jarry H. et al Planta Medica 1885; 1:46-49.
4.   Newall C. Black Cohosh Herbal Medicines. Pharmaceutical Press 1996; 80:81.
5.   The Complete German Commission E Monographs. Ed. M. Blumenthal Amer Botanical Council 1998.

BLESSED THISTLE

Trade: Blessed Thistle
Can/Aus/UK:
Uses: Anorexic, antidiarrheal, febrifuge
LRC: L3
AAP: Not reviewed

Blessed thistle contains an enormous array of chemicals, polyenes, steroids, terpenoids, and volatile oils. It is believed useful for diarrhea, hemorrhage, fevers, expectorant, bacteriostatic, and other antiseptic properties. Traditionally it has been used for loss of appetite, flatulence, cough and congestion, gangrenous ulcers, and dyspepsia. It has been documented to be antibacterial against: *B. subtilis, Brucella abortus, B. bronchiseptica, E. coli, Proteus species, P. aeruginosa, Staph. aureus*, and *Strep. faecalis*. The antibacterial and anti-inflammatory properties are due to its cnicin component.[1] While it is commonly used as a galactagogue, no data could be found suggesting this application. It is virtually nontoxic, and there are only occasional suggestions that high doses may induce GI symptoms.[2]

Pregnancy Risk Category:

Lactation Risk Category: L3

Adult Concerns: Virtually nontoxic

Pediatric Concerns: None reported via milk.

Drug Interactions:

Theoretic Infant Dose:

Relative Infant Dose:

Adult Dose:

Alternatives:

References:
1. Vanhaelen-Fastre R. Cnicus benedictus: Seperation of antimicrobial constituents. Plant Med Phytother 1968; 2:294-299.
2. Newall C. Black Cohosh Herbal Medicines. Pharmaceutical Press 1996; 80:81.

BLUE COHOSH
Trade: Blue Ginseng, Squaw Root, Papoose Root, Yellow Ginseng
Can/Aus/UK:
Uses: Uterine stimulant
LRC: L5
AAP: Not reviewed

Blue Cohosh is also known as blue ginseng, squaw root, papoose root, or yellow ginseng. It is primarily used as a uterotonic drug to stimulate uterine contractions. In one recent paper, an infant born of a mother who ingested Blue Cohosh root for 3 weeks prior to delivery, suffered from severe cardiogenic shock and congestive heart failure.[1] Blue Cohosh root contains a number of chemicals, including the alkaloid methylcytosine and the glycosides caulosaponin and caulophyllosaponin. Methylcytosine is pharmacologically similar to nicotine and may result in elevated blood pressure, gastric stimulation, and hyperglycemia. Caulosaponin and caulophyllosaponin are uterine stimulants. They also, apparently, produce severe ischemia of the myocardium due to intense coronary vasoconstriction. This product should not be used in pregnant women. No data are available as to its transfer into human milk. It is primarily used prior to delivery.

Pregnancy Risk Category: X

Lactation Risk Category: L5

Adult Concerns: The leaves and seeds contain alkaloids and glycosides that can cause severe stomach pain when ingested. Poisoning has been reported.

Pediatric Concerns: One case of severe congestive heart failure in newborn.

Drug Interactions:

Theoretic Infant Dose:

Relative Infant Dose:

Adult Dose:

Alternatives:

References:
1. Jones TK, Lawson BM. Profound neonatal congestive heart failure caused by maternal consumption of blue cohosh herbal medication. J Pediatr 1998; 132(3 Pt 1):550-552.

BOTULISM
Trade:
Can/Aus/UK:
Uses: Botulism poisoning
LRC: L4
AAP: Not reviewed

Botulism is a syndrome produced by the deadly toxin secreted by clostridium botulinum. This same toxin is sometimes used for the treatment of ophthalmic conditions such as strabismus and blepharospasm (Botox). Although the bacteria is wide spread, its colonization in food or the intestine of infants produces a deadly toxin. The syndrome is characterized by GI distress, weakness, malaise, lightheadedness, sore throat, and nausea. Dry mouth is almost universal.

In most adult poisoning the bacteria is absent; only the toxin is present. In most pediatric poisonings, the stomach is colonized by the bacterium, often from contaminated honey. In one published report, a woman severely poisoned by botulism toxin continued to breastfeed her infant throughout[1]. Four hours after admission, her milk was tested and was free of botulinum toxin and C. botulinum bacteria although she was still severely ill. The infant showed no symptoms of poisoning. It is apparent from this case that neither botulinum bacteria nor the toxin is secreted in breastmilk.

Pregnancy Risk Category:

Lactation Risk Category: L4

Adult Concerns: GI distress, weakness, malaise, lightheadedness, sore throat, nausea, dry mouth

Pediatric Concerns: None reported in one case.

Drug Interactions:

Theoretic Infant Dose:

Relative Infant Dose:

Adult Dose: 1.25-5 units IM injection

Alternatives:

References:
1. Middaugh J. Botulism and breastmilk. N Engl J Med 1978; 298(6):343.

BROMIDES

Trade:
Can/Aus/UK:
Uses: Sedatives
LRC: L5
AAP: Maternal Medication Usually Compatible with Breastfeeding

Small amounts are known to be secreted in milk[1]. May cause persistent rash, drowsiness, or weakness in infants. Secretion in milk has been known for many years. Bromide preparations are no longer available in the US. They are poorly effective products and have no place in modern medicine. Contraindicated in nursing mothers.

Pregnancy Risk Category: D

Lactation Risk Category: L5

Adult Concerns: Rash, sedation

Pediatric Concerns: Rash, drowsiness, weakness

Drug Interactions:

Theoretic Infant Dose:

Relative Infant Dose:

Adult Dose: 3-6 g daily

Alternatives:

References:
1. Van der Bogert F. Bromine poisoning through mother's milk. Am J Dis Child 1921; 21:167.

BROMOCRIPTINE MESYLATE

Trade: Parlodel
Can/Aus/UK: Parlodel, Apo-Bromocriptine, Kripton, Bromolactin
Uses: Inhibits prolactin secretion
LRC: L5 (milk suppression)
AAP: Drugs associated with significant side effects and should be given with caution

Bromocriptine is an anti-parkinsonian, synthetic ergot alkaloid which inhibits prolactin secretion and hence physiologic lactation. Most of the dose of bromocriptine is absorbed first-pass by the liver, leaving less than 6% to remain in the plasma. Maternal serum prolactin levels remain suppressed for up to 14 hrs after a single dose. The FDA approved indication for lactation suppression has been withdrawn and it is no longer approved for this purpose due to numerous maternal deaths, seizures, and strokes.

Observe for transient hypotension or vomiting. It is sometimes used in hyperprolactinemic patients who have continued to breastfeed although the incidence of maternal side-effects is significant and newer products are preferred.[1,2] In one breastfeeding patient who received 5 mg/day for a pituitary tumor, continued lactation produced no untoward effects in her infant.[3] Caution is recommended as profound postpartum hypotension has been reported. While bromocriptine is no longer recommended for suppression of lactation, a newer product cabergoline (Dostinex) is considered much safer for suppression of prolactin production.

Pregnancy Risk Category: C

Lactation Risk Category: L5 (milk suppression)

Adult Concerns: Most frequent side effects include nausea (49%), headache (19%), and dizziness (17%), peripheral vasoconstriction. Rarely, significant hypotension, shock, myocardial infarction. Transient hypotension and hair loss. A number of deaths have been associated with this product and it is no longer cleared for postpartum use to inhibit lactation.

Pediatric Concerns: No reports of direct toxicity to infant via milk but use with caution. Inhibits lactation.

Drug Interactions: Amitriptyline, butyrophenones, imipramine, methyldopa, phenothiazines, reserpine, may decrease efficacy of bromocriptine at reducing serum prolactin. My increase toxicity of other ergot alkaloids.

Theoretic Infant Dose:

Relative Infant Dose:

Adult Dose: 1.25-2.5 mg BID-TID

Alternatives: Cabergoline

T½ =	50 hours	M/P =	
PHL =		PB =	90-96%
T_max =	1-3 hours	Oral =	< 28%
MW =	654	pKa =	
Vd =	3.4		

References:
1. Meese MG. Reassessment of bromocriptine use for lactation suppression. P and T 1992; 17:1003-1004.
2. Spalding G. Bromocriptine (Parlodel) for suppression of lactation. Aust N Z J Obstet Gynaecol 1991; 31(4):344-345.
3. Canales ES, Garcia IC, Ruiz JE, Zarate A. Bromocriptine as prophylactic therapy in prolactinoma during pregnancy. Fertil Steril 1981; 36(4):524-526.

BROMPHENIRAMINE

Trade: Dimetane, Brombay, Dimetapp, Bromfed
Can/Aus/UK: Dimetane, Dimotane
Uses: Antihistamine
LRC: L3
AAP: Not reviewed

Brompheniramine is a popular antihistamine sold as Dimetane by itself or in combination with phenylpropanolamine as Dimetapp or with d-isoephedrine as Bromfed. Although untoward effects appear limited, some reported side effects from Dimetapp preparations are known. Although only insignificant amounts appear to be secreted into breastmilk, there are a number of reported cases of irritability, excessive crying, and sleep disturbances that have been reported in breastfeeding infants.[1] While in the USA, phenylpropanolamine is no longer used in cold remedies, it is still used in certain countries. Only modest amounts of phenylpropanolamine (PPA, Propadrine) are believed to be secreted into breastmilk. See phenylpropanolamine.

Pregnancy Risk Category: C

Lactation Risk Category: L3

Adult Concerns: Drowsiness, dry mucosa, excessive crying, irritability, sleep disturbances

Pediatric Concerns: Irritability, excessive crying, and sleep disturbances have been reported.

Drug Interactions: May enhance toxicity of other CNS depressants, MAO inhibitors, alcohol and tricyclic depressants.

Theoretic Infant Dose:

Relative Infant Dose:

Adult Dose: 4 mg q 4-6 hours

Alternatives: Loratadine, Cetirizine

$T^{1/2}$ =	24.9 hours	M/P =	
PHL =		PB =	
T_{max} =	3.1 hours	Oral =	Complete
MW =	319	pKa =	
Vd =	11.7		

References:
1. Paton DM, Webster DR. Clinical pharmacokinetics of H1-receptor antagonists (the antihistamines). Clin Pharmacokinet 1985; 10(6):477-497.

BUDESONIDE

Trade: Rhinocort, Pulmicort Respules
Can/Aus/UK: Entocort, Pulmicort, Rhinocort
Uses: Corticosteroid
LRC: L3
AAP: Not reviewed

Budesonide is a new and potent corticosteroid primarily used intranasally for allergic rhinitis. As such, the systemic bioavailability is minimal with less than 20% of the intranasal dose ever reaching systemic circulation.[1] Once absorbed systemically budesonide is a weak systemic steroid and should not be used to replace other steroids. In one 5 year study of children aged 2-7 years, no changes in linear growth, weight, and bone age were noted.[2] Adrenal suppression at these doses is extremely remote. Using normal doses, it is unlikely that clinically relevant concentrations of budesonide would ever reach the milk nor be systemically bioavailable to a breastfed infant.

Pregnancy Risk Category: C

Lactation Risk Category: L3

Adult Concerns: Adverse effects following intranasal use include irritation, pharyngitis, cough, bleeding, candidiasis, dry mouth. No adrenal suppression has been reported.

Pediatric Concerns: None reported via milk. Pediatric use down to age six is permitted.

Drug Interactions:

Theoretic Infant Dose:

Relative Infant Dose:

Adult Dose: 200-400 µg BID

Alternatives:

$T\frac{1}{2}$ =	2.8 hours	M/P =	
PHL =		PB =	
T_{max} =	2-4 hours (oral)	Oral =	10.7% (oral)
MW =	430	pKa =	
Vd =	4.3		

References:

1. Pharmaceutical Manufacturer Prescribing Information. 1999.
2. Volovitz B, Amir J, Malik H, Kauschansky A, Varsano I. Growth and pituitary-adrenal function in children with severe asthma treated with inhaled budesonide. N Engl J Med 1993; 329(23):1703-1708.

BUMETANIDE

Trade: Bumex
Can/Aus/UK: Burinex
Uses: Loop diuretic
LRC: L3
AAP: Not reviewed

Bumetanide is a potent loop diuretic similar to Lasix.[1]   As with all diuretics, some reduction in breastmilk production may result but it is rare. It is not known if bumetanide transfers into human milk.   If needed furosemide may be a better choice, as the oral bioavailability of furosemide in neonates is minimal.

Pregnancy Risk Category: D

Lactation Risk Category: L3

Adult Concerns: Dehydration, hepatic cirrhosis, ototoxicity, potassium loss. See furosemide.

Pediatric Concerns: None reported via milk.

Drug Interactions: Numerous interactions exist, this is a partial list of the most important.   NSAIDS may block the diuretic effect. Lithium excretion may be reduced.   Increased effect with other antihypertensives.   Bumetanide may induce hypoglycemia when added to sulfonylurea users.   Clofibrate may induce an exaggerated diuresis. Increased ototoxicity with aminoglycoside antibiotics.   Increased anticoagulation with anticoagulants.

Theoretic Infant Dose:

Relative Infant Dose:

Adult Dose: 0.5-2 mg daily-TID

Alternatives: Furosemide

$T\frac{1}{2}$ =	1-1.5	M/P =	
PHL =	2.5 hours (neonate)	PB = 95%	
T_{max} =	1 hour (oral)	Oral =	
MW =	364	pKa =	
Vd =			

References:
1.   Pharmaceutical Manufacturer Prescribing Information. 1999.

BUPIVACAINE

Trade: Marcaine
Can/Aus/UK: Marcaine, Marcain
Uses: Epidural, local anesthetic
LRC: L2
AAP: Not reviewed

Bupivacaine is the most commonly employed regional anesthetic used in delivery because its concentrations in the fetus are the least of the local anesthetics. In one study of five patients, levels of bupivacaine in breastmilk were below the limits of detection (< 0.02 mg/L) at 2 to 48 hrs postpartum[1]. These authors concluded that bupivacaine is a safe drug for perinatal use in mothers who plan to breastfeed.

In a study of 27 parturients who received an average of 183.3 mg lidocaine and 82.1 mg bupivacaine via an epidural catheter, lidocaine milk levels at 2, 6 , and 12 hours post administration were 0.86 , 0.46, and 0.22 mg/L respectively.[2] Levels of bupivacaine in milk at 2, 6, and 12 hours were 0.09, 0.06, 0.04 mg/L respectively. The milk/serum ratio bases upon area under the curve values (AUC) were 1.07 and 0.34 for lidocaine and bupivacaine respectively. Based on AUC data of lidocaine and bupivacaine milk levels, the average milk concentration of these agents over 12 hours was 0.5 and 0.07 mg/L. Most of the infants had a maximal APGAR score.

Pregnancy Risk Category: C

Lactation Risk Category: L2

Adult Concerns: Sedation, bradycardia, respiratory depression

Pediatric Concerns: None reported via milk.

Drug Interactions: Increases effect of hyaluronidase, beta blockers, MAO inhibitors, tricyclic antidepressants, phenothiazines, and vasopressors.

Theoretic Infant Dose: 0.014 mg/kg/day

Relative Infant Dose: 1.15%

Adult Dose: 25-100 mg once

Alternatives:

$T\frac{1}{2}$ =	2.7 hours	M/P =		
PHL =	8.1 hours	PB =	95%
T_{max} =	30-45 minutes	Oral =		
MW =	288	pKa =	8.1
Vd =	0.4-1.0			

References:
1. Naulty JS. Bupivacaine in breastmilk following epidural anesthesia for vaginal delivery. Regional Anesthesia 1983; 8(1):44-45.
2. Ortega D, Viviand X, Lorec AM, Gamerre M, Martin C, Bruguerolle B. Excretion of lidocaine and bupivacaine in breastmilk following epidural anesthesia for cesarean delivery. Acta Anaesthesiol Scand 1999; 43(4):394-397.

BUPRENORPHINE

Trade: Buprenex
Can/Aus/UK: Temgesic, Subutex
Uses: Narcotic analgesic
LRC: L3
AAP: Not reviewed

Buprenorphine is a potent, long-acting narcotic agonist and antagonist and may be useful as a replacement for methadone treatment in addicts. While its elimination half-life is short, it is retained on the opiate receptor site for long periods and may produce effects longer than the elimination half-life would suggest.

In one patient who received 4 mg/day to facilitate withdrawal from other opiates, the amount of buprenorphine transferred via milk was only 3.28 micrograms per day, an amount that was clinically insignificant.[1] No symptoms were noted in this breastfed infant. In another study of continuous extradural bupivacaine and buprenorphine in postcesarean women for 3 days[2], it was suggested that buprenorphine may suppress the production of milk (and infant weight gain) although this was not absolutely clear. As with most opiates, breastmilk levels are probably low, but sustained exposure should be avoided.

Pregnancy Risk Category: C

Lactation Risk Category: L3

Adult Concerns: Typical opiate side effects include pruritus, sedation, analgesia, hallucinations, euphoria, dizziness, respiratory depression.

Pediatric Concerns: Low weight gain and reduced breastmilk levels in one study, and no effects in another study.

Drug Interactions: May enhance effects of other opiates, benzodiazepines, and barbiturates.

Theoretic Infant Dose: 3.28 μg/day

Relative Infant Dose:

Adult Dose: 0.3 mg q 6 hours PRN

Alternatives:

T½ =	1.2-7.2 hours	M/P =	
PHL =		PB =	96%
T$_{max}$ =	15-30 minutes	Oral =	31%
MW =		pKa =	8.24, 9.92
Vd =	97		

References:

1. Marquet P, Chevrel J, Lavignasse P, Merle L, Lachatre G. Buprenorphine withdrawal syndrome in a newborn. Clin Pharmacol Ther 1997; 62(5):569-571.
2. Hirose M, Hosokawa T, Tanaka Y. Extradural buprenorphine suppresses breast feeding after caesarean section. Br J Anaesth 1997; 79(1):120-121.

BUPROPION

Trade: Wellbutrin, Zyban
Can/Aus/UK: Wellbutrin, Zyban
Uses: Antidepressant, smoking deterrent
LRC: L3
AAP: Drugs whose effect on nursing infants is unknown but may be of concern

Bupropion is an older antidepressant with a structure unrelated to tricyclics. It may be teratogenic in pregnant women. One report in the literature indicates that bupropion probably accumulates in human milk although the absolute dose transferred appears minimal.

Following one 100 mg dose in a mother, the milk/plasma ratio ranged from 2.51 to 8.58, clearly suggesting a concentrating mechanism for this drug in human milk.[1] However, plasma levels of bupropion (or its metabolites) in the infant were undetectable, indicating that the dose transferred to the infant was low, and accumulation in infant plasma apparently did not occur under these conditions (infant was fed 7.5 to 9.5 hours after dosing). The peak milk bupropion level (0.189 mg/L) occurred two hours after a 100 mg dose. This milk level would provide 0.66% of the maternal dose, a dose that is likely to be clinically insignificant to a breastfed infant. A new formulation is currently recommended for smoking cessation therapy and is called Zyban. I have received a number of patient reports (personnal communication) of reduced milk supply in patients receiving bupropion. Some caution concerning milk supply is in order.

Pregnancy Risk Category: B

Lactation Risk Category: L3

Adult Concerns: Seizures, restlessness, agitation, sleep disturbances. Probably contraindicated in patients with seizure disorders.

Pediatric Concerns: None reported in one study, but this infant was only breastfed but twice daily. Observe for a reduction in milk production.

Drug Interactions: May increase clearance of diazepam, carbamazepine, phenytoin. May increase effects of MAO inhibitors.

Theoretic Infant Dose: 0.028 mg/kg/d

Relative Infant Dose: 0.66%

Adult Dose: 100 mg TID

Alternatives: Sertraline, Paroxetine

$T\frac{1}{2}$ =	8-24 hours	M/P =	2.51-8.58
PHL =		PB =	75-88%
T_{max} =	2 hours	Oral =	
MW =	240	pKa =	8.0
Vd =	40		

References:
1. Briggs GG, Samson JH, Ambrose PJ, Schroeder DH. Excretion of bupropion in breastmilk. Ann Pharmacother 1993; 27(4):431-433.

BUSPIRONE
Trade: BuSpar
Can/Aus/UK: BuSpar, Apo-Buspirone, Novo-Buspirone
Uses: Antianxiety medication
LRC: L3
AAP: Not reviewed

No data exists on excretion into human milk. It is secreted into animal milk, so the same would be expected in human milk.[1] BuSpar is mg for mg equivalent to diazepam (Valium) in its anxiolytic properties but does not produce significant sedation or addiction as the benzodiazepine family. Its metabolite is partially active but has a brief half-life (4.8 hrs) as well. Compared to the benzodiazepine family, this product would be a better choice for treatment of anxiety in breastfeeding women. But without accurate breastmilk levels, it is not known if the product is safe for breastfeeding women or the levels the infant would ingest daily. The rather brief half-life of this product and its metabolite would not likely lead to buildup in the infants plasma.

Pregnancy Risk Category: B

Lactation Risk Category: L3

Adult Concerns: Dizziness, nausea, drowsiness, fatigue, excitement, euphoria

Pediatric Concerns: None reported.

Drug Interactions: Cimetidine may increase the effect of buspirone. Increased toxicity may occur when used with MAO inhibitors, phenothiazines, CNS depressants, digoxin and haloperidol.

Theoretic Infant Dose:

Relative Infant Dose:

Adult Dose: 5 mg TID

Alternatives:

T½ =	2-3 hours	M/P =	
PHL =		PB =	95%
T$_{max}$ =	60-90 minutes	Oral =	90%
MW =	386	pKa =	
Vd =	5.3		

References:
1.   Pharmaceutical Manufacturer Prescribing Information. 1996.

BUSULFAN
Trade: Myleran
Can/Aus/UK: Myleran
Uses: Antineoplastic, anticancer drug.
LRC: L5
AAP: Not reviewed

Busulfan is a potent antineoplastic agent that can produce severe bone marrow suppression, anemia, loss of blood cells, and elevated risk of infection[1]. It is not known if busulfan is distributed to human milk. No data are available concerning breastmilk concentrations, but this agent would be extremely toxic to growing infants and continued breastfeeding would not be justified. Use of this drug during breastfeeding is definitely not recommended.

Pregnancy Risk Category: D

Lactation Risk Category: L5

Adult Concerns: Severe bone marrow suppression, anemia, leukopenia, pulmonary fibrosis, cholestatic jaundice

Pediatric Concerns: Extremely cytotoxic, use is not recommended in nursing women.

Drug Interactions:

Theoretic Infant Dose:

Relative Infant Dose:

Adult Dose: 1 mg/kg/dose q 6 hours (16 doses total)

Alternatives:

T½ =	2.6 hours	M/P =	
PHL =		PB =	14%
T$_{max}$ =	0.5-2 hours	Oral =	Complete
MW =	246	pKa =	
Vd =	1.0		

References:
1. McEvoy GE. (ed):AFHS Drug Information. New York, NY: 2003.

BUTABARBITAL
Trade: Butisol, Butalan, Ampyrox
Can/Aus/UK:
Uses: Sedative, hypnotic
LRC: L3
AAP: Not reviewed

Butabarbital is an intermediate acting barbiturate similar to phenobarbital. Small amounts are secreted in breastmilk.[1] No harmful effects have been reported. Watch for drowsiness and sedation.

Pregnancy Risk Category: D

Lactation Risk Category: L3

Adult Concerns: Sedation, weakness

Pediatric Concerns: None reported but observe for sedation.

Drug Interactions: May have a decreased effect when used with phenothiazines, haloperidol, cyclosporin, tricyclic antidepressants, doxycycline, and beta-blockers. May increase effects of benzodiazepines, CNS depressants, valproic acid, methylphenidate, and chloramphenicol.

Theoretic Infant Dose:

Relative Infant Dose:

Adult Dose: 15-30 mg TID or QID

Alternatives:

T½ =	100 hours	M/P =	
PHL =		PB =	
T$_{max}$ =	3-4 hours	Oral =	Complete
MW =	232	pKa =	7.9
Vd =			

References:
1. Tyson RM, Shrader EA, Perlman HH. Drugs transmitted through breastmilk. II Barbiturates. J Pediatr 1938; 14:86-90.

BUTALBITOL COMPOUND
Trade: Fioricet, Fiorinal, Bancap, Two-Dyne
Can/Aus/UK: Tecnal, Fiorinal
Uses: Mild analgesic, sedative
LRC: L3
AAP: Not reviewed

Mild analgesic with acetaminophen (325mg) or aspirin, caffeine (40mg), and butalbital (50mg). Butalbital is a mild, short-acting barbiturate that probably transfers into breastmilk to a limited degree although it is unreported[1]. No data are available on the transfer of butalbital to breastmilk, but it is likely minimal.

Pregnancy Risk Category: D

Lactation Risk Category: L3

Adult Concerns: Sedation

Pediatric Concerns: Sedation

Drug Interactions: Decreased effect when used with phenothiazines, haloperidol, cyclosporin, tricyclic antidepressants, and oral contraceptives. Increased effect when used with alcohol, benzodiazepines, CNS depressants, valproic acid, and methylphenidate.

Theoretic Infant Dose:

Relative Infant Dose:

Adult Dose: 50-100 mg q 4 hours

Alternatives:

$T^{1/2}$ =	40-140 hours	M/P =		
PHL =		PB =	26%	
T_{max} =	40-60 minutes	Oral =	Complete	
MW =	224	pKa =		
Vd =	0.8			

References:
1. McEvoy GE. (ed):AFHS Drug Information. New York, NY: 2003.

BUTORPHANOL

Trade: Stadol
Can/Aus/UK: Stadol
Uses: Potent narcotic analgesic
LRC: L3
AAP: Maternal Medication Usually Compatible with Breastfeeding

Butorphanol is a potent narcotic analgesic. It is available both by IV, IM, and a nasal spray. Butorphanol passes into breastmilk in low to moderate concentrations (estimated 4 μg/L of milk following 2 mg IM 4 times daily).[1] Levels produced in infants are considered very low to insignificant. Butorphanol undergoes first-pass extraction by the liver, hence only 17% of the oral dose reaches the plasma. Butorphanol has been frequently used in labor and delivery in women who subsequently nursed their infants. Although, it has been noted to produce a sinusoidal fetal heart rate pattern and dysphoric or psychotomimetic responses in postpartum women.

Pregnancy Risk Category: B during 1st and 2nd trimester
                                     D during 3rd trimester

Lactation Risk Category: L3

Adult Concerns: Sedation, respiratory depression

Pediatric Concerns: None reported via milk but sedation is possible in newborns.

Drug Interactions: May produce increase toxicity when used with CNS depressants, other opiates, phenothiazines, barbiturates, benzodiazepines, MAO inhibitors.

Theoretic Infant Dose: 0.6 μg/kg/day

Relative Infant Dose: 0.5%

Adult Dose: 1-4 mg IM q 3-4 hours OR 0.5-2 mg IV q 3-4 hours

Alternatives:

$T\frac{1}{2}$ =	3-4 hours	M/P =		
PHL =		PB =	80%	
T_{max} =	1 hour	Oral =	17 %	
MW =	327	pKa =	8.6	
Vd =	5			

References:
1. Pittman KA, Smyth RD, Losada M, Zighelboim I, Maduska AL, Sunshine A. Human perinatal distribution of butorphanol. Am J Obstet Gynecol 1980; 138(7 Pt 1):797-800.

CABERGOLINE
Trade: Dostinex
Can/Aus/UK: Dostinex
Uses: Antiprolactin
LRC: L4
AAP: Not reviewed

Cabergoline is a long-acting synthetic ergot alkaloid derivative which produces a dopamine agonist effect similar but much safer than bromocriptine (Parlodel). Cabergoline directly inhibits prolactin secretion by the pituitary.[1] It is primarily indicated for pathological hyperprolactinemia but in several European studies it has been used for inhibition of post-partum lactation. In several European countries, cabergoline is indicated for the inhibition or suppression of physiologic lactation.[2] The dose regimen used for the inhibition of physiologic lactation is cabergoline 1 mg administered as a single dose on the first day post-partum. For the suppression of established lactation, cabergoline 0.25 mg is taken every 12 hours for 2 days for a total of 1 mg. Single doses of 1 mg have been found to completely inhibit postpartum lactation. Transfer into human milk is not reported.

In patients with hyperprolactinemia, it is possible to carefully administered doses to lower the prolactin to safe ranges, but high enough to retain lactation. In such cases, the infant should be observed for potential ergot side effects, if any.

Pregnancy Risk Category: B

Lactation Risk Category: L4

Adult Concerns: Headache, dizziness, fatigue, orthostatic hypotension, nose bleed, inhibition of lactation

Pediatric Concerns: Transfer via milk is unknown. Will completely and irreversibly suppress lactation and should not be used in mothers who are breastfeeding.

Drug Interactions: Do not use with other dopamine antagonists such as the phenothiazines (Thorazine,etc), butyrophenones (Haldol), thioxanthines, and metoclopramide (Reglan).

Theoretic Infant Dose:

Relative Infant Dose:

Adult Dose: 0.25-1 mg twice a week

Alternatives:

T½ =	80 hours	M/P =	
PHL =		PB =	
T_{max} =	2-3 hours	Oral =	Complete
MW =	451	pKa =	
Vd =			

References:

1. Caballero-Gordo A, Lopez-Nazareno N, Calderay M, Caballero JL, Mancheno E, Sghedoni D. Oral cabergoline. Single-dose inhibition of puerperal lactation. J Reprod Med 1991; 36(10):717-721.
2. Single dose cabergoline versus bromocriptine in inhibition of puerperal lactation: randomised, double blind, multicentre study. European Multicentre Study Group for Cabergoline in Lactation Inhibition BMJ 1991; 302(6789):1367-1371.

CAFFEINE

Trade: Vivarin, Nodoz, Coffee
Can/Aus/UK:
Uses: CNS stimulant
LRC: L2
AAP: Maternal Medication Usually Compatible with Breastfeeding

Caffeine is a naturally-occurring CNS stimulant present in many foods and drinks. While the half-life in adults is 4.9 hours, the half-life in neonates is as high as 97.5 hours. The half-life decreases with age to 14 hours at 3-5 months and 2.6 hours at 6 months and older. The average cup of coffee contains 100-150 mg of caffeine depending on preparation and country of origin. Peak levels of caffeine are found in breastmilk 60-120 minutes after ingestion.

In a study of 5 patients following an ingestion of 150 mg caffeine, peak concentrations of caffeine in serum ranged from 2.39 to 4.05 µg/mL, and peak concentrations in milk ranged from 1.4 to 2.41 mg/L with a milk/serum ratio of 0.52.[1] The average milk concentration at 30, 60, and 120 minute post dose was 1.58, 1.49, and 0.926 mg/L respectively.

In another study of 7 breastfeeding mothers who consumed 750 mg caffeine/day for 5 days, and were 11-22 days postpartum, the average milk concentration was 4.3 mg/L.[2] Values ranged significantly from non detectable to 15.7 mg/L. The mean concentration of caffeine in sera of the infants on day 5 was 1.4 µg/mL (range non detectable to 2.8 µg/mL). In two patients whose milk levels were 13.4 and 28 mg/L the respective infant serum levels were 0.25 and 3.2 µg/mL.

In a study of 6 breastfeeding mothers who received one dose of 100 mg PO, peak levels (C_{max}) in maternal serum ranged from 0.5 to 1 hour and 0.75 to 2 hours in milk.[3] The maternal plasma C_{max} ranged from 3.6 to 6.15 µg/mL, while the C_{max} for their milk ranged from 1.98 to 4.3 mg/L. The average concentration of caffeine in milk was 2.45 mg/L at 1 hour. The average milk/plasma ratio (AUC) was 0.812 for both breasts. This elegant study shows that caffeine rapidly enters milk and that the decay of caffeine in milk is similar to that of plasma. In infants from 4 to 7 kg body weight, the estimated dose to the infant would be 1.77 to 3.10 mg/d following a 100 mg maternal dose.

In a group of mothers who ingested from 35 to 336 mg of caffeine daily, the level of caffeine in milk ranged from 2.09 to 7.17 mg/L.[4] The author estimates the dose to infant at 0.01 to 1.64 mg/d or 0.06% to 1.5% of the maternal dose.

An interesting review of the nutritional effects of caffeine ingestion on infants is provided by Nehlig.[5] There is some evidence that chronic coffee drinking may reduce the iron content of milk. Irritability and insomnia may occur and have been reported. Occasional use of caffeine is not contraindicated, but persistent, chronic use may lead to high plasma levels in the infant particularly during the neonatal period.

Pregnancy Risk Category: B

Lactation Risk Category: L2

Adult Concerns: Agitation, irritability, poor sleeping patterns

Pediatric Concerns: Rarely, irritability, and insomnia

Drug Interactions: Reduces vasodilation of adenosine. Reduces bioavailability of alendronate by 60%. Cimetidine reduces caffeine clearance by 50%. Fluoroquinolone antibiotics increases half-life of caffeine by 5 to 8 hours.

Theoretic Infant Dose: 0.6 mg/kg/day

Relative Infant Dose: 6.0%

Adult Dose:

Alternatives:

$T\frac{1}{2}$ =	4.9 hours	M/P =	0.52 - 0.76
PHL =	80-97.5 hours	PB =	36%
T_{max} =	60 minutes	Oral =	100%
MW =	194	pKa =	0.8
Vd =	0.4-0.6		

References:

1. Tyrala EE, Dodson WE. Caffeine secretion into breastmilk. Arch Dis Child 1979; 54(10):787-800.
2. Ryu JE. Caffeine in human milk and in serum of breast-fed infants. Dev Pharmacol Ther 1985; 8(6):329-337.
3. Stavchansky S, Combs A, Sagraves R, Delgado M, Joshi A. Pharmacokinetics of caffeine in breastmilk and plasma after single oral

administration of caffeine to lactating mothers. Biopharm Drug Dispos 1988; 9(3):285-299.

4. Berlin CM, Jr., Denson HM, Daniel CH, Ward RM. Disposition of dietary caffeine in milk, saliva, and plasma of lactating women. Pediatrics 1984; 73(1):59-63.

5. Nehlig A, Debry G. Consequences on the newborn of chronic maternal consumption of coffee during gestation and lactation: a review. J Am Coll Nutr 1994; 13(1):6-21.

CALCIPOTRIENE

Trade: Dovonex
Can/Aus/UK: Dovonex
Uses: Synthetic Vitamin D3 used for treatment of psoriasis
LRC: L3
AAP: Not reviewed

Calcipotriene is a synthetic vitamin D3 derivative used topically for the treatment of plaque psoriasis. Only approximately 5-6% is transcutaneously absorbed into the systemic circulation (via ointment). It is rapidly bound to plasma proteins and excreted by the liver via bile. Less than 1% is absorbed from the scalp when the solution is used. It is unlikely plasma levels of calcipotriene would be elevated at all, and milk levels would be virtually nil because vitamin D transport to milk is normally quite low. Calcipotriene is active, however, and used over wide areas of the body could (but unlikely) lead to significant absorption. However, hypercalcemia in treated patients has been reported by only rarely.

Pregnancy Risk Category: C

Lactation Risk Category: L3

Adult Concerns: Adverse events include skin irritation, rare but reversible hypercalcemia, rash, pruritus, and worsening of psoriasis.

Pediatric Concerns: None reported via milk but no studies are available. Adverse effects in a breastfed infant are unlikely if the surface area treated is moderate to low.

Drug Interactions:

Theoretic Infant Dose:

Relative Infant Dose:

Adult Dose: Apply to skin lesions twice daily.

Alternatives:

$T\frac{1}{2}$ =		M/P =	
PHL =		PB =	
T_{max} =		Oral =	Variable
MW =	430	pKa =	
Vd =			

References:
1. Pharmaceutical Manufacturers Package Insert, 2003.

CALCITONIN

Trade: Calcimar, Salmonine, Osteocalcin, Miacalcin
Can/Aus/UK: Caltine, Calcimar, Calcitare, Calsynar, Miacalcic
Uses: Calcium metabolism
LRC: L3
AAP: Not reviewed

Calcitonin is a large polypeptide hormone (32 amino acids) secreted by the parafollicular cells of the thyroid that inhibits osteoclastic bone resorption, thus, maintaining calcium homeostasis in mammals.[1] It is used for control of postmenopausal osteoporosis and other calcium metabolic diseases. Calcitonins are destroyed by gastric acids, requiring parenteral (SC, IM) or intranasal dosing.   Calcitonin is unlikely to penetrate human milk due to its large molecular weight. Further, its oral bioavailability is nil due to destruction in the GI tract. It has been reported to inhibit lactation in animals although this has not been reported in humans.[2]

Pregnancy Risk Category: C

Lactation Risk Category: L3

Adult Concerns: Nausea, facial flushing, shivering, edema, metallic taste, and increased urinary frequency

Pediatric Concerns: None reported via milk. Unlikely to enter milk. Calcitonins have been reported to inhibit lactation in animals.

Drug Interactions: It is reported that ketoprofen inhibits the calciuric and uricosuric effect of porcine calcitonin. May have additive effect with plicamycin.

Theoretic Infant Dose:

Relative Infant Dose:

Adult Dose: 50-100 units (salmon) three times weekly

Alternatives:

$T\frac{1}{2}$ =	1 hour	M/P =	
PHL =		PB =	
T_{max} =	2 hours	Oral =	None
MW =		pKa =	
Vd =			

References:
1. Pharmaceutical Manufacturer Prescribing Information. 1997.
2. Fiore CE, Petralito A, Mazzarino MC, Liuzzo A, Malaponte G, Mangiafico RA, Gibiino S. Effects of ketoprofen on the calciuric and uricosuric activities of calcitonin in man. J Endocrinol Invest 1981; 4(1):81-84.

CALCITRIOL

Trade: Rocaltrol
Can/Aus/UK: Rocaltrol
Uses: Vitamin D analog
LRC: L3
AAP: Not reviewed

Vitamin D typically undergoes a series of metabolic steps to become active. Calcitriol (1,25 dihydro cholecalciferol) is believed to be the active metabolite of vitamin D metabolism. Calcitriol is the most potent of the synthetic vitamin D analogs. It is indicated for treatment of hypocalcemia in patients undergoing chronic renal dialysis and renal osteodystrophy. Calcitriol is also indicated in patients with severe liver dysfunction and who are unable to hydroxylate dihydrotachysterol to its active form. Because calcitriol works more quickly, it is useful in treatment of patients with severe hypocalcemia. Calcitriol is well absorbed from the GI tract with a peak at 3-6 hours.[1] It is 99.9% protein bound to a specific alpha-globulin vitamin D binding protein. The elimination half-life is about 5-8 hours in adults and 27 hours in pediatric age patients. However, plasma levels are quite low, averaging approximately 40 picograms/mL. No data are available on the transfer of calcitriol into human milk. It is not likely that normal doses of this vitamin D analog would lead to clinically relevant levels in human milk, particularly since vitamin D transfers only minimally into human milk anyway. While plasma levels of vitamin D are normally quite low in human milk (< 20 IU/L), at least one study now suggests that supplementing a mother with high levels of vitamin D2 can significantly elevate milk levels and subsequently lead to hypercalcemia in a breastfed infant.[2] Some caution is recommended.

Pregnancy Risk Category: C

Lactation Risk Category: L3

Adult Concerns: Overdosage of any form of vitamin D is dangerous and could lead to severe hypercalcemia, hypercalciuria, and hyperphosphatemia. Hypercalcemia may subsequently lead to vascular calcification, nephrocalcinosis, and other soft-tissue calcification.

Pediatric Concerns: None reported via milk, but caution recommended at higher doses.

Drug Interactions: Cholestyramine and colestipol may reduce the oral absorption of calcitriol. Hypercalcemia may result from adding thiazide diuretics in patients receiving calcitriol. Ketoconazole may reduce calcitriol concentrations in plasma. A functional antagonism can occur by adding corticosteroids to calcitriol. Avoid high-dose calcium supplements.

Theoretic Infant Dose:

Relative Infant Dose:

Adult Dose: Variable, but 0.25-0.5 µg/day initially.

Alternatives: Vitamin D

T½ =	5-8 hours	M/P =	
PHL =	27 hour	PB =	99.9%
Tmax =	3-6 hours	Oral =	Complete
MW =	416	pKa =	
Vd =			

References:
1. Pharmaceutical Manufacturers prescribing information, 2003.
2. Greer FR, Hollis BW, Napoli JL. High concentrations of vitamin D2 in human milk associated with pharmacologic doses of vitamin D2. J Pediatr 1984; 105(1):61-64.

CALENDULA

Trade: Calendula, Marigold, Garden Marigold, Holligold, Gold Bloom, Marybud
Can/Aus/UK:
Uses: Herbal wound healing
LRC: L3
AAP: Not reviewed

Calendula, grown worldwide, has been used topically to promote wound healing and to alleviate conjunctivitis and other ocular inflammations. It consists of a number of flavonol glycosides and saponins, but the active ingredients are unknown.[1]   Despite these claims, there are almost no studies regarding its efficacy in any of these disorders. Further, there are no suggestions of overt toxicity, with the exception of allergies.   Although it may have some uses externally, its internal use as an antiphlogistic and spasmolytic is largely obsolete.

Pregnancy Risk Category:

Lactation Risk Category: L3

Adult Concerns: Allergies, anaphylactoid shock.

Pediatric Concerns: None reported via milk.

Drug Interactions:

Theoretic Infant Dose:

Relative Infant Dose:

Adult Dose:

Alternatives:

References:
1. Bissett NG. In: Herbal Drugs and Phytopharmaceuticals. Medpharm Scientific Publishers, CRC Press, Boca Raton, 1994.

CANDESARTAN

Trade: Atacand
Can/Aus/UK:
Uses: Antihypertensive agent
LRC: L4
AAP: Not reviewed

Candesartan is a specific blocker of the receptor site (AT1) for angiotensin II. It is typically used as an antihypertensive similar to the ACE inhibitor family.[1] Both the ACE inhibitor family and the specific AT1 inhibitors such as candesartan are contraindicated in the 2nd and 3rd trimesters of pregnancy due to severe hypotension, neonatal skull hypoplasia, irreversible renal failure, and death in the newborn infant. However, some of ACE inhibitors can be used in breastfeeding mothers 2-3 weeks postpartum without major risk in some cases with due caution. However, no data are available on candesartan in human milk although the manufacturer states that it is present in rodent milk. Extreme caution is recommended in the neonatal period.

Pregnancy Risk Category: **C during 1st trimester**
                                     D during 2nd and 3rd trimester
Lactation Risk Category: **L4**

Adult Concerns: Headache, back pain, pharyngitis, and dizziness have been reported. The use of ACE inhibitors and angiotensin receptor blockers during pregnancy or the neonatal period is extremely dangerous and has resulted in hypotension, neonatal skull hypoplasia, anuria, renal failure, and death.

Pediatric Concerns: None reported via milk. Caution is recommended in the early postpartum period.

Drug Interactions: None have been reported.

Theoretic Infant Dose:

Relative Infant Dose:

Adult Dose: 4-32 mg daily

Alternatives: Captopril, Enalapril

$T\frac{1}{2}$ =	9 hours	M/P =	
PHL =		PB =	> 99%
T_{max} =	3-4 hours	Oral =	15%
MW =	611	pKa =	
Vd =	0.13		

References:
1. Pharmaceutical Manufacturer Prescribing Information. 1999.

CANNABIS
Trade: Marijuana
Can/Aus/UK:
Uses: Sedative, hallucinogen
LRC: L5
AAP: Contraindicated by the American Academy of Pediatrics in Breastfeeding Mothers

Commonly called marijuana, the active component delta-9-THC is rapidly distributed to the brain and adipose tissue. It is stored in fat tissues for long periods (weeks to months). Small to moderate secretion into breastmilk has been documented[1]. Analysis of breastmilk in chronic heavy user revealed an eight fold accumulation in breastmilk compared to plasma although the dose received is insufficient to produce significant side effects in the infant. Studies have shown significant absorption and metabolism in infants although long term sequela have not been shown. Marijuana could produce sedation and growth delay, but it is highly dose dependent. In one study of 27 women who smoked marijuana during breastfeeding, no differences were noted in outcomes on growth, mental, and motor development[2]. Studies in animals suggests that marijuana inhibits prolactin production and could inhibit lactation. Contraindicated in nursing mothers. Infants exposed to marijuana via breastmilk will test positive in urine screens for long periods (2-3 weeks).

Pregnancy Risk Category: C

Lactation Risk Category: L5

Adult Concerns: Sedation, weakness, poor feeding patterns. Possible decreased milk production.

Pediatric Concerns: Sedation

Drug Interactions:

Theoretic Infant Dose:

Relative Infant Dose:

Adult Dose:

Alternatives:

$T^{1/2}$ =	25-57 hours	M/P =	8
PHL =		PB =	99.9%
T_{max} =		Oral =	Complete
MW =		pKa =	
Vd =	High		

References:

1. Perez-Reyes M, Wall ME. Presence of delta9-tetrahydrocannabinol in human milk. N Engl J Med 1982; 307(13):819-820.
2. Tennes K, Avitable N, Blackard C, Boyles C, Hassoun B, Holmes L, Kreye M. Marijuana: prenatal and postnatal exposure in the human. NIDA Res Monogr 1985; 59:48-60.

CAPSAICIN

Trade: Zostrix, Axsain, Capsin, Capzasin-P, No-Pain, Absorbine Jr. Arthritis, Arthricare
Can/Aus/UK: Zostrix, Axsain, Capsig, Natraflex
Uses: Analgesic, topical.
LRC: L3
AAP: Not reviewed

Capsaicin is an alkaloid derived from peppers from the Solanaceae family. After topical absorption it increases, depletes, and then suppresses substance P release from sensory neurons, thus preventing pain sensation. Substance P is the principal chemomediator of pain from the periphery to the CNS.[1,2] After repeated application (days to weeks), it depletes substance P and prevents reaccumulation in the neuron. Very little or nothing is known about the kinetics of this product. It is approved for use in children > 2 years of age. No data are available on transfer into human milk.

Pregnancy Risk Category: C

Lactation Risk Category: L3

Adult Concerns: Local irritation, burning, stinging, erythema. Cough and infrequently neurotoxicity. Avoid use near eyes.

Pediatric Concerns: None reported. Avoid transfer to eye and other sensitive surfaces via hand contact.

Drug Interactions: May increase risk of cough with ACE inhibitors.

Theoretic Infant Dose:

Relative Infant Dose:

Adult Dose:

Alternatives:

T½ =	Several hours	M/P =	
PHL =		PB =	
T$_{max}$ =		Oral =	
MW =	305	pKa =	
Vd =			

References:
1. Bernstein JE. Capsaicin in dermatologic disease. Semin Dermatol 1988; 7(4):304-309.
2. Watson CP, Evans RJ, Watt VR. The post-mastectomy pain syndrome and the effect of topical capsaicin. Pain 1989; 38(2):177-186.

CAPTOPRIL
Trade: Capoten
Can/Aus/UK: Capoten, Apo-Capto, Novo-Captopril, Acenorm, Enzace, Acepril
Uses: Antihypertensive drug (ACE inhibitor)
LRC: L3 if used after 30 days
AAP: Maternal Medication Usually Compatible with Breastfeeding

Captopril is a typical angiotensin converting enzyme inhibitor (ACE) used to reduce hypertension. Small amounts are secreted (4.7 μg/L milk). In one report of 12 women treated with 100 mg three times daily, maternal serum levels averaged 713 μg/L while breastmilk levels averaged 4.7 μg/L at 3.8 hrs after administration[1]. Data from this study suggest that an infant would ingest approximately 0.002% of the free captopril consumed by its mother (300mg) on a daily basis. No adverse effects have been reported in this study. Use only if determined to be important to mother's health.

Pregnancy Risk Category: D

Lactation Risk Category: L3 if used after 30 days

Adult Concerns: Hypotension, bradycardia, decreased urine output, and possible seizures. A decrease in taste acuity or metallic taste.

Pediatric Concerns: None reported but observe for hypotension.

Drug Interactions: Probenecid increases plasma levels of captopril. Captopril and diuretics have additive hypotensive effects. Antacids reduce bioavailability of ACE inhibitors. NSAIDS reduce hypotension of ACE inhibitors. Phenothiazines increase effects of ACEi. Allopurinol may increase risk of Steven-Johnson's syndrome when admixed with captopril. ACEi increase digoxin and lithium plasma levels. May elevate potassium levels when potassium supplementation is added.

Theoretic Infant Dose: 0.70 μg/kg/day

Relative Infant Dose: 0.0165%

Adult Dose: 50 mg TID

Alternatives: Enalapril

T½ =	2.2 hours	M/P =	0.012
PHL =		PB =	30%
T$_{max}$ =	1 hour	Oral =	60-75%
MW =	217	pKa =	3.7, 9.8
Vd =	0.7		

References:
1. Devlin R. Selective resistance to the passage of captopril into human milk. Clin Pharmacol Ther 27:250, 1980.

CARBAMAZEPINE

Trade: Tegretol, Epitol, Carbatrol
Can/Aus/UK: Apo-Carbamazepine, Mazepine, Tegretol, Teril
Uses: Anticonvulsant
LRC: L2
AAP: Maternal Medication Usually Compatible with Breastfeeding

Carbamazepine (CBZ) is a unique anticonvulsant commonly used for grand mal, clonic-tonic, simple and complex seizures. It is also used in manic depression and a number of other neurologic syndromes. It is one of the most commonly used anticonvulsants in pediatric patients.

In a brief study by Kaneko, with maternal plasma levels averaging 4.3 μg/mL, milk levels were 1.9 mg/L.[1] In a study of 3 patients who received from 5.8 to 7.3 mg/kg/day carbamazepine, milk levels were reported to vary from 1.3 to 1.8 mg/L while the epoxide metabolite varied from 0.5 to 1.1 mg/L.[2] No adverse effects were noted in any of the infants. In another study by Niebyl, breastmilk levels were 1.4 mg/L in the lipid fraction and 2.3 mg/L in the skim fraction in a mother receiving 1000 mg daily of carbamazepine[3]. Niebyl estimated that the daily intake of 2 mg carbamazepine daily (0.5 mg/kg) in an infant ingesting 1 Liter of milk per day.

In a study of CBZ and its epoxide metabolite (ECBZ) in milk, 16 patients received an average dose of 13.8 mg/kg/d.[4] The average maternal serum levels of CBZ and ECBZ were 7.1 and 2.6 μg/mL respectively. The average milk levels of CBZ and ECBZ were 2.5 and 1.5 mg/L respectively. The relative percent of CBZ and ECBZ in milk were 36.4% and 53% of the maternal serum levels. A total of 50 milk samples in 19 patients were analyzed. Of these, the lowest CBZ concentration in milk was 1.0 mg/L; the highest was 4.8 mg/L. The CBZ level was determined in 7 infants 4-7 days postpartum. All infants have CBZ levels below 1.5 μg/mL.

In a study of 7 women receiving 250-800 mg/d carbamazepine, the CBZ level ranged from 2.8-4.5 mg/L in milk to 3.2-15.0 mg/L in plasma.[5]   The levels of ECBZ ranged from 0.5-1.7 mg/L in milk to 0.8-4.8 mg/L in plasma.

The amount of CBZ transferred to the infant is apparently quite low. Although the half-life of CBZ in infants appears shorter than in adults, infants should still be monitored for sedative effects.

Pregnancy Risk Category: C

Lactation Risk Category: L2

Adult Concerns: Sedation,   nausea,   respiratory depression, tachycardia, vomiting, diarrhea, blood dyscrasias

Pediatric Concerns: None reported via milk.

Drug Interactions: Carbamazepine may induce the metabolism of warfarin, cyclosporin, doxycycline, oral contraceptives, phenytoin, theophylline, benzodiazepines, ethosuximide, valproic acid, corticosteroids, and thyroid hormones. Macrolide antibiotics, isoniazid, verapamil, danazol, and diltiazem may inhibit metabolism of carbamazepine and increase plasma levels.

Theoretic Infant Dose: 0.6 mg/kg/day

Relative Infant Dose: 4.35%

Adult Dose: 800-1200 mg daily divided TID or QID

Alternatives:

$T^{1/2}$	=	18-54 hours	M/P	=	0.69
PHL	=	8-28 hours	PB	=	74%
T_{max}	=	4-5 hours	Oral	=	100%
MW	=	236	pKa	=	7.0
Vd	=	0.8-1.8			

References:
1.   Kaneko S, Sato T, Suzuki K. The levels of anticonvulsants in breastmilk. Br J Clin Pharmacol 1979; 7(6):624-627.
2.   Pynnonen S, Kanto J, Sillanpaa M, Erkkola R. Carbamazepine: placental transport, tissue concentrations in foetus and newborn, and level in milk. Acta Pharmacol Toxicol (Copenh) 1977; 41(3):244-253.
3.   Niebyl JR, Blake DA, Freeman JM, Luff RD. Carbamazepine levels in pregnancy and lactation. Obstet Gynecol 1979; 53(1):139-140.
4.   Froescher W, Eichelbaum M, Niesen M, Dietrich K, Rausch P. Carbamazepine levels in breastmilk. Ther Drug Monit 1984; 6(3):266-271.
5.   Shimoyama R, Ohkubo T, Sugawara K. Monitoring of carbamazepine and carbamazepine 10,11-epoxide in breastmilk and plasma by high-performance liquid chromatography. Ann Clin Biochem 2000; 37 (Pt 2):210-215.

CARBAMIDE PEROXIDE

Trade: Gly-Oxide, Debrox, Auro Otic, Teeth Whiteners
Can/Aus/UK: Exterol
Uses: Antibacterial, whitening agent
LRC: L1
AAP: Not reviewed

Carbamide peroxide is stable while immersed in glycerin, but upon contact with moisture, releases hydrogen peroxide and nascent oxygen, both strong oxidizing agents. It is used to disinfect infected lesions and for whitening of teeth and dental appliances. Hydrogen peroxide is rapidly metabolized by hydroperoxidases, peroxidases, and catalase present in all tissues, plasma, and saliva. Its transfer to the plasma is minimal if at all. It would be all but impossible for any to reach breastmilk unless under extreme overdose.

Pregnancy Risk Category: C

Lactation Risk Category: L1

Adult Concerns: Dermal irritation, mucous membrane irritation, inflammation. Overgrowth of candida and other opportunistic infections.

Pediatric Concerns: Toxic in major overdose. Exposure to small amounts may lead to inflamed membranes.

CARBENICILLIN

Trade: Geopen, Geocillin, Carindacillin
Can/Aus/UK: Geopen, Carbapen
Uses: Extended spectrum penicillin antibiotic
LRC: L1
AAP: Not reviewed

Carbenicillin is an extended spectrum penicillin antibiotic. Only limited levels are secreted into breastmilk (0.26 mg/liter or about 0.001% of adult dose).[1] In a study of 2-3 women who received 1000 mg I.M., the maximum milk level occurred at 4 hours and averaged 0.24 mg/L.[2] The average milk/plasma ratio reported was 0.045 at 4 hours. Due to its poor oral absorption (< 10%) the amount absorbed by a nursing infant would be minimal.

Pregnancy Risk Category: B

Lactation Risk Category: L1

Adult Concerns: Rash, thrush, headache, hyperthermia, or diarrhea

Pediatric Concerns: None reported via milk.

Drug Interactions: Coadministration of aminoglycosides (within 1 hr) may inactivate both drugs. Increased half-life with probenecid.

Theoretic Infant Dose: 36 µg/kg/day

Relative Infant Dose: 0.25%

Adult Dose: 382-764 mg q 6 hours

Alternatives:

T½ =	1 hour	M/P =	0.02
PHL =	0.8-1.8 hours	PB =	26-60%
T$_{max}$ =	1-3 hours	Oral =	< 10-30%
MW =	378	pKa =	
Vd =			

References:
1. Pharmaceutical Manufacturer Prescribing Information. 1996.
2. Matsuda S. Transfer of antibiotics into maternal milk. Biol Res Pregnancy Perinatol 1984; 5(2):57-60.

CARBIDOPA

Trade: Lodosyn
Can/Aus/UK: Sinemet, Kinson, Sinacarb
Uses: Inhibits levodopa metabolism
LRC: L3
AAP: Not reviewed

Carbidopa inhibits the metabolism of levodopa in parkinsonian patients therefore extending the half-life of levodopa. Its effect on lactation is largely unknown, but skeletal malformations have occurred in pregnant rabbits.[1,2] Use discretion in administering to pregnant or lactating women.

Pregnancy Risk Category: C

Lactation Risk Category: L3

Adult Concerns: GI distress, nausea, vomiting, diarrhea

Pediatric Concerns:

Drug Interactions: May interact with tricyclic antidepressants leading to hypertensive reactions.

Theoretic Infant Dose:

Relative Infant Dose:

Adult Dose: 70-100 mg daily

Alternatives:

T½ =	1-2 hours	M/P =	
PHL =		PB =	36%
T$_{max}$ =		Oral =	40-70%
MW =	244	pKa =	
Vd =			

References:
1. Pharmaceutical Manufacturer Prescribing Information. 1996.
2. McEvoy GE. (ed):AFHS Drug Information. New York, NY: 2003 .

CARBIMAZOLE
Trade:
Can/Aus/UK: Neo-Mercazole
Uses: Thyroid inhibitor
LRC: L3
AAP: Maternal Medication Usually Compatible with Breastfeeding

Carbimazole, a prodrug of methimazole, is rapidly and completely converted to the active methimazole in the plasma. Only methimazole is detected in plasma, urine, and thyroid tissue. See breastfeeding specifics for methimazole. Data from Rylance suggests that subclinical levels of methimazole enter milk subsequent to administration of 30 mg/day carbimazole.[1] Free methimazole measured in milk on 10 occasions averaged 43 µg/L. Plasma methimazole in twins was 45 to 52 ng/mL. Thyroid suppression is believed to occur only when plasma levels exceed 50-100 ng/mL. No thyroid suppression was noted in these two twins. Peak transfer into milk occurred at 2-4 hours and the lowest at 6 hours after the dose. The authors suggest that breastfeeding is permissible if the maternal dose is less than 30 mg/day. See propylthiouracil as alternative.

In another study of 5 five lactating women receiving 40 mg/d, the mean concentration of methimazole in milk was 182 µg/K.[2] The reported milk/plasma ratio was 0.98. The mean total amount of methimazole excreted in milk over 8 hours was 34 µg (or 0.14% of the dose).[2]

The limited data above suggest that the transfer of carbimazole is too low to affect thyroid function in breastfeeding infants. However, close monitoring of infant thyroid function is probably advisable.

Pregnancy Risk Category: D

Lactation Risk Category: L3

Adult Concerns: Hypothyroidism, hepatic dysfunction, bleeding, drowsiness, skin rash, nausea, vomiting, fever

Pediatric Concerns: None reported via milk, but propylthiouracil is generally preferred in breastfeeding women.

Drug Interactions: Use with iodinated glycerol, lithium, and potassium iodide may increase toxicity.

Theoretic Infant Dose: 6.45 µg/kg/day

Relative Infant Dose: 1.5%

Adult Dose: < 30 mg daily

Alternatives: Propylthiouracil

$T\frac{1}{2}$ =	6-13 hours	M/P =	0.3-0.7
PHL =		PB =	0%
T_{max} =	4 hour	Oral =	Complete
MW =	186	pKa =	
Vd =			

References:
1. Rylance GW, Woods CG, Donnelly MC, Oliver JS, Alexander WD. Carbimazole and breastfeeding. Lancet 1987; 1(8538):928.
2. Johansen K, Andersen AN, Kampmann JP, Molholm Hansen JM, Mortensen HB. Excretion of methimazole in human milk. Eur J Clin Pharmacol 1982; 23(4):339-341.

CARBOPROST TROMETHAMINE
Trade: Hemabate
Can/Aus/UK: Hemabate
Uses: Oxytocic prostaglandin for postpartum hemorrhage
LRC: L3
AAP: Not reviewed

Carboprost is a prostaglandin analogue (15-methyl prostaglandin F2-alpha) that stimulates the gravid uterus myometrial contractions similar to labor. It is a commonly used oxytocic agent used to prevent postpartum hemorrhage. No data are available on its transfer to human milk. Prostaglandins have brief half-lives and little distribution out of the plasma compartment. Even then, rather large intramuscular doses only produce picogram concentrations in the plasma of recipients. It is not likely it will penetrate milk in clinically relevant amounts.

Pregnancy Risk Category: C

Lactation Risk Category: L3

Adult Concerns: Adverse events include vomiting, diarrhea, leukocytosis, hypertension, headache, dystonic reactions, fever, uterine rupture, bronchoconstriction, and flushing of the skin.

Pediatric Concerns: None reported via milk. Commonly used in obstetrics without complication in breastfeeding mothers.

Drug Interactions: May augment other oxytocics.

Theoretic Infant Dose:

Relative Infant Dose:

Adult Dose: 100-250 mg initially

Alternatives:

$T\frac{1}{2}$ =	< 1 hour	M/P =	
PHL =		PB =	
T_{max} =	15-30 minutes	Oral =	
MW =	489	pKa =	
Vd =			

References:
1. Pharmaceutical Manufacturers prescribing information, 2003.

CARISOPRODOL

Trade: Soma Compound, Solol
Can/Aus/UK: Soma, Carisoma
Uses: Muscle relaxant, CNS depressant
LRC: L3
AAP: Not reviewed

Carisoprodol is a commonly used skeletal muscle relaxant that is a CNS depressant. It is metabolized to an active metabolite called meprobamate. As Soma Compound it also contains 325 mg of aspirin. In a study of one breastfeeding mother receiving 2100 mg/d, the average milk concentration of carisoprodol and meprobamate was 0.9 mg/L and 11.6 mg/L respectively.[1] Based on these combined values, the relative infant dose for carisoprodol and meprobamate would be 4.1% of the weight-adjusted maternal dose. No adverse effects on the infant were noted.

Pregnancy Risk Category: C

Lactation Risk Category: L3

Adult Concerns: Nausea, vomiting, hiccups, sedation, weakness, mild withdrawal symptoms after chronic use

Pediatric Concerns: None reported, but observe for sedation.

Drug Interactions: Increased toxicity when added to alcohol, CNS depressants, MAO inhibitors.

Theoretic Infant Dose:

Relative Infant Dose:

Adult Dose: 350 mg TID-QID

Alternatives:

T½ =	8 hours	M/P =	2-4
PHL =		PB =	
T$_{max}$ =		Oral =	Complete
MW =	260	pKa =	
Vd =			

References:
1. Nordeng H, Zahlsen K, Spigset O. Transfer of carisoprodol to breastmilk. Ther Drug Monit 2001; 23(3):298-300.

CARTEOLOL

Trade: Cartrol
Can/Aus/UK: Teoptic
Uses: Beta-adrenergic antihypertensive
LRC: L3
AAP: Not reviewed

Carteolol is a typical beta blocker used for hypertension. Carteolol is reported to be excreted in breastmilk of lactating animals[1]. No data available on human milk.

Pregnancy Risk Category: C

Lactation Risk Category: L3

Adult Concerns: Hypotension, bradycardia, lethargy, and sedation

Pediatric Concerns: None reported but observe for hypoglycemia, hypotension, bradycardia, lethargy.

Drug Interactions: Decreased effect when used with aluminum salts, barbiturates, calcium salts, cholestyramine, NSAIDs, ampicillin, rifampin, and salicylates. Beta blockers may reduce the effect of oral sulfonylureas (hypoglycemic agents). Increased toxicity/effect when used with other antihypertensives, contraceptives, MAO inhibitors, cimetidine, and numerous other products. See drug interaction reference for complete listing.

Theoretic Infant Dose:

Relative Infant Dose:

Adult Dose: 2.5-5 mg daily

Alternatives: Propranolol, Metoprolol

T½ =	6 hours	M/P =	
PHL =		PB =	23-30%
T$_{max}$ =		Oral =	80%
MW =	292	pKa =	
Vd =			

References:
1. Pharmaceutical Manufacturer Prescribing Information. 1996.

CARVEDILOL
Trade: Coreg
Can/Aus/UK: Coreg, Eucardic, Proreg, Dilatrend
Uses: Antihypertensive
LRC: L3
AAP: Not reviewed

Carvedilol is a nonselective beta-adrenergic blocking agent (and partial alpha-1 blocking activity) with high lipid solubility and no intrinsic sympathomimetic activity.[1] There are no data available on the transfer of this drug into human milk. However, due to its high lipid solubility, some may transfer. As with any beta blocker, some caution is recommended until milk levels are reported.

Pregnancy Risk Category: C

Lactation Risk Category: L3

Adult Concerns: Postural hypotension, fatigue, dizziness, lightheadedness, bradycardia, bronchospasm. Use with caution in asthmatics.

Pediatric Concerns: None reported via milk. Observe for hypotension, bradycardia, hypoglycemia.

Drug Interactions: Severe bradycardia may result when used with amiodarone. Digoxin may prolong AV conduction time. Severe hypotension when added with calcium channel blockers. Severe hypertension, bradycardia when used with epinephrine.

Theoretic Infant Dose:

Relative Infant Dose:

Adult Dose: 6.25-12.5 mg BID

Alternatives: Propranolol, metoprolol.

T½ =	7-10 hours	M/P =	
PHL =		PB =	98%
T$_{max}$ =	1-1.5 hours	Oral =	25-35%
MW =		pKa =	
Vd =	1.88		

References:
1. Pharmaceutical Manufacturer Prescribing Information.

CASCARA SAGRADA

Trade: Cascara Sagrada
Can/Aus/UK: Cascara Sagrada
Uses: Laxative
LRC: L3
AAP: Maternal Medication Usually Compatible with Breastfeeding

Trace amounts appear to be secreted into breastmilk[1,2]. No exact estimates have been published. May cause loose stools and diarrhea in neonates.

Pregnancy Risk Category: C

Lactation Risk Category: L3

Adult Concerns: Diarrhea, GI cramping

Pediatric Concerns: May loosen stools in infants

Drug Interactions: Decreased effect of oral anticoagulants

Theoretic Infant Dose:

Relative Infant Dose:

Adult Dose: 5 mL daily

Alternatives:

References:
1. O'Brien TE. Excretion of drugs in human milk. Am J Hosp Pharm 1974; 31(9):844-854.
2. Vorherr H. Drug excretion in breastmilk. Postgrad Med 1974; 56(4):97-104.

CASPOFUNGIN ACETATE

Trade: Cancidas
Can/Aus/UK:
Uses: Antifungal
LRC: L3
AAP: Not reviewed

Caspofungin is a unique semisynthetic lipopeptide that is active against Aspergillus fumigatus. It has a large polycyclic structure with a molecular weight of 1213 daltons. The half-life of this product is unique with a polyphasic elimination curve with 3 distinct phases. The half-life varies from 11 hours in one phase to 40-50 hours in the last phase. This is a new product and limited data are available on its use, particularly in pediatrics. The pharmaceutical manufacture states that it was found in rodent milk; no data are available for human milk. Regardless, the oral bioavailability is reported as poor and it is unlikely an infant would absorb enough to be clinically relevant, but this is only speculative.

Pregnancy Risk Category: C

Lactation Risk Category: L3

Adult Concerns: Fever, nausea, vomiting, flushing, phlebitis, anemia, headache, etc.

Pediatric Concerns: None reported via milk. Not cleared for pediatric patients.

Drug Interactions: Cyclosporin increases AUC of Cancidas. Do not use with cyclosporin unless potential benefits outweigh risk. Cancidas reduces plasma levels of tacrolimus.

Theoretic Infant Dose:

Relative Infant Dose:

Adult Dose: 70 mg STAT, 50 mg/d

Alternatives:

$T\frac{1}{2}$ =	> 11 hours	M/P =	
PHL =		PB =	97%
T_{max} =		Oral =	Poor
MW =	1213	pKa =	5.1, 10.7
Vd =			

References:
1. Pharmaceutical Manufacturer Prescribing Information.

CASTOR OIL

Trade: Alphamul, Neoloid, Emulsoil
Can/Aus/UK: Castrol Oil, Seda-rash, Exzem Oil
Uses: Laxative
LRC: L3
AAP: Not reviewed

Castor oil is converted to ricinoleic acid in the gut. Its transfer into milk is unknown. Caution should be used. Excess amounts could produce diarrhea, insomnia, and tremors in exposed infants.

Pregnancy Risk Category: X

Lactation Risk Category: L3

Adult Concerns: Insomnia, tremors, diarrhea

Pediatric Concerns: Observe for diarrhea, insomnia, tremors in infants.

Drug Interactions:

Theoretic Infant Dose:

Relative Infant Dose:

Adult Dose: N/A

Alternatives:

$T\frac{1}{2}$ =		M/P =	
PHL =		PB =	
T_{max} =	2-3 hours	Oral =	Unknown
MW =	932	pKa =	
Vd =			

References:

CEFACLOR

Trade: Ceclor
Can/Aus/UK: Ceclor, Apo-Cefaclor, Keflor, Distaclor
Uses: Cephalosporin antibiotic
LRC: L2
AAP: Not reviewed

Cefaclor is a commonly used pediatric cephalosporin antibiotic. Small amounts are known to be secreted into human milk. Following a 500 mg oral dose, milk levels averaged 0.16 to 0.21 mg/L.[1] See cephalosporins.

Pregnancy Risk Category: B

Lactation Risk Category: L2

Adult Concerns: Diarrhea, GI irritation, rash, penicillin allergy, delayed serum sickness at 14 days.

Pediatric Concerns: None reported via milk.

Drug Interactions: Probenecid may increase levels of cephalosporins by reducing renal clearance.

Theoretic Infant Dose: 31.5 µg/kg/day

Relative Infant Dose: 0.44%

Adult Dose: 250-500 mg q 8 hours

Alternatives:

T½ =	0.5-1 hour	M/P =	
PHL =		PB =	25%
T$_{max}$ =	0.5-1 hour	Oral =	100%
MW =	386	pKa =	
Vd =			

References:
1. Takase Z. Clinical and laboratory studies of cefaclor in the field of obstetrics and gynecology. Chemotherapy 1979; 27:(Suppl)668.

CEFADROXIL

Trade: Ultracef, Duricef
Can/Aus/UK: Duricef, Baxan
Uses: Cephalosporin antibiotic
LRC: L1
AAP: Maternal Medication Usually Compatible with Breastfeeding

Cefadroxil is a typical first-generation, cephalosporin antibiotic. Small amounts are known to be secreted into milk. Milk concentrations following a 1000 mg oral dose were 0.10 mg/L at 1 hour and 1.24 mg/L at 5 hours[1]. Milk/serum ratios were 0.009 at 1 hour and 0.019 at 3 hours.

In a study of 2-3 patients who received an oral dose of 500 mg cefadroxil, milk levels peaked at 4 hours at an average of 0.4 mg/L.[2] The milk/plasma ratio was 0.085.

Pregnancy Risk Category: B

Lactation Risk Category: L1

Adult Concerns: Diarrhea, allergic rash

Pediatric Concerns: None reported via milk. Observe for GI symptoms such as diarrhea.

Drug Interactions: Probenecid may decrease clearance. Furosemide, aminoglycosides may enhance renal toxicity.

Theoretic Infant Dose: 186 µg/kg/day

Relative Infant Dose: 1.3%

Adult Dose: 0.5-1 g BID

Alternatives:

T½ =	1.5 hours	M/P =	0.009-0.019
PHL =		PB =	20%
T$_{max}$ =	1-2 hours	Oral =	100%
MW =	381	pKa =	
Vd =			

References:
1. Kafetzis DA, Siafas CA, Georgakopoulos PA, Papadatos CJ. Passage of cephalosporins and amoxicillin into the breastmilk. Acta Paediatr Scand 1981; 70(3):285-288.
2. Matsuda S. Transfer of antibiotics into maternal milk. Biol Res Pregnancy Perinatol 1984; 5(2):57-60.

CEFAZOLIN

Trade: Ancef, Kefzol
Can/Aus/UK: Ancef, Kefzol, Cefamezin
Uses: Cephalosporin antibiotic
LRC: L1
AAP: Maternal Medication Usually Compatible with Breastfeeding

Cefazolin is a typical first-generation, cephalosporin antibiotic that has adult and pediatric indications. It is only used IM or IV, never orally. In 20 patients who received a 2 gm STAT dose over 10 minutes, the average concentration of cefazolin in milk 2, 3, and 4 hours after the dose was 1.25, 1.51, and 1.16 mg/L respectively[1]. A very small milk/plasma ratio (0.023) indicates insignificant transfer into milk. Cefazolin is poorly absorbed orally; therefore, the infant would absorb a minimal amount. Plasma levels in infants are reported to be too small to be detected.

Pregnancy Risk Category: B

Lactation Risk Category: L1

Adult Concerns: Allergic rash, thrush, diarrhea

Pediatric Concerns: None reported via milk. Observe for GI symptoms such as diarrhea.

Drug Interactions: Probenecid may decrease clearance. Furosemide, aminoglycosides may enhance renal toxicity.

Theoretic Infant Dose: 226 µg/kg/day

Relative Infant Dose: 0.79%

Adult Dose: 250-2000 mg TID

Alternatives:

$T\frac{1}{2}$ =	1.2-2.2 hours	M/P =	0.023
PHL =		PB =	89%
T_{max} =	1-2 hours	Oral =	Poor
MW =	455	pKa =	
Vd =			

References:
1. Yoshioka H, Cho K, Takimoto M, Maruyama S, Shimizu T. Transfer of cefazolin into human milk. J Pediatr 1979; 94(1):151-152.

CEFDINIR
Trade: Omnicef
Can/Aus/UK:
Uses: Antibiotic
LRC: L2
AAP: Not reviewed

Cefdinir is a broad spectrum cephalosporin antibiotic. Following administration of a 600 mg oral dose, no cefdinir was detected in human milk.

Pregnancy Risk Category: B

Lactation Risk Category: L2

Adult Concerns: Similar for other cephalosporins, and include diarrhea, vaginal moniliasis, nausea, and rash. Allergic reactions are possible.

Pediatric Concerns: None reported via milk. Milk levels virtually undetectable.

Drug Interactions: Reduced oral absorption following use of antacids. Probenecid will decrease renal excretion and a 54% increase in peak levels, and a 50% prolongation of clearance.

Theoretic Infant Dose:

Relative Infant Dose:

Adult Dose: 14 mg/kg/day

Alternatives:

T½ =	1.7 hours	M/P =	
PHL =		PB =	70%
Tmax =	3 hours	Oral =	21%
MW =	395	pKa =	
Vd =	0.35		

References:
1. Pharmaceutical Manufacturer Prescribing Information.

CEFDITOREN

Trade: Spectracef
Can/Aus/UK:
Uses: Cephalosporin antibiotic
LRC: L3
AAP: Not reviewed

Cefditoren is a new third generation cephalosporin antibiotic that is indicated in the treatment of acute bacterial exacerbations of chronic bronchitis, pharyngitis, tonsillitis, and uncomplicated skin infections. It is moderately active against resistant penicillin-resistant pneumococcus. It is cleared for use in children < 12 years of age. No data on breastmilk levels are available.

Pregnancy Risk Category: B

Lactation Risk Category: L3

Adult Concerns: Diarrhea, nausea, headache, vaginal moniliasis

Pediatric Concerns: None reported.

Drug Interactions:

Theoretic Infant Dose:

Relative Infant Dose:

Adult Dose:

Alternatives: Cephalexin

$T\frac{1}{2}$ =	1.3-2 hours	M/P =	
PHL =		PB =	88%
T_{max} =	1-3 hours	Oral =	14%
MW =	620	pKa =	
Vd =	9.3		

References:
1. Pharmaceutical Manufacturer Prescribing Information.

CEFEPIME

Trade: Maxipime
Can/Aus/UK: Maxipime
Uses: Cephalosporin antibiotic
LRC: L2
AAP: Not reviewed

Cefepime is a new 'fourth-generation' parenteral cephalosporin. Cefepime is secreted in human milk in small amounts averaging 0.5

mg/L.[1,2]   In a mother consuming 2 gm/d, an infant would ingest approximately 75 µg/kg/d or only approximately 0.3 % of the maternal dose. This amount is too small to produce any clinical symptoms other than possible changes in gut flora.

Pregnancy Risk Category: B

Lactation Risk Category: L2

Adult Concerns: Headache, blurred vision, dyspepsia, diarrhea, transient elevation of liver enzymes

Pediatric Concerns: None reported via milk.

Drug Interactions: May produce additive nephrotoxic effects when used with aminoglycosides.

Theoretic Infant Dose: 75 µg/kg/day

Relative Infant Dose: 0.26%

Adult Dose: 1-2 g BID

Alternatives:

$T\frac{1}{2}$ =	2 hours	M/P =	0.8
PHL =		PB =	16-19%
T_{max} =	0.5-1.5 hours	Oral =	Poor
MW =	571	pKa =	
Vd =	0.3		

References:
1.   Pharmaceutical Manufacturer Prescribing Information. 1997.
2.   Sanders CC. Cefepime: the next generation? Clin Infect Dis 1993; 17(3):369-379.

CEFIXIME

Trade: Suprax
Can/Aus/UK: Suprax
Uses: Cephalosporin antibiotic
LRC: L2
AAP: Not reviewed

Cefixime is an oral, third-generation cephalosporin used in treating infections.   It is poorly absorbed (30-50%) by the oral route.   It is secreted to a limited degree in the milk although in one study of a mother receiving 100 mg, it was undetected in the milk from 1-6 hours after the dose.[1]

Pregnancy Risk Category: B

Lactation Risk Category: L2

Adult Concerns: Allergic rash, diarrhea, thrush

Pediatric Concerns: None reported. Observe for GI symptoms such as diarrhea.

Drug Interactions: Probenecid may decrease clearance. Furosemide, aminoglycosides may enhance renal toxicity.

Theoretic Infant Dose:

Relative Infant Dose:

Adult Dose: 200 mg BID

Alternatives:

T½ =	7 hours	M/P =	
PHL =		PB =	70%
T$_{max}$ =	2-6 hours	Oral =	30-50%
MW =	453	pKa =	
Vd =			

References:
1. Pharmaceutical Manufacturer Prescribing Information. 1996.

CEFOPERAZONE SODIUM

Trade: Cefobid
Can/Aus/UK: Cefobid, Dicapen
Uses: Cephalosporin antibiotic
LRC: L2
AAP: Not reviewed

Cefoperazone is a broad spectrum, third-generation cephalosporin antibiotic. It is poorly absorbed from GI tract and is only available via IV and I.M. injection. Cefoperazone is extremely labile in acid environments which would account both for its destruction and its lack of absorption via the GI tract. Following an IV dose of 1000 mg, milk levels ranged from 0.4 to 0.9 mg/L.[1] In a study of 2-3 women who received 1000 mg IV, the maximum milk concentration was 0.4 mg/L at 6 hours.[2] The average milk/plasma ratio was 0.12 at 4 hours. Cefoperazone is extremely acid labile and would be destroyed in the GI tract of an infant. It is unlikely that significant absorption would occur.

Pregnancy Risk Category: B

Lactation Risk Category: L2

Adult Concerns: Diarrhea, allergic rash, thrush

Pediatric Concerns: None reported. Observe for GI symptoms such as diarrhea.

Drug Interactions: Probenecid may decrease clearance. Furosemide, aminoglycosides may enhance renal toxicity.

Theoretic Infant Dose: 0.06 mg/kg/day

Relative Infant Dose: 0.42%

Adult Dose: 1-2 g BID

Alternatives:

T½ =	2 hours	M/P =	0.12
PHL =	6-10 hours (neonatal)	PB =	82-93%
T$_{max}$ =	73-153 minutes (IV)	Oral =	Poor
MW =	645	pKa =	
Vd =			

References:
1. Pfizer/Roerig Laboratories. Personal Communication. 1996.
2. Matsuda S. Transfer of antibiotics into maternal milk. Biol Res Pregnancy Perinatol 1984; 5(2):57-60.

CEFOTAXIME

Trade: Claforan
Can/Aus/UK: Claforan
Uses: Cephalosporin antibiotic
LRC: L2
AAP: Maternal Medication Usually Compatible with Breastfeeding

Cefotaxime is poorly absorbed orally and is only used via IV or IM administration. Milk levels following a 1000 mg IV maternal dose were 0.26 mg/L at 1 hour, 0.32 mg/L at 2 hours, and 0.30 mg/L at 3 hours.[1] No effect on infant or lactation were noted. Milk/serum ratio at 3 hours was 0.160.

In a group of 2-3 patients receiving 1000 mg IV, none to trace amounts were found in milk after 6 hours.[2]

Pregnancy Risk Category: B

Lactation Risk Category: L2

Adult Concerns: Diarrhea, allergic rash, thrush

Pediatric Concerns: None reported. Observe for GI symptoms such as diarrhea.

Drug Interactions: Probenecid may decrease clearance. Furosemide, aminoglycosides may enhance renal toxicity.

Theoretic Infant Dose: 0.048 mg/kg/day

Relative Infant Dose: 0.34%

Adult Dose: 1-2 g q BID

Alternatives:

T½ =	< 0.68 hour	M/P =	0.027 - 0.17
PHL =	2-3.5 hours	PB =	40%
T$_{max}$ =	30 minutes	Oral =	Poor
MW =	455	pKa =	
Vd =			

References:
1. Kafetzis DA, Lazarides CV, Siafas CA, Georgakopoulos PA, Papadatos CJ. Transfer of cefotaxime in human milk and from mother to foetus. J Antimicrob Chemother 1980; 6 Suppl A:135-141.
2. Matsuda S. Transfer of antibiotics into maternal milk. Biol Res Pregnancy Perinatol 1984; 5(2):57-60.

CEFOTETAN

Trade: Cefotan
Can/Aus/UK: Cefotan, Apatef
Uses: Cephalosporin antibiotic
LRC: L2
AAP: Not reviewed

Cefotetan is a third generation cephalosporin that is poorly absorbed orally and is only available via IM and IV injection. The drug is distributed into human milk in low concentrations. Following a maternal dose of 1000mg IM every 12 hours in 5 patients, breastmilk concentrations ranged from 0.29 to 0.59 mg/L.[1] Plasma concentrations were almost 100 times higher.

In a group of 2-3 women who received 1000 mg IV, the maximum average milk level reported was 0.2 mg/L at 4 hours with a milk/plasma ratio of 0.02.[2]

Pregnancy Risk Category: B

Lactation Risk Category: L2

Adult Concerns: Diarrhea, allergic rash, thrush

Pediatric Concerns: None reported. Observe for GI symptoms such as diarrhea.

Drug Interactions: Probenecid may decrease clearance. Furosemide, aminoglycosides may enhance renal toxicity.

Theoretic Infant Dose: 88.5 µg/kg/day

Relative Infant Dose: 0.31%

Adult Dose: 1-2 g BID

Alternatives:

T½ =	3-4.6 hours	M/P =	
PHL =		PB =	76-91%
T$_{max}$ =	1.5-3 hours	Oral =	Poor
MW =	576	pKa =	
Vd =			

References:
1. Novelli A. The penetration of intramuscular cefotetan disodium into human esta-vascular fluid and maternal milk secretion. Chemoterapia 1983; 11(5):337-342.
2. Matsuda S. Transfer of antibiotics into maternal milk. Biol Res Pregnancy Perinatol 1984; 5(2):57-60.

CEFOXITIN
Trade: Mefoxin
Can/Aus/UK: Mefoxin
Uses: Cephalosporin antibiotic
LRC: L1
AAP: Maternal Medication Usually Compatible with Breastfeeding

Cefoxitin is a cephalosporin antibiotic with a spectrum similar to the second generation family. It is transferred into human milk in very low levels. In a study of 18 women receiving 2000-4000 mg doses, only one breastmilk sample contained cefoxitin (0.9 mg/L), all the rest were too low to be detected.[1] In a study of 2-3 women who received 1000 mg IV, only trace amounts were reported in milk over 6 hours.[2] In a group of 5 women who received an I.M. injection of 2000 mg, the highest milk levels were reported at 4 hours after dose.[3] The maternal plasma levels varied from 22.5 at 2 hours to 77.6 µg/mL at 4 hours. Maternal milk levels ranged from < 0.25 to 0.65 mg/L.

Pregnancy Risk Category: B

Lactation Risk Category: L1

Adult Concerns: Diarrhea, allergic rash, thrush

Pediatric Concerns: None reported. Observe for GI symptoms such as diarrhea.

Drug Interactions: Probenecid may decrease clearance. Furosemide, aminoglycosides may enhance renal toxicity.

Theoretic Infant Dose: 135 µg/kg/day

Relative Infant Dose: 0.24%

Adult Dose: 1-2 g TID

Alternatives:

T½ =	0.7-1.1 hour	M/P =	
PHL =		PB =	85-99%
T$_{max}$ =	20-30 minutes (IM)	Oral =	Poor
MW =	427	pKa =	
Vd =			

References:
1. Roex AJ, van Loenen AC, Puyenbroek JI, Arts NF. Secretion of cefoxitin in breastmilk following short-term prophylactic administration in caesarean section. Eur J Obstet Gynecol Reprod Biol 1987; 25(4):299-302.
2. Matsuda S. Transfer of antibiotics into maternal milk. Biol Res Pregnancy Perinatol 1984; 5(2):57-60.
3. Dresse A, Lambotte R, Dubois M, Delapierre D, Kramp R. Transmammary passage of cefoxitin: additional results. J Clin Pharmacol 1983; 23(10):438-440.

CEFPODOXIME PROXETIL
Trade: Vantin
Can/Aus/UK: Orelox
Uses: Cephalosporin antibiotic
LRC: L2
AAP: Not reviewed

Cefpodoxime is a cephalosporin antibiotic that is subsequently metabolized to an active metabolite. Only 50% is orally absorbed. In a study of 3 lactating women, levels of cefpodoxime in human milk were 0%, 2%, and 6% of maternal serum levels at 4 hours following a 200 mg oral dose[1]. At 6 hours post-dosing, levels were 0%, 9%, and 16% of concomitant maternal serum levels. Pediatric indications down to 6 months of age are available.

Pregnancy Risk Category: B

Lactation Risk Category: L2

Adult Concerns: Diarrhea, allergic rash, thrush

Pediatric Concerns: None reported. Observe for GI symptoms such as diarrhea.

Drug Interactions: Probenecid may decrease clearance. Furosemide and aminoglycosides may enhance renal toxicity. Antacids and H2 blockers reduce GI absorption of cefpodoxime.

Theoretic Infant Dose:

Relative Infant Dose:

Adult Dose: 100-400 mg BID

Alternatives:

T½ =	2.09-2.84 hours	M/P =	0-0.16
PHL =		PB =	22-33%
T$_{max}$ =	2-3 hours	Oral =	50%
MW =	558	pKa =	
Vd =			

References:
1. Pharmaceutical Manufacturer Prescribing Information. 1996.

CEFPROZIL

Trade: Cefzil
Can/Aus/UK:
Uses: Oral cephalosporin antibiotic
LRC: L1
AAP: Maternal Medication Usually Compatible with Breastfeeding

Cefprozil is a typical second-generation, cephalosporin antibiotic. Following an oral dose of 1000 mg, the breastmilk concentrations were 0.7, 2.5, and 3.4 mg/L at 2, 4, and 6 hours post-dose respectively. The peak milk concentration occurred at 6 hours and was lower thereafter.[1] Milk/plasma ratios varied from 0.05 at 2 hours to 5.67 at 12 hours. However, the milk concentration at 12 hours was small (1.3 µg/mL). Using the highest concentration found in breastmilk (3.5 mg/L), an infant consuming 800 mL of milk daily would ingest about 2.8 mg of cefprozil daily. Because the dose used in this study is approximately twice that normally used, it is reasonable to assume that an infant would ingest less than 1.7 mg per day, an amount clinically insignificant. Pediatric indications for infants 6 months and older are available.

Pregnancy Risk Category: C

Lactation Risk Category: L1

Adult Concerns: Diarrhea, allergic rash, and thrush

Pediatric Concerns: None reported. Observe for GI symptoms such as diarrhea.

Drug Interactions: Probenecid may decrease clearance. Furosemide, aminoglycosides may enhance renal toxicity.

Theoretic Infant Dose: 0.51 mg/kg/day

Relative Infant Dose: 3.5%

Adult Dose: 250 mg BID

Alternatives:

T½ =	78 minutes	M/P =	0.05 - 5.67
PHL =		PB =	36 %
T$_{max}$ =	1.5 hours	Oral =	Complete
MW =		pKa =	
Vd =			

References:

1. Shyu WC, Shah VR, Campbell DA, Venitz J, Jaganathan V, Pittman KA, Wilber RB, Barbhaiya RH. Excretion of cefprozil into human breastmilk. Antimicrob Agents Chemother 1992; 36(5):938-941.

CEFTAZIDIME

Trade: Ceftazidime, Fortaz, Tazidime, Ceptaz
Can/Aus/UK: Fortaz, Ceptaz, Fortum
Uses: Cephalosporin antibiotic
LRC: L1
AAP: Maternal Medication Usually Compatible with Breastfeeding

Ceftazidime is a broad spectrum, third-generation, cephalosporin antibiotic. Is has poor oral absorption (<10%). In lactating women who received 2000 mg (IV) every 8 hours for 5 days, concentrations of ceftazidime in milk averaged 3.8 mg/L before the dose and 5.2 mg/L at 1 hour after the dose and 4.5 mg/L 3 hours after the dose.[1] There is, however, no progressive accumulation of ceftazidime in breastmilk, as evidenced by the similar levels prior to and after seven doses. The therapeutic dose for neonates is 30-50 mg/kg every 12 hours.

Pregnancy Risk Category: B

Lactation Risk Category: L1

Adult Concerns: Diarrhea, allergic rash, thrush

Pediatric Concerns: None reported. Observe for GI symptoms such as diarrhea.

Drug Interactions: Probenecid may decrease clearance. Furosemide, aminoglycosides may enhance renal toxicity.

Theoretic Infant Dose: 0.78 mg/kg/day

Relative Infant Dose: 0.9%

Adult Dose: 500-2000 mg BID

Alternatives:

T½ =	1.4-2 hours	M/P =	
PHL =	2.2-4.7 hours (neonates)	PB =	5-24%
T$_{max}$ =	69-90 minutes	Oral =	< 10%
MW =	547	pKa =	
Vd =			

References:
1. Blanco JD, Jorgensen JH, Castaneda YS, Crawford SA. Ceftazidime levels in human breastmilk. Antimicrob Agents Chemother 1983; 23(3):479-480.

CEFTIBUTEN
Trade: Cedax
Can/Aus/UK: Cedax
Uses: Cephalosporin antibiotic
LRC: L2
AAP: Not reviewed

Ceftibuten is a broad spectrum, third generation oral cephalosporin antibiotic. No data yet available on penetration into human breastmilk.[1] Small to moderate amounts may penetrate into milk, but ceftibuten is cleared for pediatric use.[2] Its strength is in activity against gram negative species. Its weakness is in staphylococci and strep. pneumonia coverage (which causes many inner ear infections).

Pregnancy Risk Category: B

Lactation Risk Category: L2

Adult Concerns: Diarrhea, vomiting, loose stools, abdominal pain

Pediatric Concerns: None reported. Observe for GI symptoms such as diarrhea.

Drug Interactions: Probenecid may decrease clearance. Furosemide and aminoglycosides may enhance renal toxicity.

Theoretic Infant Dose:

Relative Infant Dose:

Adult Dose: 400 mg daily

Alternatives:

T½ =	2.4 hours	M/P =	
PHL =	2-3 hours	PB =	65%
Tmax =	2.6 hours	Oral =	High
MW =	410	pKa =	
Vd =			

References:
1. Pharmaceutical Manufacturer Prescribing Information. 1996.
2. Barr WH, Affrime M, Lin CC, Batra V. Pharmacokinetics of ceftibuten in children. Pediatr Infect Dis J 1995; 14(7 Suppl):S93-101.

CEFTRIAXONE

Trade: Rocephin
Can/Aus/UK: Rocephin
Uses: Cephalosporin antibiotic
LRC: L2
AAP: Maternal Medication Usually Compatible with Breastfeeding

Ceftriaxone is a very popular third-generation broad spectrum cephalosporin antibiotic. Small amounts are transferred into milk (3-4% of maternal serum level). Following a 1 gm IM dose, breastmilk levels were approximately 0.5-0.7 mg/L at between 4-8 hours.[1,2] The estimated mean milk levels at steady state were 3-4 mg/L. Another source indicates that following a 2 g/d dose and at steady state, approximately 4.4 % of dose penetrates into milk.[3] In this study, the maximum breastmilk concentration was 7.89 mg/L after prolonged therapy (7days). Poor oral absorption of ceftriaxone would further limit systemic absorption by the infant. The half-life of ceftriaxone in human milk varies from 12.8 to 17.3 hrs (longer than maternal serum). Even at this high dose, no adverse effects were noted in the infant.

Ceftriaxone levels in breastmilk are probably too low to be clinically relevant, except for changes in GI flora. Ceftriaxone is commonly used in neonates.

Pregnancy Risk Category: B

Lactation Risk Category: L2

Adult Concerns: Diarrhea, allergic rash, pseudomembranous colitis, thrush

Pediatric Concerns: None reported. Observe for GI symptoms such as diarrhea.

Drug Interactions: Probenecid may decrease clearance. Furosemide, aminoglycosides may enhance renal toxicity.

Theoretic Infant Dose: 0.6 mg/kg/day

Relative Infant Dose: 4.2%

Adult Dose: 1-2 g daily-BID

Alternatives:

$T\frac{1}{2}$ =	7.3 hours	M/P =	0.03
PHL =		PB =	95%
T_{max} =	1 hour	Oral =	Poor
MW =	555	pKa =	
Vd =			

References:
1. Kafetzis DA, Siafas CA, Georgakopoulos PA, Papadatos CJ. Passage of cephalosporins and amoxicillin into the breastmilk. Acta Paediatr Scand 1981; 70(3):285-288.
2. Kafetzis DA, Brater DC, Fanourgakis JE, Voyatzis J, Georgakopoulos P. Ceftriaxone distribution between maternal blood and fetal blood and tissues at parturition and between blood and milk postpartum. Antimicrob Agents Chemother 1983; 23(6):870-873.
3. Bourget P, Quinquis-Desmaris V, Fernandez H. Ceftriaxone distribution and protein binding between maternal blood and milk postpartum. Ann Pharmacother 1993; 27(3):294-297.

CEFUROXIME

Trade: Ceftin, Zinacef, Kefurox
Can/Aus/UK: Zinacef, Ceftin, Zinnat
Uses: Cephalosporin antibiotic
LRC: L2
AAP: Not reviewed

Cefuroxime is a broad spectrum, second generation cephalosporin antibiotic that is available orally and IV. The manufacturer states that it is secreted into human milk in small amounts, but the levels are not available[1]. Thus far, no untoward effects in infants have been reported. Cefuroxime has a very bitter taste. The IV salt form, cefuroxime sodium, is very poorly absorbed orally. Only the axetil salt form is orally bioavailable.

Pregnancy Risk Category: B

Lactation Risk Category: L2

Adult Concerns: Nausea, vomiting, diarrhea, GI distress, skin rash, allergies

Pediatric Concerns: None reported. Observe for GI symptoms such as diarrhea.

Drug Interactions: Probenecid may decrease clearance. Furosemide and aminoglycosides may enhance renal toxicity.

Theoretic Infant Dose:

Relative Infant Dose:

Adult Dose: 250-500 mg BID

Alternatives:

T½ =	1.4 hours	M/P =	
PHL =		PB =	33-50%
T$_{max}$ =		Oral =	30-50%
MW =	424	pKa =	
Vd =			

References:
1. Pharmaceutical Manufacturer Prescribing Information. 1995.

CELECOXIB
Trade: Celebrex
Can/Aus/UK: Celebrex
Uses: NSAID antiinflammatory
LRC: L2
AAP: Not reviewed

Celecoxib is a new anti-inflammatory NSAID that specifically blocks the cycyclooxygenase-2 (COX-2) enzyme. It is primarily used for arthritic or inflammatory pain.

In a recent case report of a patient receiving 100 mg twice daily, the authors report a milk level of 133 and 101 ng/mL in left and right breasts 4.75 hours after the dose.[1] They estimated (using the C_{max} levels) the M/P ratio to be 0.27 to 0.59 and that the infant's exposure would be approximately 20 µg/kg/day.

In unpublished data from our laboratories in 5 women receiving 200 mg once daily, the mean milk/plasma AUC ratio was 0.23.[2] The average concentration of celecoxib (AUC) in milk was 66 µg/L. The absolute infant dose averaged 9.9 µg/kg/day. Using this data, the relative infant dose was 0.34% of the maternal dose. Plasma levels of celecoxib in two infants studied were undetectable.

Pregnancy Risk Category: C

Lactation Risk Category: L2

Adult Concerns: GI distress, diarrhea, dyspepsia, headache, aggravated hypertension and asthma

Pediatric Concerns: None reported via milk. Plasma levels in 2 infants were undetectable. Milk levels are very low.

Drug Interactions: Celecoxib may significantly diminish antihypertensive effects of ACE inhibitors, and the natruretic effect of furosemide. Fluconazole may increase plasma levels of celecoxib two-fold. Celecoxib may increase lithium levels by 17%.

Theoretic Infant Dose: 9.9 µg/kg/day

Relative Infant Dose: 0.34%

Adult Dose: 100-400 mg daily

Alternatives: Ibuprofen

$T\frac{1}{2}$ =	11.2 hours	M/P =	1.0 (rodent)
PHL =		PB =	97%
T_{max} =	2.8 hours	Oral =	99%
MW =	381	pKa =	
Vd =	5.71		

References:
1. Knoppert DC, Stempak D, Baruchel S, Koren G. Celecoxib in human milk: a case report. Pharmacotherapy 2003; 23(1):97-100.
2. Hale TW, McDonald R, Boger J. Transfer of celecoxib into human milk. Submitted, 2003.

CEPHALEXIN

Trade: Keflex
Can/Aus/UK: Apo-Cephalex, Ceporex, Novo-Lexin, Ibilex, Keflex
Uses: Cephalosporin antibiotic
LRC: L1
AAP: Not reviewed

Cephalexin is a typical first-generation, cephalosporin antibiotic. Only minimal concentrations are secreted into human milk. Following a 1000 mg maternal oral dose, milk levels at 1, 2, 3, 4, and 5 hours ranged from 0.20, 0.28, 0.39, 0.50, and 0.47 mg/L respectively.[1] Milk/serum ratios varied from 0.008 at 1 hour to 0.140 at 3 hours. These levels are probably too low to be clinically relevant.

In a group of 2-3 patients who received 500 mg orally, milk levels averaged 0.7 mg/L at 4 hours although the average milk level was 0.36 mg/L over 6 hours.[2] The milk/plasma ratio was 0.25.

Pregnancy Risk Category: B

Lactation Risk Category: L1

Adult Concerns: Diarrhea, allergic rash, thrush

Pediatric Concerns: None reported. Observe for diarrhea.

Drug Interactions: Probenecid may decrease clearance. Furosemide, aminoglycosides may enhance renal toxicity.

Theoretic Infant Dose: 75 µg/kg/day

Relative Infant Dose: 0.5%

Adult Dose: 250-1000 mg q 6 hours

Alternatives:

T½ =	50-80 minutes	M/P =	0.008-0.14
PHL =		PB =	10%
T$_{max}$ =	1 hour	Oral =	Complete
MW =	347	pKa =	
Vd =			

References:
1. Kafetzis DA, Siafas CA, Georgakopoulos PA, Papadatos CJ. Passage of cephalosporins and amoxicillin into the breastmilk. Acta Paediatr Scand 1981; 70(3):285-288.
2. Matsuda S. Transfer of antibiotics into maternal milk. Biol Res Pregnancy Perinatol 1984; 5(2):57-60.

CEPHALOTHIN
Trade: Keflin
Can/Aus/UK: Ceporacin, Keflin
Uses: Cephalosporin antibiotic
LRC: L2
AAP: Not reviewed

Cephalothin is a first-generation, cephalosporin antibiotic for use by IM or IV administration. Following a 1000 mg IV maternal dose, milk levels varied from 0.27, 0.41, 0.47, 0.36, and 0.28 mg/L at 0.5, 1, 2, 3, and 4 hours respectively.[1] Milk/serum ratios varied from 0.06 at 1 hour to 0.51 at 3 hours.

Pregnancy Risk Category: B

Lactation Risk Category: L2

Adult Concerns: Diarrhea, allergic rash, thrush

Pediatric Concerns: None reported. Observe for diarrhea.

Drug Interactions: Probenecid may decrease clearance. Furosemide, aminoglycosides may enhance renal toxicity.

Theoretic Infant Dose: 70.5 μg/kg/day

Relative Infant Dose: 0.49%

Adult Dose: 500-2000 mg q 4-6 hours

Alternatives:

T½ =	30-50 minutes	M/P =	0.06-0.5 1
PHL =		PB =	70%
T$_{max}$ =	1-2 hours	Oral =	Poor
MW =	396	pKa =	
Vd =			

References:
1. Kafetzis DA, Siafas CA, Georgakopoulos PA, Papadatos CJ. Passage of cephalosporins and amoxicillin into the breastmilk. Acta Paediatr Scand 1981; 70(3):285-288.

CEPHAPIRIN
Trade: Cefadyl
Can/Aus/UK: Cefadyl
Uses: Cephalosporin antibiotic
LRC: L1
AAP: Not reviewed

Cephapirin is a typical first-generation, cephalosporin antibiotic for IM or IV administration. Following a 1000 mg IV maternal dose, milk levels varied from 0.26, 0.41, 0.43, 0.33, and 0.27 mg/L at 0.5, 1, 2, 3, and 4 hours respectively.[1] These are too low to be clinically relevant. Milk/serum ratios varied from 0.068 at 1 hour to 0.48 at 3 hours.

Pregnancy Risk Category: B

Lactation Risk Category: L1

Adult Concerns: Diarrhea, allergic rash, thrush

Pediatric Concerns: None reported. Observe for GI symptoms such as diarrhea.

Drug Interactions: Probenecid may decrease clearance. Furosemide and aminoglycosides may enhance renal toxicity.

Theoretic Infant Dose: 64.5 µg/kg/day

Relative Infant Dose: 0.45%

Adult Dose: 500-1000 mg q 6 hours

Alternatives:

$T\frac{1}{2}$ =	24-36 minutes	M/P =	0.068-0.48
PHL =		PB =	54%
T_{max} =	1-2 hours	Oral =	Poor
MW =	445	pKa =	
Vd =			

References:
1. Kafetzis DA, Siafas CA, Georgakopoulos PA, Papadatos CJ. Passage of cephalosporins and amoxicillin into the breastmilk. Acta Paediatr Scand 1981; 70(3):285-288.

CEPHRADINE

Trade: Velosef, Anspor
Can/Aus/UK: Velosef, Nicef
Uses: Cephalosporin antibiotic
LRC: L1
AAP: Not reviewed

Cephradine is typical first-generation cephalosporin antibiotic. In a group of 6 lactating women receiving 500 mg orally every 6 hours for 2 days, milk levels averaged about 0.6 mg/L.[1] In another study group by this same author, the average milk level was 1.0 mg/L.[2] These levels are too low to be clinically relevant.

Pregnancy Risk Category: B

Lactation Risk Category: L1

Adult Concerns: Diarrhea, allergic rash, thrush, liver dysfunction

Pediatric Concerns: None reported. Observe for GI symptoms such as diarrhea.

Drug Interactions: Probenecid may decrease clearance. Furosemide and aminoglycosides may enhance renal toxicity.

Theoretic Infant Dose: 0.09 mg/kg/day

Relative Infant Dose: 0.32%

Adult Dose: 250-500 mg q 6-12 hours

Alternatives:

$T\frac{1}{2}$ =	0.7-2 hours	M/P =	0.2
PHL =		PB =	8-17%
T_{max} =	1 hour	Oral =	Complete
MW =	349	pKa =	
Vd =			

References:
1. Mischler TW, Corson SL, Larranaga A, Bolognese RJ, Neiss ES, Vukovich RA. Cephradine and epicillin in body fluids of lactating and pregnant women. J Reprod Med 1978; 21(3):130-136.
2. Mischler TW. et.al. Presence of cephradine in body fluids of lactating and pregnant women. Clin Pharmacol Ther 1974; 15:214.

CERIVASTATIN
Trade: Baycol
Can/Aus/UK: Kazak, Lipobay
Uses: Anti-cholesterol drug.
LRC: L3
AAP: Not reviewed

Cerivastatin is a typical HMG Co-A reductase inhibitor for lowering plasma cholesterol levels. Based on preclinical data , cerivastatin is present in breastmilk at levels slightly higher than maternal plasma levels.[1] Milk/plasma ratio was 1.3. Atherosclerosis is a chronic process and discontinuation of lipid-lowering drugs during pregnancy and lactation should have little to no impact on the outcome of long-term therapy of primary hypercholesterolemia. Cholesterol and other products of cholesterol biosynthesis are essential components for fetal and neonatal development, and the use of cholesterol-lowering drugs would not be advisable under any circumstances.

Pregnancy Risk Category: X

Lactation Risk Category: L3

Adult Concerns: Transient increases in liver enzymes have been reported. Liver function tests are required prior to use. Rare cases of rhabdomyolysis with acute renal failure secondary to myoglobinuria have been reported with other HMG-CoA reductase inhibitors.

Pediatric Concerns: None reported via milk, but use is not recommended.

Drug Interactions:

Theoretic Infant Dose:

Relative Infant Dose:

Adult Dose: 0.3 mg daily

Alternatives:

$T\frac{1}{2}$ =	2-3 hours	M/P =	1.3	
PHL =		PB =	99%	
T_{max} =	2.5 hours	Oral =	60%	
MW =	481	pKa =		
Vd =	0.3			

References:
1.   Pharmaceutical Manufacturer Prescribing Information. 1999.

CETIRIZINE
Trade: Zyrtec
Can/Aus/UK: Reactine, Zyrtec, Zirtek
Uses: Antihistamine
LRC: L2
AAP: Not reviewed

Cetirizine is a popular new antihistamine useful for seasonal allergic rhinitis. It is a metabolite of hydroxyzine and is one of the most potent of the antihistamines. It is rapidly and extensively absorbed orally and due to a rather long half-life is used only once daily. It penetrates the CNS poorly and therefore produces minimal sedation. Compared to other new antihistamines, cetirizine is not very toxic in overdose and produces few cardiovascular changes at higher doses.[1] Further, as with many other antihistamines, cetirizine has very few drug interactions, alcohol being the main one. Studies in dogs suggests that only 3% of the dose is transferred into milk.[2]

Pregnancy Risk Category: B

Lactation Risk Category: L2

Adult Concerns: Sedation, fatigue, dry mouth

Pediatric Concerns: None reported but observe for sedation.

Drug Interactions: Increased sedation with other CNS sedatives, alcohol.

Theoretic Infant Dose:

Relative Infant Dose:

Adult Dose: 5-10 mg daily

Alternatives:

$T\frac{1}{2}$ =	8.3 hours	M/P =	
PHL =	6.2 hours	PB =	93%
T_{max} =	1.7 hour	Oral =	70%
MW =	389	pKa =	
Vd =			

References:
1. Pharmaceutical Manufacturer Prescribing Information. 1996.
2. Pharmaceutical Manufacturer. Personal Communication. 1996.

CEVIMELINE
Trade: Evoxac
Can/Aus/UK:
Uses: Treatment of dry mouth; Alzheimer's disease
LRC: L3
AAP: Not reviewed

Cevimeline is a cholinergic agonist agent which binds to muscarinic receptors and can increase secretion of exocrine glands such as salivary and sweat glands and increase tone in the GI and urinary tracts. It is indicated for the treatment of patients with Sjögren's Syndrome. This drug has a large volume of distribution which suggests that most of the compound is stored in peripheral tissues, not the plasma compartment. Many such drugs produce lower milk levels. No data are available on transfer into human milk. Due to the strong cholinergic effects, some caution is recommended in breastfeeding mothers. Observe closely for excess salivation, diarrhea, excess sweating, nausea, and urinary frequency and infection.

Pregnancy Risk Category: C

Lactation Risk Category: L3

Adult Concerns: Diaphoresis (excessive perspiration), nausea, rhinitis, urinary frequency, headache, diarrhea, and gastric cramping are reported.

Pediatric Concerns: No reports in breastfeeding mothers available.

Drug Interactions: None reported.

Theoretic Infant Dose:

Relative Infant Dose:

Adult Dose: 30 mg TID

Alternatives: Oral pilocarpine

$T\frac{1}{2}$ =	3-5 hours	M/P =	
PHL =		PB =	< 20%
T_{max} =	1-2 hours	Oral =	Complete
MW =	244	pKa =	
Vd =	6		

References:
1.   Pharmaceutical Manufacturers Prescribing Information, 2003.

CHAMOMILE, GERMAN
Trade: Hungarian Chamomile, Sweet False, Wild Chamomile
Can/Aus/UK:
Uses: Anti-inflammatory, carminative
LRC: L3
AAP: Not reviewed

Chamomile has been used since Roman times and is primarily used for its anti-inflammatory, carminative, antispasmodic, mild sedative, and antiseptic properties. It has been used for flatulent dyspepsia, travel sickness, diarrhea, and GI irritation.[1] It has been used topically for hemorrhoids and mastitis. Chamomile contains coumarins, flavonoids such as quercetin, rutin, and others. Anti-allergic and anti-inflammatory have been well documented and are due to the azulene components of the volatile oil which inhibit histamine release.[2] Matricin is reported to be a significant anti-inflammatory agent. In humans, German chamomile has been reported to exhibit anti-inflammatory, antipeptic, and anti-spasmodic effects on the stomach.[2] Reports of allergic reactions to chamomile are common, including two cases of anaphylaxis.[3,4,5] Asthmatics should avoid this product. German chamomile is reported to be uterotonic and teratogenic in rats, rabbits, and dogs although the dose in these studies was high.[6] This product should be avoided in pregnant and lactating patients.[7]

Pregnancy Risk Category:

Lactation Risk Category: L3

Adult Concerns: Reports of allergic reactions to chamomile are common including two cases of anaphylaxis. Asthmatics should avoid this product. German chamomile is reported to be uterotonic and teratogenic in rats, rabbits, and dogs. This product should be avoided in pregnant and lactating patients.

Pediatric Concerns: None reported via milk, but hypersensitization is possible.

Drug Interactions:

Theoretic Infant Dose:

Relative Infant Dose:

Adult Dose:

Alternatives:

References:
1. Berry M. The chamomiles. Pharm J 1995; 254:191-193.
2. Mann C, Staba EJ. The chemistry, pharmacology, and commercial formulations of chamomile. In: Herbs, spices, and medicinal plants: Recent advances in botany, horticulture, and pharmacology. Vol. 1. Arizona: Oryx Press, 1986.

3. Hausen BM. The sensitizing capacity of Compositae plants. Planta Med 1984; 50:229-234.
4. Casterline CL. Allergy to chamomile tea. JAMA 1980; 244(4):330-331.
5. Benner MH, Lee HJ. Anaphylactic reaction to chamomile tea. J Allergy Clin Immunol 1973; 52(5):307-308.
6. Habersang S, Leuschner F, Isaac O, Thiemer K. Pharmacological studies with compounds of chamomile. IV. Studies on toxicity of (-)-alpha-bisabolol (author's transl)]. Planta Med 1979; 37(2):115-123.
7. Newall C, Anderson LA, Phillipson JD. Chamomile, German. In. Herbal Medicine. A guide for the healthcare professionals. The Pharmaceutical Press, London, 1996.

CHLORAL HYDRATE

Trade: Aquachloral, Noctec
Can/Aus/UK: Nortec, Novo-Chlorhydrate, Dormel, Elix-Noctec
Uses: Sedative, hypnotic
LRC: L3
AAP: Maternal Medication Usually Compatible with Breastfeeding

Chloral Hydrate is a sedative hypnotic. Small to moderate amounts are known to be secreted into milk. Mild drowsiness was reported in one infant following administration of dichloralphenazone (1300 mg/d), which is metabolized to the same active metabolite as chloral hydrate. Infant growth and development were reported to be normal. In a study of 50 postpartum women using a 1.3 gm rectal suppository, the average milk concentration of chloral hydrate at 1 hour was 3.2 mg/L.[1] The maximum level found in this study was 15 mg/L in one patient. The oral pediatric sedative dose of chloral hydrate is generally 5-15 mg/kg/dose every 8 hours.[2]

Pregnancy Risk Category: C

Lactation Risk Category: L3

Adult Concerns: Irritating to mucous membrane, laryngospasm, GI irritation, paradoxical excitement, delirium, hypotension, respiratory depression, and sedation

Pediatric Concerns: None reported via milk, but observe for sedation.

Drug Interactions: May potentiate effects of warfarin, CNS depressants such as alcohol, etc. Use with furosemide (IV) may induce flushing, hypotension.

Theoretic Infant Dose: 0.48 mg/kg/day

Relative Infant Dose: 2.5%

Adult Dose: 250 mg TID

Alternatives: Alprazolam, Midazolam

T½ =	7-10 hours	M/P =	
PHL =		PB =	35-41%
T$_{max}$ =	30-60 minutes	Oral =	Complete
MW =	165	pKa =	10.0
Vd =	0.6		

References:

1. Bernstine JB, Meyer AE, Bernstine RL. Maternal blood and breastmilk estimation following the administration of chloral hydrate during the puerperium. J Obstet Gynaecol Br Emp 1956; 63(2):228-231.
2. Johnson KB. ed. The Harriet Lane Handbook, Thirteenth Edition. Mosey, 1993.

CHLORAMBUCIL

Trade: Leukeran
Can/Aus/UK: Leukeran
Uses: Antineoplastic compound
LRC: L5
AAP: Not reviewed

Chlorambucil is an antineoplastic, anticancer agent.[1] No data are available on concentrations secreted into human milk. This product would be extremely dangerous to growing infants and is probably contraindicated in nursing mothers.

Pregnancy Risk Category: D

Lactation Risk Category: L5

Adult Concerns: Hepatoxicity with jaundice, pulmonary fibrosis, seizures, pneumonia

Pediatric Concerns: None reported via milk, but due to overt toxicity, breastfeeding is discouraged.

Drug Interactions:

Theoretic Infant Dose:

Relative Infant Dose:

Adult Dose: 0.1-0.2 mg/kg daily

Alternatives:

T½ =	1.3 hours	M/P =	
PHL =		PB =	99%
T$_{max}$ =	1 hour	Oral =	80%
MW =	304	pKa =	
Vd =	0.14-0.24		

References:

1. Drug Facts and Comparisons 1995 ed. ed. St. Louis: 2003.

CHLORAMPHENICOL

Trade: Chloromycetin
Can/Aus/UK: Ak-Chlor, Chloromycetin, Chloroptic,
Sopamycetin, Chlorsig, Biocetin
Uses: Antibiotic
LRC: L4
AAP: Drugs whose effect on nursing infants is unknown but may
be of concern

Chloramphenicol is a broad spectrum antibiotic. In one study of 5 women receiving 250 mg PO four times daily, the concentration of chloramphenicol in milk ranged from 0.54 to 2.84 mg/L.[1] In the same study but in another group receiving 500 mg four times daily, the concentration of chloramphenicol in milk ranged from 1.75 to 6.10 mg/L. In a group of patients being treated for typhus, milk levels were lower than maternal plasma levels.[2] With maternal plasma levels of 49 and 26 mg/L in two patients, the milk levels were 26 and 16 mg/L respectively.

In a study of 2-3 patients who received a single 500 mg oral dose, the average milk concentration at 4 hours was 4.1 mg/L.[3] The milk/plasma ratio at 4 hours was 0.84. Safety in infants is highly controversial. Milk levels are too low to produce overt toxicity in infants but could produce allergic sensitization to subsequent exposures. Generally, chloramphenicol is considered contraindicated in nursing mothers although it is occasionally used in infants. This antibiotic can be extremely toxic, particularly in newborns, and should not be used for trivial infections. Blood levels should be constantly monitored and kept below 20 μg/mL.

Pregnancy Risk Category: C

Lactation Risk Category: L4

Adult Concerns: Numerous blood dyscrasias, aplastic anemia, fever, skin rashes

Pediatric Concerns: None reported via milk.

Drug Interactions: Phenobarbital and rifampin may reduce plasma levels of chloramphenicol. Chloramphenicol inhibits metabolism of chlorpropamide, phenytoin, and oral anticoagulants.

Theoretic Infant Dose: 0.9 mg/kg/day

Relative Infant Dose: 3.2%

Adult Dose: 50-100 mg/kg daily divided q 6 hours

Alternatives:

T½ =	4 hours	M/P =	0.5-0.6
PHL =	22 hours (neonates)	PB =	53%
T$_{max}$ =	1 hour	Oral =	Complete
MW =	323	pKa =	5.5
Vd =	0.57		

References:
1. Havelka J, Hejzlar M, Popov V, Viktorinova D, Prochazka J. Excretion of chloramphenicol in human milk. Chemotherapy 1968; 13(4):204-211.
2. Smadel JE. et.al. Chloramphenicol in the treatment of tsutsugamushi disease. J Clin Invest 1949; 28:1196-1215.
3. Matsuda S. Transfer of antibiotics into maternal milk. Biol Res Pregnancy Perinatol 1984; 5(2):57-60.

CHLORDIAZEPOXIDE

Trade: Apo-Chlordiazepoxide, Librium, Libritabs, Solium
Can/Aus/UK: Apo-Chlordiazepoxide, Librium, Medilium, Amitrol
Uses: Antianxiety, benzodiazepine sedative
LRC: L3
AAP: Not reviewed

Chlordiazepoxide is an older benzodiazepine that belongs to Valium family. It is secreted in breastmilk in moderate but unreported levels.[1] See Diazepam.

Pregnancy Risk Category: D

Lactation Risk Category: L3

Adult Concerns: Sedation

Pediatric Concerns: Observe for sedation.

Drug Interactions: Increased CNS sedation when used with other sedative-hypnotics. May increase risk when used with anticoagulants, alcohol, tricyclic antidepressants, MAO inhibitors.

Theoretic Infant Dose:

Relative Infant Dose:

Adult Dose: 15-100 mg q 6-8 hours

Alternatives: Alprazolam

T½ =	5-30 hours	M/P =	
PHL =		PB =	90-98%
T$_{max}$ =	1-4 hours	Oral =	Complete
MW =	300	pKa =	4.8
Vd =	0.3-0.5		

References:
1. Pharmaceutical Manufacturer Prescribing Information. 1996.

CHLORHEXIDINE

Trade: Peridex, Bactoshield, Betasept, Dyna-Hex, Hibiclens
Can/Aus/UK: Peridex, Hibitane, Hexol, Savlon, Bactigras
Uses: Lozenge antimicrobial
LRC: L2
AAP: Not reviewed

Chlorhexidine is a topical antimicrobial used in oral lozenges. It is poorly absorbed in humans and is not likely to cause untoward effects in nursing infant due to poor oral absorption by mother and infant as well.[1]

Pregnancy Risk Category: B

Lactation Risk Category: L2

Adult Concerns: Staining of teeth and dentures, changes in taste, increased plaque, staining of tongue, keep out of eyes

Pediatric Concerns: None reported via milk.

Drug Interactions:

Theoretic Infant Dose:

Relative Infant Dose:

Adult Dose: N/A

Alternatives:

T½ =	< 4 hours	M/P =	
PHL =		PB =	
T$_{max}$ =		Oral =	Poor
MW =	505	pKa =	
Vd =			

References:
1. Lacy C. Drug information handbook. Lexi-Comp Inc. Cleveland, OH, 1996.

CHLOROQUINE

Trade: Aralen, Novo-Chloroquin
Can/Aus/UK: Aralen, Chlorquin, Avloclor
Uses: Antimalarial
LRC: L3
AAP: Maternal Medication Usually Compatible with Breastfeeding

Chloroquine is an antimalarial drug. Following 5 mg/kg IM injection in lactating mothers 17 days postpartum, milk levels averaged 0.227 mg/L.[1] In this study the milk level of chloroquine in 6 patients ranged from 0.192 to 0.319 mg/L. Based on these levels, the infant would consume approximately 34 µg/kg/day, an amount considered safe.

Other studies have shown absorption to vary from 2.2 to 4.2% of maternal dose.[2] The breastmilk concentration of chloroquine in this study averaged 0.58 mg/L following a single dose of 600 mg. Current recommended pediatric dose for patients exposed to malaria is 8.3 mg/kg per week. Pediatric patients are exceedingly sensitive to chloroquine. If used, children should be closely monitored.

Pregnancy Risk Category: C

Lactation Risk Category: L3

Adult Concerns: Ocular disturbances including blindness, skin lesions, headache, fatigue, nervousness, hypotension, neutropenia, aplastic anemia

Pediatric Concerns: None reported but close observation is required. Observe for diarrhea, GI distress, hypotension.

Drug Interactions: Decreased oral absorption if used with kaolin and magnesium trisilicate. Increased toxicity if used with cimetidine.

Theoretic Infant Dose: 34.05 µg/kg/day

Relative Infant Dose: 0.68%

Adult Dose: 300-600 mg q day

Alternatives:

$T\frac{1}{2}$ =	72-120 hours	M/P =	0.358
PHL =		PB =	61%
T_{max} =	1-2 hours	Oral =	Complete
MW =	320	pKa =	8.4, 10.8
Vd =	116-285		

References:
1. Akintonwa A, Gbajumo SA, Mabadeje AF. Placental and milk transfer of chloroquine in humans. Ther Drug Monit 1988; 10(2):147-149.
2. Edstein MD, Veenendaal JR, Newman K, Hyslop R. Excretion of chloroquine, dapsone and pyrimethamine in human milk. Br J Clin Pharmacol 1986; 22(6):733-735.

CHLOROTHIAZIDE

Trade: Hydrodiuril
Can/Aus/UK: Chlotride, Saluric
Uses: Diuretic
LRC: L3
AAP: Maternal Medication Usually Compatible with Breastfeeding

Chlorothiazide is a typical thiazide diuretic. In one study of 11 lactating women, each receiving 500 mg of chlorothiazide, the concentrations in milk samples taken one, two, and three hours after the dose were all less than 1 mg/L with a milk/plasma ratio of 0.05.[1] Although thiazide diuretics are reported to produce thrombocytopenia in nursing infants, it is remote and unsubstantiated. Most thiazide diuretics are considered compatible with breastfeeding if doses are kept low and milk production is unaffected.

Pregnancy Risk Category: D

Lactation Risk Category: L3

Adult Concerns: Fluid loss, dehydration, lethargy

Pediatric Concerns: None reported but observe for reduced milk production.

Drug Interactions: NSAIDs may reduce hypotensive effect of chlorothiazide. Cholestyramine resins may reduce absorption of chlorothiazide. Diuretics reduce efficacy of oral hypoglycemics. May reduce lithium clearance leading to high levels. May elevate digoxin levels.

Theoretic Infant Dose: 0.15 mg/kg/day

Relative Infant Dose: 2.1%

Adult Dose: 500-2000 mg q 12-24 hours

Alternatives:

T½ =	1.5 hours	M/P =	0.05
PHL =		PB =	95%.
T$_{max}$ =	1 hour	Oral =	20%
MW =	296	pKa =	6.7, 9.5
Vd =			

References:
1. Werthmann MW, Jr., Krees SV. Excretion of chlorothiazide in human breastmilk. J Pediatr 1972; 81(4):781-783.

CHLORPHENIRAMINE

Trade: Aller Chlor, Chlor-Tripolon, Chlor-Trimeton
Can/Aus/UK: Chlor-Tripolon, Demazin, Alunex, Piridon
Uses: Antihistamine
LRC: L3
AAP: Not reviewed

Chlorpheniramine is a commonly used antihistamine. Although no data are available on secretion into breastmilk, it has not been reported to produce side effects. Sedation is the only likely side effect.[1]

Pregnancy Risk Category: B

Lactation Risk Category: L3

Adult Concerns: Sedation, dry mouth

Pediatric Concerns: None reported but observe for sedation.

Drug Interactions: May increase sedation when used with other CNS depressants such as opiates, tricyclic antidepressants, MAO inhibitors.

Theoretic Infant Dose:

Relative Infant Dose:

Adult Dose: 4 mg q 4-6 hours

Alternatives: Cetirizine, Loratadine

$T\frac{1}{2}$ =	12-43 hours	M/P =	
PHL =	9.5-13 hours	PB =	70%
T_{max} =	2-6 hours	Oral =	25-45%
MW =	275	pKa =	9.2
Vd =	5.9		

References:
1. Paton DM, Webster DR. Clinical pharmacokinetics of H1-receptor antagonists (the antihistamines). Clin Pharmacokinet 1985; 10(6):477-497.

CHLORPROMAZINE

Trade: Thorazine, Ormazine
Can/Aus/UK: Chlorpromanyl, Largactil, Novo-Chlorpromazine, Chloractil
Uses: Tranquilizer
LRC: L3
AAP: Drugs whose effect on nursing infants is unknown but may be of concern

Chlorpromazine is a powerful CNS tranquilizer. Small amounts are known to be secreted into milk. Following a 1200 mg oral dose, samples were taken at 60, 120, and 180 minutes.[1] Breastmilk concentrations were highest at 120 minutes and were 0.29 mg/L at that time. The milk/plasma ratio was less than 0.5. Ayd suggests that in one group of 16 women who took chlorpromazine during and after pregnancy, while breastfeeding, the side effects were minimal and infant development was normal. [2] In a group of 4 breastfeeding mothers receiving unspecified amounts of chlorpromazine, milk levels varied from 7 to 98 μg/L.[3] Maternal serum levels ranged from 16 to 52 μg/L. Only the infant who ingested milk with a chlorpromazine level of 92 μg/L showed drowsiness and lethargy.

Chlorpromazine has a long half-life and is particularly sedating. Long term use of this product in a lactating mother may be risky to the breastfed infant. Observer for sedation and lethargy.

Pregnancy Risk Category: C

Lactation Risk Category: L3

Adult Concerns: Sedation, lethargy, extrapyramidal jerking motion

Pediatric Concerns: One report of lethargy and sedation.

Drug Interactions: Additive effects when used with other CNS depressants. May increase valproic acid plasma levels.

Theoretic Infant Dose: 0.04 mg/kg/day

Relative Infant Dose: 0.25%

Adult Dose: 200 mg daily

Alternatives:

$T^{1/2}$ =	30 hours	M/P =	< 0.5
PHL =		PB =	95%
T_{max} =	1-2 hours	Oral =	Complete
MW =	319	pKa =	9.3
Vd =	10-35		

References:

1. Blacker KH, Weinstein BJ. et. al. Mothers milk and chlorpromazine. Am J Psychol 1962; 114:178-179.
2. Ayd FJ. Excretion of psychotropic drugs in breastmilk. In: International Drug Therapy Newsletter.Ayd Medical Communications 8[November-December]. 1973.
3. Wiles DH, Orr MW, Kolakowska T. Chlorpromazine levels in plasma and milk of nursing mothers. Br J Clin Pharmacol 1978; 5(3):272-273.

CHLORPROPAMIDE

Trade: Diabenese
Can/Aus/UK: Apo-Chlorpropamide, Diabinese, Novopropamide, Melitase
Uses: Oral hypoglycemic
LRC: L3
AAP: Drugs whose effect on nursing infants is unknown but may be of concern

Chlorpropamide stimulates the secretion of insulin in some patients. Following one 500 mg dose, the concentration of chlorpropamide in milk after 5 hours was approximately 5 mg/L of milk.[1] May cause hypoglycemia in infant although effects are largely unknown and unreported.

Pregnancy Risk Category: D

Lactation Risk Category: L3

Adult Concerns: Hypoglycemia, diarrhea, edema

Pediatric Concerns: None actually reported, but observe for hypoglycemia although unlikely.

Drug Interactions: Thiazides and hydantoins reduce hypoglycemic effect of chlorpropamide. Chlorpropamide may increase disulfiram effects when used with alcohol. Increases anticoagulant effect when used with warfarin. Sulfonamides may decrease chlorpropamide clearance.

Theoretic Infant Dose: 0.75 mg/kg/day

Relative Infant Dose: 10.5%

Adult Dose: 250-500 mg daily

Alternatives:

T½ =	33 hours	M/P =		
PHL =		PB =	96%	
T$_{max}$ =	3-6 hours	Oral =	Complete	
MW =	277	pKa =	4.8	
Vd =	0.1-0.3			

References:
1. Pharmaceutical Manufacturer Prescribing Information. 1986

CHLORPROTHIXENE

Trade: Taractan
Can/Aus/UK: Tarasan, Taractan
Uses: Sedative, tranquilizer
LRC: L3
AAP: Drugs whose effect on nursing infants is unknown but may be of concern

Sedative commonly used in psychotic or disturbed patients. Chlorprothixene is poorly absorbed orally (< 40%) and has been found to increase serum prolactin levels in mothers. Although the milk/plasma ratios are relatively high, only modest levels of chlorprothixene are actually secreted into human milk. In one patient taking 200 mg/day, maximum milk concentrations of the parent and metabolite were 19 μg/L and 28.5 μg/L respectively.[1] This is approximately 0.1% of the maternal dose.

Pregnancy Risk Category: C

Lactation Risk Category: L3

Adult Concerns: Sedation, hypotension, pseudoparkinsonian jerking, constipation

Pediatric Concerns: None reported, but observe for sedation.

Drug Interactions: May reduce effect of guanethidine. May increase effects of alcohol and other CNS sedatives.

Theoretic Infant Dose: 4.2 μg/kg/day

Relative Infant Dose: 0.15%

Adult Dose:

Alternatives:

T½ =	8-12 hours	M/P =	1.2-2.6
PHL =		PB =	
T$_{max}$ =	4.25 hours	Oral =	< 40%
MW =	316	pKa =	8.8
Vd =	11-23		

References:
1. Matheson I, Evang A, Overo KF, Syversen G. Presence of chlorprothixene and its metabolites in breastmilk. Eur J Clin Pharmacol 1984; 27(5):611-613.

CHLORTHALIDONE

Trade: Hydroton
Can/Aus/UK: Apo-Chlorthalidone, Hygrotin, Novo-Thalinode, Hygroton
Uses: Diuretic
LRC: L3
AAP: Maternal Medication Usually Compatible with Breastfeeding

See hydrochlorothiazide. Avoid if possible. May reduce milk production.

Pregnancy Risk Category: D

Lactation Risk Category: L3

Adult Concerns: Thrombocytopenia, hypotension, reduction of milk supply

Pediatric Concerns: None reported via milk, but may reduce milk supply.

Drug Interactions: Reduces hypoglycemic effect of oral sulfanurias used in diabetics. Increases digoxin related arrhythmias. May increase lithium levels.

Theoretic Infant Dose:

Relative Infant Dose:

Adult Dose: 50-100 mg daily
Alternatives:

T½ =	54 hours	M/P =	
PHL =		PB =	75%
T$_{max}$ =		Oral =	Complete
MW =	339	pKa =	
Vd =			

References:
1. McEvoy GE. (ed):AFHS Drug Information. New York, NY: 2003 .

CHOLERA VACCINE

Trade: Cholera Vaccine
Can/Aus/UK:
Uses: Cholera vaccination.
LRC: L3
AAP: Not reviewed

Cholera vaccine is a sterile solution containing equal parts of phenol inactivated Ogawa and Inaba serotypes of Vibrio cholerae bacteria. Maternal immunization with cholera vaccine significantly increases levels of anti-cholera antibodies (IgA, IgG) in their milk.[1]   It is not contraindicated in nursing mothers. Breastfed infants are generally protected from cholera transmission. Immunization is approved from the age of 6 months and older.

Pregnancy Risk Category: C

Lactation Risk Category: L3

Adult Concerns: Malaise, fever, headache, pain at injection site

Pediatric Concerns: None reported.

Drug Interactions: Decreased effect when used with yellow fever vaccine. Wait at least 3 weeks between.

Theoretic Infant Dose:

Relative Infant Dose:

Adult Dose: 2 0.5 mL injections (IM or SC) 1 week-month apart

Alternatives:

References:
1.   Merson MH, Black RE, Sack DA, Svennerholm AM, Holmgren J. Maternal cholera immunisation and scecretory IgA in breastmilk. Lancet 1980; 1(8174):931-932.

CHOLESTYRAMINE

Trade: Questran, Cholybar
Can/Aus/UK: Questran, Novo-Cholamine
Uses: Cholesterol binding resin
LRC: L1
AAP: Not reviewed

Cholestyramine is a bile salt chelating resin. Used orally in adults, it binds bile salts and prevents reabsorption of bile salts in the gut, thus reducing cholesterol plasma levels[1].   This resin is not absorbed from the maternal GI tract. Therefore, it is not secreted into breastmilk.

Pregnancy Risk Category: C

Lactation Risk Category: L1

Adult Concerns: Constipation, skin rash, nausea, vomiting, malabsorption, intestinal obstruction

Pediatric Concerns: None reported via milk.

Drug Interactions: Decreases oral absorption of digoxin, warfarin, thyroid hormones, thiazide diuretics, propranolol, phenobarbital, amiodarone, methotrexate, NSAIDs, and many other drugs.

Theoretic Infant Dose:

Relative Infant Dose:

Adult Dose: 16-32 grams/day

Alternatives:

T½ =		M/P =	
PHL =		PB =	
T_{max} =		Oral =	0%
MW =		pKa =	
Vd =			

References:
1. Pharmaceutical Manufacturer Prescribing Information. 1995.

CHONDROITIN SULFATE

Trade: Viscoat
Can/Aus/UK:
Uses: Biologic polymer used for arthritis
LRC: L3
AAP: Not reviewed

Chondroitin is a biological polymer that acts as a flexible connecting matrix between the protein filaments in cartilage. It is derived largely from natural sources such as shark or bovine cartilage and chemically is composed of a high-viscosity mucopolysaccharide (glycosaminoglycan) polymer found in most mammalian cartilaginous tissues.[1] Thus far, chondroitin has been found to be nontoxic. Its molecular weight averages 50,000 daltons which is far too large to permit its entry into human milk. Combined with a poor oral bioavailability and large molecular weight, it is unlikely to pose a problem for a breastfed infant.

Pregnancy Risk Category:

Lactation Risk Category: L3

Adult Concerns: Virtually nontoxic and poorly absorbed orally.

Pediatric Concerns: None reported via milk.

Drug Interactions:

Theoretic Infant Dose:

Relative Infant Dose:

Adult Dose:

Alternatives:

$T\frac{1}{2}$ =		M/P =	
PHL =		PB =	
T_{max} =		Oral =	0-13%
MW =	50,000	pKa =	
Vd =			

References:
1. Review of Natural Products Facts and Comparisons, St Louis, MO 1996.

CHORIONIC GONADOTROPIN

Trade: A.P.L., Chorex-5, Profasi, Gonic, Pregnyl, Novarel
Can/Aus/UK: Humegon, Profasi HP, Pregnyl, Profasik, APL
Uses: Placental hormone
LRC: L3
AAP: Not reviewed

Human chorionic gonadotropin (HCG) is a large polypeptide hormone produced by the human placenta with functions similar to luteinizing hormone (LH). Its function is to stimulate the corpus luteum of the ovary to produce progesterone, thus sustaining pregnancy.[1,2] During pregnancy, HCG secreted by the placenta maintains the corpus luteum, supporting estrogen and progesterone secretion and preventing menstruation. It is used for multiple purposes including pediatric cryptorchidism, male hypogonadism, and ovulatory failure. HCG has no known effect on fat mobilization, appetite, sense of hunger, or body fat distribution. HCG has NOT been found to be effective in treatment of obesity.

Due to the large molecular weight (47,000) of HCG, it would be extremely unlikely to penetrate into human milk. Further, it would not be orally bioavailable due to destruction in the GI tract.

Choriogonadotropin alfa (Ovidrel) is a biosynthetic form of the human chorionic gonadotropin.

Pregnancy Risk Category: X

Lactation Risk Category: L3

Adult Concerns: Headache, irritability, restlessness, depression, fatigue, edema, gynecomastia, pain at injection site

Pediatric Concerns: None reported via milk. Absorption unlikely due to gastric digestion and poor penetration into milk.

Drug Interactions:

Theoretic Infant Dose:

Relative Infant Dose:

Adult Dose: 5000-10000 units X 1

Alternatives:

$T\frac{1}{2}$ =	5.6 hours	M/P =		
PHL =		PB =		
T_{max} =	6 hours	Oral =	0%	
MW =	47,000	pKa =		
Vd =				

References:
1. Drug Facts and Comparisons 1996 ed. ed. St. Louis: 1996.
2. Pharmaceutical Manufacturer Prescribing Information. 1997.

CHROMIUM

Trade: Chromium Picrolinate
Can/Aus/UK:
Uses: Metal supplement
LRC: L3
AAP: Not reviewed

Trace metal, required in glucose metabolism. Less than 1% is absorbed following oral administration. Chromium levels are depleted in multiparous women. Chromium levels in neonate are approximately 2.5 times that of mother due to concentrating mechanism during gestation. Because chromium is difficult to measure, levels reported vary widely.

One article reports that breastmilk levels are less than 2% of the estimated safe and adequate daily intake of 10 μg (which is probably excessive and needs review)[1]. Most importantly, breastmilk levels are independent of dietary intake in mother and do not apparently increase with increased maternal intake. Chromium is apparently secreted into breastmilk by a well controlled pumping mechanism. Hence, breastmilk levels of chromium are independent of maternal plasma levels. Increased maternal plasma levels may not alter milk chromium levels.

Pregnancy Risk Category: C

Lactation Risk Category: L3

Adult Concerns: Chromium poisoning if used in excess.

Pediatric Concerns: None reported.

Drug Interactions:

Theoretic Infant Dose:

Relative Infant Dose:

Adult Dose: 200 µg/day

Alternatives:

T½ =		M/P =	
PHL =		PB =	
T$_{max}$ =		Oral =	< 1%
MW =	52	pKa =	
Vd =			

References:
1. Anderson RA, Bryden NA, Patterson KY, Veillon C, Andon MB, Moser-Veillon PB. Breastmilk chromium and its association with chromium intake, chromium excretion, and serum chromium. Am J Clin Nutr 1993; 57(4):519-523.

CICLOPIROX OLAMINE
Trade: Loprox
Can/Aus/UK: Loprox
Uses: Antifungal
LRC: L3
AAP: Not reviewed

Ciclopirox is a broad spectrum antifungal and is active in numerous species including tinea, candida albicans, and trichophyton rubrum. An average of 1.3% ciclopirox is absorbed when applied topically.[1] Topical application produces minimal systemic absorption; it is unlikely that topical use would expose the nursing infant to significant risks. The risk to a breastfeeding infant associated with application directly on the nipple is not known; only small amounts should be used. Ciclopirox and miconazole are comparable in treatment of vaginal candida.

Pregnancy Risk Category: B

Lactation Risk Category: L3

Adult Concerns: Pruritus and burning following topical therapy.

Pediatric Concerns: None via milk.

Drug Interactions:

Theoretic Infant Dose:

Relative Infant Dose:

Adult Dose: Apply topical BID

Alternatives: Fluconazole, Miconazole.

T½ =	1,7 hours	M/P =	
PHL =		PB =	98%
T$_{max}$ =	6 hours	Oral =	
MW =		pKa =	
Vd =			

References:
1.   Pharmaceutical Manufacturer Prescribing Information.

CIMETIDINE

Trade: Tagamet
Can/Aus/UK: Apo-Cimetidine, Novo-Cimetine, Peptol,
Tagamet, Magicul,Sigmetadine,Peptimax, Zita
Uses: Reduces gastric acid production
LRC: L2
AAP: Maternal Medication Usually Compatible with Breastfeeding

Cimetidine is an antisecretory, histamine-2 antagonist that reduces stomach acid secretion. Cimetidine is apparently actively transported into human milk as evidenced by a higher milk/plasma ratio. In a study of 12 women who received single oral doses of 100, 600, and 1200 mg cimetidine, the observed milk/serum ratio was 5.65, 5.84, and 5.83 respectively.[1] The reported maximum concentration in milk were 2.5, 16.2, and 37.2 mg/L respectively.

In another study of one patient ingesting 600 mg daily, the reported milk level was 5.6 mg/L.[2] The potential dose from lactation would be approximately 5.8 mg/kg/d, which is still quite small. The pediatric dose administered IV for therapeutic treatment of pediatric gastroesophageal reflux averages 8-20 mg/kg/24 hours. Other choices for breastfeeding mothers should preclude the use of this drug however. See famotidine, nizatidine. Short term use (days) would not be incompatible with breastfeeding.

Pregnancy Risk Category: B

Lactation Risk Category: L2

Adult Concerns: Headache, dizziness, somnolence

Pediatric Concerns: None reported via milk. Frequently used in pediatric patients.

Drug Interactions: Cimetidine inhibits the metabolism of many drugs and may potentially increase their plasma levels. Such drugs include: lidocaine, theophylline, phenytoin, metronidazole, triamterene, procainamide, quinidine, propranolol, warfarin, tricyclic antidepressants, diazepam, cyclosporin.

Theoretic Infant Dose: 5.58 mg/kg/day

Relative Infant Dose: 32.5%

Adult Dose: 800 mg q HS

Alternatives: Famotidine, Nizatidine

T½ =	2 hours	M/P =	4.6-11.76
PHL =	3.6 hours (neonate)	PB =	19%
T$_{max}$ =	0.75-1.5 hours	Oral =	60-70%
MW =	252	pKa =	
Vd =			

References:
1. Oo CY, Kuhn RJ, Desai N, McNamara PJ. Active transport of cimetidine into human milk. Clin Pharmacol Ther 1995; 58(5):548-555.
2. Somogyi A, Gugler R. Cimetidine excretion into breastmilk. Br J Clin Pharmacol 1979; 7(6):627-629.

CIPROFLOXACIN

Trade: Cipro, Ciloxan
Can/Aus/UK: Cipro, Ciloxan, Ciproxin
Uses: Fluoroquinolone antibiotic
LRC: L3
AAP: Maternal Medication Usually Compatible with Breastfeeding

Ciprofloxacin is a fluoroquinolone antibiotic primarily used for gram negative coverage and is presently the drug of choice for anthrax treatment and prophylaxis. Because it has been implicated in arthropathy in newborn animals, it is not normally used in pediatric patients. Levels secreted into breastmilk (2.26 to 3.79 mg/L) are somewhat conflicting. They vary from the low to moderate range to levels that are higher than maternal serum up to 12 hours after a dose. In one study of 10 women who received 750 mg every 12 hours, milk levels of ciprofloxacin ranged from 3.79 mg/L at 2 hours post-dose to 0.02 mg/L at 24 hours.[1]

In another study of a single patient receiving one 500 mg tablet daily at bedtime, the concentrations in maternal serum and breastmilk were 0.21 µg/mL and 0.98 µg/mL respectively[2]. Plasma levels were undetectable (< 0. 03 µg/mL) in the infant. The dose to the 4 month old infant was estimated to be 0.92 mg/day or 0.15 mg/kg/day. No adverse effects were noted in this infant.

There has been one reported case of severe pseudomembranous colitis in an infant of a mother who self-medicated with ciprofloxacin for 6 days(3). In a patient 17 days postpartum, who received 500 mg orally, ciprofloxacin levels in milk were 3.02, 3.02, 3.02 and 1.98 mg/L 4, 8, 12, and 16 hours post dose respectively.[4]

If used in lactating mothers, observe the infant closely for GI symptoms. Current studies seem to suggest that the amount of ciprofloxacin present in milk is quite low. Ciprofloxacin was recently approved by the American Academy of Pediatrics for use in breastfeeding women and it is becoming increasingly popular for use in pediatric patients.[5] Ciprofloxacin is available in several ophthalmic preparations (Ciloxan). As the absolute dose presented to the nursing mother is minimal, they would not be contraindicated in breastfeeding mothers.

Pregnancy Risk Category: C

Lactation Risk Category: L3

Adult Concerns: Nausea, vomiting, diarrhea, abdominal cramps, GI bleeding. Several cases of tendon rupture have been noted.

Pediatric Concerns: Pseudomembranous colitis in one infant. Observe for diarrhea. Tooth discoloration in several infants reported.

Drug Interactions: Decreased absorption with antacids. Quinolones cause increased levels of caffeine, warfarin, cyclosporine, theophylline. Cimetidine, probenecid, azlocillin increase ciprofloxacin levels. Increased risk of seizures when used with foscarnet.

Theoretic Infant Dose: 0.56 mg/kg/day

Relative Infant Dose: 2.65%

Adult Dose: 250 mg BID

Alternatives: Norfloxacin, Ofloxacin

T½ =	4.1 hours	M/P =	> 1
PHL =	2.5 hours	PB =	40%
T_{max} =	0.5-2.3 hours	Oral =	50-85%
MW =	331	pKa =	7.1
Vd =	1.4		

References:
1. Giamarellou H, Kolokythas E, Petrikkos G, Gazis J, Aravantinos D, Sfikakis P. Pharmacokinetics of three newer quinolones in pregnant and lactating women. Am J Med 1989; 87(5A):49S-51S.
2. Gardner DK, Gabbe SG, Harter C. Simultaneous concentrations of ciprofloxacin in breastmilk and in serum in mother and breast-fed infant. Clin Pharm 1992; 11(4):352-354.
3. Harmon T, Burkhart G, Applebaum H. Perforated pseudomembranous colitis in the breast-fed infant. J Pediatr Surg 1992; 27(6):744-746.
4. Cover DL, Mueller BA. Ciprofloxacin penetration into human breastmilk: a case report. DICP 1990; 24(7-8):703-704.

5.   Ghaffar F, McCracken GH. Quinolones in Pediatrics. In: Hooper DC, Rubinstein E, editors. Quinolone Antimicrobial Agents. Washington, D.C.: ASM Press, 2003: 343-354.

CISAPRIDE

Trade: Propulsid
Can/Aus/UK: Propulsid, Prepulsid
Uses: Gastrointestinal tract stimulant
LRC: L2
AAP: Not reviewed

Cisapride is a gastrointestinal stimulant used to increase lower esophageal sphincter pressure and increase the rate of gastric emptying. It is frequently used in gastroesophageal reflux[1]. It is often preferred over metoclopramide (Reglan) due to the lack of CNS side effects. CNS concentrations are generally 2-3 fold less than the serum levels. It is frequently used in pediatric patients and neonates.

Breastmilk levels following a maternal dose of 60 mg/day for 4 days averaged 6.2 μg/L while maternal plasma levels averaged 137 μg/L[2]. The dose of cisapride absorbed in breastfeeding infants would be expected to be 600-800 times lower than the usual therapeutic dose. Manufacturers internal data suggest that breastmilk levels are less than 5% of maternal plasma levels (approximately 2.2 to 3.0 μg/L)[3].

Pregnancy Risk Category: C

Lactation Risk Category: L2

Adult Concerns: Diarrhea, abdominal pain, cramping. Note many drug-drug interactions.

Pediatric Concerns: None reported via milk.

Drug Interactions: Increased effect of atropine and digoxin. Increased toxicity when used with warfarin, diazepam levels may be increased, cimetidine, ranitidine, CNS depressants. Cisapride levels may rise when used with azole antifungals such as ketoconazole, fluconazole, erythromycins.

Theoretic Infant Dose: 0.93 μg/kg/day

Relative Infant Dose: 0.10%

Adult Dose: 10 mg QID

Alternatives:

$T\frac{1}{2}$ =	7-10 hours	M/P =	0.045
PHL =		PB =	98%
T_{max} =	1-2 hours	Oral =	35-40%
MW =	466	pKa =	
Vd =			

References:

1. McCallum RW, Prakash C, Campoli-Richards DM, Goa KL. Cisapride. A preliminary review of its pharmacodynamic and pharmacokinetic properties, and therapeutic use as a prokinetic agent in gastrointestinal motility disorders. Drugs 1988; 36(6):652-681.
2. Hofmeyr GJ, Sonnendecker EW. Secretion of the gastrokinetic agent cisapride in human milk. Eur J Clin Pharmacol 1986; 30(6):735-736.
3. Janssen Pharmaceuticals, personal communication. 1996.

CISPLATIN

Trade: Platinol
Can/Aus/UK: Abiplatin, Platinol, Platinol-AQ, Cisplatin, Platosin
Uses: Anticancer drug
LRC: L4
AAP: Maternal Medication Usually Compatible with Breastfeeding

Cisplatin is a potent and very toxic anticancer medication. Plasma and breastmilk samples were collected from a 24 year old woman treated for three prior days with cisplatin (30mg/meter).[1] On the third day, 30 minutes prior to chemotherapy, platinum levels in milk were 0.9 mg/L and plasma levels were 0.8 mg/L. In another study, no cisplatin was found in breastmilk following a dose of 100 mg/meter.[2] Other studies suggest that milk levels are 10 fold lower than serum levels in an older lactating woman. Cisplatin has multiple half-lives with the terminal half-life equal to greater than 24 to 73 hours. These studies generally support the recommendation that mothers should not breastfeed while undergoing cisplatin therapy. A brief interruption of perhaps a week would significantly lower the risk to the infant.

Pregnancy Risk Category: D

Lactation Risk Category: L4

Adult Concerns: Nausea, vomiting, tinnitus, ototoxicity, renal toxicity, leukopenia, peripheral neuropathy, etc.

Pediatric Concerns: None reported via milk, but due to enormous toxicity, do not use in breastfeeding women.

Drug Interactions: Increased toxicity when used with ethacrynic acid (ototoxicity). Delayed bleomycin metabolism. Sodium thiosulfate inactivates cisplatin.

Theoretic Infant Dose: 0.135 mg/kg/day

Relative Infant Dose:

Adult Dose: 20 mg/m^2 IV daily

Alternatives:

T½ =	24-73 hours	M/P =	> 1
PHL =		PB =	90%
T$_{max}$ =	< 1 hour	Oral =	
MW =	300	pKa =	
Vd =			

References:

1. de Vries EG, van der Zee AG, Uges DR, Sleijfer DT. Excretion of platinum into breastmilk. Lancet 1989; 1(8636):497.
2. Egan PC, Costanza ME, Dodion P, Egorin MJ, Bachur NR. Doxorubicin and cisplatin excretion into human milk. Cancer Treat Rep 1985; 69(12):1387-1389.

CITALOPRAM

Trade: Celexa
Can/Aus/UK: Celexa, Cipramil, Talam, Talohexal
Uses: Antidepressant
LRC: L3
AAP: Not reviewed

Citalopram is a new SSRI antidepressant similar in effect to Prozac and Zoloft. In one study of a 21 year old patient receiving 20 mg citalopram per day, citalopram levels in milk peaked at 3-9 hours following administration.[1] Peak milk levels varied during the day, but the mean daily concentration was 298 nM (range 270-311). The milk/serum ratio was approximately 3. The metabolite, desmethylcitalopram, was present in milk in low levels (23-28 nM). The concentration of metabolite in milk varied little during the day. Assuming a milk intake of 150 mL/kg baby, approximately 272 nM (88 µg or 16 ng/kg) of citalopram was passed to the baby each day. This amounts to only 0.4% of the dose administered to the mother. At three weeks, maternal serum levels of citalopram were 185 nM, compared to the infants plasma level of just 7 nM. No untoward effects were noted in this breastfed infant. In another study[2], a milk/serum ratio of 1.16 to 1.88 was reported. This study suggests the infant would ingest 4.3 µg/kg/day and a relative dose of 0.7 to 5.9% of the weight-adjusted maternal dose.

In another study of 7 women receiving an average of 0.41 mg/kg/d citalopram, the average peak level (C$_{max}$) of citalopram was 154 µg/L and 50 µg/L for demethylcitalopram (metabolite is 8 times less potent than citalopram).[3] However, average milk concentrations (AUC) were lower and averaged 97 µg/L for citalopram and 36 µg/L for demethylcitalopram during the dosing interval. The mean peak milk/plasma AUC ratio was 1.8 for citalopram. Low concentrations of citalopram (around 2-2.3 µg/L) were detected in only three of the seven infant plasmas. No adverse effects were found in any of the infants. The authors estimate the daily intake to be approximately 3.7% of the maternal dose.

In a study of a single patient receiving 40 mg/day of citalopram, the concentration in milk and serum were 205 µg/L and 98.9 ng/mL respectively.[4] Infant serum levels were 12.7 ng/mL. This infant was noted to have 'uneasy' sleep patterns, which were reduced upon lowering the maternal dose.

Pregnancy Risk Category: C

Lactation Risk Category: L3

Adult Concerns: Diarrhea, headache, anxiety, dizziness, insomnia, constipation, nausea, vomiting, and tremor. Tachycardia, hypotension have been reported. Increased salivation, and flatulence. Amenorrhea, coughing, rash, pruritus, polyuria have been reported.

Pediatric Concerns: There have been two cases of excessive somnolence, decreased feeding, and weight loss in breastfed infants.

Drug Interactions: Increased citalopram levels when used with macrolide antibiotics (erythromycin), and azole antifungals such as fluconazole, itraconazole, ketoconazole, etc. Carbamazepine may reduce plasma levels of citalopram. Serious reactions may occur if citalopram is administered too soon after MAO use. Beta blocker (metoprolol) levels may increase by 2 fold when admixed with citalopram.

Theoretic Infant Dose: 14.55 µg/kg/day

Relative Infant Dose: 3.6%

Adult Dose: 20-40 mg daily

Alternatives: Sertraline, Paxil

T½ =	36 hours	M/P =	1.16 - 3
PHL =		PB =	80%
T$_{max}$ =	2-4 hours	Oral =	80%
MW =	405	pKa =	
Vd =	12		

References:

1. Jensen PN, Olesen OV, Bertelsen A, Linnet K. Citalopram and desmethylcitalopram concentrations in breastmilk and in serum of mother and infant. Ther Drug Monit 1997; 19(2):236-239.
2. Spigset O, Carieborg L, Ohman R, Norstrom A. Excretion of citalopram in breastmilk. Br J Clin Pharmacol 1997; 44(3):295-298.
3. Rampono J, Kristensen JH, Hackett LP, Paech M, Kohan R, Ilett KF. Citalopram and demethylcitalopram in human milk; distribution, excretion and effects in breast fed infants. Br J Clin Pharmacol 2000; 50(3):263-268.
4. Schmidt K, Olesen OV, Jensen PN. Citalopram and breast-feeding: serum concentration and side effects in the infant. Biol Psychiatry 2000; 47(2):164-165.

CLARITHROMYCIN

Trade: Biaxin
Can/Aus/UK: Biaxin, Klacid, Klaricid
Uses: Antibiotic
LRC: L2
AAP: Not reviewed

Antibiotic that belongs to erythromycin family. Clarithromycin is known to transfer into animal milk although no studies have been done on humans. This drug is a weak base and could concentrate in human milk by ion trapping[1,2]. However, it is a commonly used pediatric antibiotic, and pediatric indications down to 6 months of age are available. See azithromycin as alternative.

Pregnancy Risk Category: C

Lactation Risk Category: L2

Adult Concerns: Diarrhea, nausea, dyspepsia, abdominal pain, metallic taste

Pediatric Concerns: None reported via milk. Pediatric indications are available.

Drug Interactions: Clarithromycin increases serum theophylline by as much as 20%. Increases plasma levels of carbamazepine, cyclosporin, digoxin, ergot alkaloids, tacrolimus, triazolam, zidovudine, terfenadine, astemizole, cisapride (serious arrhythmias). Fluconazole increases clarithromycin serum levels by 25%. Numerous other drug-drug interactions are unreported, but probably occur.

Theoretic Infant Dose:

Relative Infant Dose:

Adult Dose: 250 mg BID

Alternatives:

$T\frac{1}{2}$ =	5-7 hours		M/P =	> 1
PHL =			PB =	40-70%
T_{max} =	1.7 hours		Oral =	50%
MW =	748		pKa =	
Vd =				

References:
1. Drug Facts and Comparisons 1995 ed. ed. St. Louis: 1995.
2. Pharmaceutical Manufacturer Prescribing Information. 1996.

CLEMASTINE

Trade: Tavist
Can/Aus/UK: Tavist, Tavegyl
Uses: Antihistamine
LRC: L4
AAP: Drugs associated with significant side effects and should be given with caution

Clemastine is a long-acting antihistamine. Following a maternal dose of 1 mg twice daily a 10 week old breastfeeding infant developed drowsiness, irritability, refusal to feed, and neck stiffness[1]. Levels in milk and plasma (20 hours post dose) were 5-10 µg/L(milk) and 20 µg/L (plasma) respectively.

Pregnancy Risk Category: C

Lactation Risk Category: L4

Adult Concerns: Drowsiness, headache, fatigue, nervousness, appetite increase, depression

Pediatric Concerns: Drowsiness, irritability, refusal to feed, and neck stiffness in one infant. Increased risk of seizures.

Drug Interactions: Increased toxicity when mixed with CNS depressants, anticholinergics, MAO inhibitors, tricyclic antidepressants, phenothiazines.

Theoretic Infant Dose: 1.5 µg/kg/day

Relative Infant Dose: 5.2%

Adult Dose: 1.34 to 2.68 mg BID or TID

Alternatives: Cetirazine, Loratadine

$T\frac{1}{2}$ =	10-12 hours	M/P =	0.25-0.5
PHL =		PB =	
T_{max} =	2-5 hours	Oral =	100%
MW =	344	pKa =	
Vd =			

References:
1. Kok TH, Taitz LS, Bennett MJ, Holt DW. Drowsiness due to clemastine transmitted in breastmilk. Lancet 1982; 1(8277):914-915.

CLINDAMYCIN

Trade: Cleocin
Can/Aus/UK: Dalacin, Clindatech, Cleocin
Uses: Antibiotic
LRC: L3
AAP: Maternal Medication Usually Compatible with Breastfeeding

Clindamycin is a broad spectrum antibiotic frequently used for anaerobic infections. In one study of two nursing mothers and following doses of 600 mg IV every 6 hours, the concentration of clindamycin in breastmilk was 3.1 to 3.8 mg/L at 0.2 to 0.5 hours after dosing.[1] Following oral doses of 300 mg every 6 hours, the breastmilk levels averaged 1.0 to 1.7 mg/L at 1.5 to 7 hours after dosing. In another study of 2-3 women who received a single oral dose of 150 mg, milk levels averaged 0.9 mg/L at 4 hours with a milk/plasma ratio of 0.47.[2]

An alteration of GI flora is possible even though the dose is low. One case of bloody stools (pseudomembranous colitis) has been associated with clindamycin and gentamycin therapy on day 5 postpartum, but this is considered rare[3]. In this case, the mother of a newborn infant was given 600 mg IV every 6 hours. In rare cases, pseudomembranous colitis can appear several weeks later.

In a study by Steen, in 5 breastfeeding patients who received 150 mg three times daily for 7 days, milk concentration ranged from <0.5 to 3.1 mg/L with the majority of levels < 0.5 mg/L.[4] There are a number of pediatric clinical uses of clindamycin (anaerobic infections, bacterial endocarditis, pelvic inflammatory disease, and bacterial vaginosis). The current pediatric dosage recommendation is 10-40 mg/kg/day divided every 6-8 hours[5].

Pregnancy Risk Category: B

Lactation Risk Category: L3

Adult Concerns: Diarrhea, rash, pseudomembranous colitis, nausea, vomiting, GI cramps

Pediatric Concerns: One case of pseudomembranous colitis has been reported. But this is rare. It is unlikely the levels in breastmilk would be clinically relevant. Commonly used in pediatric infections. Observe for diarrhea.

Drug Interactions: Increased duration of muscle blockade when administered with neuromuscular blockers such as tubocurarine and pancuronium.

Theoretic Infant Dose: 0.57 mg/kg/day

Relative Infant Dose: 1.6%

Adult Dose: 150-450 mg q 6 hours

Alternatives:

$T\frac{1}{2}$ =	2.9 hours	M/P =	0.47
PHL =	3.6 hours (term)	PB =	94%
T_{max} =	45-60 minutes	Oral =	90%
MW =	425	pKa =	7.45
Vd =			

References:

1. Smith JA. et.al. Clindamycin in human breastmilk. Can Med Assn J 1975; 112:806.
2. Matsuda S. Transfer of antibiotics into maternal milk. Biol Res Pregnancy Perinatol 1984; 5(2):57-60.
3. Mann CF. Clindamycin and breast-feeding. Pediatrics 1980; 66(6):1030-1031.
4. Steen B, Rane A. Clindamycin passage into human milk. Br J Clin Pharmacol 1982; 13(5):661-664.
5. Johnson KB. ed. The Harriet Lane Handbook. Thirteenth ed. Mosby Publishing, 1993.

CLINDAMYCIN VAGINAL

Trade: Cleocin Vaginal
Can/Aus/UK: Dalacin Vaginal Cream, Dalacin T
Uses: Antibiotic
LRC: L2
AAP: Maternal Medication Usually Compatible with Breastfeeding

Clindamycin when administered by IV has been found in breastmilk (see clindamycin). One case of bloody stools (pseudomembranous colitis) has been associated with oral clindamycin.

However, only about 5% of Clindamycin Vaginal (100 mg/dose) is absorbed into the maternal circulation, which would be approximately 5 mg clindamycin/day[1]. It is unlikely that clindamycin when administered via a vaginal gel would produce any significant danger to a breastfeeding infant.

Pregnancy Risk Category: B

Lactation Risk Category: L2

Adult Concerns: Diarrhea, rash, GI cramps, colitis, rarely bloody diarrhea

Pediatric Concerns:

Drug Interactions:

Theoretic Infant Dose:

Relative Infant Dose:

Adult Dose: 100 mg intravaginally q HS

Alternatives:

T½ =	2.9 hours	M/P =	
PHL =		PB =	94%
T$_{max}$ =		Oral =	90%
MW =	425	pKa =	
Vd =			

References:
1.   Pharmaceutical Manufacturer Prescribing Information. 1996.

CLOBAZAM
Trade: Frisium
Can/Aus/UK: Frisium
Uses: Benzodiazepine anxiolytic
LRC: L3
AAP: Not reviewed

Clobazam (Frisium) is a typical benzodiazepine very similar to Valium[1]. It is primarily an anxiolytic, but it is sometimes used to treat refractory seizures. The median half-life for tolerance is only 3.5 months, so it would not be suitable for long term therapy of seizures. It has a rather long half-life averaging 17-31 hours for the parent drug in young adults and 11-77 hours for the active metabolite desmethylclobazam. As with Valium, it would probably reach relatively high levels in a breastfeeding infant.   No data are available on breastmilk concentrations.   See diazepam.

Pregnancy Risk Category: C

Lactation Risk Category: L3

Adult Concerns: Sedation, drowsiness, hangover, weakness, insomnia

Pediatric Concerns: Typical benzodiazepine,   use caution.   See Diazepam.

Drug Interactions: May increase effects of opiates, CNS depressants. Macrolide (erythromycin) antibiotics may increase levels of clobazam. Clobazam may increase levels of carbamazepine.

Theoretic Infant Dose:

Relative Infant Dose:

Adult Dose: 20-30 mg/day

Alternatives: Alprazolam

T½ =	17-31 hours	M/P =	
PHL =		PB =	90%
T$_{max}$ =	1-2 hours	Oral =	87%
MW =	301	pKa =	
Vd =	0.87-1.8		

References:

1. Pharmaceutical Manufacturer Prescribing Information. 1995.

CLOFAZIMINE

Trade: Lamprene
Can/Aus/UK: Lamprene
Uses: Antimicrobial for leprosy
LRC: L3
AAP: Drugs whose effect on nursing infants is unknown but may be of concern

Clofazimine exerts a slow bacteriocidal effect on M. Leprae. In a study of 8 female leprosy patients on clofazimine (50 mg/day or 100 mg on alternate days) for 1-18 months, blood samples were take at 4-6 hours after the dose.[1] Average plasma and milk levels were 0.9 µg/mL and 1.33 µg/mL (1.33 mg/Liter) respectively. The milk/plasma ratio varied from 1.0 to 1.7 with a mean of 1.48. A red tint and pigmentation has been reported in breastfed infants.[2,3]

Pregnancy Risk Category: C

Lactation Risk Category: L3

Adult Concerns: Reversible red-brown discoloration of skin and eyes. Gastrointestinal effects include nausea, abdominal cramps and pain, nausea and vomiting. Splenic infarction, crystalline deposits of clofazimine in multiple organs and tissues.

Pediatric Concerns: Reddish discoloration of milk and infant.

Drug Interactions:

Theoretic Infant Dose: 0.19 mg/kg/day

Relative Infant Dose: 13.9%

Adult Dose: 100-200 mg daily

Alternatives:

T½ =	70 days	M/P =	1.7
PHL =		PB =	
T$_{max}$ =		Oral =	45-70%
MW =	473	pKa =	
Vd =			

References:

1. Venkatesan K, Mathur A, Girdhar A, Girdhar BK. Excretion of clofazimine in human milk in leprosy patients. Lepr Rev 1997; 68(3):242-246.
2. Farb H, West DP, Pedvis-Leftick A. Clofazimine in pregnancy complicated by leprosy. Obstet Gynecol 1982; 59(1):122-123.
3. Freerksen E, Seydel JK. Critical comments on the treatment of leprosy and other mycobacterial infections with clofazimine. Arzneimittelforschung 1992; 42(10):1243-1245.

CLOMIPHENE

Trade: Clomid, Serophene, Milophene
Can/Aus/UK: Clomid, Serophene
Uses: Ovulation stimulator for ovulatory failure
LRC: L4
AAP: Not reviewed

Clomiphene appears to stimulate the release of the pituitary gonadotropins, follicle-stimulating hormone (FSH), and luteinizing hormone (LH), which result in development and maturation of the ovarian follicle, ovulation, and subsequent development and function of the corpus luteum. It has both estrogenic and anti-estrogenic effects. LH and FSH peak at 5-9 days after completing clomiphene therapy.

In a study of 60 postpartum women (1-4 days postpartum), clomiphene was effective in totally inhibiting unestablished lactation and in suppressing established lactation (day 4)[1]. Only 7 of 40 women receiving clomiphene to inhibit lactation had signs of congestion or discomfort. In the 20 women who received clomiphene to suppress established lactation (on day 4), a rapid amelioration of breast engorgement and discomfort was produced. After 5 days of treatment no signs of lactation were present. In another study of 177 postpartum women, clomiphene was very effective at inhibiting lactation[2].

Clomiphene appears to be very effective in suppressing lactation when used up to 4 days postpartum. However, its efficacy in reducing milk production in women, months after lactation has been established, is unknown but believed to be minimal.[3]

Pregnancy Risk Category: X

Lactation Risk Category: L4

Adult Concerns: Dizziness, insomnia, lightheadedness, hot flashes, ovarian enlargement, depression, headache, alopecia. May inhibit lactation early postpartum.

Pediatric Concerns: Transfer and effect on infant is unreported, but may suppress early lactation.

Drug Interactions:

Theoretic Infant Dose:

Relative Infant Dose:

Adult Dose: 50 mg daily

Alternatives:

T½ =	5-7 days	M/P =	
PHL =		PB =	
T$_{max}$ =		Oral =	Complete
MW =	406	pKa =	
Vd =			

References:
1. Masala A, Delitala G, Alagna S, Devilla L, Stoppelli I, Lo DG. Clomiphene and puerperal lactation. Panminerva Med 1978; 20(3):161-163.
2. Zuckerman H, Carmel S. The inhibition of lactation by clomiphene. J Obstet Gynaecol Br Commonw 1973; 80(9):822-823.
3. J.N. Personal communication. 2001.

CLOMIPRAMINE

Trade: Anafranil
Can/Aus/UK: Anafranil, Apo-Clomipramine, Placil
Uses: Antiobsessional, antidepressant drug
LRC: L2
AAP: Drugs whose effect on nursing infants is unknown but may be of concern

Clomipramine is a tricyclic antidepressant frequently used for obsessive-compulsive disorder[1].   In one patient taking 125 mg/day, on the 4th and 6th day postpartum, milk levels were 342.7 and 215.8 µg/L respectively[2]. Maternal plasma levels were 211 and 208.4 µg/L at day 4 and 6 respectively. milk/plasma ratio varies from 1.62 to 1.04 on day 4 to 6 respectively. Neonatal plasma levels continued to drop from a high of 266.6 ng/mL at birth to 127.6 ng/mL at day 4, to 94.8 ng/mL at day 6, to 9.8 ng/mL at 35 days.   In a study of four breastfeeding women who received doses of 75 to 125 mg/day, plasma levels of clomipramine in the breastfed infants were below the limit of detection, suggesting minimal transfer to the infant via milk[3]. No untoward effects were noted in any of the infants.

Pregnancy Risk Category: C

Lactation Risk Category: L2

Adult Concerns: Drowsiness, fatigue, dry mouth, seizures, constipation, sweating, reduced appetite

Pediatric Concerns: None reported in several studies.

Drug Interactions: Decreased effect when used with barbiturates, carbamazepine and phenytoin. Increased sedation when used with alcohol, CNS depressants (hypnotics). Increased dangers when used with MAO inhibitors. Additive anticholinergic effects when used with other anticholinergics.

Theoretic Infant Dose: 51.4 µg/kg/day

Relative Infant Dose: 2.8%

Adult Dose: 50 mg BID

Alternatives:

T½ =	19-37 hours	M/P =	0.84- 1.62
PHL =	92.8 hours	PB =	96%
T$_{max}$ =		Oral =	Complete
MW =	315	pKa =	9.5
Vd =	17		

References:
1. Pharmaceutical Manufacturer Prescribing Information. 1996.
2. Schimmell MS, Katz EZ, Shaag Y, Pastuszak A, Koren G. Toxic neonatal effects following maternal clomipramine therapy. J Toxicol Clin Toxicol 1991; 29(4):479-484.
3. Wisner KL, Perel JM, Foglia JP. Serum clomipramine and metabolite levels in four nursing mother-infant pairs. J Clin Psychiatry 1995; 56(1):17-20.

CLONAZEPAM

Trade: Klonopin
Can/Aus/UK: Rivotril, Apo-Clonazepam, PMS-Clonazepam, Paxam
Uses: Benzodiazepine anticonvulsant
LRC: L3
AAP: Not reviewed

Clonazepam is a typical benzodiazepam sedative, anticonvulsant. In one case report, milk levels varied between 11 and 13 µg/L (the maternal dose was omitted).[1] Milk/maternal serum ratio was approximately 0.33. In this report, the infant's serum level of clonazepam dropped from 4.4 µg/L at birth to 1.0 µg/L at 14 days while continuing to breastfeed.

Pregnancy Risk Category: C

Lactation Risk Category: L3

Adult Concerns: Apnea, sedation, ataxia, hypotonia. Behavioral disturbances (in children) include aggressiveness, irritability, agitation.

Pediatric Concerns: None reported via milk. Observe for sedation.

Drug Interactions: Phenytoin and barbiturates may increase clearance of clonazepam. CNS depressants may increase sedation.

Theoretic Infant Dose: 1.95 μg/kg/day

Relative Infant Dose:

Adult Dose: 0.5-1 mg TID

Alternatives:

T½ =	18-50 hours	M/P =	0.33
PHL =		PB =	50-86%
T_{max} =	1-4 hours	Oral =	Complete
MW =	316	pKa =	1.5, 10.5
Vd =	1.5-4.4		

References:
1. Fisher JB, Edgren BE, Mammel MC, Coleman JM. Neonatal apnea associated with maternal clonazepam therapy: a case report. Obstet Gynecol 1985; 66(3 Suppl):34S-35S.

CLONIDINE

Trade: Catapres
Can/Aus/UK: Catapres, Dixarit, Apo-Clonidine, Novo-Clonidine
Uses: Antihypertensive
LRC: L3
AAP: Not reviewed

Clonidine is an antihypertensive that reduces sympathetic nerve activity from the brain. Clonidine is excreted in human milk. In a study of 9 nursing women receiving between 241.7 and 391.7 μg/day of clonidine, milk levels varied from approximately 1.8 μg/L to as high as 2.8 μg/L on postpartum day 10-14.[1] In another report following a maternal dose of 37.5 μg twice daily, maternal plasma was determined to be 0.33 ng/mL and milk level was 0.60 μg/L.[2] Clinical symptoms of neonatal toxicity are unreported and are unlikely in normal full term infants. Clonidine may reduce prolactin secretion and could conceivably reduce milk production early postpartum. Transdermal patches produce maternal plasma levels of 0.39, 0.84, and 1.12 ng/mL using the 3.5, 7, and 10.5 cm square patches respectively. The 3.7 square cm patch would produce maternal plasma levels equivalent to the 37.5 μg oral dose and would likely produce milk levels equivalent to the above study.

Pregnancy Risk Category: C

Lactation Risk Category: L3

Adult Concerns: Drowsiness, dry mouth, hypotension, constipation, dizziness

Pediatric Concerns: None reported, but may induce hypotension in infant. May reduce milk production by reducing prolactin secretion.

Drug Interactions: Tricyclic antidepressants inhibit hypotensive effect of clonidine. Beta blockers may potentiate slow heart rate when administered with clonidine. Discontinue beta blockers several days to week prior to using clonidine.

Theoretic Infant Dose: 0.42 µg/kg/day

Relative Infant Dose: 7.5%

Adult Dose: 0.1-0.3 mg BID

Alternatives:

T½ =	20-24 hours	M/P =	2
PHL =		PB =	20-40 %
T$_{max}$ =	3-5 hours	Oral =	75-100%
MW =	230	pKa =	8.3
Vd =	3.2-5.6		

References:
1. Hartikainen-Sorri AL, Heikkinen JE, Koivisto M. Pharmacokinetics of clonidine during pregnancy and nursing. Obstet Gynecol 1987; 69(4):598-600.
2. Bunjes R, Schaefer C, Holzinger D. Clonidine and breast-feeding. Clin Pharm 1993; 12(3):178-179.

CLOPIDOGREL
Trade: Plavix
Can/Aus/UK: Plavix
Uses: Platelet aggregation inhibitor
LRC: L4
AAP: Not reviewed

Clopidogrel selectively inhibits platelet adenosine diphosphate-induced platelet aggregation. It is used to prevent ischemic events in patients at risk (e.g. cardiovascular disease, strokes, myocardial infarct). Aspirin is generally preferred as it is less expensive, quite tolerable, and very effective. Clopidogrel is only used in those patients who are aspirin-intolerant. It is not known if it transfers into human milk, but it does enter rodent milk.[1] Although the plasma half-life is rather brief (8 hrs), it's metabolite covalently bonds to platelet receptors with a half-life of 11 days. Because it produces an irreversible inhibition of platelet aggregation, any present in milk could inhibit an infant's platelet function for a prolonged period. Because aspirin affects platelet aggregation similarly, and its milk levels are quite low, it would appear to be an ideal alternative. However, aspirin also inhibits platelet aggregation for long periods as well and may increase the risk of Reye's syndrome in infants. The choice between using clopidogrel and aspirin must be made on clinical grounds until we know more about the levels secreted into human milk.

Pregnancy Risk Category: B

Lactation Risk Category: L4

Adult Concerns: Contraindicated in individuals with bleeding phenomenon.

Pediatric Concerns: None reported via milk. The transfer of clinically relevant amounts to the infant is remote, but we do not have any data thus far suggesting milk levels and clinical dose transferred to the infant.

Drug Interactions: At high concentrations, clopidogrel inhibits Cytochrome P450 2C9, and may inhibit metabolism of phenytoin, tamoxifen, tolbutamide, warfarin, torsemide, fluvastatin, and many NSAIDs.

Theoretic Infant Dose:

Relative Infant Dose:

Adult Dose: 75 mg daily

Alternatives:

T½ =	8 hours	M/P =	
PHL =		PB =	9%
T_{max} =	1 hour	Oral =	50%
MW =	420	pKa =	
Vd =			

References:
1. Pharmaceutical Manufacturer Prescribing Information. 1999.

CLORAZEPATE
Trade: Tranxene, Transene-Sd
Can/Aus/UK: Apo-Clorazepate, Novo-Clopate
Uses: Benzodiazepine sedative.
LRC: L3
AAP: Not reviewed

Clorazepate is a typical benzodiazepine. The primary metabolite, nordiazepam, is the same as from diazepam(Valium). Clorazepate has a brief half-life of less than 2 hours, and is rapidly converted to the active drug, nordiazepam, and oxazepam. The active metabolite has a prolonged half-life of 40-50 hours. No data are available on clorazepate and its transfer to human milk, but this drug should be evaluated the same as for diazepam. Check the monograph on diazepam for specifics.

Pregnancy Risk Category: D

Lactation Risk Category: L3

Adult Concerns: Adverse reactions include drowsiness, dizziness, blurred vision, dry mouth, headache, fatigue, ataxia, slurred speech, and mental confusion.

Pediatric Concerns: Poor suckling, sedation, lethargy, constipation have been reported for diazepam.

Drug Interactions: This drug is additive for most all CNS sedatives. The may prolong the sleeping time after hexobarbital, ethyl alcohol, and other hypnotic sedatives including barbiturates, narcotics, phenothiazines, monoamine oxidase inhibitors, etc. Cimetidine may increase plasma levels of clorazepate.

Theoretic Infant Dose:

Relative Infant Dose:

Adult Dose: 15-60 mg/day

Alternatives: Lorazepam, midazolam

T½ =	40-50 hours(metab)	M/P =	
PHL =		PB =	98%
T$_{max}$ =	1 hour	Oral =	97%
MW =	408	pKa =	3.5; 12.5
Vd =	1.7		

References:

1. Pharmaceutical Manufacturers prescribing information, 2003.

CLOTRIMAZOLE

Trade: Gyne-Lotrimin, Mycelex, Lotrimin, Femcare, Trivaqizole
Can/Aus/UK: Canesten, Clotrimaderm, Myclo, Clonea, Hiderm
Uses: Antifungal
LRC: L1
AAP: Not reviewed

Clotrimazole is a broad spectrum antifungal agent. It is generally used for candidiasis and various tinea species (athletes foot, ring worm). Clotrimazole is available in oral lozenges, topical creams, intravaginal tablets and creams. No data are available on penetration into breastmilk. However, after intravaginal administration, only 3-10% of the drug is absorbed (peak serum level= 0.01 to 0.03 μg/mL) and even less by oral lozenge[1]. Hence, from vaginal administration it seems very unlikely that levels absorbed by a breastfeeding infant would be high enough to produce untoward effects. Safety of clotrimazole lozenges in children younger than 3 years of age has not been established. The risk of contact dermatitis with this agent may be higher.[1]

Pregnancy Risk Category: **B during 1st and 2nd trimester**
                                C during 3rd trimester

Lactation Risk Category: **L1**

Adult Concerns: Nausea, vomiting from oral administration. Itching, burning , and stinging following topical application. Elevated liver enzymes in > 10% of treated.

Pediatric Concerns: None reported via milk.   Limited oral absorption probably limits clinical relevance in breastfed infants.

Drug Interactions: May inhibit amphotericin activity. Clotrimazole is reported to increase cyclosporin plasma levels.   May enhance hypoglycemic effect of oral hypoglycemic agents. Clotrimazole inhibits cytochrome P450 IIIA and may inhibit metabolism of any number of other medications.

Theoretic Infant Dose:

Relative Infant Dose:

Adult Dose: 500 mg intravaginally q HS

Alternatives: Fluconazole, Miconazole

$T\frac{1}{2}$ =	3.5-5 hours	M/P =	
PHL =		PB =	
T_{max} =	3 hours (oral)	Oral =	Poor
MW =	345	pKa =	
Vd =			

References:
1. McEvoy GE. (ed):AFHS Drug Information. New York, NY: 2003.
2. Newman J. Personal communication. 1999.

CLOXACILLIN
Trade: Tegopen, Cloxapen
Can/Aus/UK: Apo-Cloxi, Novo-Cloxin, Orbenin, Alclox, Kloxerate-DC
Uses: Penicillin antibiotic
LRC: L2
AAP: Not reviewed

Cloxacillin is an oral penicillinase-resistant penicillin frequently used for peripheral (non CNS) Staphylococcus aureus and S. epidermidis infections, particularly mastitis. Following a single 500 mg oral dose of cloxacillin in lactating women, milk concentrations of the drug were zero to 0.2 mg/L one and two hours after the dose respectively and 0.2 to 0.4 mg/L after 6 hours[1]. Usual dose for adults is 250-500 mg four times daily for at least 10-14 days[2].   As with most penicillins, it is unlikely these levels would be clinically relevant.

Pregnancy Risk Category: B

Lactation Risk Category: L2

Adult Concerns: Rash, diarrhea, nephrotoxicity, fever, shaking, chills

Pediatric Concerns: None reported but observe for GI symptoms such as diarrhea.

Drug Interactions: Efficacy of oral contraceptives may be reduced. Disulfiram, probenecid may increase cloxacillin levels. Increased effect of oral anticoagulants.

Theoretic Infant Dose: 60 µg/kg/day

Relative Infant Dose: 0.21%

Adult Dose: 250-500 mg q 6 hours

Alternatives:

$T\frac{1}{2}$ =	0.7-3 hours	M/P =	
PHL =	0.8-1.5 hours	PB =	90-96%
T_{max} =	0.5-2 hours	Oral =	37-60%
MW =	436	pKa =	
Vd =	6.6-10.8		

References:
1. Matsuda S. Transfer of antibiotics into maternal milk. Biol Res Pregnancy Perinatol 1984; 5(2):57-60.
2. McEvoy GE. (ed):AFHS Drug Information. New York, NY: 2003.

CLOZAPINE

Trade: Clozaril
Can/Aus/UK: Clozaril
Uses: Antipsychotic, sedative
LRC: L3
AAP: Drugs whose effect on nursing infants is unknown but may be of concern

Clozapine is an atypical antipsychotic, sedative drug somewhat similar to the phenothiazine family. In a study of one patient receiving 50 mg/d clozapine at delivery, the maternal and fetal plasma were reported to be 14.1 ng/mL and 27 ng/mL respectively. After 24 hours postpartum, the maternal plasma level was 14.7 ng/mL and maternal milk levels were 63.5 ng/mL. On day 7 postpartum and receiving a dose of 100 mg/d clozapine, the maternal plasma and milk levels were 41.1 ng/mL and 115.6 µg/L respectively. From this data it is apparent that clozapine concentrates in milk with a milk/plasma ratio of 4.3 at a dose of 50 mg/d and 2.8 at a dose of 100 mg/d. The change from day one to seven suggests that clozapine entry into mature milk is less. From this data, the weight-adjusted relative infant dose would be 1.2% of the maternal dose.

Pregnancy Risk Category: C

Lactation Risk Category: L3

Adult Concerns: Drowsiness, salivation, constipation, dizziness, tachycardia, nausea, GI distress, agranulocytosis

Pediatric Concerns: None reported.

Drug Interactions: Decreased effect of epinephrine, phenytoin. Increased sedation with CNS depressants.   Increased effect with guanabenz, anticholinergics.   Increased toxicity with cimetidine, MAO inhibitors, tricyclic antidepressants.

Theoretic Infant Dose: 17.3 µg/kg/day

Relative Infant Dose: 1.2%

Adult Dose: 300-600 mg daily

Alternatives:

T½ =	8-12 hours	M/P =	2.8-4.3
PHL =		PB =	95%
T$_{max}$ =	2.5 hours	Oral =	90%
MW =	327	pKa =	
Vd =	5		

References:

1.   Barnas C, Bergant A, Hummer M, Saria A, Fleischhacker WW. Clozapine concentrations in maternal and fetal plasma, amniotic fluid, and breastmilk. Am J Psychiatry 1994; 151(6):945.

COAGULATION FACTOR VIIa

Trade: Novoseven
Can/Aus/UK: NovoSeven
Uses: Promotes coagulation in hemophilia
LRC: L2
AAP: Not reviewed

NovoSeven is recombinant human coagulation Factor VIIa (rFVIIa), intended for promoting coagulation by activating the extrinsic pathway of the coagulation cascade. It is a vitamin K-dependent glycoprotein consisting of 406 amino acids and a molecular weight of 50 K Dalton. NovoSeven is structurally similar to human plasma-derived Factor VIIa normally found in human plasma.

This is a large molecular weight protein (50,000 daltons) which is very unlikely to enter milk. It is structurally similar to human plasma derived factor VIIa normally found in humans anyway.

Pregnancy Risk Category: C

Lactation Risk Category: L2

Adult Concerns: Adverse reactions include fever, allergic reaction, purpura, rash, hemorrhage , hemarthrosis, and hypertension.

Pediatric Concerns: None reported via milk. Unlikely to enter milk.

Drug Interactions: Do not use simultaneously with activated prothrombin complex.

Theoretic Infant Dose:

Relative Infant Dose:

Adult Dose: 90 µg/kg/2 hours until hemostasis is achieved.

Alternatives:

T½ =	1.7-2.7 hours	M/P =		
PHL =		PB =		
T$_{max}$ =		Oral =	Nil	
MW =	50,000	pKa =		
Vd =	0.103			

References:
1. Pharmaceutical Manufacturers prescribing information, 2003.

COCAINE

Trade: Crack
Can/Aus/UK:
Uses: Powerful CNS stimulant, local anesthetic
LRC: L5
AAP: Contraindicated by the American Academy of Pediatrics in Breastfeeding Mothers

Cocaine is a local anesthetic and a powerful central nervous system stimulant. It is well absorbed from all locations including the stomach, nasal passages, intrapulmonary tissues via inhalation, and even via ophthalmic instillation. Adverse effects include agitation, nervousness, restlessness, euphoria, hallucinations, tremors, tonic-clonic seizures, and myocardial arrhythmias. Although the pharmacologic effects of cocaine are relatively brief (20-30 minutes) due to redistribution out of the brain, cocaine is slowly metabolized and excreted over a prolonged period. Urine samples can be positive for cocaine metabolites for up to 7 days or longer in adults. Breastfeeding infants will likewise become urine positive for cocaine for even longer periods. Even after the clinical effects of cocaine have subsided, the breastmilk will still probably contain significant quantities of benzoecgonine, the inactive metabolite of cocaine. The infant could still test positive for urine cocaine metabolites for long periods (days). The ingestion of small amounts of cocaine by infants via inhalation of smoke (environmental) is likely.

Studies of exact estimates of cocaine transmission to breastmilk have not been reported. Significant secretion into breastmilk is suspected with a probable high milk/plasma ratio. A number of case reports in the literature clearly indicate the transmission of maternal cocaine to the infant via milk with significant agitation in the breastfeeding infant resulting[1,2]. In one case study, a woman who applied topical cocaine to her nipples and breastfed her infant, produced extreme toxicity in the infant. Topical application to nipples is EXTREMELY dangerous and is definitely contraindicated. Oral, intranasal, and smoking of crack cocaine is dangerous and definitely contraindicated. In those individuals who have ingested cocaine, a minimum pump and dump period of 24 hours is recommended for clearance.

Pregnancy Risk Category: **C during 1st and 2nd trimester**
                                              X during 3rd trimester

Lactation Risk Category: **L5**

Adult Concerns: Nausea, vomiting, CNS excitement, hypertension, tachycardia, arrhythmias

Pediatric Concerns: Choking, vomiting, diarrhea, tremulousness, hyperactive startle reflex, gasping, agitation, irritability, hypertension, tachycardia. Extreme danger.

Drug Interactions: Increased toxicity when used with MAO inhibitors.

Theoretic Infant Dose:

Relative Infant Dose:

Adult Dose: N/A

Alternatives:

T½ =	0.8 hour	M/P =	
PHL =		PB =	91%
T$_{max}$ =	15 minutes	Oral =	Complete
MW =	303	pKa =	8.6
Vd =	1.6-2-7		

References:
1. Chaney NE, Franke J, Wadlington WB. Cocaine convulsions in a breast-feeding baby. J Pediatr 1988; 112(1):134-135.
2. Chasnoff IJ, Lewis DE, Squires L. Cocaine intoxication in a breast-fed infant. Pediatrics 1987; 80(6):836-838.

CODEINE

Trade: Empirin #3, #4, Tylenol #3, #4
Can/Aus/UK: Paveral, Penntuss, Actacode, Codalgin, Codral, Panadeine, Veganin, Kaodene, Teropin
Uses: Analgesic
LRC: L3
AAP: Maternal Medication Usually Compatible with Breastfeeding

Codeine is considered a mild opiate analgesic whose action is probably due to its metabolism to small amounts of morphine. The amount of codeine secreted into milk is low and dose dependent. Infant response is higher during neonatal period (first or second week). Four cases of neonatal apnea have been reported following administration of 60 mg codeine every 4-6 hours to breastfeeding mothers although codeine was not detected in serum of the infants tested.[1] Apnea resolved after discontinuation of maternal codeine. Number 3 tablets contain 30 mg and 4 tablets contain 60 mg of codeine.

In another study, following a dose of 60 mg, milk concentrations averaged 140 µg/L of milk with a peak of 455 µg/L at 1 hour.[2] Following 12 doses in 48 hours, the authors estimate the dose of codeine in milk (2000 mL milk) was 0.7 mg. There are few reported side effects following codeine doses of 30 mg, and it is believed to produce only minimal side effects in newborns. But some infants may be sedated.

Pregnancy Risk Category: C

Lactation Risk Category: L3

Adult Concerns: Sedation, respiratory depression, constipation

Pediatric Concerns: Several rare cases of neonatal apnea have been reported, but at higher doses. Codeine analgesics are so commonly used postpartum, that side effect are extremely rare and seldom reported. Observe for sedation, apnea in premature or weakened infants.

Drug Interactions: Cigarette smoking increases effect of codeine. Increased toxicity/sedation when used with CNS depressants, phenothiazines, tricyclic antidepressants, other opiates, guanabenz, MAO inhibitors, neuromuscular blockers.

Theoretic Infant Dose: 68 µg/kg/day

Relative Infant Dose: 7.9%

Adult Dose: 15-60 mg q 4-6 hours

Alternatives:

T½ =	2.9 hours	M/P =	1.3-2.5
PHL =		PB =	7%
T$_{max}$ =	0.5-1 hour	Oral =	Complete
MW =	299	pKa =	8.2
Vd =	3.5		

References:
1. Davis JM, Bhutari VK. Neonatal apnea and maternal codeine use. Ped Res 2004; 19(4):170A abstract.
2. Findlay JW, DeAngelis RL, Kearney MF, Welch RM, Findlay JM. Analgesic drugs in breastmilk and plasma. Clin Pharmacol Ther 1981; 29(5):625-633.

COENZYME Q10

Trade: Ubiquinone, CoQ10, Ubidecarenone
Can/Aus/UK:
Uses: Cofactor in electron transport chain
LRC: L3
AAP: Not reviewed

Coenzyme Q10, also known as ubiquinone and ubidecarenone, is a cofactor in the mitochondrial electron-transport chain in the synthesis of ATP within the cell. It may also possess antioxidant and membrane-stabilizing properties. Although it is a naturally occurring cofactor, it is generally synthesized within the cell. Those cells that have the highest metabolic activity are most sensitive to deficiencies.

The clinical uses of ubiquinone are quite interesting and include congestive heart disease, hypertension, periodontal disease, obesity, immune deficiencies, and angina.[1]

Ubiquinone is slowly absorbed requiring 5-10 hours to reach a peak. Following oral doses of 100 mg, peak blood levels of 1 µg/mL have been reported.[2] With doses of 300 mg/d, mean plasma levels were 5.4 µg/mL after 4 days. No data are available on ubiquinone levels in milk. However, ubiquinone is very lipid soluble and has a long plasma half-life; transfer to milk is likely. If one were to assume a milk/plasma ratio of 1.0 and a significant maternal dose of 300 mg/d, then the average daily intake via milk in an infant would be approximately 16% of the weight-adjusted maternal dose. Were these numbers correct, it is not likely that this dose would be overtly toxic to an infant. Although ubiquinone is relatively non-toxic in adults, there are no data on the relative toxicity of this substance in infants. Most references suggest that pregnant and lactating women should avoid supplementation with this cofactor.

Pregnancy Risk Category:

Lactation Risk Category: L3

Adult Concerns: Caution when using in patient with biliary obstruction. Caution when using with hypolipidemic agents, oral hypoglycemic agents, insulin, in patients with hepatic and renal insufficiency. Most common adverse effects include nausea, epigastric pain, diarrhea, heartburn, appetite suppression.

Pediatric Concerns: None reported but caution recommended.

Drug Interactions: Do not use with oral hypoglycemics, hypolipidemic agents. May decrease INR in patients taking warfarin.

Theoretic Infant Dose:

Relative Infant Dose:

Adult Dose:

Alternatives:

T½ =	34 hours	M/P =	
PHL =		PB =	
T_max =	5-10 hours	Oral =	Complete
MW =		pKa =	
Vd =			

References:
1. Gaby AR. Coenzyme Q10, in Pizzorno JE. Churchill Livingstone(eds): Textbook of Natural Medicine. 1999.
2. Greenberg S, Frishman WH. Co-enzyme Q10: a new drug for cardiovascular disease. J Clin Pharmacol 1990; 30(7):596-608.

COLCHICINE

Trade: Colchicine
Can/Aus/UK: Colchicine, Colgout
Uses: Analgesic in gouty arthritis
LRC: L4
AAP: Maternal Medication Usually Compatible with Breastfeeding

Colchicine is an old product primarily used to reduce pain associated with inflammatory gout. Although it reduces the pain, it is not a true analgesic but simply reduces the inflammation associated with uric acid crystals by inhibiting leukocyte and other cellular migration into the region. However, it is quite toxic, and routine CBCs should be done while under treatment. Blood dyscrasias, hepatomegaly, and bone marrow depression are all possible, particularly in infants. Although the plasma half-life is only 20 minutes, it deposits in blood leukocytes and many other tissues thereby extending the elimination half-life to over 60 hours.

Little or no consistent data on breastmilk levels are available. In the one study published, even the authors questioned the percent recovery in the breastmilk, so the data must be considered questionable. Nevertheless, the milk concentration varied from 1.2 to 2.5 µg/L (16-19 days postpartum) in one patient receiving 0.6 mg of colchicine twice daily.[1]

Pregnancy Risk Category: D

Lactation Risk Category: L4

Adult Concerns: Nausea, vomiting, diarrhea, myopathy, leukopenia, bone marrow suppression

Pediatric Concerns: None reported in one case reviewed.

Drug Interactions: Colchichine reduces vitamin B-12 absorption. Avoid alcohol.

Theoretic Infant Dose: 0.375 µg/kg/day

Relative Infant Dose: 4.3%

Adult Dose: 0.5-0.6 mg 1-4 times a week

Alternatives:

T½ =	12-30 minutes	M/P =	
PHL =		PB =	10-31%
T$_{max}$ =	1-2 hours	Oral =	Complete
MW =	399	pKa =	1.7, 12.4
Vd =	10-12		

References:
1.   Milunsky JM. Breast-feeding during colchicine therapy for familial Mediterranean fever. J Pediatr 1991; 119(1 (Pt 1)):164.

COLESEVELAM HCL
Trade: Welchol
Can/Aus/UK:
Uses: Cholesterol lower agent
LRC: L1
AAP: Not reviewed

Colesevelam is a non-absorbed, polymeric, lipid-lowering agent that prevents the absorption of bile acids from the intestines. As bile acids are the precursors for cholesterol production, hepatic cholesterol production is lowered. Colesevelam is almost totally unabsorbed from the GI tract (only 0.05%) and is unlikely to enter milk at all (see cholestyramine). The only potential problem of using this product in breastfeeding mothers is the lowering of maternal plasma cholesterol levels, and any possible lowering of milk cholesterol levels.   Milk cholesterol is particularly important in infant neurodevelopment.

Pregnancy Risk Category: B

Lactation Risk Category: L1

Adult Concerns: Constipation, dyspepsia and myalgia are the most commonly reported.

Pediatric Concerns: None reported via milk. It is totally unabsorbed so none would penetrate milk.

Drug Interactions: Apparently does not inhibit absorption of many drugs tested (as is seen with cholestyramine). May decrease absorption of verapamil.

Theoretic Infant Dose:

Relative Infant Dose:

Adult Dose: Three to six 625 mg tablets daily

Alternatives: Cholestyramine

T½ =		M/P =	
PHL =		PB =	
T$_{max}$ =		Oral =	None
MW =		pKa =	
Vd =			

References:
1. Pharmaceutical Manufacturers prescribing information, 2003.

COMFREY

Trade: Russian Comfrey, Knitbone, Bruisewort, Blackwort, Slippery Root
Can/Aus/UK:
Uses: Herbal poultice
LRC: L5
AAP: Not reviewed

Comfrey has been claimed to heal gastric ulcers, hemorrhoids, and suppress bronchial congestion and inflammation.[1] The product contains allantoin, tannin, and a group of dangerous pyrrolizidine alkaloids. Ointments containing Comfrey have been found to be antiinflammatory, probably due to the allantoin content. However, when administered orally to animals, most members of this family (Boraginaceae) have been noted to induce severe liver toxicity including elevated liver enzymes and liver tumors (hepatocellular adenomas).[2,3] Bladder tumors were noted at low concentrations. Russian Comfrey has been found to induce liver damage and pancreatic islet cell tumors.[4] A number of significant human toxicities have been reported including several deaths, all associated with the ingestion of Comfrey teas or yerba mate tea.[5]   Even when applied to the skin, pyrrolizidine alkaloids were noted in the urine of rodents.   Lactating rats excreted pyrrolizidine alkaloids into breastmilk.

Comfrey and members of this family are exceedingly dangerous and should not be used topically, ingested orally, or used in any form in breastfeeding mothers.

Pregnancy Risk Category: X

Lactation Risk Category: L5

Adult Concerns: Liver toxicity, hepatic carcinoma, hepatocellular adenomas, hepatonecrosis

Pediatric Concerns: Passes into animal milk.   Too dangerous for breastfeeding mothers and infants.

Drug Interactions:

Theoretic Infant Dose:

Relative Infant Dose:

Adult Dose:

Alternatives:

References:
1.   Review of Natural Products Facts and Comparisons, St Louis, MO 1996.
2.   Hirono I, Mori H, Haga M. Carcinogenic activity of Symphytum officinale. J Natl Cancer Inst 1978; 61(3):865-869.
3.   Yeong ML, Wakefield SJ, Ford HC. Hepatocyte membrane injury and bleb formation following low dose comfrey toxicity in rats. Int J Exp Pathol 1993; 74(2):211-217.
4.   Yeong ML, Clark SP, Waring JM, Wilson RD, Wakefield SJ. The effects of comfrey derived pyrrolizidine alkaloids on rat liver. Pathology 1991; 23(1):35-38.
5.   McGee J, Patrick RS, Wood CB, Blumgart LH. A case of veno-occlusive disease of the liver in Britain associated with herbal tea consumption. J Clin Pathol 1976; 29(9):788-794.

COPPER-64

Trade: Copper-64
Can/Aus/UK:
Uses: Radioisotope
LRC: L4
AAP: Radioactive compound that requires temporary cessation of breastfeeding

Copper-64 is a radioactive compound.   Radioactivity is present in milk after 50 hours.   Pump and discard until radioactivity has decayed (approximately 5 half-lives = 64 hrs).   Radioactive half-life is 12.7 hours.

Pregnancy Risk Category:

Lactation Risk Category: L4

Adult Concerns:

Pediatric Concerns:

Drug Interactions:

Theoretic Infant Dose:

Relative Infant Dose:

Adult Dose:

Alternatives:

$T\frac{1}{2}$ =	12.7 hours	M/P =	
PHL =		PB =	
T_{max} =		Oral =	
MW =	64	pKa =	
Vd =	2.0		

References:

CORTICOTROPIN
Trade: ACT, ACHTAR ACTH
Can/Aus/UK: ACTHAR
Uses: Stimulates cortisol release
LRC: L3
AAP: Not reviewed

ACTH is secreted by the anterior pituitary in the brain and stimulates the adrenal cortex to produce and secrete adrenocortical hormones (cortisol, hydrocortisone). As a peptide product, ACTH is easily destroyed in the infants GI tract. None would be absorbed by the infant. ACTH stimulates the endogenous production of cortisol, which theoretically can transfer to the breastfed infant. However, the use of ACTH in breastfeeding mothers largely depends on the dose and duration of exposure and the risks to the infant. Brief exposures are probably not contraindicated.

Pregnancy Risk Category: C

Lactation Risk Category: L3

Adult Concerns: Hypersensitivity reactions, increased risk of infection, embryocidal effects, other symptoms of hypercorticalism

Pediatric Concerns: None reported via milk.

Drug Interactions:

Theoretic Infant Dose:

Relative Infant Dose:

Adult Dose: 80 U injection (IM or SC)

Alternatives:

References :

CO-TRIMOXAZOLE
Trade: TMP-SMZ, Bactrim, Cotrim, Septra
Can/Aus/UK: Novo-Trimel, Septrin, Bactrim, Respax, Trimogal
Uses: Sulfonamide antibiotic
LRC: L3
AAP: Maternal Medication Usually Compatible with Breastfeeding

Co-trimoxazole is the mixture of trimethoprim and sulfamethoxazole. See individual monographs for each of these products.

Pregnancy Risk Category:

Lactation Risk Category: **L3**

References:

CROMOLYN SODIUM
Trade: Nasalcrom, Gastrocrom, Intal
Can/Aus/UK: Intral, Nalcrom, Opticrom, Rhynacrom, Vistacrom, Cromese
Uses: Antiasthmatic, antiallergic
LRC: L1
AAP: Not reviewed

Cromolyn is an extremely safe drug that is used clinically as an antiasthmatic, antiallergic, and to suppress mast cell degranulation and allergic symptoms. No data on penetration into human breastmilk are available, but it has an extremely low pKa, and minimal levels would be expected.[1]   Less than 0.001% of a dose is distributed into milk of the monkey.   No harmful effects have been reported on breastfeeding infants. Less than 1% of this drug is absorbed from the maternal (and probably the infant's) GI tract, so it is unlikely to produce untoward effects in nursing infants.   This product is frequently used in pediatric patients.

Pregnancy Risk Category: **B**

Lactation Risk Category: **L1**

Adult Concerns: Headache, itching, nausea, diarrhea, allergic reactions, hoarseness, coughing

Pediatric Concerns: None reported via milk. Probably quite safe.

Drug Interactions:

Theoretic Infant Dose:

Relative Infant Dose:

Adult Dose: 20 mg QID via inhalation

Alternatives:

T½ =	80-90 minutes	M/P =	
PHL =		PB =	
T$_{max}$ =	< 15 minutes	Oral =	< 1%
MW =	468	pKa =	Low
Vd =			

References:
1. McEvoy GE. (ed):AFHS Drug Information. New York, NY: 2003.

CYCLIZINE

Trade: Marezine
Can/Aus/UK: Marzine, Migral, Diconal, Valoid
Uses: Antihistamine, antiemetic
LRC: L3
AAP: Not reviewed

Cyclizine is an antihistamine frequently used as an antiemetic and for antimotion-sickness. In past years, this drug was frequently used for nausea and vomiting of pregnancy although it is no longer used for this purpose. No reports concerning its secretion into human milk are available.

Pregnancy Risk Category: B

Lactation Risk Category: L3

Adult Concerns: Sedation, dry mouth

Pediatric Concerns: None reported via milk.

Drug Interactions: Increased sedation with CNS depressants such as alcohol, barbiturates.

Theoretic Infant Dose:

Relative Infant Dose:

Adult Dose: 50 mg q 4-6 hours

Alternatives:

T½ =		M/P =	
PHL =		PB =	
T$_{max}$ =		Oral =	
MW =	266	pKa =	7.7
Vd =			

References:

CYCLOBENZAPRINE

Trade: Flexeril, Cycoflex
Can/Aus/UK: Flexeril, Novo-Cycloprine
Uses: Muscle relaxant, CNS depressant
LRC: L3
AAP: Not reviewed

Cyclobenzaprine is a centrally acting skeletal muscle relaxant that is structurally and pharmacologically similar to the tricyclic antidepressants. Cyclobenzaprine is used as an adjunct to rest and physical therapy for the relief of acute, painful musculoskeletal conditions.[1] Studies have not conclusively shown whether the skeletal muscle relaxation properties are due to the sedation or placebo effects. At least one study has found it no more effective than placebo. It is not known if cyclobenzaprine is secreted in milk, but one must assume that its secretion would be similar to the tricyclics (see amitriptyline, desipramine). There are no pediatric indications for this product.

Pregnancy Risk Category: B

Lactation Risk Category: L3

Adult Concerns: Drowsiness, dry mouth, dizziness, nausea, vomiting, unpleasant taste sensation. Tachycardia, hypotension, arrhythmias.

Pediatric Concerns: None reported, but caution is urged.

Drug Interactions: Do not use with 14 days of MAO inhibitor. Additive effect with tricyclic antidepressants. Enhances effect of alcohol, barbiturates, and other CNS depressants.

Theoretic Infant Dose:

Relative Infant Dose:

Adult Dose: 20-60 mg daily

Alternatives:

T½ =	24-72 hours	M/P =	
PHL =		PB =	93%
T$_{max}$ =	3-8 hours	Oral =	Complete
MW =	275	pKa =	
Vd =	High		

References:
1. McEvoy GE. (ed):AFHS Drug Information. New York, NY: 2003.

CYCLOPENTOLATE
Trade: Ak-Pentolate, Cyclogyl, Cylate, Ocu-Pentolate, Pentolair
Can/Aus/UK: Ak-Pentolate, Diopentolate, Cyclogyl, Minims Cyclopentolate
Uses: Anticholinergic for the induction of mydriasis
LRC: L3 after 6 hours
AAP: Not reviewed

Cyclopentolate is use to dilate the pupils to facilate refraction, eye examinations, and other diagnostic purpose in the eye. Cyclopentolate is commonly used by ophthalmologists and optometrists because it works rapidly and briefer than atropine. It is a potent anticholinergic and some is absorbed systemically. Children and particularly infants would be extremely susceptible to this agent. Several cases of pediatric seizures[1] and one case of necrotizing enterocolitis[2] have been reported following the ophthalmic use of this agent in children and an infant respectively. While no data are available on the transfer of this agent into human milk, it is rather unlikely that significant quantities would enter as plasma levels are so low, and milk levels would be even lower.

Plasma levels are approximately 3000 times lower than ophthalmic levels. Only 3-18% of muscarinic receptors were occupied after 55-124 minutes following administration. In healthy volunteers, peak plasma concentrations of cyclopentolate, 2.06 nM, occurred at 53 minutes, maximum receptor occupancy being 5.9%.[3] After topical application, plasma receptor occupancy was not high enough to cause any significant changes in heart rate and in PQ time. None of the subjects experienced subjectively or objectively adverse effects to be attributed to cyclopentolate. In another study, peak plasma drug concentrations of about 3 ng/mL occurred within 30 min after all formulations.[4] The mean elimination half-life of cyclopentolate was 111 min when all subjects and formulations were considered together.

Some caution is recommended with this product. A waiting period of perhaps 6 hours following its use would be sufficient to reduce risks.

Pregnancy Risk Category: C

Lactation Risk Category: L3 after 6 hours

Adult Concerns: While systemic side effects are rare, children, expecially infants, are more susceptible than adults. Systemic effects are consistent with other anticholinergics and include: blurred vision, dry mouth, dry eye, urinary retention, seizures in infants and children, sedation, drowsiness, and hyperpyrexia have all been reported.

Pediatric Concerns: None via milk, but caution is recommended. A brief interruption of breastfeeding is advised to reduce risk.

Drug Interactions: Additive with belladonna alkaloids and procainamide. May negate effects of cisapride on peristaltic contractions.

Theoretic Infant Dose:

Relative Infant Dose:

Adult Dose: 1-2 drops in each eye.

Alternatives: Atropine

T½ =	111 minutes	M/P =
PHL =		PB =
T$_{max}$ =	15 minutes	Oral =
MW =		pKa =
Vd =		

References:
1. Fitzgerald DA, Hanson RM, West C, Martin F, Brown J, Kilham HA. Seizures associated with 1% cyclopentolate eyedrops. J Paediatr Child Health 1990; 26(2):106-107.
2. Isenberg SJ, Abrams C, Hyman PE. Effects of cyclopentolate eyedrops on gastric secretory function in pre-term infants. Ophthalmology 1985; 92(5):698-700.
3. Haaga M, Kaila T, Salminen L, Ylitalo P. Systemic and ocular absorption and antagonist activity of topically applied cyclopentolate in man. Pharmacol Toxicol 1998; 82(1):19-22.
4. Lahdes K, Huupponen R, Kaila T, Monti D, Saettone MF, Salminen L. Plasma concentrations and ocular effects of cyclopentolate after ocular application of three formulations. Br J Clin Pharmacol 1993; 35(5):479-483.

CYCLOPHOSPHAMIDE

Trade: Neosar, Cytoxan
Can/Aus/UK: Cytoxan, Procytox, Cycloblastin, Endoxan, Endoxana
Uses: Antineoplastic
LRC: L5
AAP: Contraindicated by the American Academy of Pediatrics in Breastfeeding Mothers

Cyclophosphamide is a powerful and toxic antineoplastic drug. A number of reports in the literature indicate that cyclophosphamide can transfer into human milk as evidenced by the production of leukopenia and bone marrow suppression in at least 3 breastfed infants. In one case of a mother who received 800 mg/week of cyclophosphamide, her infant was significantly neutropenic following 6 weeks of exposure via breastmilk.[1]   Major leukopenia was also reported in a second breastfed infant following only a brief exposure.[2]   Thus far, no reports have provided quantitative estimates of cyclophosphamide in milk.   This agent should not be used in breastfeeding mothers.

Pregnancy Risk Category: D

Lactation Risk Category: L5

Adult Concerns: Leukopenia, infections, anemia, GI distress, nausea, vomiting, diarrhea, hemorrhagic colitis

Pediatric Concerns: Leukopenia and bone marrow suppression in at least 3 breastfed infants.

Drug Interactions: Cyclophosphamide may reduce digoxin serum levels. Increased bone marrow suppression when used with allopurinol, and cardiotoxicity when used with doxorubicin. May prolong effect of neuromuscular blocking agents.   Chloramphenicol increases half-life of cyclophosphamide. Numerous others, see complete review.

Theoretic Infant Dose:

Relative Infant Dose:

Adult Dose: 1-5 mg/kg daily
Alternatives:

$T\frac{1}{2}$ =	7.5 hours	M/P =	
PHL =		PB =	13%
T_{max} =	2-3 hours	Oral =	75%
MW =	261	pKa =	
Vd =			

References:
1.   Amato D, Niblett JS. Neutropenia from cyclophosphamide in breastmilk. Med J Aust 1977; 1(11):383-384.
2.   Durodola JI. Administration of cyclophosphamide during late pregnancy and early lactation: a case report. J Natl Med Assoc 1979; 71(2):165-166.

CYCLOSERINE
Trade: Seromycin
Can/Aus/UK: Closina, Cycloserine
Uses: Anti-tuberculosis drug
LRC: L3
AAP: Maternal Medication Usually Compatible with Breastfeeding

Cycloserine is an antibiotic primarily used for treating tuberculosis. It is also effective against various staphylococcal infections. It is a small molecule with a structure similar   to the amino acid,   D-alanine.

Following a 250 mg oral dose given four times daily to mothers, milk levels ranged from 6 to 19 mg/L, an average of 72% of maternal serum levels.[1]

Pregnancy Risk Category: C

Lactation Risk Category: L3

Adult Concerns: Drowsiness, CNS confusion, dizziness, headache, lethargy, depression, seizures.   Precautions urged in epilepsy, depression, severe anxiety.

Pediatric Concerns: None reported.

Drug Interactions: Increased toxicity with alcohol, isoniazid. Phenytoin levels may be elevated due to inhibition of metabolism.

Theoretic Infant Dose: 2.85 mg/kg/day

Relative Infant Dose: 19.9%

Adult Dose: 250 mg BID

Alternatives:

T½ =	12+ hours	M/P =	0.72
PHL =		PB =	
Tmax =	3-4 hours	Oral =	70-90%
MW =	102	pKa =	
Vd =			

References:
1. Charles E, McKenna MH, Morton RF. Studies on the absorption, diffusion, and excretion of cycloserine. Antibiot Annu 1955; 3:169-172.

CYCLOSPORINE

Trade: Sandimmune, Neoral
Can/Aus/UK: Sandimmune, Neoral
Uses: Immunosuppressant
LRC: L3
AAP: Cytotoxic drug that may interfere with cellular metabolism of the nursing infant

Cyclosporine is an immunosuppressant used to reduce organ rejection following transplant and in autoimmune syndromes such as arthritis, etc.   In a recent report of 7 breastfeeding mothers treated with cyclosporine, the levels of cyclosporine in breastmilk ranged from 50 to 227 µg/L.   Corresponding plasma levels in the breastfed infants were undetectable (<30 ng/mL) in all infants.   In this study, the infants received less than 300 µg per day via breastmilk.[1]   In another, following a dose of 320 mg/d, the milk level at 22 hours post dose was 16 µg/L and the milk/plasma ratio was 0.28.[2]   In another report of a mother receiving 250 mg twice daily, the maternal plasma level of cyclosporine was measured at 187 μg/L, and the breastmilk level was 167 μg/L.[3] None was detected in the plasma of the infant.

In a study of a breastfeeding transplant patient who received 300 mg twice daily, maternal serum levels were 193, 273, and 123 ng/mL at 23 days, 6.5 and 9.7 weeks postpartum.[4] Corresponding milk cyclosporine levels were 160, 286, and 79 μg/L respectively. Using the higher milk level, an infant would receive less than 0.4% of the weight-adjusted maternal dose. All these studies suggest that the clinical dose transferred to the infant via milk is miniscule.

In another mother receiving cyclosporine (3 mg/kg/d), the concentration of cyclosporine in milk averaged 596 μg/L or a dose of about <0.1 mg/kg to the infant.[5] The infant's trough blood level was always < 3 μg/L while the mother's was 260 μg/L. No untoward effects were noted in the infant.

In a more recent study of 5 patients receiving 5.3, 4.0, 5, 4.11, and 5 mg/kg/day cyclosporine respectively[6] the average concentration of cyclosporine in the mothers milk was 403 μg/L, 465 μg/L, 97.6 μg/L, 117.7 μg/L, and 84-144 μg/L(range) respectively. Hindmilk levels were much higher in one case, probably due to the high lipid content. In mother 1, the cyclosporine blood levels in the infant were 131 μg/L and 117 μg/L on two occasions which were near a therapeutic trough. In none of the other infants were blood levels of cyclosporine determinable (< 25 μg/L). This study clearly suggests that some infants could potentially attain near-therapeutic levels from ingesting breastmilk. From this data the relative infant dose would be approximately 0.78% of the weight-normalized maternal dose.

These studies together suggest cyclosporine transfer to milk is generally low, but the latter study suggests that some infants may receive more than has been expected from the prior studies. Therefore cyclosporine use in breastfeeding mothers should be followed by close observation of the infant.

Pregnancy Risk Category: C

Lactation Risk Category: L3

Adult Concerns: Kidney toxicity, edema, tremor, seizures, elevated liver enzymes, hypertension, hirsutism. Use during pregnancy does not pose a major risk. Infections and possible lymphomas may result.

Pediatric Concerns: None reported, but caution is recommended.

Drug Interactions: Rifampin, phenytoin, phenobarbital decrease plasma concentrations of cyclosporine. Ketoconazole, fluconazole, and itraconazole increase plasma concentrations of cyclosporine.

Theoretic Infant Dose: 42.9 μg/kg/day

Relative Infant Dose: 0.5%

Adult Dose: 5-15 mg/kg daily

Alternatives:

T½ =	5.6 hours	M/P =	0.28-0.4
PHL =		PB =	93%
Tmax =	3.5 hours	Oral =	28% pediatric
MW =		pKa =	
Vd =	3.1-4.3		

References:

1. Nyberg G, Haljamae U, Frisenette-Fich C, Wennergren M, Kjellmer I. Breast-feeding during treatment with cyclosporine. Transplantation 1998; 65(2):253-255.
2. Flechner SM, Katz AR, Rogers AJ, Van Buren C, Kahan BD. The presence of cyclosporine in body tissues and fluids during pregnancy. Am J Kidney Dis 1985; 5(1):60-63.
3. K.D.T. Personal communication. 1997.
4. Munoz-Flores-Thiagarajan KD, Easterling T, Davis C, Bond EF. Breast-feeding by a cyclosporine-treated mother. Obstet Gynecol 2001; 97(5 Pt 2):816-818.
5. Thiru Y, Bateman DN, Coulthard MG. Successful breast feeding while· mother was taking cyclosporin. BMJ 1997; 315(7106):463.
6. Moretti ME, Sgro M, Johnson DW, Sauve RS, Woolgar MJ, Taddio A, Verjee Z, Giesbrecht E, Koren G, Ito S. Cyclosporine excretion into breastmilk. Transplantation 2003; 75(12):2144-2146.

CYPROHEPTADINE

Trade: Periactin
Can/Aus/UK: PMS-Cyproheptadine, Periactin
Uses: Antihistamine
LRC: L3
AAP: Not reviewed

Cyproheptadine is a serotonin and histamine antagonist with anticholinergic and sedative effects. It has been used as an appetite stimulant in children and for rashes and pruritus (itching).[1] No data are available on its transfer to human milk.

Pregnancy Risk Category: B

Lactation Risk Category: L3

Adult Concerns: Sedation, nausea, vomiting, diarrhea

Pediatric Concerns: None reported. Observe for sedation.

Drug Interactions: Additive sedation when used with other antihistamines and CNS depressants. Increased toxicity (hallucinations) when used with MAO inhibitors.

Theoretic Infant Dose:

Relative Infant Dose:

Adult Dose: 4 mg TID-QID

Alternatives: Hydroxyzine

T½ =	16 hours	M/P =	
PHL =		PB =	
T$_{max}$ =		Oral =	
MW =	287	pKa = 9.3	
Vd =			

References:
1. Pharmaceutical Manufacturers prescribing information, 2003.

CYTARABINE
Trade: Cytosar
Can/Aus/UK: Cytosar, Alexan
Uses: Antineoplastic
LRC: L5
AAP: Not reviewed

Cytarabine is converted intracellularly to a nucleotide that interrupts DNA synthesis. No data has been reported on transfer into breastmilk.[1] The compound is poorly absorbed orally and is therefore used IM or IV only. This drug would be extremely toxic to an infant and is generally contraindicated in breastfeeding mothers.

Pregnancy Risk Category: D

Lactation Risk Category: L5

Adult Concerns: Anemia, bone marrow suppression, nausea, vomiting, diarrhea, GI hemorrhage, elevated liver enzymes.

Pediatric Concerns: None reported via milk. But due to toxicity, this product should never be used in a breastfeeding mother.

Drug Interactions: Decreases effect of gentamycin flucytosine, digoxin. Increases toxicity of alkylating agents, radiation, purine analogs, methotrexate.

Theoretic Infant Dose:

Relative Infant Dose:

Adult Dose: 100 mg/m(2) IV daily
Alternatives:

T½ =	1-3 hours	M/P =	
PHL =		PB =	13%.
T$_{max}$ =		Oral =	< 20%
MW =	243	pKa =	
Vd =			

References:
1. Drug Facts and Comparisons 2003 ed. ed. St. Louis: 2003.

CYTOMEGALOVIRUS
Trade: Human Cytomegalovirus, CMV
Can/Aus/UK:
Uses: Viral infection
LRC:
AAP: Not reviewed

Cytomegalovirus is one of the family of herpes viruses that is rather ubiquitous. Many infants have been exposed in utero and later in day care centers.[1] Maternal cervical infection is very common. CMV is found in breastmilk of virtually all CMV positive women using the newer PCR techniques.[2] The timing of maternal infection is important. If the mother seroconverts early in gestation, the infant is likely to be affected in utero. Symptoms include: small for gestational age, jaundice, microcephaly, petechia, hepatosplenomegaly, hearing loss. If the mother seroconverts late in gestation, the infant is less likely to be severely affected. In most infants from seropositive mothers, the CMV found in breastmilk is not overtly dangerous, and these mothers can breastfeed successfully.[3] However, infants who are not provided with maternal antibodies to CMV (those who convert during lactation) may be exceedingly susceptible to CMV in breastmilk. Breastmilk from CMV positive mothers should never be fed to unprotected infants.

Pregnancy Risk Category:

Lactation Risk Category:

Adult Concerns: Asymptomatic to Hepatosplenomegaly. Fever, mild hepatitis.

Pediatric Concerns: CMV transfer into breastmilk is known but of low risk to infants born of CMV positive mothers. Breastmilk from CMV positive mothers should never be fed to unprotected non-immune infants.

Drug Interactions:

Theoretic Infant Dose:

Relative Infant Dose:

Adult Dose:

Alternatives:

References:

1. Dworsky M, Yow M, Stagno S, Pass RF, Alford C. Cytomegalovirus infection of breastmilk and transmission in infancy. Pediatrics 1983; 72(3):295-299.
2. Hotsubo T, Nagata N, Shimada M, Yoshida K, Fujinaga K, Chiba S. Detection of human cytomegalovirus DNA in breastmilk by means of polymerase chain reaction. Microbiol Immunol 1994; 38(10):809-811.
3. Lawrence RA. Breastfeeding: A guide for the medical profession. St. Louis: Mosby Publishers, 1994.

DACTINOMYCIN

Trade: Cosmegen
Can/Aus/UK: Cosmegen
Uses: Antibiotic used in cancer chemotherapy
LRC: L5
AAP: Not reviewed

Dactinomycin is an antineoplastic antibiotic that inhibits DNA and RNA synthesis. It is extremely dangerous and very toxic. Transfer into breastmilk is unreported.[1] Although its oral absorption is very poor, it is extremely irritating to tissues and must be administered IV only. Definitely contraindicated in nursing mothers.

Pregnancy Risk Category: C

Lactation Risk Category: L5

Adult Concerns: Anemia, bone marrow suppression, skin lesions and rashes, alopecia, malaise, fatigue, fever, liver toxicity

Pediatric Concerns: None reported but could be extremely toxic. Caution urged.

Drug Interactions: Dactinomycin potentiates the toxicity of radiation therapy.

Theoretic Infant Dose:

Relative Infant Dose:

Adult Dose: 0.5 mg IV daily

Alternatives:

T½ =	36 hours	M/P =	
PHL =		PB =	
T$_{max}$ =		Oral =	Poor
MW =	1255	pKa =	
Vd =			

References:

1. Drug Facts and Comparisons 2003 ed. ed. St. Louis: 2003.

DALTEPARIN SODIUM

Trade: Fragmin, Low Molecular Weight Heparin
Can/Aus/UK: Fragmin
Uses: Anticoagulant
LRC: L2
AAP: Not reviewed

Dalteparin is a low molecular weight polysaccharide fragment of heparin used clinically as an anticoagulant.

In a study of two patients who received 5000-10,000 IU of dalteparin, none was found in human milk.[1]

In another study of 15 post-caesarian patients early postpartum(mean = 5.7 days), blood and milk levels of dalteparin were determined 3-4 hours post-treatment.[2]   Following subcutaneous doses of 2500 IU, maternal plasma levels averaged 0.074 to 0.308 IU/mL.   Breastmilk levels of dalteparin ranged from < 0.005 to 0.037 IU/mL of milk. The milk/plasma ratio ranged from 0.025 to 0.224. Using this data, an infant ingesting 150 mL/kg/day would ingest approximately 5.5 IU/kg/day. Due to the polysaccharide nature of this production, oral absorption is unlikely. Further, because this study was done early postpartum, it is possible that the levels in 'mature' milk would be lower. The authors suggest that "it appears highly unlikely that puerperal thromboprophylaxis with LMWH has any clinically relevant effect on the nursing infant". Although the RID appears high, it would be largely unabsorbable.

Pregnancy Risk Category: B

Lactation Risk Category: L2

Adult Concerns: Anticoagulant effects in adults when administered subcutaneously.

Pediatric Concerns: Transfer to milk is low. Oral bioavailability is minimal. Side effects remote. No adverse effects were reported.

Drug Interactions:

Theoretic Infant Dose: 5.5 IU/kg/d

Relative Infant Dose: 2-35.7% (unabsorbable)

Adult Dose: 2500 units daily

Alternatives: Enoxaparin.

$T\frac{1}{2}$ =	2.3 hours	M/P =	0.025-0.224
PHL =		PB =	
T_{max} =	2-4 hours (SC)	Oral =	None
MW =	4000	pKa =	
Vd =	0.06		

References:
1. Harenberg J, Leber G, Zimmermann R, Schmidt W. [Prevention of thromboembolism with low-molecular weight heparin in pregnancy]. Geburtshilfe Frauenheilkd 1987; 47(1):15-18.
2. Richter C, Sitzmann J, Lang P, Weitzel H, Huch A, Huch R. Excretion of low molecular weight heparin in human milk. Br J Clin Pharmacol 2001; 52(6):708-710.

DANAZOL

Trade: Danocrine
Can/Aus/UK: Cyclomen, Azol, Danocrine, Danol
Uses: Synthetic androgen, antigonadotropic agent
LRC: L5
AAP: Not reviewed

Danazol suppresses the pituitary-ovarian axis by inhibiting output of pituitary and hypothalamic hormones. It also appears to inhibit the synthesis of sex steroids and provides antiestrogenic effects.[1] It is primarily used for treating endometriosis. Due to its effect on pituitary hormones and its androgenic effects, it may reduce the rate of breastmilk production although this has not been documented. No data on its transfer to human milk are available.

Pregnancy Risk Category: X

Lactation Risk Category: L5

Adult Concerns: Breast size reduction. Androgenic effects, hirsutism, acne, weight gain, edema, testicular atrophy, thrombocytopenia, thrombocytosis, hot flashes, breakthrough menstrual bleeding.

Pediatric Concerns: None reported, but caution is urged.

Drug Interactions: Decreased insulin requirements. May increase anticoagulation with warfarin therapy.

Theoretic Infant Dose:

Relative Infant Dose:

Adult Dose: 50-200 mg BID

Alternatives:

$T\frac{1}{2}$ =	4.5 hours	M/P =	
PHL =		PB =	
T_{max} =	2 hours	Oral =	Complete
MW =	337	pKa =	
Vd =			

References:
1. Pharmaceutical Manufacturers prescribing information, 2003.

DANTROLENE

Trade: Dantrium
Can/Aus/UK: Dantrium
Uses: Skeletal muscle relaxant
LRC: L4
AAP: Not reviewed

Dantrolene produces a direct skeletal muscle relaxation and is indicated for spasticity resulting from upper motor neuron disorders such as multiple sclerosis, cerebral palsy, etc.[1] It is not indicated for rheumatic disorders or musculoskeletal trauma. No data on transfer into human milk are available.

Pregnancy Risk Category: C

Lactation Risk Category: L4

Adult Concerns: Adverse effects are quite common and include weakness, dizziness, diarrhea, slurred speech, drooling, and nausea. Significant risk for hepatotoxicity. Visual and auditory hallucinations.

Pediatric Concerns: None reported, but caution is urged.

Drug Interactions: Increased toxicity with estrogens, CNS sedatives, MAO inhibitors, phenothiazines, calcium channel blockers, warfarin, and tolbutamide.

Theoretic Infant Dose:

Relative Infant Dose:

Adult Dose: 1-2 mg/kg TID-QID

Alternatives:

$T\frac{1}{2}$ =	8.7 hours	M/P =	
PHL =	7.3 hours	PB =	
T_{max} =	5 hours	Oral =	35%
MW =	314	pKa =	
Vd =			

References:
1. Pharmaceutical Manufacturer Prescribing Information. 1997.

DAPSONE

Trade: Dapsone
Can/Aus/UK: Avlosulfon, Maloprim
Uses: Sulfone antibiotic
LRC: L4
AAP: Maternal Medication Usually Compatible with Breastfeeding

Dapsone is a sulfone antibiotic useful for treating leprosy, tuberculoid leprosy, dermatitis herpetiformis, and pneumocystis carinii pneumonia. In one case report of a mother consuming 50 mg daily while breastfeeding, both the mother and infant had symptoms of hemolytic anemia.[1] Plasma levels of dapsone in mother and infant were 1622 ng/mL and 439 ng/mL respectively. Breastmilk levels were reported to be 1092 μg/L. In another study of 3 patients receiving 100 mg/day, milk levels averaged 580 μg/L, but these were not at steady state levels.[2] The authors estimated the dose via milk was 4.6 to 14.3% of the maternal dose.

Dapsone is one of those drugs which apparently has all the proper kinetic parameters to enter milk: high lipophilicity, low molecular weight, high volume of distribution, high pKa, etc. While it is approved by the AAP, this is one exception that should be used very cautiously, if at all.

Pregnancy Risk Category: C

Lactation Risk Category: L4

Adult Concerns: Adverse effects reported include hemolytic anemia (particularly in G6PD deficient persons), methemoglobinemia, aplastic anemia, psychotic episodes, peripheral neuropathy, acute renal failure, nephrotic syndrome, hepatotoxicity, exfoliative dermatitis, erythema multiforme, toxic epidermal necrolysis, and hypersensitivity reactions

Pediatric Concerns: Hemolytic anemia in one breastfeeding patient. Caution is recommended.

Drug Interactions: Increased dapsone levels when taken with Amprenavir, trimethoprim, delavirdine, and probenecid. Dapsone may increase chloramphenicol plasma levels. Rifampin may decrease plasma levels of dapsone. Concomitant administration of zidovudine with drugs like dapsone which are cytotoxic or suppress bone marrow function may increase the risk of hematologic toxicity

Theoretic Infant Dose: 163.8 μg/kg/day

Relative Infant Dose: 22.9%

Adult Dose: 100 mg daily

Alternatives:

T½ =	28 hours	M/P =	
PHL =		PB =	70-90%
T$_{max}$ =	4-8 hours	Oral =	86-100%
MW =	248	pKa =	
Vd =	1-2		

References:
1. Sanders SW, Zone JJ, Foltz RL, Tolman KG, Rollins DE. Hemolytic anemia induced by dapsone transmitted through breastmilk. Ann Intern Med 1982; 96(4):465-466.
2. Edstein MD, Veenendaal JR, Newman K, Hyslop R. Excretion of chloroquine, dapsone and pyrimethamine in human milk. Br J Clin Pharmacol 1986; 22(6):733-735.

DAPTOMYCIN
Trade: Cubicin
Can/Aus/UK:
Uses: Antibiotic for resistant staphylococcus infections.
LRC: L3
AAP: Not reviewed

Daptomycin is used intravenously for the treatment of complicated skin and skin structure infections caused by susceptible strains of Staphylococcus aureus (including methicillin-resistant or MRSA strains), Streptococcus pyogenes, S. agalactiae, S. dysgalactiae, Equisimilis, and Enterococcus faecalis.[1] While no data are available on its use in breastfeeding mothers or its transfer into human milk, it is rather unlikely this antibiotic will enter the milk compartment in clinically relevant amounts. Its molecular weight is large, and it is not likely to be orally bioavailable in an infant.

Pregnancy Risk Category: B

Lactation Risk Category: L3

Adult Concerns: Elevations of creatinine kinase have been reported suggesting skeletal muscle toxicity and blood tests are required weekly during treatment. Gastrointestinal disorders, injection site reactions, fever, headache, insomnia, dizziness, and rash have been infrequently reported.

Pediatric Concerns: None reported via milk. It is rather unlikely to penetrate mature milk due to its large molecular weight. It is not likely to be orally bioavailable. However some diarhea and overgrowth of C. difficle is possible.

Drug Interactions: When used with tobramycin, a small increase (12.7%) in plasma concentration of daptomycin was produced.

Theoretic Infant Dose:

Relative Infant Dose:

Adult Dose: 4 mg/kg infusions once every 24 hours for 7-14 days.

Alternatives: Nafcillin

T½ =	9 hours	M/P =		
PHL =		PB =	92%	
T$_{max}$ =	0.5 hours	Oral =	Unlikely	
MW =	1620	pKa =		
Vd =	0.9			

References:
1.   Pharmaceutical Manufacturer Prescribing Information. 2003.

DEFEROXAMINE
Trade: Desferal, Desferrioxamine
Can/Aus/UK: Desferal
Uses: Iron chelator
LRC: L3
AAP: Not reviewed

Deferoxamine is an iron-chelating agent, commonly used to facilitate the increased clearance of iron from the plasma compartment.   It is indicated for the treatment of acute iron intoxication and of chronic iron overload due to transfusion-dependent anemias.[1] No data are available on its transfer into human milk, but it is very unlikely. Further, oral bioavailability of this product is virtually nil, and it is not likely to harm a breastfeeding infant.

Pregnancy Risk Category: C

Lactation Risk Category: L3

Adult Concerns: Adverse events include flushing, pain at injection site, erythema, urticaria, hypotension and shock.   Other side effects which occur with chronic administration include allergy-type reactions, pruritus, rahs, anaphylactoid reactions, ocular and otic effects, abdominal discomfort, leg cramps, etc.

Pediatric Concerns: None reported via milk but no studies are available. Oral bioavailability is low to nil so it is not likely to be hazardous. However, observe for iron deficiency anemia.

Drug Interactions: Temporary loss of consciousness has been reported when used with prochlorperazine.   Vitamin C is commonly added to deferoxamine therapy to enhance availability of iron for absorption.

Theoretic Infant Dose:

Relative Infant Dose:

Adult Dose: 1 gm followed by 500 mg every 4 hours times two. Highly variable.

Alternatives:

$T\frac{1}{2}$ =	3-6 hours	M/P =	
PHL =		PB =	
T_{max} =		Oral =	Nil
MW =	656	pKa =	
Vd =	1.33		

References:
1.   Pharmaceutical Manufacturer Prescribing Information. 2003.

DESIPRAMINE
Trade: Pertofrane, Norpramin
Can/Aus/UK: Norpramin, Pertofrane, Novo-Desipramine
Uses: Tricyclic antidepressant
LRC: L2
AAP: Drugs whose effect on nursing infants is unknown but may be of concern

Desipramine is a prototypical tricyclic antidepressant.   In one case report, a mother taking 200 mg of desipramine at bedtime had milk/plasma ratios of 0.4 to 0.9 with milk levels ranging between 17-35 µg/L.[1] Desipramine was not found in the infant's blood although these levels are probably too low to measure. In another study of a mother consuming 300 mg of desipramine daily, the milk levels were 30% higher than the maternal serum.[2]   The milk concentrations of desipramine were reported to be 316 to 328 µg/L with peak concentrations occurring at 4 hours post-dose.   Assuming an average milk concentration of 280 µg/L an infant would receive approximately 42 µg/kg/day. No untoward effects have been reported.

Pregnancy Risk Category: C

Lactation Risk Category: L2

Adult Concerns: Anticholinergic side effects such as drying of secretions, dilated pupil, sedation, constipation, fatigue, peculiar taste.

Pediatric Concerns: None reported in several studies.

Drug Interactions: Do not use with MAO inhibitors or within two weeks of therapy. Increased effects occur following use with stimulants and benzodiazepines.   Decreased effects occur with barbiturates, carbamazepine, and phenytoin use.

Theoretic Infant Dose: 42 µg/kg/day

Relative Infant Dose: 0.98%

Adult Dose: 100-200 mg daily

Alternatives: Amoxapine, Imipramine

T½ =	7-60 hours	M/P =	0.4-0.9
PHL =		PB =	82%
T$_{max}$ =	4-6 hours	Oral =	90%
MW =	266	pKa =	9.5
Vd =	22-59		

References:
1. Sovner R, Orsulak PJ. Excretion of imipramine and desipramine in human breastmilk. Am J Psychiatry 1979; 136(4A):451-452.
2. Stancer HC, Reed KL. Desipramine and 2-hydroxydesipramine in human breastmilk and the nursing infant's serum. Am J Psychiatry 1986; 143(12):1597-1600.

DESLORATADINE
Trade: Clarinex
Can/Aus/UK: Clarinex
Uses: Antihistamine
LRC: L2
AAP: Not reviewed

Desloratadine is the active metabolite of loratadine(Claritin) and its half-life is longer than the parent compound. While we do not have specific data on desloratadine, we do have a good report on the prodrug loratadine. During 48 hours following administration of 'loratadine', the amount of loratadine transferred via milk was 4.2 µg, which was 0.01% of the administered dose.[1]   Through 48 hours, only 6.0 µg of desloratadine (active metabolite) (7.5 µg loratadine equivalents) were excreted into breastmilk, or 0.029% of the administered dose of loratadine or its active metabolite were transferred via milk to the infant. A 4 kg infant would receive only 0.46% of the loratadine dose received by the mother on a mg/kg basis (2.9 µg/kg/day). It is very unlikely this dose would present a hazard to infants. Desloratadine does not transfer into the CNS of adults, so it is unlikely to induce sedation even in infants. The half-life in neonates is not known although it is likely quite long. Pediatric formulations are available.

Note, the AAP approves the use of loratadine in breastfeeding mothers. It has not yet reviewed desloratadine.

Pregnancy Risk Category: C

Lactation Risk Category: L2

Adult Concerns: Sedation, dry mouth, fatigue, nausea, tachycardia, palpitations

Pediatric Concerns: None reported via milk. Levels of loratadine have been reported and are low. No adverse effects have been reported in breastfeeding infants with loratadine or desloratadine.

Drug Interactions: Clarithromycin, erythromycin, and ketoconazole may increase plasma levels of desloratadine but they do not appear to be hazardous.

Theoretic Infant Dose:

Relative Infant Dose: 0.029%

Adult Dose: 5 mg daily

Alternatives: Loratadine

T½ =	27 hours	M/P =	
PHL =		PB =	87%
T$_{max}$ =	3 hours	Oral =	Good
MW =	310	pKa =	
Vd =			

References:
1. Hilbert J, Radwanski E, Affrime MB et al. Excretion of loratadine in human breastmilk. J Clin Pharmacol 28:234-9, 1988.

DESMOPRESSIN ACETATE
Trade: DDAVP, Stimate
Can/Aus/UK: DDAVP, Rhinyle, Minirin, Desmospray
Uses: Synthetic antidiuretic hormone.
LRC: L2
AAP: Not reviewed

Desmopressin (DDAVP) is a small synthetic octapeptide antidiuretic hormone.[1] Desmopressin increases reabsorption of water by the collecting ducts in the kidneys resulting in decreased urinary flow (ADH effect). Generally used in patients who lack pituitary vasopressin, it is primarily used intranasally or intravenous. Unlike natural vasopressin, desmopressin has no effect on growth hormone, prolactin, or leuteinizing hormone.

Following intranasal administration, less than 10-20% is absorbed through the nasal mucosa. This peptide has been used in lactating women without effect on nursing infants.[2,3] In a study of one breastfeeding mother receiving 10 µg twice daily of DDAVP (desmopressin), maternal plasma levels peaked at 40 minutes after the dose at approximately 7 ng/L, while milk levels were virtually unchanged at 1-1.5 ng/L.[4] Because DDAVP is easily destroyed in the gastrointestinal tract by trypsin, the oral absorption of these levels in milk would be nil.

Pregnancy Risk Category: B

Lactation Risk Category: L2

Adult Concerns: Reduced urine production, edema, fluid retention

Pediatric Concerns: None reported. It is probably not absorbed orally.

Drug Interactions: Lithium, demeclocycline may decrease ADH effect. Chlorpropamide, fludrocortisone may increase ADH effect.

Theoretic Infant Dose: 0.225 ng/kg/day

Relative Infant Dose: 0.075%

Adult Dose: 10-40 μg intranasally daily

Alternatives:

T½ =	75.5 minutes	M/P =	0.2
PHL =		PB =	
T_{max} =	40 minutes	Oral =	0.16%
MW =	1069	pKa =	
Vd =			

References:
1. McEvoy GE. (ed): AFHS Drug Information. 1992.
2. Hime MC, Richardson JA. Diabetes insipidus and pregnancy. Case report, incidence and review of literature. Obstet Gynecol Surv 1978; 33(6):375-379.
3. Hadi HA, Mashini IS, Devoe LD. Diabetes insipidus during pregnancy complicated by preeclampsia. A case report. J Reprod Med 1985; 30(3):206-208.
4. Burrow GN, Wassenaar W, Robertson GL, Sehl H. DDAVP treatment of diabetes insipidus during pregnancy and the post-partum period. Acta Endocrinol (Copenh) 1981; 97(1):23-25.

DESOGESTREL + ETHINYL ESTRADIOL

Trade: Mircette, Cyclessa
Can/Aus/UK:
Uses: Low dose oral contraceptive
LRC: L3
AAP: Not reviewed

Mircette is a somewhat atypical lower-dose estrogen/progestin oral contraceptive. It contains a potent progestin desogestrel in combination with 10 or 20 micrograms/day of ethinyl estradiol (EE).[1] While most oral contraceptives contain 40 micrograms of EE or more, the reduced level estrogen in this product may be less inhibitory of milk production as is occasionally seen with the higher dose products. Small amounts of estrogens and progestins are known to pass into milk, but long-term follow-up of children whose mothers used combination hormonal contraceptives while breastfeeding has shown no deleterious effects on infants. Estrogen-containing contraceptives may interfere with milk production by decreasing the quantity and quality of milk production.

Cyclessa contains 100-150 µg desogestrel and 25 µg of ethinyl estradiol.

Pregnancy Risk Category: X

Lactation Risk Category: L3

Adult Concerns: Observe for reduced milk production. Breakthrough bleeding is more common with this product. Fluid retention has been reported. See typical oral contraceptive contraindications.

Pediatric Concerns: Reduced milk supply is possible. Do not use early postpartum.

Drug Interactions: Reduced efficacy when used with rifampin, barbiturates, phenytoin, carbamazepine, griseofulvin, ampicillin, and tetracyclines.

Theoretic Infant Dose:

Relative Infant Dose:

Adult Dose:

Alternatives: Norethindrone

References:
1. Pharmaceutical Manufacturer package insert, 2003.

DEXAMETHASONE

Trade: Decadron, AK-Dex, Maxidex
Can/Aus/UK: AK-Dex
Uses: Corticosteroid anti-inflammatory
LRC: L3
AAP: Not reviewed

Dexamethasone is a long-acting corticosteroid similar in effect to prednisone although more potent. Dexamethasone 0.75 mg is equivalent to a 5 mg dose of prednisone.[1] While the elimination half-life is brief, only 3-6 hours in adults, its metabolic effects last for up to 72 hours. No data are available on the transfer of dexamethasone into human milk. It is likely similar to that of prednisone which is extremely low. Doses of prednisone as high as 120 mg fail to produce clinically relevant milk levels. This product is commonly used in pediatrics for treating immune syndromes such as arthritis and, particularly, acute onset asthma or other bronchoconstrictive diseases. It is not likely that the amount in milk would produce clinical effects unless used in high doses over prolonged periods.

Pregnancy Risk Category: C

Lactation Risk Category: L3

Adult Concerns: In pediatrics: shortened stature, GI bleeding, GI ulceration, edema, osteoporosis, glaucoma, and other symptoms of hyperadrenalism.

Pediatric Concerns: None reported via milk. Avoid high doses over prolonged periods of time.

Drug Interactions: Barbiturates, phenytoin, rifampin may reduce the corticosteroid effect of dexamethasone. Dexamethasone may decrease effects of vaccines, salicylates, and toxoids.

Theoretic Infant Dose:

Relative Infant Dose:

Adult Dose: 0.5-9 mg daily

Alternatives: Prednisone

$T\frac{1}{2}$ =	3.3 hours	M/P =	
PHL =		PB =	
T_{max} =	1-2 hours	Oral =	78%
MW =	392	pKa =	
Vd =	2		

References:
1. Pharmaceutical Manufacturer Prescribing Information. 1999.

DEXFENFLURAMINE

Trade: Redux
Can/Aus/UK: Adifax
Uses: Anorexigenic, diet pill
LRC: L4
AAP: Not reviewed

Dexfenfluramine is the dextrostereoisomer of fenfluramine (Pondimin) and is used for its anorexiant effect in weight reduction. It is both a serotonin reuptake inhibitor and releasing agent. It is metabolized to d-norfenfluramine (active), which has a half-life of 32 hours. Its transfer to human milk has not been reported although it is secreted in animal milk.[1,2] Due to the low molecular weight and high CNS penetration, it is likely that this product may attain moderate levels in breastmilk. Further, its long half-life and active metabolite could possibly induce higher steady state plasma levels in the neonate with corresponding anorexia and weight loss after prolonged therapy. Risk assessment with this product may not justify exposure of a breastfeeding infant.

Pregnancy Risk Category: C

Lactation Risk Category: L4

Adult Concerns: Adverse effects include diarrhea, drowsiness, dizziness, mood disorders, sleep disorders, tiredness, dry mouth, nausea, constipation, polyuria, suicide ideations, impaired concentration and memory(18%), pulmonary hypertension (1 per 22-44,000).

Pediatric Concerns: None reported, but caution urged.

Drug Interactions: Increased risk of serotonin syndrome when used with sumatriptan, dihydroergotamine, and tricyclic antidepressants. Increased toxicity when used with MAO inhibitors. Allow at least 14 days after MAOI use. May cause false positive results on urine drug screens.

Theoretic Infant Dose:

Relative Infant Dose:

Adult Dose: 15 mg BID

Alternatives:

$T\frac{1}{2}$ =	17-20 hours	M/P =	
PHL =		PB =	36%
T_{max} =	2 hours	Oral =	68%
MW =	231	pKa =	
Vd =	10		

References:
1.   Drug Facts and Comparisons 1996 ed. ed. St. Louis: 1996.
2.   Pharmaceutical Manufacturer Prescribing Information. 1997.

DEXTROAMPHETAMINE

Trade: Dexedrine, Amphetamine, Oxydess, Adderall
Can/Aus/UK: Dexedrine, Dexamphetamine, Dexten
Uses: Powerful CNS stimulant
LRC: L4
AAP: Drugs of abuse for which adverse effects have been
reported

The only data available are on racemic amphetamines. Following a 20 mg daily dose of racemic amphetamine administered at 1000, 1200, 1400, and 1600 hours each day (total= 80 mg/d) to a breastfeeding mother, amphetamine concentrations were determined in milk at 10 days and 42 days postpartum.   Samples were taken at 20 min prior to the 1000 dose and immediately prior to the 1400 hour dose. Milk levels were 55 and 118 µg/L respectively.[1] Corresponding maternal plasma levels were 20 and 40 ng/mL at the same times.   Milk/plasma ratios at these times were 2.8 and 3.0 respectively. At 42 days, breastmilk levels of amphetamine were 68 and 138 µg/L while maternal plasma levels were 9 and 21 ng/mL respectively. Milk/plasma ratios in the 42 day samples were 7.5 and 6.6 respectively. Although the milk/plasma ratios appear high, using a daily milk intake of 150 mL/kg/d, the relative infant dose would be only 1.8% of the weight-normalized maternal dose, which probably accounts for the fact that the infant in this study was unaffected.

Pregnancy Risk Category: C

Lactation Risk Category: L4

Adult Concerns: Nervousness, insomnia, anorexia, hyperexcitability

Pediatric Concerns: Possible insomnia, irritability, anorexia, or poor sleeping patterns in infants. However in this study, the infant was unaffected.

Drug Interactions: May precipitate hypertensive crisis in patients on MAO inhibitors and arrhythmias in patients receiving general anesthetics. Increased effect/toxicity with tricyclic antidepressants, phenytoin, phenobarbital, norepinephrine, meperidine.

Theoretic Infant Dose: 20.7 µg/kg/day

Relative Infant Dose: 1.8%

Adult Dose: 5-60 mg daily

Alternatives:

T½ =	6-8 hours	M/P =	2.8-7.5	
PHL =		PB =	16-20%	
T$_{max}$ =	1-2 hours	Oral =	Complete	
MW =	368	pKa =	9.9	
Vd =	3.2-5.6			

References:
1. Steiner E, Villen T, Hallberg M, Rane A. Amphetamine secretion in breastmilk. Eur J Clin Pharmacol 1984; 27(1):123-124.

DEXTROMETHORPHAN
Trade: DM, Benylin, Delsym, Pertussin, Robitussin DM
Can/Aus/UK: Balminil-DM, Delsym, Benylin DM, Cosylan
Uses: Antitussive, Cough preparation
LRC: L1
AAP: Not reviewed

Dextromethorphan is a weak antitussive commonly used in infants and adults. It is a congener of codeine and appears to elevate the cough threshold in the brain. It does not have addictive, analgesic, or sedative actions, and it does not produce respiratory depression at normal doses.[1] It is the safest of the antitussives and is routinely used in children and infants. No data on its transfer to human milk are available. It is very unlikely that enough would transfer via milk to provide clinically significant levels in a breastfed infant.

Pregnancy Risk Category: C

Lactation Risk Category: L1

Adult Concerns: Drowsiness, fatigue, dizziness, hyperpyrexia

Pediatric Concerns: None reported.

Drug Interactions: May interact with MAO inhibitors producing hypotension, hyperpyrexia, nausea, coma.

Theoretic Infant Dose:

Relative Infant Dose:

Adult Dose: 10-20 mg q 4 hours

Alternatives: Codeine

$T\frac{1}{2}$ =	< 4 hours	M/P =	
PHL =		PB =	
T_{max} =	1-2 hours	Oral =	Complete
MW =	271	pKa =	8.3
Vd =			

References:
1. Pender ES, Parks BR. Toxicity with dextromethorphan-containing preparations: a literature review and report of two additional cases. Pediatr Emerg Care 1991; 7(3):163-165.

DIAZEPAM

Trade: Valium
Can/Aus/UK: Apo-Diazepam, Meval, Novo-Dipam, Vivol, Antenex, Ducene, Sedapam
Uses: Sedative, anxiolytic drug
LRC: L3
   L4 if used chronically
AAP: Drugs whose effect on nursing infants is unknown but may be of concern

Diazepam is a powerful CNS depressant and anticonvulsant. Published data on milk and plasma levels are highly variable and many are poor studies. In 3 mothers receiving 10 mg three times daily for up to 6 days, the maternal plasma levels of diazepam averaged 491 ng/mL (day 4) and 601 ng/mL (day 6).[1] Corresponding milk levels were 51 ng/mL (day 4) and 78 ng/mL (day6). The milk/plasma ratio was approximately 0.1.

In a case report of a patient taking 6-10 mg of diazepam daily, her milk levels varied from 7.5 to 87 µg/L.[2] In a study of 9 mothers receiving diazepam postpartum, milk levels of diazepam varied from approximately 0.01 to 0.08 mg/L.[3] Other reports suggest slightly higher values. Taken together, most results suggest that the dose of diazepam and its metabolite, desmethyldiazepam, to a suckling infant will be on average < 9 of the weight-adjusted maternal dose of diazepam.[4] The active metabolite, desmethyldiazepam, in general has a much longer half-life in adults and pediatric patients and may tend to accumulate on longer therapy. Some reports of lethargy, sedation, and poor suckling have been found. The acute use such as in surgical procedures is not likely to lead to significant accumulation. Long-term, sustained therapy may prove troublesome. The benzodiazepine family as a rule, are not ideal for breastfeeding mothers due to relatively long half-lives and the development of dependence. However, it is apparent that the shorter-acting benzodiazepines (lorazepam, alprazolam) are safest during lactation provided their use is short-term or intermittent, low dose, and after the first week of life.[5]

Pregnancy Risk Category: **D**

Lactation Risk Category: **L3**
                                                  L4 if used chronically

Adult Concerns: Adverse reactions include drowsiness, dizziness, blurred vision, dry mouth, headache, fatigue, ataxia, slurred speech, and mental confusion.

Pediatric Concerns: Some reports of lethargy, sedation, poor suckling have been found.

Drug Interactions: May increase sedation when used with CNS depressants such as alcohol, barbiturates, opioids. Cimetidine may decrease metabolism and clearance of diazepam. Cisapride can dramatically increase plasma levels of diazepam. Valproic may displace diazepam from binding sites, thus increasing sedative effects. SSRIs (fluoxetine, sertraline, paroxetine) can dramatically increase diazepam levels by altering clearance, thus leading to sedation .

Theoretic Infant Dose: 13 µg/kg/day

Relative Infant Dose: < 9.13%

Adult Dose: 2-10 mg BID to QID

Alternatives: Lorazepam, Midazolam

$T^{1/2}$ =	43 hours	M/P =	0.2-2.7
PHL =	20-50hours(full-term neonate)	PB =	99%
T_{max} =	1-2 hours	Oral =	Complete
MW =	285	pKa =	3.4
Vd =	0.7-2.6		

References:

1. Erkkola R, Kanto J. Diazepam and breast-feeding. Lancet 1972; 1(7762):1235-1236.
2. Wesson DR, Camber S, Harkey M, Smith DE. Diazepam and desmethyldiazepam in breastmilk. J Psychoactive Drugs 1985; 17(1):55-56.
3. Cole AP, Hailey DM. Diazepam and active metabolite in breastmilk and their transfer to the neonate. Arch Dis Child 1975; 50(9):741-742.
4. Spigset O. Anaesthetic agents and excretion in breastmilk. Acta Anaesthesiol Scand 1994; 38(2):94-103.
5. Maitra R, Menkes DB. Psychotropic drugs and lactation. N Z Med J 1996; 109(1024):217-218.

DIBUCAINE
Trade: Nupercainal
Can/Aus/UK: Nupercainal, Cinchocaine, Nupercaine, Ultraproct, Dermacaine
Uses: Local anesthetic
LRC: L3
AAP: Not reviewed

Dibucaine is a long-acting local anesthetic generally used topically. It is primarily used topically in creams and ointments, and due to toxicity, has been banned in the USA for IV or IM injections.[1]   No data are available on transfer to breastmilk. Dibucaine is effective for sunburn, topical burns, rash, rectal hemorrhoids, and other skin irritations. Long-term use and use over large areas of the body are discouraged. Although somewhat minimal, some dibucaine can be absorbed from irritated skin.

Pregnancy Risk Category: C

Lactation Risk Category: L3

Adult Concerns: Rash or allergic symptoms

Pediatric Concerns: None reported via milk.

Drug Interactions:

Theoretic Infant Dose:

Relative Infant Dose:

Adult Dose: 10-30 g daily
Alternatives:

T½ =		M/P =
PHL =		PB =
T$_{max}$ =		Oral =
MW =	379	pKa =
Vd =		

References:
1. Pharmaceutical Manufacturer Prescribing Information. 1995.

DICLOFENAC

Trade: Cataflam, Voltaren
Can/Aus/UK: Voltaren, Apo-Diclo, Novo-Difenac, Fenac, Voltarol
Uses: NSAID analgesic for arthritis
LRC: L2
AAP: Not reviewed

Diclofenac is a typical nonsteroidal analgesic (NSAID). Voltaren is a sustained release product whereas Cataflam is an immediate release product. In one study of six postpartum mothers receiving three 50 mg doses on day 1, followed by two 50 mg doses on day 2, the levels of diclofenac in breastmilk were approximately 5 ng/mL of milk although the limit of detection was reported as < 19 ng/mL.[1]

In another patient on long-term treatment with diclofenac, milk levels of 0.1 μg/mL milk were reported which would amount to 0.015 mg/kg/d ingested.[2] These amounts are probably far too low to affect an infant.

Pregnancy Risk Category: B

Lactation Risk Category: L2

Adult Concerns: GI distress, diarrhea, nausea, vomiting

Pediatric Concerns: None reported via milk. Milk levels are extremely low.

Drug Interactions: May prolong prothrombin time when used with warfarin. Antihypertensive effects of ACEi family may be blunted or completely abolished by NSAIDs. Some NSAIDs may block antihypertensive effect of beta blockers, diuretics. Used with cyclosporin, may dramatically increase renal toxicity. May increase digoxin, phenytoin, lithium levels. May increase toxicity of methotrexate. May increase bioavailability of penicillamine. Probenecid may increase NSAID levels.

Theoretic Infant Dose: 0.015 mg/kg/day

Relative Infant Dose: 1%

Adult Dose: 75 mg BID

Alternatives: Ibuprofen

T½ =	1.1 hours	M/P =	
PHL =		PB =	99.7%
Tmax =	1 hour (Cataflam)	Oral =	Complete
MW =	318	pKa =	4.0
Vd =	0.55		

References:
1. Sioufi A. et.al. Recent findings concerning clinically relevant pharmacokinetics of diclofenac sodium. In: Kass(ed), Voltaren-new findings. Hans Huber Publishers, Bern, 1982.
2. Pharmaceutical Manufacturer Prescribing Information.

DICLOXACILLIN
Trade: Pathocil, Dycill, Dynapen
Can/Aus/UK: Dynapen, Diclocil, Dicloxsig
Uses: Penicillin antibiotic
LRC: L1
AAP: Not reviewed

Dicloxacillin is an oral penicillinase-resistant penicillin frequently used for peripheral (non CNS) infections caused by Staph. aureus and Staph. epidermidis infections, particularly mastitis. Following oral administration of a 250 mg dose, milk concentrations of the drug were 0.1, and 0.3 mg/L at 2 and 4 hours after the dose respectively.[1] Levels were undetectable after 6 hours.

Pregnancy Risk Category: B

Lactation Risk Category: L1

Adult Concerns: Elimination is delayed in neonates. Rash, diarrhea.

Pediatric Concerns: None reported via milk.

Drug Interactions: May increase effect of oral anticoagulants. Disulfiram, probenecid may increase levels of penicillin. May reduce efficacy of oral contraceptives.

Theoretic Infant Dose: 45 µg/kg/day

Relative Infant Dose: 1.2%

Adult Dose: 125-250 mg q 6 hours

Alternatives:

T½ =	0.6-0.8 hour	M/P =	
PHL =	1.9 hours	PB =	96%
Tmax =	0.5-2 hours	Oral =	35-76%
MW =	470	pKa =	
Vd =			

References:
1. McEvoy GE. (ed):AFHS Drug Information. New York, NY: 2003.

DICYCLOMINE

Trade: Bentyl, Antispas, Spasmoject
Can/Aus/UK: Bentylol, Formulex, Lomine, Merbentyl
Uses: Anticholinergic, drying agent.
LRC: L4
AAP: Not reviewed

Dicyclomine is a tertiary amine antispasmodic. It belongs to the family of anticholinergics such as atropine and the belladonna alkaloids. It was previously used for infant colic but due to overdoses and reported apnea, it is seldom recommended for this use. Infants are exceedingly sensitive to anticholinergics, particularly in the neonatal period.

Following a dose of 20 mg in a lactating woman, a 12 day old infant reported severe apnea. The manufacturer reports milk levels of 131 μg/L with corresponding maternal serum levels of 59 μg/L.[1] The reported milk/plasma level was 2.22.

Pregnancy Risk Category: B

Lactation Risk Category: L4

Adult Concerns: Apnea, dry secretions, urinary hesitancy, dilated pupils

Pediatric Concerns: Severe apnea in one 12 day old infant. Observe for anticholinergic symptoms, drying, constipation, rapid heart rate.

Drug Interactions: Decreased effect with antacids, phenothiazines, haloperidol. Increased toxicity when used with other anticholinergics, amantadine, opiates, antiarrhythmics, antihistamines, tricyclic antidepressants.

Theoretic Infant Dose: 19.65 μg/kg/day

Relative Infant Dose: 6.8%

Adult Dose: 20-40 mg QID

Alternatives:

$T\frac{1}{2}$ =	9-10 hours	M/P =	2.22
PHL =		PB =	
T_{max} =	1-1.5 hours	Oral =	67%
MW =	345	pKa =	
Vd =			

References:
1. Pharmaceutical Manufacturer Prescribing Information. 1999.

DIETHYL ETHER
Trade: Diethyl Ether, Ether
Can/Aus/UK:
Uses: Anesthetic
LRC: L4
AAP: Not reviewed

Ether is seldom used today. Although some would be transferred into human milk, it would rapidly redistribute back to the blood and be eliminated, particularly if the mother were to withhold breastmilk for at least 12 or more hours after administration.

Pregnancy Risk Category:

Lactation Risk Category: **L4**

Adult Concerns: GI distress, unique ether odor

Pediatric Concerns:

Drug Interactions:

Theoretic Infant Dose:

Relative Infant Dose:

Adult Dose:

Alternatives:

T½ =		M/P =	
PHL =		PB =	
Tmax =	10-20 minutes	Oral =	
MW =		pKa =	
Vd =			

References:

DIETHYLPROPION
Trade: Tepanil, Tenuate
Can/Aus/UK: Tenuate, Dospan
Uses: Anorexiant
LRC: L5
AAP: Not reviewed

Diethylpropion belongs to the amphetamine family and is typically used to reduce food intake. No data available other than manufacturer states this medication is secreted into breastmilk.[1] Diethylpropion's structure is similar to amphetamines. Upon withdrawal, significant withdrawal symptoms have been reported in adults. Such symptoms could be observed in breastfeeding infants of mothers using this product. The use of this medication during lactation is simply unrealistic and not justified.

Pregnancy Risk Category: B

Lactation Risk Category: L5

Adult Concerns: Overstimulation, insomnia, anorexia, jitteriness, rapid heart rate, elevated blood pressure

Pediatric Concerns: None reported, but observe for anorexia, agitation, insomnia.

Drug Interactions: Increased toxicity with MAO inhibitors, CNS depressants, general anesthetics (arrhythmias), other adrenergics.

Theoretic Infant Dose:

Relative Infant Dose:

Adult Dose: 25 mg TID

Alternatives:

T½ =	8 hours	M/P =		
PHL =		PB =		
T$_{max}$ =	2 hours	Oral =	70%	
MW =	205	pKa =		
Vd =				

References:
1. Pharmaceutical Manufacturer Prescribing Information. 1995.

DIETHYLSTILBESTROL
Trade: DES
Can/Aus/UK: Honvol, Fosfestrol, Apstil
Uses: Synthetic estrogen
LRC: L5
AAP: Not reviewed

Diethylstilbestrol is a synthetic estrogen that is seldom used today. It is known to produce a high risk of cervical cancer in female infants exposed during pregnancy.[1,2] It has been shown to cause anatomical abnormalities in males and females, neoplasia, reduced fertility, and immunologic changes. Its effect in the breastfeeding infant is unknown but should be absolutely avoided. DES would probably inhibit milk production. Strongly suggest using other estrogens during breastfeeding if absolutely mandatory. Contraindicated.

Pregnancy Risk Category: X

Lactation Risk Category: **L5**

Adult Concerns: Decreased breastmilk production

Pediatric Concerns: None reported via milk, but this product is too dangerous for use in breastfeeding mothers.

Drug Interactions:

Theoretic Infant Dose:

Relative Infant Dose:

Adult Dose: 15 mg daily
Alternatives:

$T\frac{1}{2}$ =		M/P =	
PHL =		PB =	
T_{max} =		Oral =	Complete
MW =	268	pKa =	
Vd =			

References:
1. O'Brien TE. Excretion of drugs in human milk. Am J Hosp Pharm 1974; 31(9):844-854.
2. Shapiro S, Slone D. The effects of exogenous female hormones on the fetus. Epidemiol Rev 1979; 1:110-123.

DIFLUNISAL

Trade: Dolobid
Can/Aus/UK: Apo-Diflunisal, Dolobid, Novo-Diflunisal
Uses: Nonsteroidal anti-inflammatory analgesic
LRC: L3
AAP: Not reviewed

Diflunisal is a derivative of salicylic acid. Diflunisal is excreted into human milk in concentrations 2-7% of the maternal plasma levels.[1] No reports of side-effects have been located. This product is potentially a higher risk NSAID and other less toxic compounds should be used.

Pregnancy Risk Category: C in 1st and 2nd trimester
D in 3rd trimester

Lactation Risk Category: **L3**

Adult Concerns: Prolonged bleeding time, headache, GI distress, diarrhea, GI cramping, fluid retention. Ulcer complications. Worsening hypertension.

Pediatric Concerns: None reported but alternatives are suggested.

Drug Interactions: Antacids reduce effect. Increased toxicity of digoxin, methotrexate, anticoagulants, phenytoin, sulfonylureas, lithium, acetaminophen.

Theoretic Infant Dose:

Relative Infant Dose:

Adult Dose: 500 mg BID or TID

Alternatives: Ibuprofen, celecoxib

T½ =	8-12 hours	M/P =	
PHL =		PB =	99%
T$_{max}$ =	2-3 hours	Oral =	Complete
MW =	250	pKa =	
Vd =	0.1-0.2		

References:
1.   Pharmaceutical Manufacturer Prescribing Information. 1995.

DIGITOXIN
Trade: Crystodigin
Can/Aus/UK: Digitaline
Uses: Cardiac stimulant
LRC: L3
AAP: Not reviewed

No data available on digitoxin and its transfer to human milk.[1] Digitoxin is occasionally given to infants. High lipid solubility and good oral bioavailability would suggest some transfer into breastmilk.   See digoxin.

Pregnancy Risk Category: C

Lactation Risk Category: L3

Adult Concerns: Nausea, vomiting, anorexia, cardiac arrhythmias

Pediatric Concerns: None reported thus far.

Drug Interactions: Reduced plasma levels when used with antacids, penicillamine, bran fiber, sucralfate, cholestyramine, rifampin, etc. Increased toxicity when used with diltiazem, ibuprofen, cimetidine, omeprazole, etc.

Theoretic Infant Dose:

Relative Infant Dose:

Adult Dose: 0.15 mg daily

Alternatives:

T½ =	6.7 days	M/P =	
PHL =		PB =	97%
T$_{max}$ =	4 hours	Oral =	90-100%
MW =	765	pKa =	
Vd =	7 (variable)		

References:
1. Levy M, Granit L, Laufer N. Excretion of drugs in human milk. N Engl J Med 1977; 297(14):789.

DIGOXIN

Trade: Lanoxin, Lanoxicaps
Can/Aus/UK: Lanoxin, Novo-Digoxin
Uses: Cardiac stimulant
LRC: L2
AAP: Maternal Medication Usually Compatible with Breastfeeding

Digoxin is a cardiac stimulant used primarily to strengthen the contractile process. In one mother receiving 0.25 mg digoxin daily, the amount found in breastmilk ranged from 0.96 to 0.61 μg/L at 4 and 6 hours post-dose respectively.[1] Mean peak breastmilk levels varied from 0.78 μg/L in one patient to 0.41 μg/L in another. Plasma levels in the infants were undetectable. In another study of 5 women receiving digoxin therapy, the average breastmilk concentration was 0.64 μg/L.[2] From these studies, it is apparent that a breastfeeding infant would receive less than 1 μg/day of digoxin, too low to be clinically relevant. The small amounts secreted into breastmilk have not produced problems in nursing infants. Poor and erratic GI absorption could theoretically reduce absorption in nursing infant.

Pregnancy Risk Category: C

Lactation Risk Category: L2

Adult Concerns: Nausea, vomiting, bradycardia, arrhythmias

Pediatric Concerns: None reported in several studies.

Drug Interactions: Too numerous to list all. Decreased digoxin effect when used with antacids, bran fiber, sucralfate, sulfasalazine, diuretics, phenytoin, cholestyramine, aminoglutethimide. Increase digoxin effects may result when used with diltiazem, ibuprofen, cimetidine, omeprazole, bepridil, reserpine, amphotericin B, erythromycin, quinine, tetracycline, cyclosporine, etc.

Theoretic Infant Dose: 0.096 μg/kg/day

Relative Infant Dose: 2.6%

Adult Dose: 0.125-0.5 mg daily

Alternatives:

$T\frac{1}{2}$ =	39 hours	M/P =	< 0.9
PHL =	20-180 hours	PB =	25%
T_{max} =	1.5-3 hours	Oral =	65-85%
MW =	781	pKa =	
Vd =	5.1-7.4		

References:

1. Loughnan PM. Digoxin excretion in human breastmilk. J Pediatr 1978; 92(6):1019-1020.
2. Levy M, Granit L, Laufer N. Excretion of drugs in human milk. N Engl J Med 1977; 297(14):789.

DILTIAZEM HCL

Trade: Cardizem SR, Dilacor-XR, Cardizem CD
Can/Aus/UK: Cardizem, Apo-Diltiazem, Apo-Diltiaz, Cardcal, Coras, Dilzem, Adizem, Britiazim, Tildiem
Uses: Antihypertensive, calcium channel blocker
LRC: L3
AAP: Maternal Medication Usually Compatible with Breastfeeding

Diltiazem is an typical calcium channel blocker antihypertensive.[1] In a report of a single patient receiving 240 mg/d on day 14 postpartum, levels in milk were parallel those of serum (Milk/plasma ratio is approximately 1.0).[2] Peak level in milk (and plasma) was slightly higher than 200 µg/L and occurred at 8 hours. While nifedipine is probably a preferred choice calcium channel blocker because of our experience with it, the relative infant dose with this agent is quite small and it is not likely to be problematic.

Pregnancy Risk Category: C

Lactation Risk Category: L3

Adult Concerns: Hypotension, bradycardia

Pediatric Concerns: Hypotension, bradycardia is possible. See nifedipine.

Drug Interactions: H-2 blockers may increase bioavailability of diltiazem. Beta blockers may increase cardio depressant effect. May increase cyclosporine, and carbamazepine levels. Fentanyl may increase hypotension.

Theoretic Infant Dose: 30 µg/kg/day

Relative Infant Dose: 0.87%

Adult Dose: 30-90 mg QID

Alternatives: Nifedipine, Nimodipine, Verapamil

T½ =	3.5-6 hours	M/P =	1.0
PHL =		PB =	78%
T$_{max}$ =	2-3 hours	Oral =	40-60%
MW =	433	pKa =	
Vd =	1.7		

References:
1. Pharmaceutical Manufacturer Prescribing Information. 1995.
2. Okada M, Inoue H, Nakamura Y, Kishimoto M, Suzuki T. Excretion of diltiazem in human milk. N Engl J Med 1985; 312(15):992-993.

DIMENHYDRINATE

Trade: Marmine, Dramamine
Can/Aus/UK: Gravol, Traveltabs, Andrumin, Travacalm, Dramamine
Uses: Antihistamine for vertigo and motion sickness
LRC: L2
AAP: Not reviewed

Consists of 55% diphenhydramine and 45% of 8-chlorotheophylline. Diphenhydramine (Benadryl) is considered to be the active ingredient. See Benadryl.

Pregnancy Risk Category: B

Lactation Risk Category: L2

Adult Concerns: Sedation, dry secretions

Pediatric Concerns: None reported but observe for sedation. See diphenhydramine.

Drug Interactions: May enhance CNS depressants, anticholinergics, tricyclic antidepressants, and MAO exhibitors. Increased toxicity of antibiotics, especially aminoglycosides "ototoxicity".

Theoretic Infant Dose:

Relative Infant Dose:

Adult Dose: 50-100 mg q 4-6 hours

Alternatives: Cetirizine, loratadine

$T\frac{1}{2}$ =	8.5 hours	M/P =	
PHL =		PB =	78%
T_{max} =	1-2 hours	Oral =	
MW =	470	pKa =	
Vd =			

References:
1. Pharmaceutical Manufacturer Prescribing Information. 1995.

DIMETHYLSULFOXIDE
Trade: DMSO, Rimso-50, DMSO2, MSM
Can/Aus/UK:
Uses: Solvent used for arthritis, etc.
LRC: L3
AAP: Not reviewed

Dimethyl sulfoxide (DMSO) is a solvent that has been found useful for musculo skeletal inflammation and injury and interstitial cystitis. It has been used topically, orally, and intravenously. DMSO is relatively nontoxic, requiring rather large intravenous doses to induce toxicity (20 gm). Following dermal application of 1g/kg (640 mL/70 kg), reported serum concentrations were 560 mg/L within 4-8 hours. By 48 hours only traces were detectable.[1] Daily oral doses of 32 mL/70 kg for 14 days produced peak serum levels of 1850 mg/L. DMSO penetrates to many compartment, and it would probably penetrate into milk in significant quantities. Due to the high plasma levels above, it is probable that milk levels would be quite high as well. Although the overall toxicity of this compound is quite minimal, exposing an infant to this agent, which is minimally efficacious, is probably not justified. DMSO is capable of transporting most substances across the skin. When contaminated with other solvents it can become quite dangerous. Only highly purified products should be used.

Methylsulfonylmethane (DMSO2, MSM, "Crystalline DMSO") is the normal oxidation product of DMSO. No data are available on this product, but it is probably distributed and eliminated the same as DMSO above.

Pregnancy Risk Category: C

Lactation Risk Category: L3

Adult Concerns: DMSO imparts a garlic-like breath, taste and body odor to all users. GI disturbances including vomiting and nausea, drowsiness, sedation, neuropathy, dizziness, headache, and dermatologic rash have been reported. Heapatotoxicity, milk jaundice, and heaptic precoma was reported in two elderly patients receiving IV infusions of 100 g of 20% DMSO.

Pediatric Concerns: None reported. This agent is not particularly effective therefore the risks do not justify its use in breastfeeding mothers.

Drug Interactions:

Theoretic Infant Dose:

Relative Infant Dose:

Adult Dose: Variable

Alternatives:

T½ =	11-14 hours (dermal)	M/P =	
PHL =		PB =	
T$_{max}$ =	4-8 hours(topically)	Oral =	Complete
MW =		pKa =	
Vd =	0.53		

References:
1   Baselt RC. Disposition of toxic drugs and chemicals in man. Foster City, CA: Chemical Toxicology Institute, 2000: 282-283.

DINOPROSTONE

Trade: Prostin E2, Prepidil, Cervidil
Can/Aus/UK: Cervidil, Propress
Uses: Prostaglandin E-2
LRC: L3
AAP: Not reviewed

Dinoprostone is a naturally occurring prostaglandin E2 that is primarily used for induction of labor, for cervical ripening, as an abortifacient, for postpartum bleeding, and for uterine atony.[1]   Available as a vaginal gel or insert, it is slowly absorbed into the plasma where it is rapidly cleared and metabolized by most tissues and the lung. Its half-life is a brief 2.5 to 5 minutes although absorption from the vaginal mucosa is slow. Neonatal effects from maternal dinoprostone include fetal heart rate abnormalities and neonatal jaundice.   The amount of dinoprostone entering milk is not known, but a brief wash out period would preclude any possible side effects.

However, dinoprostone has been used to suppress lactation.   When used orally (Prostin E2, 2 mg orally/d on day 3 and 4; then 6 mg/d thereafter) it has been found to significantly suppress milk production.[2,3]   However, the use of prostaglandin E2 products for cervical ripening (during delivery) is generally brief and probably does not clinically impact the production of breastmilk many hours or days later.

Pregnancy Risk Category: **C in 1st & 2nd trimester**
                            X in 3rd trimester

Lactation Risk Category: **L3**

Adult Concerns: Side effects of vaginal dinoprostone are numerous and include: abortion, labor induction, blood loss, hypotension, syncope, tachycardia, dizziness, hyperthermia, nausea, vomiting, diarrhea, and taste disorders.

Pediatric Concerns: None reported via milk, but a washout period is suggested.

Drug Interactions:

Theoretic Infant Dose:

Relative Infant Dose:

Adult Dose: 10-20 mg X 1-2

Alternatives:

$T^{1/2}$ =	2.5-5 minutes	M/P =	
PHL =		PB =	High
T_{max} =	0.5-1 hour	Oral =	
MW =		pKa =	
Vd =			

References:
1. Pharmaceutical Manufacturer Prescribing Information. 1999.
2. Caminiti F, De Murtas M, Parodo G, Lecca U, Nasi A. Decrease in human plasma prolactin levels by oral prostaglandin E2 in early puerperium. J Endocrinol 1980; 87(3):333-337.
3. Nasi A, De Murtas M, Parodo G, Caminiti F. Inhibition of lactation by prostaglandin E2. Obstet Gynecol Surv 1980; 35(10):619-620.

DIPHENHYDRAMINE
Trade: Benadryl, Cheracol
Can/Aus/UK: Allerdryl, Benadryl, Insomnal, Nytol, Delixir, Paedamin
Uses: Antihistamine, antitussive
LRC: L2
AAP: Not reviewed

Small but unreported levels are thought to be secreted into breastmilk.[1,2] In rodents, the milk/plasma ratio has been reported to be 3.85-9.54, although the total transfer was minimal. At present we do not have data on levels in breastmilk. However, the use of this sedating antihistamine in breastfeeding mothers is not ideal. Non-sedating antihistamines are generally preferred.

Pregnancy Risk Category: C

Lactation Risk Category: **L2**

Adult Concerns: Sedation, drowsiness

Pediatric Concerns: None reported, but observe for sedation. Some suggestions of reduced milk supply but these are unsubstantiated.

Drug Interactions: Increased sedation when used with other CNS depressants. MAO inhibitors may increase anticholinergic side effects.

Theoretic Infant Dose:

Relative Infant Dose:

Adult Dose: 25-50 mg TID or QID

Alternatives: Cetirizine, Loratadine

T½ =	4.3 hours	M/P =	
PHL =		PB =	78%
T$_{max}$ =	2-3 hours	Oral =	43-61%
MW =	255	pKa =	8.3
Vd =	3-4		

References:
1. O'Brien TE. Excretion of drugs in human milk. Am J Hosp Pharm 1974; 31(9):844-854.
2. Paton DM, Webster DR. Clinical pharmacokinetics of H1-receptor antagonists (the antihistamines). Clin Pharmacokinet 1985; 10(6):477-497.

DIPHENOXYLATE

Trade: Lomotil, Lofene
Can/Aus/UK: Lofenoxal, Lomotil, Tropergen
Uses: Antidiarrheal
LRC: L3
AAP: Not reviewed

Lomotil is a combination product of diphenoxylate and atropine.[1] Diphenoxylate belongs to the opiate family (meperidine) and acts on the intestinal tract inhibiting GI motility and excessive GI propulsion. The drug has no analgesic activity. Although no reports on its transfer to human milk are available, it is probably secreted in breastmilk in very small quantities.[2] Some authors consider diphenoxylate to be contraindicated, but this is questionable.

Pregnancy Risk Category: C

Lactation Risk Category: L3

Adult Concerns: Anticholinergic effects such as drying, constipation, and sedation

Pediatric Concerns: None reported, but observe for dryness, constipation, sedation.

Drug Interactions: Increased toxicity when used with MAO inhibitors, CNS depressants, anticholinergics.

Theoretic Infant Dose:

Relative Infant Dose:

Adult Dose: 5 mg QID

Alternatives:

T½ =	2.5 hours	M/P =	
PHL =		PB =	
T$_{max}$ =	2 hours	Oral =	90%
MW =	453	pKa =	7.1
Vd =	3.8		

References:
1. Drug Facts and Comparisons 1994 ed. ed. St. Louis: 1994.
2. Stewart JJ. Gastrointestinal drugs. In Wilson, J.T., ed. Drugs in Breastmilk. Balgowlah, Australia ADIS Press 1981;71.

DIPHTHERIA AND TETANUS TOXOID
Trade: DT, TD
Can/Aus/UK: ADT, CDT, Triple Antigen
Uses: Vaccine
LRC: L3
AAP: Not reviewed

Diphtheria and tetanus toxoid contains large molecular weight protein toxoids. It is extremely unlikely proteins of this size would be secreted in breastmilk. No data are available on its transfer to human milk.

Pregnancy Risk Category: C

Lactation Risk Category: L3

Adult Concerns: Swelling, fretfulness, drowsiness, anorexia, vomiting

Pediatric Concerns: None reported via breastmilk exposure.

Drug Interactions:

Theoretic Infant Dose:

Relative Infant Dose:

Adult Dose: 0.5 mL injection (IM)

Alternatives:

References:

DIPHTHERIA-TETANUS-PERTUSSIS

Trade: DTAP, Acel-Imune, Tripedia, Tetramune, DPT
Can/Aus/UK:
Uses: Vaccine
LRC: L2
AAP: Not reviewed

DTP injections come in two forms: one including acellular pertussis (Acel-Imune, Tripedia) and one including whole-cell pertussis and Haemophilus Influenzae Type B Conjugate (Tetramune).[1] Both are inactivated bacterial vaccines or toxoids.

The use of pertussis vaccinations in individuals over 7 years of age is generally contraindicated. Hence there is no indication for administering this vaccine to adult mothers. Because these are inactivated bacterial products, there is no specific contraindication in breastfeeding following injection with these vaccines. The CDC states that all vaccines are safe for breastfeeding mothers.

Pregnancy Risk Category: B

Lactation Risk Category: L2

Adult Concerns: Pain, fever, swelling

Pediatric Concerns: None reported via breastmilk.

Drug Interactions: Immunosuppressive agents, high dose corticosteroids, may reduce immunogenicity.

Theoretic Infant Dose:

Relative Infant Dose:

Adult Dose: N/A

Alternatives:

References:
1. Pharmaceutical Manufacturer Prescribing Information. 1996.

DIPIVEFRIN
Trade: AK-Pro, Propine
Can/Aus/UK: PSM-Dipivefrin, Propine
Uses: Adrenergic for glaucoma
LRC: L2
AAP: Not reviewed

Dipivefrin is a synthetic amine prodrug that is metabolized to epinephrine. Because of its structure, it is more lipophilic and better absorbed into the eye; hence, it is more potent.[1,2] Following absorption into the eye, dipivefrin reduces interocular pressure. It is not known if dipivefrin enters milk, but small amounts may be present. It is unlikely that any dipivefrin or epinephrine present in milk would be orally bioavailable to the infant.

Pregnancy Risk Category: B

Lactation Risk Category: L2

Adult Concerns: Infrequently, tachycardia, arrhythmias, hypertension have occurred with intraocular epinephrine. Burning, itching, tearing, hyperemia of eyes, redness of the eyes, burning and stinging have been reported.

Pediatric Concerns: None via milk.

Drug Interactions: When admixed with a pilocarpine Ocusert system, a transient increase in myopia was reported.

Theoretic Infant Dose:

Relative Infant Dose:

Adult Dose: 1 drop affected eye q 12 hours

Alternatives:

$T^{1/2}$ =		M/P =	
PHL =		PB =	
T_{max} =	1 hour	Oral =	Minimal
MW =		pKa =	
Vd =			

References:
1. Pharmaceutical Manufacturer Prescribing Information. 1999.
2. McEvoy GE. (ed): AFHS Drug Information. New York, NY: 1999.

DIPYRIDAMOLE

Trade: Persantine
Can/Aus/UK: Apo-Dipyridamole, Novo-Dipiradol, Persantin
Uses: Vasodilator, antiplatelet agent
LRC: L3
AAP: Not reviewed

Dipyridamole is most commonly used in addition to coumarin anticoagulants to prevent thromboembolic complications of cardiac valve replacement. According to the manufacturer, only small amounts are believed to be secreted in human milk.[1] No reported untoward effects have been reported.

Pregnancy Risk Category: C

Lactation Risk Category: L3

Adult Concerns: Headache, dizziness, GI distress, nausea, vomiting, diarrhea, flushing

Pediatric Concerns: No untoward effects have been reported.

Drug Interactions: When used with Heparin, may increase anticoagulation. Theophylline may reduce the hypotensive effect of dipyridamole.

Theoretic Infant Dose:

Relative Infant Dose:

Adult Dose: 75-100 mg QID

Alternatives:

T½ =	10-12 hours	M/P =	
PHL =		PB =	91-99%
T$_{max}$ =	45-150 minutes	Oral =	Poor
MW =	505	pKa =	
Vd =	2-3		

References:
1. Pharmaceutical Manufacturer Prescribing Information. 1995.

DIRITHROMYCIN

Trade: Dynabac
Can/Aus/UK:
Uses: Macrolide antibiotic
LRC: L3
AAP: Not reviewed

Dirithromycin is a macrolide antibiotic similar to the erythromycins but is characterized by low serum levels and high tissue levels.[1]. Dirithromycin is metabolized to erythromycyclamine which is the active component. No data on the transfer of erythromycyclamine into human milk are available, but it is known to transfer into animal milk. Due to the kinetics of dirithromycin and its distribution largely to tissues, it is unlikely that major levels in milk will result. Suitable alternatives include erythromycin and azithromycin.

Pregnancy Risk Category: C

Lactation Risk Category: L3

Adult Concerns: GI distress, abdominal pain, diarrhea, nausea, vomiting, skin rash, headache and dizziness. Changes in liver function have been reported.

Pediatric Concerns: None reported via milk. Suitable alternatives are erythromycin and azithromycin.

Drug Interactions: Increased anticoagulant effect when used with warfarin, dicoumarol, phenindione, and anisindione. Dirithromycin may increase the level of astemizole significantly. May increase digoxin levels. Acute and dangerous toxicity have resulted following use of dirithromycin with ergot alkaloids. Increased serum levels of pimozide and triazolam may result.

Theoretic Infant Dose:

Relative Infant Dose:

Adult Dose: 500 mg daily

Alternatives: Azithromycin, erythromycin

T½ =	20-50 hours	M/P =	
PHL =		PB =	15-30%
T$_{max}$ =	3.9 hours	Oral =	6-14%
MW =		pKa =	
Vd =	11		

References:
1. Pharmaceutical Manufacturer Prescribing Information.

DISOPYRAMIDE

Trade: Norpace, Napamide
Can/Aus/UK: Norpace, Rythmodan, Isomide
Uses: Antiarrhythmic
LRC: L2
AAP: Maternal Medication Usually Compatible with Breastfeeding

Disopyramide is used for treating cardiac arrhythmias similar to quinidine and procainamide. Small levels are secreted into milk. Following a maternal dose of 450 mg every 8 hrs for two weeks, the milk/plasma ratio was approximately 1.06 for disopyramide and 6.24 for its active metabolite.[1] Although no disopyramide was measurable in the infant's plasma, the milk levels were 2.6-4.4 mg/L (disopyramide) and 9.6-12.3 mg/L (metabolite). Infant urine collected over an 8 hour period contained 3.3 mg/L of disopyramide. Such levels are probably too small to affect an infant. No reported side effects.

In another study, in a woman receiving 100 mg five times daily, the maternal serum level was 10.3 µmol/L and the breastmilk level was 4.0 µmol/L giving a milk/serum ratio of 0.4.[2] From these levels, an infant ingesting 1 liter of milk would receive only 1.5 mg per day. Lowest milk levels are at 6-8 hours post-dose.

Pregnancy Risk Category: C

Lactation Risk Category: L2

Adult Concerns: Dry mouth, constipation, edema, hypotension, nausea, vomiting, diarrhea

Pediatric Concerns: None reported.

Drug Interactions: Increased side effects with drugs such as phenytoin, phenobarbital, rifampin. Increased effects/toxicity with rifamycin. Increased plasma levels of digoxin.

Theoretic Infant Dose: 0.66 mg/kg/day

Relative Infant Dose: 3.42%

Adult Dose: 150 mg q 6 hours

Alternatives:

T½ =	8.3-11.65 hours	M/P =	0.4-1.06
PHL =		PB =	50%
T$_{max}$ =	2.3 hours	Oral =	60-83%
MW =	339	pKa =	8.4
Vd =	0.6-1.3		

References:

1. MacKintosh D, Buchanan N. Excretion of disopyramide in human breastmilk. Br J Clin Pharmacol 1985; 19(6):856-857.

2. Ellsworth AJ, Horn JR, Raisys VA, Miyagawa LA, Bell JL. Disopyramide and N-monodesalkyl disopyramide in serum and breastmilk. DICP 1989; 23(1):56-57.

DISULFIRAM

Trade: Antabuse
Can/Aus/UK: Antabuse
Uses: Inhibitor of alcohol metabolism.
LRC: L5
AAP: Not reviewed

Disulfiram is an old product that is occasionally used to prevent alcohol consumption in chronic alcoholics.[1,2] Disulfiram inhibits the enzyme, aldehyde dehydrogenase, (ADH) which is one of two enzymes responsible for the metabolism of alcohol. Patients receiving disulfiram, and who ingest alcohol, become extremely nauseated due to elevated plasma levels of acetaldehyde. This also results in flushing, thirst, palpitations, chest pain, vertigo, and hypotension. All sources of alcohol should be avoided including mouthwash, cough syrups, and after shave. There are no data on the transfer of disulfiram into human milk, but due to its small molecular weight, it likely penetrates milk to some degree. Because it produces an irreversible inhibition of aldehyde dehydrogenase, any absorbed via milk could potentially produce long-lasting inhibition of the infants ADH. With the ingestion of any alcohol containing product, the infant could become seriously ill. Further, because the enzyme is permanently inhibited, the individual will be susceptible to alcohol toxicity for up to 2 weeks following discontinuing of the medication. Because so many products contain small amounts of alcohol (cough syrups, etc.), the use of this product in breastfeeding mothers is extremely risky and probably does not justify continued breastfeeding unless the mother is warned and compliant.

Pregnancy Risk Category: C

Lactation Risk Category: L5

Adult Concerns: Symptoms primarily occur following ingestion of alcohol, and include: ectopic heartbeats, tachycardia, chest pain, angina, palpitations, hypertension, headache, severe nausea and vomiting, leg and muscle cramps, dyspnea and shortness of breath.

Pediatric Concerns: None reported via milk but with ingestion of alcohol could produce profound symptoms in infant.

Drug Interactions: Severe reactions may occur with any product containing alcohol. Concomitant therapy with amitriptyline or metronidazole has resulted in a confusional and psychotic mental state. When used with anisindione or dicumarol, an increased hypoprothrombinemic effect has been documented. Use with bacampicillin has resulted in an disulfiram-type reaction. Significantly increased plasma levels of chlordiazepoxide and diazepam, phenytoin and fosphenytoin when coadministered with disulfiram. An increased half-life and plasma level of desipramine.

Theoretic Infant Dose:

Relative Infant Dose:

Adult Dose: 250 mg daily

Alternatives:

T½ =		M/P =	
PHL =		PB =	96%
T$_{max}$ =	1-2 hours	Oral =	80-90%
MW =	296	pKa =	
Vd =			

References:
1. Pharmaceutical Manufacturer Prescribing Information. 1999.
2. McEvoy GE. (ed): AFHS Drug Information. New York, NY: 1999.

DOCUSATE
Trade: Colace, Docusate, Softgels, Dialose, Surfak
Can/Aus/UK: Albert Docusate, Colax-C, Colace, Surfak, Coloxyl, Rectalad, Waxsol, Audinorm, Diocotyl-medo
Uses: Laxative, stool softener
LRC: L2
AAP: Not reviewed

Docusate is a detergent commonly used as a stool softener. The degree of oral absorption is poor, but some is known to be absorbed and re-secreted in the bile. Although some drug is absorbed by mother via her GI tract, transfer into breastmilk is unknown but probably minimal. Watch for loose stools in infant. It is not likely this would be overly detrimental to a breastfed infant.

Pregnancy Risk Category: C

Lactation Risk Category: L2

Adult Concerns: Nausea, diarrhea

Pediatric Concerns: None reported. Observe for loose stools.

Drug Interactions: Decreased effect of Coumadin with high doses of docusate. Increased toxicity with mineral oil, phenolphthalein.

Theoretic Infant Dose:

Relative Infant Dose:

Adult Dose: 50-200 mg daily

Alternatives:

T½ =		M/P =	
PHL =		PB =	
T$_{max}$ =		Oral =	Poor
MW =	444	pKa =	
Vd =			

References:
1. Pharmaceutical Manufacturer Prescribing Information, 2003.

DOLASETRON MESYLATE
Trade: Anzemet
Can/Aus/UK:
Uses: Antinauseant and antiemetic
LRC: L3
AAP: Not reviewed

Dolasetron and its active metabolite, hydrodolasetron, are selective serotonin 5-HT3 receptor antagonists, primarily in the chemoreceptor trigger zone responsible for control of nausea and vomiting. It is believed that chemotherapeutic agents release serotonin in the gastrointestinal tract that then activates the 5-HT3 receptors on the vagus nerve that initiates the vomiting reflex. This product is used prior to cancer treatment chemotherapeutic agents or prior to surgery and general anesthesia.[1]

No data are available on its transfer to milk. The maximum concentration in maternal plasma would be 556 ng/mL, which is quite low. At this plasma level, an infant would likely receive far less than a milligram daily. It has been safely used in children 2 years of age at doses of 1.2 mg/kg.

Pregnancy Risk Category: B

Lactation Risk Category: L3

Adult Concerns: Changes in ECG intervals (PR, QT,JT prolongation, and QRS widening) have been reported but are dose related. Use cautiously in patients with hypokalemia or hypomagnesemia, patients on diuretics, or patients on other antiarrhythmics. Side effects include: headache, fatigue, diarrhea, bradycardia.

Pediatric Concerns: None reported via milk.

Drug Interactions: Drug-drug interactions are few but include rifampin and cimetidine.

Theoretic Infant Dose:

Relative Infant Dose:

Adult Dose: 100 mg orally

Alternatives:

$T\frac{1}{2}$ =	8.1 hours	M/P =		
PHL =		PB =	77%	
T_{max} =	1 hour	Oral =	75%	
MW =	438	pKa =		
Vd =	5.8			

References:
1.   Pharmaceutical Manufacturer Prescribing Information.

DOMPERIDONE

Trade: Motilium
Can/Aus/UK: Motilium, Motilidone
Uses: Gastrokinetic agent, galactagogue
LRC: L1
AAP: Maternal Medication Usually Compatible with Breastfeeding

Domperidone (Motilium) is a peripheral dopamine antagonist (similar to Reglan) generally used for controlling nausea and vomiting, dyspepsia, and gastric reflux. It blocks peripheral dopamine receptors in the GI wall and in the CTZ (nausea center) in the brain stem and is currently used in Canada as an antiemetic.[1] Unlike metoclopramide (Reglan), it does not enter the brain compartment, and it has few CNS effects such as depression.

It is also known to produce significant increases in prolactin levels and has proven useful as a galactagogue.[1] Serum prolactin levels have been found to increase from 8.1 ng/mL to 124.1 ng/mL in non-lactating women after one 20 mg dose.[2] Concentrations of domperidone reported in milk vary according to dose. But following a dose of 10 mg three times daily, the average concentration in milk was only 2.6 µg/L.[3]

In a study by da Silva, 16 mothers with premature infants and low milk production (mean= 112.8 mL/d in domperidone group; 48.2 mL/d in placebo group) were randomly chosen to receive placebo (n=9) or domperidone (10mg TID) (n = 7) for 7 days.[4] Milk volume increased from 112.8 to 162.2 mL/d in the domperidone group and 48.2 to 56.1 mL/d in the placebo group. Prolactin levels increased from 12.9 to 119.3 µg/L in the domperidone group and 15.6 to 18.1 µg/L in the placebo group. On day 5, the mean domperidone concentration was 6.6 ng/mL in plasma and 1.2 µg/L in breastmilk of the treated group (n=6). No adverse effects were reported in infants or mothers.

The usual oral dose for controlling GI distress is 10-20 mg three to four times daily although for nausea and vomiting the dose can be higher (up to 40 mg). The galactagogue dose is suggested to be 10-20 mg orally 3-4 times daily. At present, this product is unavailable in the USA but is available in compounding pharmacies.

Pregnancy Risk Category:

Lactation Risk Category: L1

Adult Concerns: Dry mouth, skin rash, itching, headache, thirst, abdominal cramps, diarrhea, drowsiness. Seizures have occurred rarely.

Pediatric Concerns: None reported. Considered the ideal galactalogue.

Drug Interactions: Cimetidine, famotidine, nizatidine, ranitidine (H-2 blockers) reduce absorption of domperidone. Prior use of bicarbonate reduces absorption of domperidone.

Theoretic Infant Dose: 0.18 µg/kg/day

Relative Infant Dose: 0.042%

Adult Dose: 10-20 mg 3-4 times daily

Alternatives: Metoclopramide, Cisapride

$T\frac{1}{2}$ =	7-14 hours	M/P =	0.25
PHL =		PB =	93%
T_{max} =	30 minutes	Oral =	13-17%
MW =	426	pKa =	
Vd =			

References:
1. Hofmeyr GJ, van Iddekinge B. Domperidone and lactation. Lancet 1983; 1(8325):647.
2. Brouwers JR, Assies J, Wiersinga WM, Huizing G, Tytgat GN. Plasma prolactin levels after acute and subchronic oral administration of domperidone and of metoclopramide: a cross-over study in healthy volunteers. Clin Endocrinol (Oxf) 1980; 12(5):435-440.
3. Hofmeyr GJ, van Iddekinge B, Blott JA. Domperidone: secretion in breastmilk and effect on puerperal prolactin levels. Br J Obstet Gynaecol 1985; 92(2):141-144.
4. da Silva OP, Knoppert DC, Angelini MM, Forret PA. Effect of domperidone on milk production in mothers of premature newborns: a randomized, double-blind, placebo-controlled trial. CMAJ 2001; 164(1):17-21.

DONEPEZIL

Trade: Aricept
Can/Aus/UK: Aricept
Uses: Cholinesterase inhibitor in Alzheimer's disease
LRC: L3
AAP: Not reviewed

Donepezil is a reversible inhibitor of acetylcholinesterase which ultimately increases synaptic levels of acetylcholine by inhibition of its breakdown. It is believed to improve mild to moderate dementia and cognitive function in patients with Alzheimer's disease. While this agent is only 'cleared' for treatment of patients with Alzheimer's disease, numerous other applications probably exist. No data are available on its transfer to human milk. Due to its long half-life and its ability to affect cholinergic function in all mammals, some caution is recommended in breastfeeding women until data are available.

Pregnancy Risk Category: C

Lactation Risk Category: L3

Adult Concerns: May impede bladder emptying. Seizures and convulsions have been reported. Increase gastric acid secretion. Patients at risk would be those subject to ulcers using concurrent NSAIDs. Diarrhea, nausea, vomiting, muscle cramps, fatigue, and loss of appetite have been reported. Should be used cautiously in patients with pulmonary diseases such as asthma.

Pediatric Concerns: None reported via milk.

Drug Interactions: Use cautiously with NSAIDs. Interfere with activity of anticholinergics such as atropine.

Theoretic Infant Dose:

Relative Infant Dose:

Adult Dose: 5-10 mg daily
Alternatives:

$T^{1/2}$ =	70 hours	M/P =		
PHL =		PB =	96%	
T_{max} =	3-4 hours	Oral =	100%	
MW =	415	pKa =		
Vd =	12			

References:
1. Pharmaceutical Manufacturer Prescribing Information.

DOPAMINE-DOBUTAMINE
Trade: Intropin
Can/Aus/UK: Intropin, Revimine, Dobutrex
Uses: Adrenergic stimulants
LRC: L2
AAP: Not reviewed

Dopamine and dobutamine are catecholamine pressor agents used in shock and severe hypotension.[1] They are rapidly destroyed in the GI tract and are only used IV. It is not known if they transfer into human milk, but the half-life is so short they would not last long. Dopamine, while in the plasma, significantly (> 60%) inhibits prolactin secretion and would likely inhibit lactation while being used.

Pregnancy Risk Category: C

Lactation Risk Category: L2

Adult Concerns: Stimulation, agitation, tachycardia

Pediatric Concerns: None reported. No GI absorption.

Drug Interactions: Increased effect when used with monoamine oxidase inhibitors MAO, alpha and beta adrenergic blockers, general anesthetics, and phenytoin.

Theoretic Infant Dose:

Relative Infant Dose:

Adult Dose: 5-50 µg/kg/min IV

Alternatives:

T½ =	2 minutes	M/P =	
PHL =	7 minutes	PB =	
T$_{max}$ =	5 minutes	Oral =	Poor
MW =	153	pKa =	
Vd =			

References:
1. McEvoy GE. (ed):AFHS Drug Information. New York, NY: 2003.

DORNASE
Trade: Pulmozyme
Can/Aus/UK: Pulmozyme
Uses: Mucolytic enzyme
LRC: L2
AAP: Not reviewed

Dornase is a mucolytic enzyme used in the treatment of cystic fibrosis. It is a large molecular weight peptide (260 amino acids, 37,000 daltons) that selectively digests DNA.[1] It is poorly absorbed by the pulmonary tissues. Serum levels are undetectable. Even if it were to reach the milk, it would not be orally bioavailable in the infant.

Pregnancy Risk Category: B

Lactation Risk Category: L2

Adult Concerns: Hoarseness, sore throat, facial edema

Pediatric Concerns: None reported.

Drug Interactions:

Theoretic Infant Dose:

Relative Infant Dose:

Adult Dose: 2.5 mg via inhalation

Alternatives:

T½ =		M/P =	
PHL =		PB =	
T$_{max}$ =		Oral =	None
MW =		pKa =	
Vd =			

References:
1. Pharmaceutical Manufacturer Prescribing Information. 1995.

DORZOLAMIDE
Trade: Trusopt
Can/Aus/UK: Trusopt
Uses: Glaucoma treatment
LRC: L4
AAP: Not reviewed

Dorzolamide is a carbonic anhydrase-II inhibitor used for treatment of increased intraocular pressure in glaucoma patients. It reduces intraocular pressure by reducing the production of aqueous humor.[1]

Some systemic absorption of dorzolamide is known and is primarily associated with red blood cell carbonic anhydrase. It produces sustained inhibition of erythrocyte carbonic anhydrase (T1/2 = 147 days). No data are available on levels in milk. This is an incredibly potent and long-lasting inhibitor of carbonic anhydrase. Transfer of small amounts into breastmilk over a sustained period could prove detrimental to breastfed infants. Exercise caution when using with breastfeeding mothers.

Pregnancy Risk Category: C

Lactation Risk Category: L4

Adult Concerns: Headache, vertigo, taste disorders, renal stones, burning, stinging, conjunctivitis

Pediatric Concerns: None reported via milk. Exercise caution.

Drug Interactions:

Theoretic Infant Dose:

Relative Infant Dose:

Adult Dose: 1 drop in affected eye TID

Alternatives:

References:
1. Pharmaceutical Manufacturer Prescribing Information. 1997.

DOTHIEPIN

Trade: Prothiaden
Can/Aus/UK: Dothep, Prothiaden
Uses: Tricyclic antidepressant
LRC: L2
AAP: Drugs whose effect on nursing infants is unknown but may be of concern

---

New analog of the older tricyclic antidepressant amitriptyline. Dothiepin appears in breastmilk in a concentration of 11 µg/L following a dose of 75 mg/day while the maternal plasma level was 33 µg/L.[1] If the infant ingests 150 mL/kg/day of milk, the total daily dose of dothiepin ingested by the infant in this case would be approximately 1.7 µg/kg/day, approximately 1/650th of the adult dose. In an outcome study of 15 mother/infant pairs 3-5 years postpartum, no overall cognitive differences were noted in dothiepin treated mothers/infants, suggesting that this medication did not alter cognitive abilities in breastfed infants.[2]

In a study by Ilett[3], dothiepin concentrations in the milk of 8 mothers was determined (dose ranged from 25-225 mg/day). The mean post-feeding milk/plasma ratio was 1.59 and the mean post-feeding dothiepin concentration in milk ranged from 20-475 µg/L(median=52 µg/L). Mean daily infant doses on a weight basis (in dothiepin equivalents) was 4.4% for dothiepin and its metabolites. Blood levels in all 5 infants were low (> 10 µg/L). No untoward effects were noted in any of the 8 infants following chronic maternal use.

Pregnancy Risk Category: D

Lactation Risk Category: L2

Adult Concerns: Anticholinergic side effects, such as drying of secretions, dilated pupil, sedation, dizziness, drowsiness, urinary retention

Pediatric Concerns: None reported in numerous studies.

Drug Interactions: Phenobarbital may reduce effect of dothiepin. Dothiepin blocks the hypotensive effect of guanethidine. May increase toxicity of dothiepin when used with clonidine. Dangerous when used with MAO inhibitors and other CNS depressants. May increase anticoagulant effect of coumadin, warfarin. SSRIs (Prozac, Zoloft,etc) should not be used with or soon after dothiepin or other TCAs due to serotonergic crisis.

Theoretic Infant Dose: 7.8 µg/kg/day

Relative Infant Dose: 4.4%

Adult Dose: 75-300 mg/day

Alternatives:

T½ =	14.4-23.9 hours	M/P =	0.3
PHL =		PB =	
T$_{max}$ =	3 hours	Oral =	30%
MW =	295	pKa =	
Vd =	20-92		

References:
1. Rees JA. Serum and breastmilk concentrations of dotheipin. Practitioner 1976; 217:686.
2. Buist A, Janson H. Effect of exposure to dothiepin and northiaden in breastmilk on child development. Br J Psychiatry 1995; 167(3):370-373.
3. Ilett KF, Lebedevs TH, Wojnar-Horton RE, Yapp P, Roberts MJ, Dusci LJ, Hackett LP. The excretion of dothiepin and its primary metabolites in breastmilk. Br J Clin Pharmacol 1992; 33(6):635-639.

DOXAZOSIN MESYLATE

Trade: Cardura
Can/Aus/UK: Cardura, Carduran
Uses: Antiadrenergic antihypertensive
LRC: L4
AAP: Not reviewed

Studies in lactating animals indicate milk levels that are 20 times that of maternal plasma levels, suggesting a concentrating mechanism in breastmilk.[1] It is not known if this occurs in human milk. Extreme caution recommended.

Pregnancy Risk Category: B

Lactation Risk Category: L4

Adult Concerns: Low blood pressure, malaise, and edema

Pediatric Concerns: None reported, but extreme caution is recommended.

Drug Interactions: Decreased antihypertensive effect with NSAIDs. Increased effect with other diuretics, antihypertensive medications, and particularly beta blockers.

Theoretic Infant Dose:

Relative Infant Dose:

Adult Dose: 2-4 mg daily

Alternatives: Propranolol, Metoprolol

$T\frac{1}{2}$ =	9-22 hours	M/P =	20
PHL =		PB =	98%
T_{max} =	2 hours	Oral =	62-69%
MW =	451	pKa =	
Vd =			

References:
1. Pharmaceutical Manufacturer Prescribing Information. 1995.

DOXEPIN

Trade: Adapin, Sinequan
Can/Aus/UK: Sinequan, Triadapin, Novo-Doxepin, Deptran
Uses: Antidepressant
LRC: L5
AAP: Drugs whose effect on nursing infants is unknown but may be of concern

Small but significant amounts are secreted in milk. Two published reports indicate absorption by infant varying from significant to modest. One report of dangerous sedation and respiratory arrest in one infant.[1] Doxepin has an active metabolite with long half-life (37 hrs). In one study, peak milk doxepin levels were 27 and 29 μg/L four-five hours after a dose of 25 mg, and the level of metabolite was 9 μg/L.[2] In this infant, the metabolite was believed responsible for the severe depression. Although the milk concentrations were low, the infant's plasma level of metabolite was similar to the maternal plasma level. It is apparent that the active metabolite of doxepin can concentrate in nursing infants and may be hazardous.

In another case report of a mother ingesting 35 mg/d, the infant was readmitted to the neonatal intensive care unit at day 9 postpartum because of poor sucking and swallowing, muscle hypotonia, vomiting, drowsiness, and jaundice.[3] Doxepin levels in the infant were found in small amounts. Breastmilk levels were reported at 60-100 μg/L with a milk/plasma ratio of 1.0-1.7. Upon discontinuing of breastfeeding the infant rapidly became lively and active.

Pregnancy Risk Category: C

Lactation Risk Category: L5

Adult Concerns: Respiratory arrest, sedation, dry mouth

Pediatric Concerns: One report of dangerous sedation and respiratory arrest in an infant. Poor sucking and swallowing, muscle hypotonia, vomiting, drowsiness and jaundice reported in a second infant.

Drug Interactions: Decreased effect of Doxepin when use with bretylium, guanethidine, clonidine, levodopa, ascorbic acid and cholestyramine. Increased toxicity when used with carbamazepine, amphetamines, thyroid preparations. Increased toxicity with fluoxetine, thyroid preparations, MAO inhibitors, albuterol, CNS depressants such as benzodiazepines and opiate analgesics, anticholinergics, cimetidine.

Theoretic Infant Dose: 4.35 μg/kg/day

Relative Infant Dose: 1.2%

Adult Dose: 75-300 mg daily

Alternatives: Sertraline, Paroxetine

T½ =	8-24 hours	M/P =	1.08-1.66
PHL =		PB =	80-85%
T$_{max}$ =	2 hours	Oral =	Complete
MW =	279	pKa =	8.0
Vd =	9-33		

References:

1.   Matheson I, Pande H, Alertsen AR. Respiratory depression caused by N-desmethyldoxepin in breastmilk. Lancet 1985; 2(8464):1124.
2.   Kemp J, Ilett KF, Booth J, Hackett LP. Excretion of doxepin and N-desmethyldoxepin in human milk. Br J Clin Pharmacol 1985; 20(5):497-499.
3.   Frey OR, Scheidt P, von Brenndorff AI. Adverse effects in a newborn infant breast-fed by a mother treated with doxepin. Ann Pharmacother 1999; 33(6):690-693.

DOXEPIN CREAM

Trade: Zonalon Cream
Can/Aus/UK: Zonalon
Uses: Antipruritic cream
LRC: L4
AAP: Drugs whose effect on nursing infants is unknown but may be of concern

Doxepin cream is an antihistamine-like cream used to treat severe itching. In one study of 19 women, plasma levels ranged from zero to 47 μg/L following transcutaneous absorption.[1]   Target therapeutic ranges in doxepin antidepressant therapy is 30-150 ng/mL.   Small but significant amounts are secreted in milk.   Two published reports indicate absorption by infant varying from significant to modest but only in mother consuming oral doses.[2,3] See doxepin.

Pregnancy Risk Category: B

Lactation Risk Category: L4

Adult Concerns: Respiratory arrest, sedation, dry mouth

Pediatric Concerns: Sedation, respiratory arrest have been reported following oral administration.

Drug Interactions: Decreased effect of Doxepin when use with bretylium, guanethidine, clonidine, levodopa, ascorbic acid, and cholestyramine.   Increased toxicity when used with carbamazepine, amphetamines, thyroid preparations.   Increased toxicity with fluoxetine, thyroid preparations, MAO inhibitors, albuterol, CNS depressants such as benzodiazepines and opiate analgesics, anticholinergics, cimetidine.

Theoretic Infant Dose:

Relative Infant Dose:

Adult Dose: 150-300 mg daily

Alternatives:

T½ =	28-52 hours	M/P =	1.08, 1.66
PHL =		PB =	80-85%
T$_{max}$ =	2 hours	Oral =	Complete
MW =	279	pKa =	
Vd =			

References:
1. Drug Facts and Comparisons 1995 ed. ed. St. Louis: 1995.
2. Kemp J, Ilett KF, Booth J, Hackett LP. Excretion of doxepin and N-desmethyldoxepin in human milk. Br J Clin Pharmacol 1985; 20(5):497-499.
3. Matheson I, Pande H, Alertsen AR. Respiratory depression caused by N-desmethyldoxepin in breastmilk. Lancet 1985; 2(8464):1124.

DOXERCALCIFEROL

Trade: Hectoral
Can/Aus/UK: Hectoral
Uses: Vitamin D analog
LRC: L3
AAP: Not reviewed

Doxercalciferol is a vitamin D analog that following metabolic activation becomes 1,25-dihydroxyvitamin D2. Coxercalciferol is indicated for the treatment of hyperparathyroidism associated with patients with chronic renal failure undergoing hemodialysis. Excessive doses may lead to dangerously elevated plasma calcium levels. No data are available on its transfer into human milk. It is not likely that normal doses would lead to clinically relevant levels in human milk, particularly since vitamin D transfers only minimally into human milk. While plasma levels of vitamin D are normally quite low in human milk (< 20 IU/L), at least one study now suggests that supplementing a mother with high levels of vitamin D2 can significantly elevate milk levels, and subsequently lead to hypercalcemia in a breastfed infant.[1] Some caution with these highly active forms of vitamin D is recommended.

Pregnancy Risk Category: B

Lactation Risk Category: L3

Adult Concerns: Adverse events include hypercalcemia, hyperphosphatemia, and oversuppression of parathyroid hormone. Additional side effects include edema, headache, malaise, dizziness, pruritus, and constipation.

Pediatric Concerns: None reported via milk, but caution is recommended in breastfeeding mothers.

Drug Interactions: Do not use with magnesium antacids, as hypermagnesemia has been reported.

Theoretic Infant Dose:

Relative Infant Dose:

Adult Dose: 4 µg three times weekly

Alternatives: Vitamin D

T½ =	32-37 hours	M/P =	
PHL =		PB =	99%
T$_{max}$ =	8 hours	Oral =	Complete
MW =		pKa =	
Vd =			

References:
1. Greer FR, Hollis BW, Napoli JL. High concentrations of vitamin D2 in human milk associated with pharmacologic doses of vitamin D2. J Pediatr 1984; 105(1):61-64.

DOXORUBICIN

Trade: Adriamycin
Can/Aus/UK: Adriamycin
Uses: Anticancer drug
LRC: L5
AAP: Contraindicated by the American Academy of Pediatrics in Breastfeeding Mothers

Doxorubicin and its metabolite are secreted in significant amounts in breastmilk. Following a dose of 70 mg/meter sq., peak milk levels of doxorubicin and metabolite occurred at 24 hrs and were 128 and 111 µg/L respectively.[1] The highest milk/plasma ratio was 4.43 at 24 hours. Due to the extraordinary toxicity of this compound, breastfeeding is not recommended.

Pregnancy Risk Category: D

Lactation Risk Category: L5

Adult Concerns: Bone marrow suppression, cardiac toxicity, arrhythmias, nausea, vomiting, stomatitis, liver toxicity

Pediatric Concerns: This product could be extremely toxic to a breastfeeding infant and is not recommended.

Drug Interactions: Doxorubicin may decrease digoxin plasma levels and renal excretion. Allopurinol and verapamil may increase cytotoxicity of doxorubicin.

Theoretic Infant Dose: 20.8 µg/kg/day

Relative Infant Dose:

Adult Dose: 20-75 mg/sq. meter IV

Alternatives:

T½ =	17-30 hours	M/P =	4.43
PHL =		PB =	85%
T$_{max}$ =	24 hours	Oral =	Poor
MW =	544	pKa =	
Vd =	25		

References:
1. Egan PC, Costanza ME, Dodion P, Egorin MJ, Bachur NR. Doxorubicin and cisplatin excretion into human milk. Cancer Treat Rep 1985; 69(12):1387-1389.

DOXYCYCLINE
Trade: Doxychel, Vibramycin, Peristat
Can/Aus/UK: Apo-Doxy, Doxycin, Vibramycin, Vibra-Tabs, Doryx, Doxylar
Uses: Tetracycline antibiotic
LRC: L3
       L4 if used chronically
AAP: Not reviewed

Doxycycline is a long half-life tetracycline antibiotic. In a study of 15 subjects, the average doxycycline level in milk was 0.77 mg/L following a 200 mg oral dose.[1] One oral dose of 100 mg was administered 24 hours later, and the breastmilk levels were 0.380 mg/L. Tetracyclines administered orally to infants are known to bind in teeth, producing discoloration and inhibit bone growth although doxycycline and oxytetracycline stain teeth the least severe. Although most tetracyclines secreted into milk are generally bound to calcium thus inhibiting their absorption, doxycycline is the least bound (20%) and may be better absorbed in a breastfeeding infant than the older tetracyclines. While the absolute absorption of older tetracyclines may be dramatically reduced by calcium salts, the newer doxycycline and minocycline analogs bind less and their overall absorption while slowed, may be significantly higher than earlier versions. Prolonged use could potentially alter GI flora and induce dental staining although doxycycline produces the least dental staining. Short term use (several weeks) is not contraindicated. No harmful effects have yet been reported in breastfeeding infants but prolonged use is not advised. For prolonged administration such as for exposure to anthrax, check the CDC web site as they have published specific dosing guidelines.

Pregnancy Risk Category: D

Lactation Risk Category: L3
L4 if used chronically

Adult Concerns: Nausea, vomiting, diarrhea, photosensitivity. Doxycycline decreased prothrombin activity.

Pediatric Concerns: None reported, but prolonged exposure may lead to dental staining and decreased bone growth.

Drug Interactions: Reduced absorption with aluminum, calcium, or magnesium salts, iron or bismuth subsalicylate. Reduced doxycycline half-life when used with barbiturates, phenytoin, and carbamazepine. Concurrent use with methoxyflurane has resulted in fatal renal toxicity. May render oral contraceptives less effective.

Theoretic Infant Dose: 0.11 mg/kg/day

Relative Infant Dose: 4.04%

Adult Dose: 100 mg daily

Alternatives:

$T\frac{1}{2}$ =	15-25 hours	M/P =	0.3-0.4
PHL =		PB =	90%
T_{max} =	1.5-4 hours	Oral =	90-100%
MW =	462	pKa =	
Vd =			

References:
1. Morganti G, Ceccarelli G, Ciaffi G. [Comparative concentrations of a tetracycline antibiotic in serum and maternal milk]. Antibiotica 1968; 6(3):216-223.

DOXYLAMINE
Trade: Unisom Nighttime
Can/Aus/UK: Dozile, Mersyndol, Panalgesic, Syndol
Uses: Antihistamine, sedative.
LRC: L4
AAP: Not reviewed

Doxylamine is an antihistamine similar in structure to Benadryl. Because it has significant sedative properties, it is primarily used in over-the-counter sleep aids. Like other antihistamines, it should not be used in infants and particularly in premature or term neonates due to paradoxical effects such as CNS stimulation or even sedation.[1,2] Levels in breastmilk are not known but caution is recommended particularly in infants with apnea or other respiratory syndromes.

Pregnancy Risk Category: B

Lactation Risk Category: L4

Adult Concerns: Sedation, paradoxical CNS stimulation, agitation

Pediatric Concerns: None reported via milk but observe for sedation and paradoxical CNS stimulation. Do not use in infants with apnea.

Drug Interactions: Increased CNS sedation when added to other antihistamines and CNS sedative-hypnotics.

Theoretic Infant Dose:

Relative Infant Dose:

Adult Dose:

Alternatives:

T½ =	10.1 hours	M/P =	
PHL =		PB =	
T$_{max}$ =	2.4 hours	Oral =	Complete
MW =	270	pKa =	9.2
Vd =	2.7		

References:
1. Friedman H, Greenblatt DJ, Scavone JM, Burstein ES, Ochs HR, Harmatz JS, Shader RI. Clearance of the antihistamine doxylamine. Reduced in elderly men but not in elderly women. Clin Pharmacokinet 1989; 16(5):312-316.
2. Friedman H, Greenblatt DJ. The pharmacokinetics of doxylamine: use of automated gas chromatography with nitrogen-phosphorus detection. J Clin Pharmacol 1985; 25(6):448-451.

DROPERIDOL

Trade: Inapsine
Can/Aus/UK: Inapsine, Droleptan
Uses: Tranquilizer, antiemetic
LRC: L3
AAP: Not reviewed

Droperidol is a powerful tranquilizer. It is sometimes used as preanesthetic medication in labor and delivery because of fewer respiratory effects in neonates. In pediatric patients 2-12 years of age, it is sometimes used as an antiemetic (20-75 micrograms/kg IM, IV).[1,2] It apparently crosses the placenta only very slowly. There are no data available on secretion into breastmilk. Due to the potent sedative properties of this medication, caution is urged.

Pregnancy Risk Category: C

Lactation Risk Category: L3

Adult Concerns: Sedation, hypotension, dizziness, chills, shivering, unusual ocular movements

Pediatric Concerns: None reported via milk but observe for sedation, hypotension.

Drug Interactions: Can cause peripheral vasodilation and hypotension when used with certain anesthesia medications. Can potentiate effects of other CNS depressants and antidepressants such as barbiturates.

Theoretic Infant Dose:

Relative Infant Dose:

Adult Dose: 2.5-10 mg injection (IM)

Alternatives: Haloperidol

T½ =	2.2 hours	M/P =		
PHL =		PB =	High	
T$_{max}$ =	10-30 minutes (IM)	Oral =		
MW =	379	pKa =		
Vd =	2.0			

References:
1. McEvoy GE. (ed): AFHS Drug Information. 1992.
2. Pharmaceutical Manufacturer Prescribing Information. 1995.

DROSPIRENONE

Trade: Yasmin
Can/Aus/UK: Yasmin
Uses: Synthetic progestin
LRC: L3
AAP: Not reviewed

Drospirenone in combination with ethinyl estradiol (30 micrograms) is marketed at Yasmin. In a study of 6 women who received 3 mg drospirenone with ethinyl estradiol (Yasmin), the time to peak in plasma and milk was 2.5 and 2.8 hour respectively.[1] Average concentrations at C$_{max}$ were 30.8 and 13.5 ng/mL of serum or milk respectively. The mean milk/serum ratios increased from 0.16 to 0.57 at 2 hours following dosing and decreased to 0.16 at 24 hours although the AUC(0-48 h) ratio was only 0.23. The mean drospirenone concentration in breastmilk over the 24 hour period was 3.7 ng/mL. Using this average, the relative infant dose would be approximately 1.2% of the maternal dose. The authors estimate in this group of 6 women, the average transfer of drospirenone was 635 ng/day. Although not clear in this study, the lower estimates could be due to lower milk production in this study.

This combination oral contraceptive also contains estinyl estradiol. Estrogens are believed to strongly inhibit milk production in some women. Some caution is recommended.

Pregnancy Risk Category: X

Lactation Risk Category: L3

Adult Concerns: Reduced milk production in some mothers has been reported with combination birth control pills containing estrogens. Thrombophlebitis, pulmonary embolism, and cerebral hemorrhage are possible but remote. Nausea, vomiting, abdominal cramping, spotting have been reported.

Pediatric Concerns: In the one study, transfer of drospirenone to milk was low. No untoward effects were noted in the infants.

Drug Interactions: Metabolism of ethinyl estradiol is increased by rifampin. St. John's Wort is believed to increase the metabolism of numerous drugs by induction of hepatic enzymes (Cy-450) and the p-glycoprotein transporter and may reduce the effectiveness of oral contraceptives as well as numerous other medications. Antibiotics have been reported to reduce effectiveness of oral contraceptives. Atorvastin may increase plasma levels significantly.

Theoretic Infant Dose: 0.55 µg/kg/day

Relative Infant Dose: 1.29%

Adult Dose: 3 mg drosprenone/day

Alternatives: Micronor

T½ =	31 hours	M/P =	0.23
PHL =		PB =	97%
Tmax =	1.7 hours	Oral =	76%
MW =	366	pKa =	
Vd =	5		

References:
1. Blode H, Foidart JM, Heithecker R. Transfer of drospirenone to breastmilk after a single oral administration of 3 mg drospirenone + 30 µg ethinylestradiol to healthy lactating women. Eur J Contracept Reprod Health Care 2001; 6(3):167-171.

DYPHYLLINE

Trade: Dilor, Lufyllin, Dyphylline
Can/Aus/UK: Broncho-Grippol, Silbephylline, Noradran
Uses: Anti-asthmatic drug
LRC: L3
AAP: Maternal Medication Usually Compatible with Breastfeeding

Dyphylline is a methylxanthine, bronchodilator similar to theophylline. It is apparently secreted into milk in small quantities. Following a 5 mg/kg dose IM, the milk/plasma ratio was 2.08. Using the kinetics provided, the average milk level at 2 hours would have been approximately 14.1 mg/L.[1] No reported untoward effects. Observe infant for irritability, insomnia, and elevated heart rate.

Pregnancy Risk Category: C

Lactation Risk Category: L3

Adult Concerns: Irritability, insomnia, tachycardia, arrhythmias, GI distress, headache, seizures, hyperglycemia

Pediatric Concerns: None reported via milk but observe for irritability, insomnia, tachycardia.

Drug Interactions: Probenecid significantly increases half-life of dyphylline and increases plasma levels.

Theoretic Infant Dose: 2.11 mg/kg/day

Relative Infant Dose: 42%

Adult Dose:

Alternatives: Theophylline

$T\frac{1}{2}$ =	3-12.8 hours	M/P =	2.08
PHL =		PB =	56%
T_{max} =	1-2 hours (oral)	Oral =	Complete
MW =	254	pKa =	
Vd =	0.6-1.1		

References:
1. Jarboe CH, Cook LN, Malesic I, Fleischaker J. Dyphylline elimination kinetics in lactating women: blood to milk transfer. J Clin Pharmacol 1981; 21(10):405-410.

ECHINACEA

Trade: Echinacea Angustifolia, Echinacea Purpurea, American Cone Flower, Black Susans, Snakeroot
Can/Aus/UK: Antifect
Uses: Herbal immunostimulant
LRC: L3
AAP: Not reviewed

Echinacea is a popular herbal remedy in the central US and has been traditionally used topically to stimulate wound healing and internally to stimulate the immune system. The plant contains a complex mixture of compounds and ,thus far, no single component appears responsible for its immunostimulant properties. A number of in vitro and animal studies have documented the activation of immunologic properties although most of these are via intraperitoneal injections, not orally. The activity of orally administered extracts is unknown. Echinacea extracts appear to stimulate phagocytosis of macrophages, increase cellular respiration, and increase the mobility of phagocytic leukocytes.[1] Extracts of E. Purpurea are highly effective in activating macrophages to engulf tumor cells, to produce tumor necrosis factor, interleukin-1, and interferon beta-2. One study suggests a radioprotective effect (antioxidant) of Echinacea. Another study in humans suggests that while single doses may stimulate the immune system, repeated daily doses may actually suppress the immune response.[2] Thus far, little is known about the toxicity of this plant; although, its use has been widespread for many years. Apparently, purified Echinacea extract is relatively non-toxic even at high doses.[3,4] No data are available on its transfer into human milk or its effect on lactation. It should not be used for more than 8 weeks.[5]

Pregnancy Risk Category:

Lactation Risk Category: L3

Adult Concerns: None reported.

Pediatric Concerns: None reported via milk.

Drug Interactions:

Theoretic Infant Dose:

Relative Infant Dose:

Adult Dose:

Alternatives:

References:

1. Steinmuller C, Roesler J, Grottrup E, Franke G, Wagner H, Lohmann-Matthes ML. Polysaccharides isolated from plant cell cultures of Echinacea purpurea enhance the resistance of immunosuppressed mice against systemic infections with Candida albicans and Listeria monocytogenes. Int J Immunopharmacol 1993; 15(5):605-614.
2. Coeugniet EG, Elek E. Immunomodulation with Viscum album and Echinacea purpurea extracts. Onkologie 1987; 10(3 Suppl):27-33.
3. Review of Natural Products Facts and Comparisons, St Louis, MO 1996.
4. Bissett NG. In: Herbal Drugs and Phytopharmaceuticals. Medpharm Scientific Publishers, CRC Press, Boca Raton, 1994.
5. The Complete German Commission E Monographs. Ed. M. Blumenthal Amer Botanical Council 1998.

ELETRIPTAN

Trade: Relpax
Can/Aus/UK: Relpax
Uses: Anti-migraine
LRC: L2
AAP: Not reviewed

Eletriptan is a selective 5-hyroxytryptamine receptor agonist specifically used to treat migraine attacks. The bioavailability of eletriptan is greater than sumatriptan(Imitrex) and is faster acting.

The manufacturer reports that in one study of 8 women given a single dose of 80 mg eletriptan, the mean total amount of eletriptan in breastmilk over 24 hours in this group was approximately 0.02% of the administered dose.[1] The milk/plasma ratio was 0.25 but there was great variability. The resulting eletriptan concentration-time profile in milk was similar to that seen in the plasma over 24 hours, with very low concentrations of drug (mean 1.7 ng/mL) still present in the milk 18-24 hours post dose. It is not likely the clinical dose delivered above would harm a breastfed infant.

Pregnancy Risk Category: C

Lactation Risk Category: L2

Adult Concerns: Nausea, asthenia, somnolence, dizziness, dry mouth, paresthesias, headache, and abdominal cramps have been reported.

Pediatric Concerns: None reported via milk in one study.

Drug Interactions: Increased plasma levels of eletriptan could occur if given concomitantly with cyclosporine, erythromycin, amiodarone, amprenavir, aprepitant, clarithromycin, delavirdine, diltiazem, etc. Enhanced vasospastic reactions when given with ergot alkaloids such as dihydroergotamine, ergotamine, or methysergide.

Theoretic Infant Dose:

Relative Infant Dose: 0.02%

Adult Dose: 20-40 mg initially for headache. One repeat dose after 2 hour if needed.

Alternatives: Sumatriptan

T½ =	4 hours	M/P =	0.25
PHL =		PB =	85%
T$_{max}$ =	2 hours	Oral =	50%
MW =	463	pKa =	
Vd =	1.97		

References:
1. Pharmaceutical manufacturers presecribing information, 2003.

ENALAPRIL MALEATE

Trade: Vasotec
Can/Aus/UK: Vasotec, Amprace, Renitec, Innovace
Uses: Antihypertensive, ACE inhibitor
LRC: L2
AAP: Maternal Medication Usually Compatible with Breastfeeding

Enalapril maleate is an ACE inhibitor used as an antihypertensive. Upon absorption, it is rapidly metabolized by the adult liver to enalaprilat, the biologically active metabolite.

In one study of 5 lactating mothers who received a single 20 mg dose, the mean maximum milk concentration of enalapril and enalaprilat was only 1.74 µg/L and 1.72 µg/L respectively.[1] The author suggests that an infant consuming 850 mL of milk daily would ingest less than 2 µg of enalaprilat daily.   The milk/plasma ratios for enalapril and enalaprilat averaged 0.013 and 0.025 respectively.   However, this was only a single dose study, and the levels transferred into milk at steady state may be slightly higher.

In a study by Rush of a patient receiving 10 mg/day, the total amount of enalapril and enalaprilat measured in milk during the 24 hour period was 81.9 ng and 36.1 ng respectively or 1.44 µg/L and 0.63 µg/L of milk respectively.[2]

Exercise caution when administering to lactating women particularly early postnatal although the data thus far indicates the levels secreted into milk are clinically insignificant.

Pregnancy Risk Category: **C in 1st trimester**
                                D in 2nd and 3rd trimesters

Lactation Risk Category: L2

Adult Concerns: Hypotension, bradycardia, headache, fatigue, diarrhea, rash, cough

Pediatric Concerns: None reported via milk but observe for hypotension.

Drug Interactions: Bioavailability of ACEIs may be decreased when used with antacids. Capsaicin may exacerbate coughing associated with ACE inhibitor treatment. Pharmacologic effects of ACE inhibitors may be increased. Increased plasma levels of digoxin may result. Increased serum lithium levels may result when used with ACE inhibitors.

Theoretic Infant Dose: 0.51 µg/kg/day

Relative Infant Dose: 0.17%

Adult Dose: 10-40 mg daily

Alternatives: Captopril, Benazepril

T½ =	35 hours(metabolite)	M/P =	
PHL =		PB =	60%
T$_{max}$ =	0.5-1.5 hours	Oral =	60%
MW =	492	pKa =	
Vd =			

References:
1.   Redman CW, Kelly JG, Cooper WD. The excretion of enalapril and enalaprilat in human breastmilk. Eur J Clin Pharmacol 1990; 38(1):99.
2.   Rush JE, Snyder BA, Barrish A. et.al. Comment. Clin Nephrol 1991; 35:234.

ENCAINIDE
Trade: Enkaid
Can/Aus/UK:
Uses: Antiarrhythmic agent.
LRC: L3
AAP: Not reviewed

Encainide is a local anesthetic-type antiarrhythmic agent.   It was voluntarily removed from the market in 1999 but is available on a limited basis for certain patients with life-threatening arrhythmias. The plasma kinetics are highly variable depending on the metabolic capabilities of the maternal liver. The oral bioavailability is extremely variable and varies from 25-65% in extensive metabolizers to 80-90% in poor metabolizers. Half-lives are variable as well according to the metabolitic capacity of the individual's liver.[1]

However, encainide and its 3 active metabolites are excreted into human milk.   In one patient receiving 50 mg four times daily,   milk concentrations of encainide and o-demethyl encainide were 200-400 µg/L and 100-200 µg/L respectively.[2] These concentrations are similar to the maternal serum levels.

Pregnancy Risk Category: B

Lactation Risk Category: L3

Adult Concerns: Arrhythmias, chest pain, congestive heart failure, abdominal pain

Pediatric Concerns: None reported, but extreme caution is recommended.

Drug Interactions: Use caution when encainide is used with any other drug that effects cardiac conduction. Cimetidine increases plasma concentrations of encainide.

Theoretic Infant Dose: 60 µg/kg/day

Relative Infant Dose: 2.1%

Adult Dose: 50-200 mg daily in 3-4 divided doses.

Alternatives:

T½	=	2-36 hours	M/P	=	1
PHL	=		PB	=	70.5-78%
T$_{max}$	=	1.7 hours	Oral	=	Variable
MW	=	352	pKa	=	
Vd	=	2.7-4.3			

References:
1. Pharmaceutical Manufacturer Prescribing Information. 1992.
2. Briggs GG, Freeman RK, Yaffee SJ. Drugs in Pregnancy and Lactation. Philadelphia: Lippincott Williams & Wilkins, 1998.

ENOXACIN

Trade: Penetrex
Can/Aus/UK: Enoxin, Comprecin
Uses: Antibiotic
LRC: L3
AAP: Not reviewed

Enoxacin is a typical fluoroquinolone antibiotic similar to ciprofloxacin, norfloxacin, and others. No data are available on the transfer of enoxacin into human milk. See ofloxacin and norfloxacin as alternatives.

Pregnancy Risk Category: C

Lactation Risk Category: L3

Adult Concerns: Nausea, vomiting, diarrhea, abdominal cramps, GI bleeding, increased intracranial pressure, tremor, restlessness, other CNS reactions, photosensitivity

Pediatric Concerns: None reported via milk but caution is urged. See norfloxacin.

Drug Interactions: Decreased absorption with antacids. Quinolones cause increased levels of caffeine, warfarin, cyclosporine, theophylline. Cimetidine, probenecid, azlocillin increase ciprofloxacin levels. Increased risk of seizures when used with foscarnet.

Theoretic Infant Dose:

Relative Infant Dose:

Adult Dose: 200-400 mg BID

Alternatives: Ofloxacin, norfloxacin, ciprofloxacin

T½ =	3-6 hours	M/P =	
PHL =		PB =	40%
T$_{max}$ =		Oral =	90%
MW =		pKa =	
Vd =	2.5		

References:

ENOXAPARIN

Trade: Lovenox, Low Molecular Weight Heparin
Can/Aus/UK: Lovenox, Clexane
Uses: Anticoagulant
LRC: L3
AAP: Not reviewed

Enoxaparin is a low molecular weight fraction of heparin used clinically as an anticoagulant. In a study of 12 women receiving 20-40 mg of enoxaparin daily for up to 5 days postpartum for venous pathology (n=4) or caesarian section (n=8), no change in anti-Xa activity was noted in the breastfed infants.[1] Because it is a peptide fragment of heparin, its molecular weight is large (2000-8000 daltons). The size alone would largely preclude its entry into human milk at levels clinically relevant. Due to minimal oral bioavailability, any present in milk would not be orally absorbed by the infant. A similar compound, dalteparin, has been studied and milk levels are extremely low as well. See dalteparin.

Pregnancy Risk Category: B

Lactation Risk Category: L3

Adult Concerns: Anticoagulant effects in adults when administered subcutaneously.

Pediatric Concerns: None reported via milk. Molecular weight is too large to produce clinically relevant milk levels.

Drug Interactions: Anticoagulants and platelet inhibitors. NSAIDS may increase risk of bleeding.

Theoretic Infant Dose:

Relative Infant Dose:

Adult Dose: 30 mg BID

Alternatives: Dalteparin

T½ =	4.5 hours	M/P =	
PHL =		PB =	
T$_{max}$ =	3-5 hours	Oral =	None
MW =	8000	pKa =	
Vd =	0.1		

References:

1. Guillonneau M, de Crepy A, Aufrant C, Hurtaud-Roux MF, Jacqz-Aigrain E. L'allaitement est possible en cas de traitement maternel par l'enoxaparien. Arch Pediatr 1996; 3(5):513-514.

EPHEDRINE

Trade: Vatronol Nose Drops
Can/Aus/UK: Amsec, Adalixin, Bethal, Anestan, Anodesyn, Cam
Uses: Adrenergic stimulant, anti-asthmatic.
LRC: L4
AAP: Not reviewed

Ephedrine is a mild stimulant that belongs to the adrenergic family and functions similar to the amphetamines. Small amounts of d-isoephedrine, a close congener of ephedrine, is believed to be secreted into milk although no data are available on ephedrine itself.[1] This product is commonly used to support blood pressure of parturients during delivery. On an acute basis, it is not likely to harm a breastfeeding infant. However, it should not be used regularly by breastfeeding mothers.

Pregnancy Risk Category: C

Lactation Risk Category: L4

Adult Concerns: Anorexia, tachycardia, arrhythmias, agitation, insomnia, hyperstimulation

Pediatric Concerns: None reported but observe for anorexia, irritability, crying, disturbed sleeping patterns, excitement.

Drug Interactions: May increase toxicity and cardiac stimulation when used with theophylline. MAO inhibitors or atropine may increase blood pressure.

Theoretic Infant Dose:

Relative Infant Dose:

Adult Dose: 25-50 mg injection

Alternatives:

T½ =	3-5 hours	M/P =	
PHL =		PB =	
Tmax =	15-60 minutes	Oral =	85%
MW =	165	pKa =	9.6
Vd =			

References:
1. Mortimer EA, Jr. Drug toxicity from breastmilk? Pediatrics 1977; 60(5):780-781.

EPINEPHRINE

Trade: Adrenalin, Sus-Phren, Medihaler, Primatene
Can/Aus/UK: Adrenalin, Bronkaid, Epi-pen, Adrenutol, Eppy, Simplene
Uses: Stimulant
LRC: L1
AAP: Not reviewed

Epinephrine is a powerful adrenergic stimulant. Although likely to be secreted in milk, it is rapidly destroyed in the GI tract.[1] It is unlikely that any would be absorbed by the infant unless in the early neonatal period or premature.

Pregnancy Risk Category: C

Lactation Risk Category: L1

Adult Concerns: Nervousness, tremors, agitation, tachycardia

Pediatric Concerns: None reported but observe for brief stimulation.

Drug Interactions: Increased cardiac irritability when used with halogenated inhaled anesthetics, alpha blocking agents. Do not use with MAO inhibitors.

Theoretic Infant Dose:

Relative Infant Dose:

Adult Dose: 0.1-0.25 mg injection (IV)

Alternatives:

T½ =	1 hour (inhalation)	M/P =	
PHL =		PB =	
T$_{max}$ =	< 1-10 minutes	Oral =	Poor
MW =	183	pKa =	
Vd =			

References:
1. Wilson J. Drugs in Breastmilk. New York: ADIS Press 1981.

EPOETIN ALFA

Trade: Epogen
Can/Aus/UK:
Uses: Stimulates red blood cell production
LRC: L3
AAP: Not reviewed

Epoetin alfa is a glycoprotein which stimulates red blood cell production. Structurally similar to the natural erythropoietin, it consists of 165 amino acids manufactured by recombinant DNA technology. It has a molecular weight of 30,400 daltons. Large molecular weight proteins in general are poorly transferred into human milk. Further, due to its protein nature, it would not likely be absorbed orally to any degree by the infant.

Pregnancy Risk Category: C

Lactation Risk Category: L3

Adult Concerns: Headache, hypertension, arthralgias, nausea, edema, vomiting, and chest pain have been reported in adults.

Pediatric Concerns: None reported via milk.

Drug Interactions: None

Theoretic Infant Dose:

Relative Infant Dose:

Adult Dose: 50-100 Units three times weekly

Alternatives:

T½ =	4-13 hours	M/P =	
PHL =	4-13 hours	PB =	
T$_{max}$ =	5-24 hours	Oral =	Nil
MW =	30,400	pKa =	
Vd =			

References:
1. Pharmaceutical Manufacturer Prescribing Information, 2003.

EPOPROSTENOL

Trade: Flolan
Can/Aus/UK:
Uses: Vasodilator, platelet function inhibitor
LRC: L3
AAP: Not reviewed

Epoprostenol (Prostacyclin; PGX; PGI-2) is a naturally occurring prostaglandin that is a potent inhibitor of platelet aggregation and a vasodilator. It is commonly used to treat primary pulmonary hypertension. It is rapidly metabolized in plasma to 6-keto-prostaglandin F1-alpha, which is biologically inactive, and has a half-life of only 3-5 minutes.[1] Prostaglandins are known to be transferred into human milk, but they are believed derived from mammary tissue and synthesis by the cellular components of breastmilk.[2] With the extraordinarily short half-life of this product, it is unlikely any would penetrate into milk, be retained for very long, or be stable in the infant's gut. Oral absorption by the infant is unlikely.

Pregnancy Risk Category: B

Lactation Risk Category: L3

Adult Concerns: Flushing, headache, nausea, vomiting, hypotension, anxiety, chest pain, dizziness, bradycardia, abdominal pain

Pediatric Concerns: None reported. Unlikely to be absorbed.

Drug Interactions: May decrease clearance of digoxin. Decreased oral clearance of furosemide.

Theoretic Infant Dose:

Relative Infant Dose:

Adult Dose: 2 ng/kg per minute

Alternatives:

$T\frac{1}{2}$ =	6 minutes	M/P =	
PHL =		PB =	
T_{max} =		Oral =	Nil
MW =	374	pKa =	
Vd =	357 mL		

References:

1. Pharmaceutical Manufacturer Prescribing Information. 2002
2. Friedman Z. Prostaglandins in breastmilk. Endocrinol Exp 1986; 20(2-3):285-291.

EPSTEIN-BARR VIRUS
Trade: Mononucleosis, EBV
Can/Aus/UK:
Uses: Herpesvirus infection (EBV)
LRC: L3
AAP: Not reviewed

The Epstein-Barr virus (EBV) is one of the causes of infectious mononucleosis. EBV belongs to the herpes virus family. Symptoms include fever, exudative pharyngitis, lymphadenopathy, hepatosplenomegaly, and atypical lymphocytosis. Close personal contact is generally required for transmission and it is not known if EBV is secreted into human milk, although it is likely. Studies by Kusuhara[1] indicate that the seroprevalence of EBV at 12-23 months was the same in bottle-fed and in breastfed infants. This data suggests that breastmilk is not a significant source of early EBV infections.

Pregnancy Risk Category:

Lactation Risk Category: **L3**

Adult Concerns:

Pediatric Concerns:

Drug Interactions:

Theoretic Infant Dose:

Relative Infant Dose:

Adult Dose:

Alternatives:

References:
1. Kusuhara K, Takabayashi A, Ueda K, Hidaka Y, Minamishima I, Take H, Fujioka K, Imai S, Osato T. Breastmilk is not a significant source for early Epstein-Barr virus or human herpesvirus 6 infection in infants: a seroepidemiologic study in 2 endemic areas of human T-cell lymphotropic virus type I in Japan. Microbiol Immunol 1997; 41(4):309-312.

ERGONOVINE MALEATE
Trade: Ergotrate, Ergometrine
Can/Aus/UK: Ergotrate, Ergometrine, Syntometrine
Uses: Postpartum uterine bleeding
LRC: L3
AAP: Not reviewed

Ergonovine and its close congener, methylergonovine maleate, directly stimulate uterine and vascula smooth muscle contractions. They are primarily used to prevent/treat postpartum hemorrhage. Although pharmacologically similar, many clinicians prefer methylergonovine because it produces less hypertension than ergonovine. In a study of 8 postpartum women receiving 0.125 mg three times daily until day 5 when a 0.25 mg tablet was introduced, measurable ergonovine was only found in 4 of 8 patients and averaged 0.8 μg/L.[1] These authors suggested that use of the drug during breastfeeding would not affect the infant.

In addition, the effect of ergonovine on prolactin levels is controversial. In one study methylergonovine did not alter postpartum maternal prolactin levels[2], while in another study[3] a significant reduction in prolactin production was produced by ergonovine. Ergonovine use in lactating women would presumably suppress lactation, whereas methylergonovine may not.

When used at doses of 0.2 mg up to 3-4 times daily, only small quantities of ergonovine are found in milk. Short-term (1 week) low-dose regimens of these agents do not apparently pose problems in nursing mothers or their infants. Methylergonovine is preferred because it does not inhibit lactation and levels in milk are minimal. The prolonged use of ergot alkaloids should be avoided and can lead to severe gangrenous manifestations.

Pregnancy Risk Category: **X**

Lactation Risk Category: **L3**

Adult Concerns: Hypertension, seizures, vomiting, diarrhea, cold extremities

Pediatric Concerns: None reported, but long term exposure is not recommended. Methyl-ergonovine is commonly recommended early postpartum for breastfeeding mothers to reduce uterine bleeding.

Drug Interactions:

Theoretic Infant Dose: 0.12 μg/kg/day

Relative Infant Dose: 2.2%

Adult Dose: 0.2 mg injection (IM) q 2-4 hours

Alternatives: Methylergonovine

T½ =	0.5-2 hours	M/P =	
PHL =		PB =	
Tmax =	30- 180 minutes	Oral =	>60%
MW =	441	pKa =	
Vd =			

References:

1. Erkkola R, Kanto J, Allonen H, Kleimola T, Mantyla R. Excretion of methylergometrine (methylergonovine) into the human breastmilk. Int J Clin Pharmacol Biopharm 1978; 16(12):579-580.

2. Del Pozo E, Brun DR, Hinselmann M. Lack of effect of methyl-ergonovine on postpartum lactation. Am J Obstet Gynecol 1975; 123(8):845-846.
3. Canales ES, Garrido JT, Zarate A, Mason M, Soria J. Effect of ergonovine on prolactin secretion and milk let-down. Obstet Gynecol 1976; 48(2):228-229.

ERGOTAMINE TARTRATE

Trade: Wigraine, Cafergot, Ergostat, Ergomar, Dhe-45
Can/Aus/UK: Ergomar, Gynergen, Cafergot, Ergodryl, Migral, Lingraine
Uses: Anti-migraine, inhibits prolactin
LRC: L4
AAP: Drugs associated with significant side effects and should be given with caution

Ergotamine is a potent vasoconstrictor generally used in acute phases of migraine headache. It is never used chronically for prophylaxis of migraine. Although early reports suggest ergotamine compounds are secreted in breastmilk[1] and cause symptoms of ergotism (vomiting, and diarrhea) in infants, other authors [2] suggest that the short term use of ergotamine (0.2 mg postpartum) generally presents no problem to a nursing infant. This is likely, due to the fact that less than 5% of ergotamine is orally absorbed in adults. However, excessive dosing and prolonged administration may inhibit prolactin secretion and hence lactation. Although the initial plasma half-life is only 2 hours, ergotamine is stored for long periods in various tissues producing long-lasting effects (terminal half-life = 21 hrs). Use during lactation should be strongly discouraged.

Pregnancy Risk Category: X

Lactation Risk Category: L4

Adult Concerns: Ergotism, peripheral artery insufficiency, nausea, vomiting, paresthesia, cold skin temperatures, headache

Pediatric Concerns: One case of ergotism reported and included symptoms such as vomiting and diarrhea. Long term exposure is contraindicated.

Drug Interactions: Rifamycin and other macrolide antibiotics may enhance ergot toxicity.

Theoretic Infant Dose:

Relative Infant Dose:

Adult Dose: 2 mg q 30 minutes

Alternatives: Propranolol, Sumatriptan

T½ =	21 hours(terminal)	M/P =	
PHL =		PB =	
T$_{max}$ =	0.5-3 hours	Oral =	< 5%
MW =	581	pKa =	
Vd =			

References:
1. Fomina PL. Untersuchungen uber den ubergang des aktiven agens des Muttrkorns in die milch stillender Mutter. Arch Gynecol 1934; 157:275.
2. White G, White M. Breastfeeding and drugs in human milk. Vet and Human Tox 1984; 26:supplement 1.

ERTAPENEM

Trade: Invanz
Can/Aus/UK: Invanz
Uses: Carbapenum antibiotic
LRC: L2
AAP: Not reviewed

The manufacturer reports the concentration of ertapenem in breastmilk from 5 lactating women with pelvic infections (5 to 14 days postpartum) was measured at random time points daily for 5 consecutive days following the last 1 g dose of intravenous therapy (3-10 days of therapy). The concentration of ertapenem in breastmilk within 24 hours of the last dose of therapy in all 5 women ranged from < 0.13 (lower limit of quantitation) to 0.38 mg/l; peak concentrations were not assessed. By day 5 after discontinuation of therapy, the level of ertapenem was undetectable in the breastmilk of 4 women and below the lower limit of quantitation (< 0.13 μg/mL) in 1 woman.[1]

The above data does not report C$_{max}$ concentrations in milk nor the time samples that were collected, so it is virtually worthless for determining infant exposure to the medication during the day and following the administration.

Using the above data and an assumed average weight of 70 kg, the mothers received about 14.28 mg/kg/day. After 24 hours, the infant would ingest about 57 μg/kg/day. The relative infant dose would be 0.4% of the maternal dose at this time. Without good data it is not possible to estimate clinical dose to the infant, but it is likely small and its oral bioavailability is poor. Most all the penicillins and the carbapenems are safe to use in breastfeeding mothers.

Pregnancy Risk Category: B
Lactation Risk Category: L2

Adult Concerns: Diarrhea, infused vein complications, nausea, headache, vaginitis in females, thrombophlebitis, vomiting, fever, abdominal pain. Do not use if penicillin allergic. Seizures, altered mental status.

Pediatric Concerns: None reported via milk. However diarrhea and perhaps less common pseudomembranous colitis could occur.

Drug Interactions: Increased levels when administered with probenecid.

Theoretic Infant Dose: 0.057 mg/kg/day

Relative Infant Dose: 0.4%

Adult Dose: 1 g IV/IM daily

Alternatives: Imipenem

T½ =	4 hours	M/P =	
PHL =		PB =	95%
T$_{max}$ =	2 hours	Oral =	Poor
MW =	497	pKa =	
Vd =	0.11		

References:
1. Pharmaceutical Manufacturer Prescribing Information.

ERYTHROMYCIN

Trade: E-Mycin, Ery-Tab, Eryc, Ilosone
Can/Aus/UK: E-mycin, Eryc, Erythromide, Novo-Rythro, PCE, Ilotyc, EMU-V, Ilosone, EES, Erythrocin, Ceplac, Erycen
Uses: Macrolide antibiotic
LRC: L1
　　　　L3 early postnatally (pyloric stenosis)
AAP: Maternal Medication Usually Compatible with Breastfeeding

Erythromycin is an older, narrow-spectrum antibiotic. In one study of patients receiving 400 mg three times daily, milk levels varied from 0.4 to 1.6 mg/L.[1] Doses as high as 2 mg per day produced milk levels of 1.6 to 3.2 mg/L. One case of hypertrophic pyloric stenosis apparently linked to erythromycin administration has been reported.[2] In a study of 2-3 patients who received a single 500 oral dose, milk levels at 4 hours ranged from 0.9 to 1.4 mg/L with a milk/plasma ratio of 0.92.[3] Newer macrolide-like antibiotics (azithromycin) may preclude the use of erythromycin. A recent and large study now suggests a strong positive correlation between the use of erythromycin in breastfeeding mothers and infantile hypertrophic pyloric stenosis in newborns.[4]

Pregnancy Risk Category: B

Lactation Risk Category: **L1**
L3 early postnatally (pyloric stenosis)

Adult Concerns: Abdominal cramping, nausea, vomiting, hepatitis, ototoxicity, and hypersensitivity

Pediatric Concerns: Pyloric stenosis has been reported associated with the use of erythromycin early postpartum.

Drug Interactions: Erythromycin may decrease clearance of carbamazepine, cyclosporin, triazolam. Erythromycin may decrease theophylline clearance by as much as 60%. May increase terfenadine plasma levels and increase Q/T intervals. May potentiate anticoagulant effect of warfarin.

Theoretic Infant Dose: 0.48 mg/kg/day

Relative Infant Dose: 1.6%

Adult Dose: 500-800 mg QID

Alternatives: Azithromycin, clarithromycin

T½ =	1.5-2 hours	M/P =	0.92
PHL =		PB =	84%
T$_{max}$ =	2-4 hours	Oral =	Variable
MW =	734	pKa =	
Vd =			

References:
1. Knowles JA. Drugs in milk. Pediatr Currents 1972; 1:28-32.
2. Stang H. Pyloric stenosis associated with erythromycin ingested through breastmilk. Minn Med 1986; 69(11):669-70, 682.
3. Matsuda S. Transfer of antibiotics into maternal milk. Biol Res Pregnancy Perinatol 1984; 5(2):57-60.
4. Sorensen HT, Skriver MV, Pedersen L, Larsen H, Ebbesen F, Schonheyder HC. Risk of infantile hypertrophic pyloric stenosis after maternal postnatal use of macrolides. Scand J Infect Dis 2003; 35(2):104-106.

ESCITALOPRAM

Trade: Lexapro
Can/Aus/UK:
Uses: Antidepressant
LRC: L3 in older infants
AAP: Not reviewed

Escitalopram is a selective serotonin reuptake inhibitor (SSRI) used in the treatment of depression. It is the active S(+)-enantiomer of citalopram (Celexa). While this agent is very specific for the serotonin receptor site, it does apparently have a number of other side effects which may be related to activities at other receptors. Antagonism of muscarinic, histaminergic, and adrenergic receptors has been hypothesized to be associated with various anticholinergic, sedative and cardiovascular side effects. Two cases of somnolence in breastfeeding infants have been reported by the manufacturer.[1] The author has had numerous cases reported as well. This may be due to its inhibition of histamine receptors.

No data are available on the transfer of escitalopram to human milk, but as this drug is identical to the active ingredient in citalopram, the kinetics of transfer should be the same as is published for citalopram. Check citalopram for details of transfer. Until we know more about the effect of this agent on breastfeeding infants, significant caution is recommended, particularly with newborns. Observe for somnolence.

Pregnancy Risk Category: C

Lactation Risk Category: L3 in older infants

Adult Concerns: Adverse events include nausea, sweating, dizziness, insomnia, somnolence, ejaculation disorder, diaphoresis, anorexia, and fatigue.

Pediatric Concerns: The manufacturer reports several cases of somnolence in newborn infants using citalopram. The author has received numerous similar reports with escitalopram.   Caution is recommended in newborn or young infants.

Drug Interactions: Increased citalopram levels when used with macrolide antibiotics (erythromycin), cimetidine, and azole antifungals such as fluconazole, itraconazole, ketoconazole, etc. Carbamazepine may reduce plasma levels of citalopram. Serious reactions may occur if escitalopram is administered too soon after MAO use. Beta blocker (metoprolol) levels may increase by 2 fold when admixed with escitalopram. The combined used of escitalopram and sumatriptan (Imitrex) have been reported to produce weakness, hyperreflexia and incoordination. Escitalopram may increase levels of desipramine.

Theoretic Infant Dose: See Celexa

Relative Infant Dose: See Celexa

Adult Dose: 10-40 mg daily

Alternatives: Sertraline, paroxetine, bupropion, venlafaxine

$T\frac{1}{2}$ =	27-32 hours	M/P =	
PHL =		PB =	56%
T_{max} =	5 hours	Oral =	80%$
MW =	414	pKa =	
Vd =	12		

References:
1.   Pharmaceutical Manufacturers prescribing information, 2003.

ESMOLOL
Trade: Brevibloc
Can/Aus/UK: Brevibloc
Uses: Beta blocker antiarrhythmic
LRC: L3
AAP: Not reviewed

Esmolol is an ultra short-acting beta blocker agent with low lipid solubility. It is of the same family as propranolol. It is primarily used for treatment of supraventricular tachycardia. It is only used IV and has an extremely short half-life. It is almost completely hydrolyzed in 30 minutes.[1,2] No data on breastmilk levels are available.

Pregnancy Risk Category: C

Lactation Risk Category: L3

Adult Concerns: Hypotension, bradycardia, dizziness, somnolence

Pediatric Concerns: None reported.

Drug Interactions: Beta blockers may decrease the effect of sulfanurias. Increased effect with calcium channel blockers, contraceptives, ciprofloxacin, MAO inhibitors, thyroid hormones, haloperidol, and numerous other medications.

Theoretic Infant Dose:

Relative Infant Dose:

Adult Dose: 100 μg/kg/minute

Alternatives: Propranolol, metoprolol

$T\frac{1}{2}$ =	9 minutes	M/P =		
PHL =	4.5 minutes	PB =	55%	
T_{max} =	15 minutes	Oral =	Poor	
MW =	295	pKa =		
Vd =				

References:
1. McEvoy GE. (ed):AFHS Drug Information. New York, NY: 2003.
2. Lacy C. Drug information handbook. Lexi-Comp Inc. Cleveland, OH, 1996.

ESOMEPRAZOLE
Trade: Nexium
Can/Aus/UK: Nexium
Uses: Reduces gastric acid secretion
LRC: L2
AAP: Not reviewed

Esomeprazole is just the L isomer of omeprazole(Prilosec) and is identical to Prilosec. See omeprazole for breastfeeding recommendations.

Pregnancy Risk Category: C

Lactation Risk Category: L2

ESTAZOLAM
Trade: Prosom
Can/Aus/UK:
Uses: Benzodiazepine sedative.
LRC: L3
AAP: Not reviewed

Estazolam is a benzodiazepine sedative hypnotic that belongs to the Valium family. Estazolam, like other benzodiazepines, is secreted into rodent milk although the levels are unpublished.[1,2] No data are available on human milk levels. It is likely that some is secreted into human milk as well.

Pregnancy Risk Category: X

Lactation Risk Category: L3

Adult Concerns: Sedation

Pediatric Concerns: None reported via milk but observe for sedation, apnea.

Drug Interactions: Certain enzyme inducers such as barbiturates may increase the metabolism of estazolam. CNS depressants may increase adverse effects of estazolam. Cimetidine may decrease metabolism of estazolam.

Theoretic Infant Dose:

Relative Infant Dose:

Adult Dose: 1-2 mg daily

Alternatives: Lorazepam, Midazolam, Alprazolam

T½ =	10-24 hours	M/P =	
PHL =		PB =	93%
T$_{max}$ =	0.5-3 hours	Oral =	Complete
MW =	295	pKa =	
Vd =			

References:
1. Pharmaceutical Manufacturer Prescribing Information. 1995.
2. Drug Facts and Comparisons 1995 ed. ed. St. Louis: 1995.

ESTROGEN-ESTRADIOL

Trade: Estratab, Premarin, Menest
Can/Aus/UK: Estrace, Estraderm, Delestrogen, Estinyl, Estring, Evorel
Uses: Estrogen hormone
LRC: L3
AAP: Maternal Medication Usually Compatible with Breastfeeding

Although small amounts may pass into breastmilk, the effects of estrogens on the infant appear minimal. Early post-partum use of estrogens may reduce volume of milk produced and the protein content, but it is variable and depends on dose and the individual.[1-4] Breastfeeding mothers should attempt to wait until lactation is firmly established (6-8 weeks) prior to use of estrogen-containing oral contraceptives. In one study of six lactating women who received 50 or 100 mg vaginal suppositories of estradiol, the plasma levels peaked at 3 hours.[5] These doses are extremely large and are not used clinically. In a study of 11 women, the mean concentration of estradiol in breastmilk was found to be 113 picograms/mL.[6] This is very close to that seen when the woman begins ovulating during lactation. If oral contraceptives are used during lactation, the transfer of estradiol to human milk will be low and will not exceed the transfer during physiologic conditions when the mother has resumed ovulation. See oral contraceptives.

Pregnancy Risk Category: X

Lactation Risk Category: L3

Adult Concerns: Estrogen use has been associated with breast tenderness, increased risk of thromboembolic disorders, headache, nausea, vomiting, etc.

Pediatric Concerns: None reported. Infantile feminization is unlikely at normal dosages.

Drug Interactions: Rifampin reduces the serum levels of estrogen. Exogenous estrogens increase toxicity of hydrocortisone, and thromboembolic events with anticoagulants such as warfarin.

Theoretic Infant Dose: 16.95

Relative Infant Dose:

Adult Dose: 10 mg TID

Alternatives: Norethindrone

T½ =	60 minutes	M/P =	0.08
PHL =		PB =	98%
T~max~ =	Rapid	Oral =	Complete
MW =	272	pKa =	
Vd =			

References:
1. Booker DE, Pahl IR. Control of postpartum breast engorgement with oral contraceptives. Am J Obstet Gynecol 1967; 98(8):1099-1101.
2. Kamal I, Hefnawi F, Ghoneim M, Abdallah M, Abdel RS. Clinical, biochemical, and experimental studies on lactation. V. Clinical effects of steroids on the initiation of lactation. Am J Obstet Gynecol 1970; 108(4):655-658.
3. Kora SJ. Effect of oral contraceptives on lactation. Fertil Steril 1969; 20(3):419-423.
4. Koetsawang S, Bhiraleus P, Chiemprajert T. Effects of oral contraceptives on lactation. Fertil Steril 1972; 23(1):24-28.
5. Laukaran VH. The effects of contraceptive use on the initiation and duration of lactation. Int J Gynaecol Obstet 1987; 25 Suppl:129-142.
6. Nilsson S, Nygren KG, Johansson ED. Transfer of estradiol to human milk. Am J Obstet Gynecol 1978; 132(6):653-657.

ETANERCEPT

Trade: Enbrel
Can/Aus/UK: Enbrel
Uses: Anti-arthritic
LRC: L3
AAP: Not reviewed

Etanercept is a dimeric fusion protein consisting of the extracellular ligand-binding portion of tumor necrosis factor bound to human IgG1. Etanercept binds specifically to tumor necrosis factor (TNF) and blocks its inflammatory and immune activity in rheumatoid arthritis patients.[1,2] Elevated levels of TNF are found in the synovial fluid of arthritis patients. No data on the transfer of etanercept to human milk are available. However, due to its enormous molecular weight (150,000 daltons), it is extremely unlikely clinically relevant amounts would transfer into milk. In addition, due to its protein structure, it would not be orally bioavailable in an infant. Infliximamide is somewhat similar and is apparently not secreted into human milk (see infliximamide).

Pregnancy Risk Category: B

Lactation Risk Category: **L3**

Adult Concerns: Etanercept may suppress the immune system and increase the risk of infections significantly.   Incidence of infections is 38%. Headache, dizziness, cough, and rhinitis have been reported.

Pediatric Concerns: None reported via milk.

Drug Interactions: Do not administer live vaccines concurrent with etanercept.

Theoretic Infant Dose:

Relative Infant Dose:

Adult Dose: 25 mg twice weekly

Alternatives: Infliximab

$T\frac{1}{2}$ =	115 hours	M/P =	
PHL =		PB =	
T_{max} =	72 hours	Oral =	Nil
MW =	150000	pKa =	
Vd =	0.24		

References:
1.   Pharmaceutical Manufacturer Prescribing Information. 1999.
2.   Drug Facts and Comparisons 1999 ed. ed. St. Louis: 1999.

ETHACRYNIC ACID
Trade: Edecrin
Can/Aus/UK: Edecrin, Edecril
Uses: Powerful loop diuretic
LRC: L3
AAP: Not reviewed

Ethacrynic acid is a potent, short-acting loop diuretic similar to Lasix. It is listed by the manufacturer as contraindicated in nursing women. A significant decrease in maternal blood pressure or blood volume may reduce milk production.   No data on transfer into human milk are available.[1,2]

Pregnancy Risk Category: **B**

Lactation Risk Category: **L3**

Adult Concerns: Diuresis, hypotension, diarrhea

Pediatric Concerns: None reported.

Drug Interactions: Increased toxicity when used with antihypertensives, other diuretics, aminoglycosides. Increased risk of arrhythmias when used with digoxin.   Probenecid reduces diuresis of this product.

Theoretic Infant Dose:

Relative Infant Dose:

Adult Dose: 50-200 mg daily

Alternatives: Furosemide

T½ =	2-4 hours	M/P =	
PHL =		PB =	90%
T$_{max}$ =	2 hours (oral)	Oral =	100%
MW =	303	pKa =	
Vd =			

References:
1. Pharmaceutical Manufacturer Prescribing Information. 1996.
2. Lacy C. Drug information handbook. Lexi-Comp Inc. Cleveland, OH, 1996.

ETHAMBUTOL
Trade: Ethambutol, Myambutol
Can/Aus/UK: Etibi, Myambutol
Uses: Antitubercular drug
LRC: L2
AAP: Maternal Medication Usually Compatible with Breastfeeding

Ethambutol is an antimicrobial used for tuberculosis. Small amounts are secreted in milk although no studies are available which clearly document levels. In one unpublished study, the mother had an ethambutol plasma level of 1.5 mg/L three hours after a dose of 15 mg/kg. Following a similar dose, the concentration in milk was 1.4 mg/L.[1] In another patient, the plasma level was 4.62 mg/L, and the corresponding milk concentration was 4.6 mg/L (no dose available).

Pregnancy Risk Category: B

Lactation Risk Category: L2

Adult Concerns: Optic neuritis, dizziness, confusion, nausea, vomiting, anorexia

Pediatric Concerns: None reported but caution is recommended.

Drug Interactions: Aluminum salts may decrease oral absorption.

Theoretic Infant Dose: 0.69 mg/kg/day

Relative Infant Dose:

Adult Dose: 15-25 mg/kg daily

Alternatives:

T½ =	3.1 hours	M/P =	1.0
PHL =		PB =	8-22%
Tmax =	2-4 hours	Oral =	80%
MW =	204	pKa =	
Vd =			

References:
1. Snider DE, Jr., Powell KE. Should women taking antituberculosis drugs breast-feed? Arch Intern Med 1984; 144(3):589-590.

ETHANOL

Trade: Alcohol
Can/Aus/UK:
Uses: Depressant
LRC: L3
AAP: Maternal Medication Usually Compatible with Breastfeeding

Significant amounts of alcohol are secreted into breastmilk although it is not considered harmful to the infant if the amount and duration are limited. The absolute amount of alcohol transferred into milk is generally low. Beer, but not ethanol, has been reported in a number of studies to stimulate prolactin levels and breastmilk production.[1-3] Thus it is presumed that the polysaccharide from barley may be the prolactin-stimulating component of beer.[4] Non-alcoholic beer is equally effective.

In a study of twelve breastfeeding mothers who ingested 0.3 g/kg of ethanol in orange juice (equivalent to 1 can of beer for the average sized woman), the mean maximum concentration of ethanol in milk was 320 mg/L.[5] This report suggests a 23% reduction (156 to 120 mL) in breastmilk production following ingestion of beer and an increase in milk odor as a function of ethanol content.

Excess levels may lead to drowsiness, deep sleep, weakness, and decreased linear growth in infant. Maternal blood alcohol levels must attain 300 mg/dl before significant side effects are reported in the infant. Reduction of letdown is apparently dose-dependent and requires alcohol consumption of 1.5 to 1.9 gm/kg body weight[6]. Other studies have suggested psychomotor delay in infants of moderate drinkers (2+ drinks daily). Avoid breastfeeding during and for 2-3 hours after drinking alcohol.

In an interesting study of the effect of alcohol on milk ingestion by infants, the rate of milk consumption by infants during the 4 hours immediately after exposure to alcohol (0.3 g/kg) in 12 mothers was significantly less.[7] Compensatory increases in intake were then observed during the 8-16 hours after exposure when mothers refrained from drinking.

Adult metabolism of alcohol is approximately 1 oz in 3 hours, so mothers who ingest alcohol in moderate amounts can generally return to breastfeeding as soon as they feel neurologically normal. Chronic or heavy consumers of alcohol should not breastfeed.

Pregnancy Risk Category: D

Lactation Risk Category: L3

Adult Concerns: Sedation, decreased milk supply, altered milk taste

Pediatric Concerns: Sedation, irritability, weak sucking, decreased milk supply, increased milk odor.

Drug Interactions: Increased CNS depression when used with barbiturates, benzodiazepines, chloral hydrate, and other CNS depressants. A disulfiram-like reaction (flushing, weakness, sweating, tachycardia, etc.) may occur when used with cephalosporins, chlorpropamide, disulfiram, furazolidone, metronidazole, procarbazine. Increased hypoglycemia when used with sulfanurias and other hypoglycemic agents. Intolerance of bromocriptine.

Theoretic Infant Dose: 48 mg/kg/day

Relative Infant Dose: 16%

Adult Dose:

Alternatives:

T½ =	0.24 hours	M/P =	1.0
PHL =		PB =	0%
T$_{max}$ =	30-90 minutes (oral)	Oral =	100%
MW =	46	pKa =	
Vd =	0.53		

References:
1. Marks V, Wright JW. Endocrinological and metabolic effects of alcohol. Proc R Soc Med 1977; 70(5):337-344.
2. De Rosa G, Corsello SM, Ruffilli MP, Della CS, Pasargiklian E. Prolactin secretion after beer. Lancet 1981; 2(8252):934.
3. Carlson HE, Wasser HL, Reidelberger RD. Beer-induced prolactin secretion: a clinical and laboratory study of the role of salsolinol. J Clin Endocrinol Metab 1985; 60(4):673-677.
4. Koletzko B, Lehner F. Beer and breastfeeding. Adv Exp Med Biol 2000; 478:23-28.
5. Mennella JA, Beauchamp GK. The transfer of alcohol to human milk. Effects on flavor and the infant's behavior. N Engl J Med 1991; 325(14):981-985.
6. Cobo E. Effect of different doses of ethanol on the milk-ejecting reflex in lactating women. Am J Obstet Gynecol 1973; 115(6):817-821.
7. Mennella JA. Regulation of milk intake after exposure to alcohol in mothers' milk. Alcohol Clin Exp Res 2001; 25(4):590-593.

ETHOSUXIMIDE

Trade: Zarontin
Can/Aus/UK: Zarontin
Uses: Anticonvulsant used in epilepsy
LRC: L4
AAP: Maternal Medication Usually Compatible with Breastfeeding

Ethosuximide is an anticonvulsant used in epilepsy. Rane's data suggest that although significant levels of ethosuximide are transferred into human milk, the plasma level in the infant is quite low.[1] A peak milk concentration of approximately 55 mg/L was reported at 1 month postpartum. Milk/plasma ratios were reported to be 1.03 on day 3 postpartum and 0.8 during the first three months of therapy. The infant's plasma reached a peak (2.9 mg/dl) at approximately 1.5 months postpartum and then declined significantly over the next 3 months suggesting increased clearance by the infant. Although these levels are considered subtherapeutic, it is suggested that the infant's plasma levels be occasionally tested.

In another study of a women receiving 500 mg twice daily, her milk levels, as estimated from a graph, averaged 60-70 mg/L.[2] A total daily exposure to ethosuximide of 3.6-11 mg/kg as a result of nursing was predicted.

In a study by Kuhnz of 10 epileptic breastfeeding mothers (and 13 infants) receiving 3.5 to 23.6 mg/kg/day, the breastmilk concentrations were similar to those of the maternal plasma (milk/serum: 0.86) and the breastfed infants maintained serum levels between 15 and 40 μg/mL.[3] Maximum milk concentration reported was 77 mg/L although the average was 49.54 mg/L. Neonatal behavior complications such as poor suckling, sedation, and hyperexcitability occurred in 7 of the 12 infants. Interestingly, one infant who was not breastfed, exhibited severe withdrawal symptoms such as tremors, kloni, restlessness, insomnia, crying and vomiting which lasted for 8 weeks causing a slow weight gain. Thus the question remains; is it safer to breastfeed and avoid these severe withdrawal reactions?

These studies clearly indicate that the amount of ethosuximide transferred to the infant is significant. With milk/plasma ratios of approximately 0.86-1.0 and relatively high maternal plasma levels, the maternal plasma levels are a good indication of the dose transferred to the infant. Milk levels are generally high. Caution is recommended.

Pregnancy Risk Category: C
Lactation Risk Category: L4

Adult Concerns: Drowsiness, ataxia, nausea, vomiting, anorexia, rash

Pediatric Concerns: Neonatal behavior complications such as poor suckling, sedation, and hyperexcitability occurred in 7 of 12 infants in one study. Milk levels are significant. Caution is recommended.

Drug Interactions: Decreased efficacy of ethosuximide when used with phenytoin, carbamazepine, primidone, phenobarbital (may reduce plasma levels). Elevated levels of ethosuximide may result when used with isoniazid.

Theoretic Infant Dose: 7.4 mg/kg/day

Relative Infant Dose: 31.4%

Adult Dose: 250-750 mg BID

Alternatives:

$T\frac{1}{2}$ =	30-60 hours	M/P =	0.94
PHL =	32-38 hours	PB =	0%
T_{max} =	4 hours	Oral =	Complete
MW =	141	pKa =	9.3
Vd =	0.72		

References:
1. Rane A, Tunell R. Ethosuximide in human milk and in plasma of a mother and her nursed infant. Br J Clin Pharmacol 1981; 12(6):855-858.
2. Koup JR, Rose JQ, Cohen ME. Ethosuximide pharmacokinetics in a pregnant patient and her newborn. Epilepsia 1978; 19(6):535-539.
3. Kuhnz W, Koch S, Jakob S, Hartmann A, Helge H, Nau H. Ethosuximide in epileptic women during pregnancy and lactation period. Placental transfer, serum concentrations in nursed infants and clinical status. Br J Clin Pharmacol 1984; 18(5):671-677.

ETHOTOIN
Trade: Peganone
Can/Aus/UK:
Uses: Anticonvulsant
LRC: L3
AAP: Not reviewed

Ethotoin is a typical phenytoin-like anticonvulsant. Although no data are available on concentrations in breastmilk, its similarity to phenytoin would suggest that some is secreted via breastmilk.[1] No data are available in the literature. See phenytoin.

Pregnancy Risk Category: D

Lactation Risk Category: L3

Adult Concerns: Drowsiness, dizziness, insomnia, headache, blood dyscrasias

Pediatric Concerns: None reported, but see phenytoin.

Drug Interactions: See phenytoin.

Theoretic Infant Dose:

Relative Infant Dose:

Adult Dose:

Alternatives:

T½ =	3-9 hours	M/P =	
PHL =		PB =	Low-41%
Tmax =	1-2 hours	Oral =	Complete
MW =	204	pKa =	
Vd =			

References:
1. McEvoy GE. (ed):AFHS Drug Information. New York, NY: 2003.

ETIDRONATE

Trade: Didronel
Can/Aus/UK: Didronel
Uses: Slows bone turnover
LRC: L3
AAP: Not reviewed

Etidronate is a bisphosphonate that slows the dissolution of hydroxyapatite crystals in the bone, thus reducing bone calcium loss in certain syndromes such as Paget's syndrome.[1] Etidronate also reduces the remineralization of bone and can result in osteomalacia over time. It is not known how the administration of this product during active lactation would effect the maternal bone porosity. It is possible that milk calcium levels could be reduced although this has not been reported. Etidronate is poorly absorbed orally (1%) and must be administered in between meals on an empty stomach. Its penetration into milk is possible due to its small molecular weight, but it has not yet been reported. However, due to the presence of fat and calcium in milk, its oral bioavailability in infants would be exceedingly low. Whereas the plasma half-life is approximately 6 hours, the terminal elimination half-life (from bone) is > 90 days.

Pregnancy Risk Category: B

Lactation Risk Category: L3

Adult Concerns: Untoward effects include loss of taste, nephrotoxicity, risk of fractures, and focal osteomalacia after prolonged use. Fever, convulsions, bone pain.

Pediatric Concerns: None reported via milk. Although unreported, it could result in reduced milk calcium levels. Oral absorption in infant would be minimal.

Drug Interactions: IV Ranitidine doubles the oral absorption of alendronate (similar to etidronate). Oral products containing calcium or magnesium will significantly reduce oral bioavailability. Take on empty stomach.

Theoretic Infant Dose:

Relative Infant Dose:

Adult Dose: 5-10 mg/kg daily

Alternatives:

T½ =	6 hours(plasma)	M/P =	
PHL =		PB =	
T$_{max}$ =	2 hours	Oral =	1-2.5%
MW =	206	pKa =	
Vd =	1.37		

References:
1. Drug Facts and Comparisons 1996 ed. ed. St. Louis: 1996.

ETODOLAC

Trade: Etodolac, Lodine
Can/Aus/UK: Lodine, Ultradol
Uses: Non-steroidal analgesic, antipyretic
LRC: L3
AAP: Not reviewed

Etodolac is a prototypical nonsteroidal antiinflammatory agent (NSAID) with analgesic, antipyretic, and antiinflammatory properties.[1] Thus far no data are available regarding its secretion into human breastmilk. Shorter half-life varieties are preferred.

Pregnancy Risk Category: C

Lactation Risk Category: L3

Adult Concerns: Dyspepsia, nausea, diarrhea, indigestion, heartburn, abdominal pain, and gastrointestinal bleeding

Pediatric Concerns: None reported via milk but observe for nausea, diarrhea, indigestion. Ibuprofen probably preferred at this time.

Drug Interactions: May prolong prothrombin time when used with warfarin. Antihypertensive effects of ACEi family may be blunted or completely abolished by NSAIDs. Some NSAIDs may block antihypertensive effect of beta blockers, diuretics. Used with cyclosporin, may dramatically increase renal toxicity. May increase digoxin, phenytoin, lithium levels. May increase toxicity of methotrexate. May increase bioavailability of penicillamine. Probenecid may increase NSAID levels.

Theoretic Infant Dose:

Relative Infant Dose:

Adult Dose: 200-400 mg q 6-8 hours

Alternatives: Ibuprofen, Voltaren

T½ =	7.3 hours	M/P =		
PHL =		PB =	95-99%	
T~max~ =	1-2 hours	Oral =	80-100%	
MW =	287	pKa =	4.7	
Vd =	0.4			

References:
1. Pharmaceutical Manufacturer Prescribing Information. 1995.

ETONOGESTREL + ETHINYL ESTRADIOL

Trade: Nuvaring
Can/Aus/UK:
Uses: Slow release vaginal ring contraceptive
LRC: L3
AAP: Not reviewed

NuvaRing is a slow release vaginal ring which releases on average 0.120 mg/day of etonogestrel and 0.015 mg/day of ethinyl estradiol over a 3 week period of use. Etonogestrel is the biologically active metabolite of desogestrel and has both high progestational activity with low intrinsic androgenicity. The bioavailability of ethinyl estradiol when administered intravaginally is approximately 55.6%, which is comparable to that when it is administered orally. Small amounts of estrogens and progestins are known to pass into milk, but long-term follow-up of children whose mothers used combination hormal contraceptives while breastfeeding has shown no deleterious effects on infants. Estrogen-containing contraceptives may interfere with milk production by decreasing the quantity and quality of milk production.

Pregnancy Risk Category: X

Lactation Risk Category: L3

Adult Concerns: Do not use in patients with: thromboplebitis or thromboembolic disorders, cerebral vascular or coronary artery disease, severe hypertension. Numerous other contraindications exist, check the package insert.

Pediatric Concerns: This is an estrogen-containing contraceptive device. Estrogens in some patients may inhibit milk production significantly and change the quality of milk components. Caution patient to observe for suppression of milk production.

Drug Interactions: Check package insert

Theoretic Infant Dose:

Relative Infant Dose:

Adult Dose:

Alternatives: Progestin-only oral contraceptives.

T½ =	29.3 hours	M/P =	
PHL =		PB =	96%
Tmax =	200 hours	Oral =	
MW =	324	pKa =	
Vd =			

References:
1. Pharmaceutical Manufacturers Package Insert, 2003.

ETONOGESTREL IMPLANT
Trade: Implanon
Can/Aus/UK: Implanon
Uses: Implantable progestin contraceptive
LRC: L2
AAP: Not reviewed

Implanon is a slow release isingle-rod contraceptive implant. It consists of a non-biodegradable rod measuring 40 mm in length and 2 mm in diameter which releases on average 40 µg/day of etonogestrel over a 3 year period of use. Etonogestrel is the biologically active metabolite of desogestrel and has both high progestational activity with low intrinsic androgenicity. Implanon does not contain estrogen, making it suitable for women who do not tolerate or are contraindicated to estrogens.

Small amounts of progestins are known to pass into milk, but long-term follow-up of children whose mothers used hormonal contraceptives while breastfeeding has shown no deleterious effects on infants. Like other progestogen-only contraceptives, the use of Implanon is associated with irregular menstrual bleeding and sometimes absence of bleeding, and counseling is required to ensure women make informed choices.[1] Of the contraceptives, progestins are generally preferred as they produce fewer changes in milk production compared to estrogen-containing products. This product is probably quite safe for use in breastfeeding mothers although all mothers should be counseled to observe for changes in milk production.

Pregnancy Risk Category: X

Lactation Risk Category: L2

Adult Concerns: Adverse events include weight gain, acne, headaches.

Pediatric Concerns: Progestins generally have minimal effect on milk production, but some mothers have reported reduced milk production following the use of progestin oral contraceptives. Some caution is recommended although changes in milk supply are very unlikely. Transfer of progestins into milk and to the infant are remote.

Drug Interactions: Check package insert.

Theoretic Infant Dose:

Relative Infant Dose:

Adult Dose: One implant every 3 years.

Alternatives: Norethindrone

T½ =	29.3 hours	M/P =
PHL =		PB =
T$_{max}$ =	200 hours	Oral =
MW =	324	pKa =
Vd =		

References:

1. Pharmaceutical Manufacturers Package Insert, 2003.

ETRETINATE

Trade: Tegison
Can/Aus/UK: Tigason
Uses: Antipsoriatic
LRC: L5
AAP: Not reviewed

Etretinate is an oral Vitamin A derivative primarily used for psoriasis and sometimes acne. It is teratogenic and should not be administered to pregnant women or women about to become pregnant. Etretinate is known to transfer into animal milk although no data are available on human milk.[1,2] Etretinate is still detectable in human serum up to 2.9 years after administration has ceased due to storage at high concentrations in adipose tissue. Mothers who wish to breastfeed following therapy with this compound should be informed of its long half-life in the human. The manufacturer considers this drug to be contraindicated in breastfeeding mothers due to the potential for serious adverse effects.

Pregnancy Risk Category: X

Lactation Risk Category: L5

Adult Concerns: Dry nose, chapped lips, nose bleeds, hair loss, peeling of skin on soles, palms, sunburns, and headaches. Elevated liver enzymes, lipids. Fatigue, headache, fever.

Pediatric Concerns: None reported but great caution is urged. Premature epiphyseal closure has been reported in children treated with this product.

Drug Interactions: Milk increases absorption of oral etretinate. Exogenous vitamin A increases toxicity.

Theoretic Infant Dose:

Relative Infant Dose:

Adult Dose: 0.5-0.75 mg/kg BID

Alternatives:

T½ =	120 days (terminal)	M/P =	
PHL =		PB =	> 99%
T$_{max}$ =	2-6 hours	Oral =	Complete
MW =	354	pKa =	
Vd =	High		

References:
1. Pharmaceutical Manufacturer Prescribing Information. 1995.
2. Lacy C. Drug information handbook. Lexi-Comp Inc. Cleveland, OH, 1996.

EVENING PRIMROSE OIL
Trade: EPO
Can/Aus/UK: Efamol
Uses: Nutritional supplement
LRC: L3
AAP: Not reviewed

Evening primrose oil is a rich source of essential polyunsaturated fatty acids (EFA) particularly gamma linoleic acid (GLA). Human milk is generally rich in 6-desaturated essential fatty acids including arachidonic, GLA, and dihomoj-GLA (DGLA), which may play an important role in development of the infants brain. The brain contains about 20% of 6-desaturated EFAs. Supplementation in pregnant women has been found to significantly increase EFA content in human breastmilk.[1] Although there is some evidence that GLA may be beneficial in syndromes such as cardiovascular disease, rheumatoid arthritis, multiple sclerosis, and atopic dermatitis, many of these studies were sponsored by the manufacturer and need independent confirmation.[2,3] Overt toxicity of this product appears quite low. A number of studies in adults using GLA at rather high doses have not been found to produce significant toxicity.

Pregnancy Risk Category:

Lactation Risk Category: **L3**

Adult Concerns: Major untoward effects are largely unreported although some patients have quit various studies for unspecified reasons.

Pediatric Concerns: None reported.

Drug Interactions:

Theoretic Infant Dose:

Relative Infant Dose:

Adult Dose:

Alternatives:

References:
1. Cant A, Shay J, Horrobin DF. The effect of maternal supplementation with linoleic and gamma-linolenic acids on the fat composition and content of human milk: a placebo-controlled trial. J Nutr Sci Vitaminol (Tokyo) 1991; 37(6):573-579.
2. Horrobin DF, Manku MS. How do polyunsaturated fatty acids lower plasma cholesterol levels? Lipids 1983; 18(8):558-562.
3. Review of Natural Products Facts and Comparisons, St Louis, MO 1996.

EZETIMIBE
Trade: Zetia
Can/Aus/UK:
Uses: Anti-cholesterol agent
LRC: L3
AAP: Not reviewed

Ezetimibe reduces blood cholesterol by inhibiting the absorption of cholesterol from the small intestine.[1] It appears to act at the brush border of the small intestine and inhibits the absorption of cholesterol leading to a direct reduction in delivery of cholesterol to the liver. No data are available on the transfer of this agent to milk. This is a very lipophilic agent but has reasonably poor oral bioavailability. It's not clear at all if it would be safe for use in a breastfed infant who needs high levels of cholesterol anyway. Some caution is recommended until data are available.

Pregnancy Risk Category: **C**

Lactation Risk Category: **L3**

Adult Concerns: Generally well tolerated but viral infection, headache, fatigue, and GI symptoms such as diarrhea and abdominal pain have been reported but these symptoms are rather low in incidence.

Pediatric Concerns: No data available on transfer to human milk. Some caution is recommended.

Drug Interactions: Additive when used with HMG CoA reductase inhibitors. Ezetimibe levels increased 12 fold in a renal transplant patient receiving cyclosporine and other agents. There is an increased risk of myopathy or rhabdomyolysis when used with fibric acid products(fenofibrate).

Theoretic Infant Dose:

Relative Infant Dose:

Adult Dose: 10 mg daily

Alternatives: Cholestyramine salts

T½ =	22 hours	M/P =	
PHL =		PB =	> 90%
T~max~ =	4-12 hours	Oral =	35-60%
MW =	409	pKa =	
Vd =			

References:
1. Pharmaceutical Manufacturers prescribing information, 2003.

FAMCICLOVIR
Trade: Famvir
Can/Aus/UK: Famvir
Uses: Antiviral for Herpes Zoster
LRC: L2
AAP: Not reviewed

Famciclovir is an antiviral use in the treatment of uncomplicated herpes zoster infection (shingles) and genital herpes. It is rapidly metabolized to the active metabolite, penciclovir. Although similar to Acyclovir, no data are available on levels in human milk. Oral bioavailability of famciclovir (77%) is much better than acyclovir (15-30%). Studies with rodents suggest that the milk/plasma ratio is greater than 1.0.[1,2] Because famciclovir provides few advantages over acyclovir, at this point acyclovir would probably be preferred in a nursing mother although the side-effect profile is still minimal with this product.

Pregnancy Risk Category: B

Lactation Risk Category: L2

Adult Concerns: Headache, dizziness, nausea, diarrhea, fever, anorexia

Pediatric Concerns: None reported via milk.

Drug Interactions: Cimetidine increases plasma levels of the active metabolite penciclovir.   Famciclovir increases digoxin plasma levels by 19%.   Probenecid significantly increase penciclovir plasma levels.

Theoretic Infant Dose:

Relative Infant Dose:

Adult Dose: 125 mg BID

Alternatives: Acyclovir

T½ =	2-3 hours	M/P =	>1
PHL =		PB =	<20%
T$_{max}$ =	0.9 hours	Oral =	77%
MW =		pKa =	
Vd =	1,13		

References:
1.   Drug Facts and Comparisons 1994 ed. ed. St. Louis: 1994.
2.   Pharmaceutical Manufacturer Prescribing Information. 1995.

FAMOTIDINE
Trade: Pepcid, Axid-Ar, Pepcid-Ac
Can/Aus/UK: Pepcid, Apo-Famotidine, Novo-Famotidine, Amfamox, Pepcidine
Uses: Reduces gastric acid secretion
LRC: L1
AAP: Not reviewed

Famotidine is a typical Histamine-2 antagonist that reduces stomach acid secretion.   In one study of 8 lactating women receiving a 40 mg/day dose, the peak concentration in breastmilk was 72 μg/L and occurred at 6 hours post-dose.[1]   The milk/plasma ratios were 0.41, 1.78, and 1.33 at 2, 6, and 24 hours respectively.   These levels are apparently much lower than other histamine H-2 antagonists (ranitidine, cimetidine) and make it a preferred choice.

Pregnancy Risk Category: B

Lactation Risk Category: L1

Adult Concerns: Headache, constipation, increased liver enzymes

Pediatric Concerns: None reported.   Pediatric indications are available.

Drug Interactions: Famotidine reduces bioavailability of ketoconazole, itraconazole due to reduced oral absorption of these two products.

Theoretic Infant Dose: 10.8 µg/kg/day

Relative Infant Dose: 1.8%

Adult Dose: 20-40 mg BID

Alternatives: Nizatidine

T½ =	2.5-3.5 hours	M/P =	0.41-1.78
PHL =		PB =	17%
T$_{max}$ =	1-3.5 hours	Oral =	50%
MW =	337	pKa =	
Vd =			

References:
1. Courtney TP, Shaw RW. et.al. Excretion of famotidine in breastmilk. Br J Clin Pharmacol 1988; 26:639.

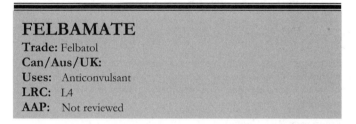

FELBAMATE
Trade: Felbatol
Can/Aus/UK:
Uses: Anticonvulsant
LRC: L4
AAP: Not reviewed

Felbamate is an oral antiepileptic agent for partial seizures and Lennox-Gastaut syndrome. Due to serious side effects, the FDA recommends that felbamate be given only to patients with serious seizures refractory to all other medications. Felbamate is known to be secreted in rodent milk and was detrimental to their offspring.[1] No data are available on human milk. Due to the incidence of severe side effects, extreme caution is recommended with this medication in breastfeeding mothers.

Pregnancy Risk Category: C

Lactation Risk Category: L4

Adult Concerns: Aplastic anemia, weight gain, flu-like symptoms, tachycardia, nausea, vomiting, headache, insomnia

Pediatric Concerns: None reported, but caution is urged.

Drug Interactions: Felbamate causes an increase in phenytoin plasma levels. Phenytoin produces a 45% decrease in felbamate levels. Carbamazepine levels may be decreased, whereas felbamate levels may drop by 40%. Valproic acid plasma levels may be increased.

Theoretic Infant Dose:

Relative Infant Dose:

Adult Dose: 1200 mg/day in 3-4 divided doses

Alternatives:

T½ =	20-23 hours	M/P =	
PHL =		PB =	25%
T$_{max}$ =	1-4 hours	Oral =	90%
MW =		pKa =	
Vd =	0.7-1.0		

References:
1.   Pharmaceutical Manufacturer Prescribing Information. 1995.

FELODIPINE

Trade: Plendil
Can/Aus/UK: Plendil, Renedil, Agon SR, Plendil ER
Uses: Calcium channel blocker, antihypertensive
LRC: L3
AAP: Not reviewed

Felodipine is a calcium channel antagonist structurally related to nifedipine.[1] Because we have numerous studies on others in this family, it is advisable to use nifedipine or others that have breastfeeding studies available.

Pregnancy Risk Category: C

Lactation Risk Category: L3

Adult Concerns: Headache, dizziness, edema, flushing, hypotension, constipation, cardiac arrhythmias

Pediatric Concerns: None reported via milk but caution is recommended.

Drug Interactions: Barbiturates may reduce bioavailability of calcium channel blockers (CCB). Calcium salts may reduce hypotensive effect.   Dantrolene may increase risk of hyperkalemia and myocardial depression. H2 blockers may increase bioavailability of certain CCBs. Hydantoins may reduce plasma levels. Quinidine increases risk of hypotension, bradycardia, tachycardia. Rifampin may reduce effects of CCBs. Vitamin D may reduce efficacy of CCBs.   CCBs may increase carbamazepine, cyclosporin, encainide, prazosin levels.

Theoretic Infant Dose:

Relative Infant Dose:

Adult Dose: 2.5-10 mg daily

Alternatives: Nifedipine, Nimodipine, Verapamil

T½ =	11-16 hours	M/P =	
PHL =		PB =	>99%
T$_{max}$ =	2.5-5 hours	Oral =	20%
MW =	384	pKa =	
Vd =			

References:
1. Pharmaceutical Manufacturer Prescribing Information. 1996.

FENNEL
Trade: Sweet Fennel, Bitter Fennel, Carosella, Florence Fennel, Finocchio, Garden Fennel, Wild fennel
Can/Aus/UK:
Uses: Estrogenic
LRC: L4
AAP: Not reviewed

Fennel is an herb native to southern Europe and Asia Minor. The oils of sweet and bitter fennel contain up to 90% trans-anethole and up to 20% fenchone and numerous other lesser oils. An acetone extract of fennel has been shown to have estrogenic effects on the genital organs of male and female rats.[1] As an herbal medicine it is reputed to increase milk secretion, promote menstruation, facilitate birth, and increased libido. The estrogenic component is believed to be a polymer of the anethole such as dianethole or photoanethole.[2] Ingestion of the volatile oil may induce nausea, vomiting, seizures, pulmonary edema, and hallucinations.[3,4] An older survey of fennel samples in Italy found viable aerobic bacteria including coliforms, fecal streptococci, and salmonella species, suggesting the plant may serve as a vector for infectious gastrointestinal diseases.[5] Fennel is a popular herb that has been used since ancient times. It is primarily believed to be estrogenic. Because estrogens are known to suppress breastmilk production, its use in lactating women is questionable.

Pregnancy Risk Category:

Lactation Risk Category: L4

Adult Concerns: Allergic reactions, photodermatitis, contact dermatitis, and bacterial contamination

Pediatric Concerns: None reported via milk. May potentially suppress milk production.

Drug Interactions:

Theoretic Infant Dose:

Relative Infant Dose:

Adult Dose:

Alternatives:

References:
1. Malini T, Vanithakumari G, Megala N, Anusya S, Devi K, Elango V. Effect of Foeniculum vulgare Mill. seed extract on the genital organs of male and female rats. Indian J Physiol Pharmacol 1985; 29(1):21-26.
2. Albert-Puleo M. Fennel and anise as estrogenic agents. J Ethnopharmacol 1980; 2(4):337-344.
3. Marcus C, Lichtenstein EP. J. Agric Food Chem 1979; 27:1217.
4. Duke JA. Handbook of Medicinal Herbs. Boca Raton, FL: CRC Press, 1985.
5. Ercolani GL. Bacteriological quality assessment of fresh marketed lettuce and fennel. Appl Environ Microbiol 1976; 31(6):847-852.

FENOFIBRATE

Trade: Tricor
Can/Aus/UK:
Uses: Cholesterol lower agent
LRC: L3
AAP: Not reviewed

Fenofibrate produces reduction in total cholesterol, LDL cholesterol, and triglycerides.[1] No data are available on its transfer into human milk, however, agents that reduce plasma cholesterol are not usually considered suitable for use in breastfeeding mothers. Milk levels of cholesterol are higher because of the newborns need for high levels of cholesterol for neurodevelopment. This and other hypocholesterolemic agents should probably not be used in breastfeeding mothers with exception of those with much older infants (>1 year).

Pregnancy Risk Category: C

Lactation Risk Category: L3

Adult Concerns: Adverse events include abdominal pain, back pain, headache, elevated liver function tests, chest pain, respiratory disorders

Pediatric Concerns: None reported via milk, but this agent should not be used in breastfeeding mothers due to the infants need for cholesterol.

Drug Interactions: Potentiates coumarin anticoagulants.

Theoretic Infant Dose:

Relative Infant Dose:

Adult Dose: 160 mg/day.

Alternatives:

T½ =	20 hours	M/P =	
PHL =		PB =	99%
Tmax =		Oral =	85%
MW =	361	pKa =	
Vd =			

References:
1. Pharmaceutical Manufacturers prescribing information, 2003.

FENOPROFEN

Trade: Nalfon
Can/Aus/UK: Nalfon, Fenopron, Progesic
Uses: NSAID, nonsteroidal analgesic
LRC: L2
AAP: Not reviewed

Fenoprofen is a typical nonsteroidal antiinflammatory and analgesic. Following 600 mg four times daily for 4 days postpartum, the milk/plasma ratio was approximately 0.017 and fenoprofen levels in milk were too low to be accurately detected and was estimated to be approximately 1/60th of the maternal plasma level.[1] Fenoprofen was undetectable in cord blood, amniotic fluid, saliva, or washed red blood cells after multiple doses.

Pregnancy Risk Category: B in 1st and 2nd trimesters
D in 3rd trimester

Lactation Risk Category: L2

Adult Concerns: GI distress and bleeding, dyspepsia, nausea, constipation, ulcers, hepatotoxicity, rash, tinnitus

Pediatric Concerns: None reported.

Drug Interactions: May prolong prothrombin time when used with warfarin. Antihypertensive effects of ACEi family may be blunted or completely abolished by NSAIDs. Some NSAIDs may block antihypertensive effect of beta blockers, diuretics. Used with cyclosporin, may dramatically increase renal toxicity. May increase digoxin, phenytoin, lithium levels. May increase toxicity of methotrexate. May increase bioavailability of penicillamine. Probenecid may increase NSAID levels.

Theoretic Infant Dose:

Relative Infant Dose:

Adult Dose: 300-600 mg q 4-6 hours

Alternatives: Ibuprofen

T½ =	2.5 hours	M/P =	0.017
PHL =		PB =	99%
T$_{max}$ =	1-2 hours	Oral =	80%
MW =	242	pKa =	4.5
Vd =	0.08-0.10		

References:
1. Rubin A. et.al. A profile of the physiological disposition and gastrointestinal effects of fenoprofen in man. Curr Med Res Opin 1974; 2:529-544.

FENTANYL

Trade: Sublimaze
Can/Aus/UK: Sublimaze, Duragesic
Uses: Opiate analgesic
LRC: L2
AAP: Maternal Medication Usually Compatible with Breastfeeding

Fentanyl is a potent narcotic analgesic used (IV, IM, transdermally) during labor and delivery. When used parenterally, its half-life is exceedingly short.[1]

The transfer of fentanyl into human milk has been documented but is low. In a group of ten women receiving a total dose of 50 to 400 µg fentanyl IV during labor, the concentration of fentanyl in milk was exceedingly low, generally below the level of detection (<0.05 ng/mL).[2] In a few samples, the levels were between 0.05 and 0.15 ng/mL. Using this data, an infant would ingest less than 3% of the weight-adjusted maternal dose per day.

In another study of 13 women who received 2 µg/kg IV after delivery and cord clamping, fentanyl concentration in colostrum was extremely low.[2] Peak colostrum concentrations occurred at 45 minutes following intravenous administration and averaged 0.4 µg/L. Colostrum levels dropped rapidly and were undetectable after 10 hours. The authors conclude that with these small concentrations and fentanyl's low oral bioavailability, intravenous fentanyl analgesia may be used safely in breastfeeding women.

The relatively low level of fentanyl found in human milk is presumably a result of the short maternal half-life, and the rather rapid redistribution out of the maternal plasma compartment. It is apparent that fentanyl transfer to milk under most clinical conditions is poor and is probably clinically unimportant.

Pregnancy Risk Category: B
Lactation Risk Category: L2

Adult Concerns: Apnea, respiratory depression, muscle rigidity, hypotension, bradycardia

Pediatric Concerns: No adverse effects reported via milk.

Drug Interactions: Increased toxicity when used with other CNS depressants, phenothiazines, tricyclic antidepressants.

Theoretic Infant Dose: 0.06 µg/kg/day

Relative Infant Dose: 3%

Adult Dose: 2-20 µg/kg injection (IV)

Alternatives:

$T\frac{1}{2}$ =	2-4 hours	M/P =	
PHL =	3-13 hours (neonates)	PB =	80-86%
T_{max} =	7-8 minutes (IV)	Oral =	25-75%
MW =	336	pKa =	8.4
Vd =	3-8		

References:
1. Madej TH, Strunin L. Comparison of epidural fentanyl with sufentanil. Analgesia and side effects after a single bolus dose during elective caesarean section. Anaesthesia 1987; 42(11):1156-1161.
2. Leuschen MP, Wolf LJ, Rayburn WF. Fentanyl excretion in breastmilk. Clin Pharm 1990; 9(5):336-337.

FENUGREEK
Trade:
Can/Aus/UK:
Uses: Herbal spice
LRC: L3
AAP: Not reviewed

Fenugreek is commonly sold as the dried, ripe seed, and extracts are used as an artificial flavor for maple syrup[1]. The seeds contain from 0.1 to 0.9% diosgenin.[2] Several coumarin compounds have been noted in the seed as well as a number of alkaloids such as trigonelline, gentianin, and carpaine. The seeds also contain approximately 8% of a foul-smelling oil.

Fenugreek has been noted to reduce plasma cholesterol in animals when 50% of their diet contained fenugreek seeds.[3] The high fiber content may have accounted for this change although it may be due to the steroid saponins. A hypoglycemic effect has also been noted. When added to the diet of diabetic dogs, a decrease in insulin dose and hyperglycemia was noted.[4] It is not known if these changes are due to the fiber content of the seeds or a chemical component. Fenugreek has been reported to increase the anticoagulant effect of warfarin.[5] One case of GI bleeding in a premature infant (30 weeks) following introduction of fenugreek to the mother has been received.[6] The implication of fenugreek in this hemorrhage is speculative.

In a group of 10 women (non-placebo controlled) with infants born between 24 to 38 weeks gestation (mean=29 weeks) who ingested 3 fenugreek capsules 3 times daily (Nature's Way) for a week, the average milk production during the week increased significantly from a mean of 207 mL/day (range 57 - 1057 mL) to 464 mL/day (range 63-1140 mL).[8] No untoward effects were reported.

When dosed in moderation, fenugreek has limited toxicity and is listed in the US as a GRAS herbal (Generally Regarded As Safe). A maple syrup odor via urine and sweat is commonly reported. Higher doses may produce hypoglycemia. A stimulant effect on the isolated uterus (guinea pig) has been reported and its use in late pregnancy may not be advisable. Fenugreek's reputation as a galactagogue is widespread but undocumented. The dose commonly employed is variable but is approximately 2-3 capsules taken three times daily. The transfer of fenugreek into milk is unknown, but untoward effects have only rarely been reported.

Pregnancy Risk Category:

Lactation Risk Category: L3

Adult Concerns: Maple syrup odor in urine and sweat. Diarrhea, hypoglycemia, dyspnea (exaggeration of asthmatic symptoms). Once case of suspected GI bleeding in a premature infant has been reported.[6] Two cases of fenugreek allergy have been reported.[7]

Pediatric Concerns: Once case of suspected GI bleeding in a premature infant has been reported.[6]

Drug Interactions:

Theoretic Infant Dose:

Relative Infant Dose:

Adult Dose:

Alternatives: Metoclopramide, domperidone

References:
1. Review of Natural Products Facts and Comparisons, St Louis, MO 1996.
2. Sauvaire Y, Baccou JC. Extraction of diosgenin, (25R)-spirost-5-ene-3beta-ol; problems of the hydrolysis of the saponins. Lloydia 1978; 41:247.
3. Valette G, Sauvaire Y, Baccou JC, Ribes G. Hypocholesterolaemic effect of fenugreek seeds in dogs. Atherosclerosis 1984; 50(1):105-111.
4. Ribes G, Sauvaire Y, Baccou JC, Valette G, Chenon D, Trimble ER, Loubatieres-Mariani MM. Effects of fenugreek seeds on endocrine pancreatic secretions in dogs. Ann Nutr Metab 1984; 28(1):37-43.

5. Lambert JP, Cormier A. Potential interaction between warfarin and boldo-fenugreek. Pharmacotherapy 2001; 21(4):509-512.
6. DH. Personal communication. 2001.
7. Patil SP, Niphadkar PV, Bapat MM. Allergy to fenugreek (Trigonella foenum graecum). Ann Allergy Asthma Immunol 1997; 78(3):297-300.
8. Swafford S, Berens P. Effect of fenugreek on breastmilk production. Abstract. ABM News and Views 2000; 6(3):2000.

FEXOFENADINE

Trade: Allegra
Can/Aus/UK: Allegra
Uses: Antihistamine
LRC: L2
AAP: Maternal Medication Usually Compatible with Breastfeeding

Fexofenadine is a non-sedating histamine-1 receptor antagonist and is the active metabolite of terfenadine (Seldane). It is indicated for symptoms of allergic rhinitis and other allergies. Unlike Seldane, no cardiotoxicity has been reported with this product.

In a study of 4 women receiving 60 mg/d terfenadine, no terfenadine was found in milk. However, the metabolite (fexofenadine) was present in small amounts. The average milk level of fexofenadine was 41 µg/L while the maternal plasma averaged 309 ng/mL. The time to peak for milk was 4.3 hours and the half-life in milk was 14.2 hours. The AUC(0-12)(ng.hr/mL) was 320 for milk and 1590 for plasma. The authors estimate that only 0.45% of the weight-adjusted maternal dose would be ingested by the infant.

Pregnancy Risk Category: C

Lactation Risk Category: L2

Adult Concerns: Drowsiness, fatigue, leukopenia, nausea, dyspepsia, dry mouth, headache, and throat irritation have been reported. Thus far, no cardiotoxicity has been reported .

Pediatric Concerns: None reported.

Drug Interactions: Erythromycin and ketoconazole (and potentially other azole antifungals and macrolide antibiotics) may elevate the plasma level of fexofenadine(82%) significantly.

Theoretic Infant Dose: 6.15 µg/kg/day

Relative Infant Dose: 0.71%

Adult Dose: 60 mg BID

Alternatives:

T½ =	14.4 hours	M/P =	0.21
PHL =		PB =	60-70%
T$_{max}$ =	2.6 hours	Oral =	Complete
MW =	538	pKa =	
Vd =			

References:
1. Lucas BD, Jr., Purdy CY, Scarim SK, Benjamin S, Abel SR, Hilleman DE. Terfenadine pharmacokinetics in breastmilk in lactating women. Clin Pharmacol Ther 1995; 57(4):398-402.

FILGRASTIM

Trade: Neupogen
Can/Aus/UK: Neupogen
Uses: Synthetic hematopoietic agent.
LRC: L2
AAP: Not reviewed

Filgrastim is a large molecular weight biosynthetic protein used to stimulate neutrophil production. It is more commonly called granulocyte colony stimulating factor (G-CSF).[1] There are no data on its entry into human milk, but due to its large molecular weight (18,800 daltons) it is extremely remote that any would enter milk. Following use, the plasma levels in most individuals is often undetectable or in the picogram range. Further, due to its protein structure, it would not likely be orally bioavailable to the infant.

Pregnancy Risk Category: C

Lactation Risk Category: L2

Adult Concerns: Transient rash, nausea and vomiting, erythema and swelling at injection site, and splenomegaly

Pediatric Concerns: None reported via milk.

Drug Interactions: Use caution with drugs such as lithium that induce release of neutrophils.

Theoretic Infant Dose:

Relative Infant Dose:

Adult Dose: 5 μg/kg daily

Alternatives:

T½ =	3.5 hours	M/P =	
PHL =		PB =	
T$_{max}$ =	2-8 hours	Oral =	None
MW =	18,800	pKa =	
Vd =	150		

References:
1. Pharmaceutical Manufacturer Prescribing Information. 1999.

FLAVOXATE
Trade: Urispas
Can/Aus/UK: Urispas
Uses: Urinary tract antispasmodic
LRC: L3
AAP: Not reviewed

Flavoxate is used as an antispasmodic to provide relief of painful urination, urgency, nocturia, urinary frequency, or incontinence.[1] It exerts a direct smooth muscle relaxation on the bladder wall and has been used in children for enuresis. No data are available on its transfer into human milk.

Pregnancy Risk Category: B

Lactation Risk Category: L3

Adult Concerns: Drowsiness, dry mouth and throat, nervousness, headache, confusion, nausea, vomiting, blurred vision. Do not use with pyloric or duodenal obstruction, GI hemorrhage, or obstructive uropathies.

Pediatric Concerns: None reported via milk.

Drug Interactions:

Theoretic Infant Dose:

Relative Infant Dose:

Adult Dose: 100-200 mg TID-QID

Alternatives:

$T\frac{1}{2}$ =	< 10 hours	M/P =	
PHL =		PB =	
T_{max} =	2 hours	Oral =	Complete
MW =	391	pKa =	
Vd =			

References:
1. Pharmaceutical Manufacturer Prescribing Information. 1997.

FLECAINIDE ACETATE

Trade: Tambocor
Can/Aus/UK: Tambocor
Uses: Antiarrhythmic agent
LRC: L3
AAP: Maternal Medication Usually Compatible with Breastfeeding

Flecainide is a potent antiarrhythmic used to suppress dangerous ventricular arrhythmias.

In a group of 11 breastfeeding mothers receiving 100 mg oral flecainide (mean =3.2 mg/kg/day) every 12 hours for 5.5 days beginning 1 day postpartum, apparent steady-state levels of flecainide in both milk and plasma were achieved in most cases by day 4 of the study.[1] Highest daily average concentration of flecainide in milk ranged from 270 to 1529 µg/L (mean= 953 µg/L) for the 11 subjects. Mean milk/plasma ratios were 3.7, 3.2, 3.5, and 2.6 on study days 2, 3, 4, and 5 respectively. After the last dose of flecainide, peak milk levels of the drug occurred at 3 to 6 hours and then declined monoexponentially. The half-life for elimination of flecainide from milk was 14.7 hours and is very similar to the plasma elimination half-life of flecainide in healthy human subjects. Based on the pharmacokinetics of flecainide in infants, the expected average steady-state plasma concentration of flecainide in a newborn infant consuming all of the milk production of its mother (approximately 700 mL/day at the highest flecainide level of 1529 µg/L), the average daily intake by the infant would be 1.07 mg. In a normal 4 kg infant, the average plasma concentration in a breastfed infant would not be expected to exceed about 62 ng/mL. The average plasma level in infants treated with therapeutic doses is 360 ng/mL.

In another study of one patient receiving 100 mg every 12 hours, milk levels of flecainide averaged 0.99 mg/L on day 4 and 5 postpartum.[2]

Pregnancy Risk Category: C

Lactation Risk Category: L3

Adult Concerns: Flecainide may induce arrhythmias in certain patients and congestive heart failure in approximately 2-5% of patients due to negative ionotropy. Dizziness, nausea, blurred vision, dyspnea, and vomiting are reported. Flecainide should be reserved for patients with life-threatening arrhythmias. Withdrawal from flecainide therapy should be gradual due to the possibility of fatal cardiac arrest.

Pediatric Concerns: No adverse effects yet reported via milk but observe for dizziness, faintness, dyspnea, headache, nausea, constipation.

Drug Interactions: Flecainide concentrations may be increased by digoxin and amiodarone. Arbutamine may exacerbate the arrhythmogenic effects of flecainide. Beta blockers, disopyramide, and verapamil may enhance the negative ionotropic effect of flecainide. Concurrent oral use of flecainide and cimetidine has been associated with a 46 to 65% increase in the elimination half-life, a 7 to 11% reduction in renal clearance and a 15 to 32% reduction in the nonrenal clearance of flecainide.

Theoretic Infant Dose: 142.9 µg/kg/day

Relative Infant Dose: 5.0%

Adult Dose: 50-100 mg BID

Alternatives:

T½ =	7-22 hours	M/P =	2.6-3.7
PHL =		PB =	50%
T$_{max}$ =	4.5 hours	Oral =	90%
MW =	414	pKa =	
Vd =			

References:
1. McQuinn RL, Pisani A, Wafa S, Chang SF, Miller AM, Frappell JM, Chamberlain GV, Camm AJ. Flecainide excretion in human breastmilk. Clin Pharmacol Ther 1990; 48(3):262-267.
2. Wagner X, Jouglard J, Moulin M, Miller AM, Petitjean J, Pisapia A. Coadministration of flecainide acetate and sotalol during pregnancy: lack of teratogenic effects, passage across the placenta, and excretion in human breastmilk. Am Heart J 1990; 119(3 Pt 1):700-702.

FLOXACILLIN

Trade: Flucil
Can/Aus/UK: Fluclox, Flucloxacillin, Flopen, Floxapen, Staphylex, Flu-Amp, Flu-Clomix, Magnapen
Uses: Penicillin antibiotic
LRC: L1
AAP: Not reviewed

Floxacillin, also called flucloxacillin, is a penicillinase-resistant penicillin frequently used for resistant staphylococcal infections. Only trace amounts are secreted into human milk.[1] Its congener, cloxacillin, is commonly used to treat mastitis in breastfeeding mothers and has been used in thousands of breastfeeding patients without problem. Changes in gut flora are possible but unlikely.

Pregnancy Risk Category: B1

Lactation Risk Category: L1

Adult Concerns: Adverse effects of FLOXACILLIN are similar to those of other penicillins and include nausea, vomiting, diarrhea, constipation, and skin rashes; hemolytic anemia and interstitial nephritis have been reported rarely. Cases of acute hepatic cholestasis related to floxacillin therapy has been reported.

Pediatric Concerns: None reported via milk.

Drug Interactions: Concomitant penicillin and aminoglycoside therapy has been reported to result in inactivation of the aminoglycoside. Small changes in methotrexate plasma levels have been reported.

Theoretic Infant Dose:

Relative Infant Dose:

Adult Dose: 250-500 mg four times daily

Alternatives: Cloxacillin, Dicloxacillin

$T^{1/2}$ =	1.5 hours	M/P =	
PHL =		PB =	94%
T_{max} =	1 hour	Oral =	50%
MW =	454	pKa =	
Vd =	0.11		

References:
1. Pharmaceutical Manufacturer Prescribing Information.

FLUCONAZOLE

Trade: Diflucan
Can/Aus/UK: Diflucan
Uses: Antifungal, particularly candida infections
LRC: L2
AAP: Maternal Medication Usually Compatible with Breastfeeding

Fluconazole is a synthetic triazole antifungal agent and is frequently used for vaginal, oropharyngeal, and esophageal candidiasis. Many of the triazole antifungals (itraconazole, terconazole) have similar mechanisms of action and are considered fungistatic in action. In vivo studies have found fluconazole to have fungistatic activity against a variety of fungal strains including C. albicans, C. tropicalis, T. glabrata, and C. neoformans.

The pharmacokinetics are similar following both oral and IV administration. The drug is almost completely absorbed orally (> 90%). Peak plasma levels occur in 1-2 hours after oral administration. Unlike ketoconazole and itraconazole, fluconazole absorption is unaffected by gastric pH and does not require an acid pH to be absorbed. Steady state plasma levels are only attained after 5-10 days of therapy but can be achieved on day two with a loading dose (twice the daily dose) on the first day. Average plasma levels are 4.12 to 8.1 µg/mL. Fluconazole is widely and evenly distributed in most tissues and fluids and is distributed in total body water. Concentrations in skin and urine may be 10 fold higher than plasma levels. CSF concentrations are 50-94% of the plasma levels. Plasma protein binding is minimal at about 11%. Fluconazole is primarily excreted renally.

Oral fluconazole is currently cleared for pediatric candidiasis for infants 6 months and older, and has an FDA Safety Profile for neonates 1 day and older. Clinical cure rate for oropharyngeal candidiasis in pediatric patients is reported at 86% with fluconazole (2-3 mg/kg/day) compared to 46% of nystatin treated patients. Fluconazole is transferred into human milk with a milk/plasma ratio of approximately 0.85.[1] Following a single 150 mg dose, milk levels at 2, 5, 24 and 48 hours were reported to be 2.93, 2.66, 1.76, and 0.98 µg/mL respectively. Plasma levels at 2, 5, 24, and 48 hours were 6.4, 2.79, 2.52, and 1.19 µg/mL respectively.[1]

Plasma Half-Life = 35 hrs   Breastmilk Half-life = 30 hours

From these data, and assuming an average milk level of 2.3 mg/L, an infant consuming 150 cc/kg/d of milk would receive an average of 0.34 mg/kg/d of fluconazole or 16% of the weight-adjusted maternal dose and less than 5.8% of the pediatric dose (6 mg/kg/d).

In another study of one patient receiving 200 mg daily (1.5 times the above dose) for 18 days, the peak milk concentration was 4.1 mg/L at 2 hours following the dose.[2] However, the mean concentration of fluconazole in milk was not reported.

Side effects: Of the antifungals, fluconazole is very well tolerated. Adverse effects have only been reported in about 5-30% of patients, and in these, only 1-2.8% of patients have required discontinuation of the medication. Although adverse hepatic effects have been reported, they are very rare, and many occur coincidentally with the administration of other medications in AIDS patients. The most common complications include vomiting, diarrhea, abdominal pain, and skin rashes.

Pediatric Indications: While fluconazole is not cleared by the FDA for neonates, it is commonly used (90% of practitioners use it). It is however, cleared for infants 6 months and older. Due to the emergence of resistance to other antifungals, particularly nystatin, the use of fluconazole in pediatrics is increasing. Numerous reports now suggest that fluconazole is an effective and safe antifungal in low birth weight infants and neonates.[3,4,5,6,10]   In one study of 40 low birth weight infants receiving fluconazole for up to 48 days,   fluconazole produced few side effects.[7]   Elevated liver enzymes were reported in only 2 of 40 serious ill LBW infants, and due to other drugs, it is not known if this was associated with fluconazole therapy.

Dosage Recommendations:

Vaginal Candidiasis: 150 mg PO-single dose.

Oropharyngeal Candidiasis: Varies, but 200 mg STAT followed by 100 mg daily for up to 14 days is recommended.   This therapy is not sufficient for ductal candidiasis in lactating women.

Ductal Candidiasis: Because symptoms of ductal candidiasis are sometimes slow to resolve, many clinicians now recommend up to two-three weeks of therapy.   For ductal candidiasis in breastfeeding mothers, doses can vary from 200-400 mg STAT followed by 100-200 mg daily depending on the severity of symptoms and resistance of organism.   The duration of therapy is variable, but a minimum of 2-3 weeks is mandatory to clear systemic infections.   For persistent or chronic infections,   fluconazole has been used prophylactically in immunocompromised patients at a dose of 150 mg weekly to prevent recurrence,[8,9] and this may be suitable for deep ductal candidiasis that is difficult to resolve.

The recommended pediatric dosing for oral candidiasis is 6 mg/kg STAT followed by 3 mg/kg/day.   For systemic candidiasis,   6-12 mg/kg/day   is   generally   recommended.[10]   These   current recommendations   are   for   infants   6   months   and   older.   The manufacturer states that a number of infants 1 day old and older have been safely treated.   One study of premature infants suggests that the dose in very low birth weight infants should be 6 mg/kg every 2 to 3 days.[11]

Fluconazole Dosage*

Indication	Day 1	Daily Therapy	Minimum Duration of Therapy
Oropharyngeal candidiasis	200 mg	100 mg	14 d
Esophageal candidiasis	200 mg	100 mg	21 d
Systemic candidiasis	400 mg	200 mg	28 d

Cryptococcal meningitis
   acute
 	
   relapse
	
	400 mg
	
	200 mg
		
		200 mg
		
		200 mg
			10-12 wk after CSF culture becomes negative

*Pharmaceutical Manufacturers Package Insert

Availability:
50, 100, 200 mg tablets.   Oral suspensions = 10 mg/mL and 40 mg/mL

Pregnancy Risk Category: C

Lactation Risk Category: L2

Adult Concerns: Side effects are minimal and usually include GI symptoms such as vomiting, diarrhea, abdominal pain. Skin rashes, liver toxicity, elevated bilirubin in neonates may occur.

Pediatric Concerns: Pediatric complications from oral ingestion include GI symptoms such as vomiting, nausea, diarrhea, abdominal pain. Nephrotoxicity has not been reported. No complications from exposure to breastmilk have found.

Drug Interactions: Decreased hepatic clearance of fluconazole results from use with cyclosporin, zidovudine, rifabutin, theophylline, oral hypoglycemics (glipizide and tolbutamide), warfarin, phenytoin, and terfenadine. Decreased plasma levels of fluconazole have resulted following administration with rifampin and cimetidine.

Theoretic Infant Dose: 0.34 mg/kg/day

Relative Infant Dose: 16.1%

Adult Dose: 50-200 mg daily

Alternatives: Ketoconazole, itraconazole

T½ =	30 hours	M/P =	0.46-0.85
PHL =	88.6 hours(neonate)	PB =	15%
T$_{max}$ =	1-2 hours	Oral =	> 90%
MW =	306	pKa =	
Vd =			

References:

1. Force RW. Fluconazole concentrations in breastmilk. Pediatr Infect Dis J 1995; 14(3):235-236.
2. Schilling CG. et.al. Excretion of fluconazole in human breastmilk (abstract 130). Pharmacotherapy 1993; 13:287.
3. Wainer S, Cooper PA, Gouws H, Akierman A. Prospective study of fluconazole therapy in systemic neonatal fungal infection. Pediatr Infect Dis J 1997; 16(8):763-767.
4. Wiest DB, Fowler SL, Garner SS, Simons DR. Fluconazole in neonatal disseminated candidiasis. Arch Dis Child 1991; 66(8):1002.
5. Gurses N, Kalayci AG. Fluconazole monotherapy for candidal meningitis in a premature infant. Clin Infect Dis 1996; 23(3):645-646.
6. Driessen M, Ellis JB, Cooper PA, Wainer S, Muwazi F, Hahn D, Gous H, De Villiers FP. Fluconazole vs. amphotericin B for the treatment of neonatal fungal septicemia: a prospective randomized trial. Pediatr Infect Dis J 1996; 15(12):1107-1112.
7. Huttova M, Hartmanova I, Kralinsky K, Filka J, Uher J, Kurak J, Krizan S, Krcmery V, Jr. Candida fungemia in neonates treated with fluconazole: report of forty cases, including eight with meningitis. Pediatr Infect Dis J 1998; 17(11):1012-1015.
8. Leen CL, Dunbar EM, Ellis ME, Mandal BK. Once-weekly fluconazole to prevent recurrence of oropharyngeal candidiasis in patients with AIDS and AIDS-related complex: a double-blind placebo-controlled study. J Infect 1990; 21(1):55-60.
9. Winston DJ, Chandrasekar PH, Lazarus HM, Goodman JL, Silber JL, Horowitz H, Shadduck RK, Rosenfeld CS, Ho WG, Islam MZ, . Fluconazole prophylaxis of fungal infections in patients with acute leukemia. Results of a randomized placebo-controlled, double-blind, multicenter trial. Ann Intern Med 1993; 118(7):495-503.
10. Viscoli C, Castagnola E, Corsini M, Gastaldi R, Soliani M, Terragna A. Fluconazole therapy in an underweight infant. Eur J Clin Microbiol Infect Dis 1989; 8(10):925-926.
11. Saxen H, Hoppu K, Pohjavuori M. Pharmacokinetics of fluconazole in very low birth weight infants during the first two weeks of life. Clin Pharmacol Ther 1993; 54(3):269-277.

FLUDEOXYGLUCOSE F 18
Trade: Fludeoxyglucose F 18
Can/Aus/UK:
Uses: PET Scanning pharmaceutical
LRC: L3
AAP: Not reviewed

Fludeoxyglucose F 18 is a positron-emitting radiopharmaceutical used in conjunction with positron emission tomography (PET Scanning) to detect alterations in tissue glucose metabolism and is useful in detecting brain tumors, certain malignancies, chronic coronary artery disease, partial epilepsy, and Alzheimer's disease.[1-3]

Fludeoxyglucose F 18 is rapidly distributed to all parts of the body that have significant glucose metabolism, including the breast. No levels in breastmilk have been reported, but it probably penetrates milk to some degree. The half-life of the F-18 is short, only 110 minutes. Due to concentration in some tissues such as the bladder, radiation exposure could be a problem and emptying of the breast at routine intervals would reduce radiation exposure to breast tissue. The USPDI(1994) recommends interruption of breastfeeding for 12-24 hours. At 9 hours, 97% of the radioisotope would be decayed away.[4] It is likely that after 12 hours, almost all radioisotope would be decayed to almost background levels. Recommend pumping and dumping of breastmilk after the procedure for at least 12-24 hours.

Pregnancy Risk Category:

Lactation Risk Category: **L3**

Adult Concerns: No untoward effects have been reported for this product.

Pediatric Concerns: None reported but possible radiation exposure if breastfed prior to 12-24 hours after dose.

Drug Interactions:

Theoretic Infant Dose:

Relative Infant Dose:

Adult Dose:

Alternatives:

T½ =	110 minutes	M/P =	
PHL =		PB =	Minimal
T$_{max}$ =	30 minutes	Oral =	Complete
MW =		pKa =	
Vd =			

References:

1. Jamieson D, Alavi A, Jolles P, Chawluk J, Reivich M. Positron emission tomography in the investigation of central nervous system disorders. Radiol Clin North Am 1988; 26(5):1075-1088.
2. Jones SC, Alavi A, Christman D, Montanez I, Wolf AP, Reivich M. The radiation dosimetry of 2 [F-18]fluoro-2-deoxy-D-glucose in man. J Nucl Med 1982; 23(7):613-617.
3. Som P, Atkins HL, Bandoypadhyay D, Fowler JS, MacGregor RR, Matsui K, Oster ZH, Sacker DF, Shiue CY, Turner H, Wan CN, Wolf AP, Zabinski SV. A fluorinated glucose analog, 2-fluoro-2-deoxy-D-glucose (F-18): nontoxic tracer for rapid tumor detection. J Nucl Med 1980; 21(7):670-675.
4. Jones SC, Alavi A, Christman D, Montanez I, Wolf AP, Reivich M. The radiation dosimetry of 2 [F-18]fluoro-2-deoxy-D-glucose in man. J Nucl Med 1982; 23(7):613-617.

FLUDROCORTISONE

Trade: Florinef, Myconef
Can/Aus/UK: Florinef
Uses: Mineralocorticoid.
LRC: L3
AAP: Not reviewed

Fludrocortisone is a halogenated derivative of hydrocortisone with very potent mineralocorticoid activity and is generally used to treat Addison's disease.[1,2] Although its glucocorticoid effect is 15 times more potent than hydrocortisone, it is primarily used for its powerful ability to retain sodium in the vascular compartment (mineralocorticoid activity). It is not known if fludrocortisone penetrates into milk but if it is similar to other corticosteroids, it is very unlikely the amounts in milk will be clinically relevant until extremely high doses are used, but caution is recommended.

Pregnancy Risk Category: C

Lactation Risk Category: L3

Adult Concerns: Hypertension, sodium retention, cardiac hypertrophy, congestive heart failure, and headache

Pediatric Concerns: None via milk.

Drug Interactions: Excessive potassium levels may result from use with amphotericin B. Use with loop diuretics may dramatically increase potassium loss. Phenytoin, rifampin, phenobarbital, and fosphenytoin may increase hepatic metabolism of fludrocortisone and reduce its efficacy. Lithium may reduce efficacy of fludrocortisone. Tuberculin reactions may be suppressed for periods up to 6 weeks in patients receiving fludrocortisone.

Theoretic Infant Dose:

Relative Infant Dose:

Adult Dose: 0.1-0.4 mg daily

Alternatives:

T½ =	3.5 hours	M/P =	
PHL =		PB =	42%
T$_{max}$ =	1.7 hours	Oral =	Complete
MW =	380	pKa =	
Vd =			

References:
1. Pharmaceutical Manufacturer Prescribing Information. 1999.
2. Drug Facts and Comparisons 1999 ed. ed. St. Louis: 1999.

FLUNARIZINE
Trade: Sibelium
Can/Aus/UK: Sibelium, Novo-Flunarizine
Uses: Antihypertensive
LRC: L4
AAP: Not reviewed

Flunarizine is a calcium channel blocker primarily indicated for use in migraine headache prophylaxis and peripheral vascular disease. It has a very long half-life and a huge volume of distribution, which contributes to the long half-life.[1]   No data are available on the transfer of this product into human milk. However, due to its incredibly long half-life and high volume of distribution, it is possible that this product, over time, could build up and concentrate in a breastfed infant. Other calcium channel blockers may be preferred. Use with extreme caution.

Pregnancy Risk Category:

Lactation Risk Category: L4

Adult Concerns: Extrapyramidal symptoms in elderly patients, depression, porphyria, thrombophlebitis, drowsiness, headache, dizziness

Pediatric Concerns: None reported via milk, but caution is advised.

Drug Interactions: Prolonged bradycardia with adenosine. Sinus arrest when used with amiodarone. Hypotension and bradycardia when used with beta blockers. Increase of carbamazepine and cyclosporin plasma levels when used with flunarizine.

Theoretic Infant Dose:

Relative Infant Dose:

Adult Dose: 10 mg daily

Alternatives: Nifedipine, Nimodipine, Verapamil

T½ =	19 days	M/P =	
PHL =	23 days	PB =	99%
T$_{max}$ =	2-4 hours	Oral =	Complete
MW =		pKa =	
Vd =	43.2		

References:
1. Pharmaceutical Manufacturer Prescribing Information.

FLUNISOLIDE

Trade: Nasalide, Aerobid
Can/Aus/UK: Bronalide, Rhinalar, PMS-Flunisolide, Syntaris
Uses: Inhaled and intranasal steroid.
LRC: L3
AAP: Not reviewed

Flunisolide is a potent corticosteroid used to reduce airway hyperreactivity in asthmatics. It is also available as Nasalide for intranasal use for allergic rhinitis. Generally, only small levels of flunisolide are absorbed systemically (about 40%) thereby reducing systemic effects and presumably breastmilk levels as well.[1,2] After inhalation of 1 mg flunisolide, systemic availability was only 40% and plasma level was 0.4-1 nanogram/mL. Adrenal suppression in children has not been documented even after therapy of 2 months with 1600 µg/day. Once absorbed, flunisolide is rapidly removed from the plasma compartment by first-pass uptake in the liver. Although no data on breastmilk levels are yet available, it is unlikely that the level secreted in milk is clinically relevant.

Pregnancy Risk Category: C

Lactation Risk Category: L3

Adult Concerns: Most common side effect is irritation, due to vehicle not drug itself. Loss of taste, nasal irritation, flu-like symptoms, sore throat, headache.

Pediatric Concerns: None reported. Can be used in children down to age 6.

Drug Interactions:

Theoretic Infant Dose:

Relative Infant Dose:

Adult Dose: 1 mg daily

Alternatives:

T½ =	1.8 hours	M/P =	
PHL =		PB =	
T$_{max}$ =	30 minutes	Oral =	21% (oral)
MW =	435	pKa =	
Vd =	1.8		

References:
1. Pharmaceutical Manufacturer Prescribing Information. 1995.
2. Drug Facts and Comparisons 1995 ed. ed. St. Louis: 1995.

FLUNITRAZEPAM
Trade: Rohypnol
Can/Aus/UK: Rohypnol, Hypnodorm
Uses: Benzodiazepine sedative
LRC: L3
      L4 if used chronically
AAP: Not reviewed

Flunitrazepam is a prototypical benzodiazepine. Frequently called the "Date Rape Pill", it induces rapid sedation and significant amnesia, particularly when admixed with alcohol.[1,2] Effects last about 8 hours. It is recommended for adult insomnia and for pediatric preanesthetic sedation.

Pregnancy Risk Category: D

Lactation Risk Category: L3
                                 L4 if used chronically

Adult Concerns: Drowsiness, amnesia, sedation, ataxia, headache, memory impairment, tremors

Pediatric Concerns: None reported via milk but observe for sedation.

Drug Interactions: Clarithromycin and other macrolide antibiotics may increase plasma levels for benzodiazepines by inhibiting metabolism. May have enhanced effect when added to fentanyl, ketamine, nitrous oxide. Addition of even small amounts of alcohol may produce profound sedation, psychomotor impairment, and amnesia. Theophylline may reduce the sedative effects of benzodiazepines.

Theoretic Infant Dose:

Relative Infant Dose:

Adult Dose: 2 mg daily

Alternatives: Lorazepam, Alprazolam

T½ =	20-30 hours	M/P =	
PHL =		PB =	80%
T$_{max}$ =	2 hours	Oral =	80-90%
MW =	313	pKa =	
Vd =	3.6		

References:
1. Kanto J, Erkkola R, Kangas L, Pitkanen Y. Placental transfer of flunitrazepam following intramuscular administration during labour. Br J Clin Pharmacol 1987; 23(4):491-494.
2. Kanto J, Kangas L, Leppanen T. A comparative study of the clinical effects of oral flunitrazepam, medazepam, and placebo. Int J Clin Pharmacol Ther Toxicol 1982; 20(9):431-433.

FLUORESCEIN
Trade: Ak-Fluor, Fluorescite, Funduscein-10, Ophthifluor, Fluorescein Sodium, Ful-Glo, FluoretsFluor-I-Strip
Can/Aus/UK:
Uses: Diagnostic dye in angiography
LRC: L3
AAP: Maternal Medication Usually Compatible with Breastfeeding

Sodium fluorescein is a yellow, water-soluble dye. A 2% fluorescein ophthalmic solution or an impregnated fluorescein strip is used topically to detect corneal abrasions, for fitting of hard contact lenses, and intravenously for fluorescein angiography. Fluorescein is used in two ways. One, in which a small amount is added directly to the eye generally by ophthalmologists and optometrists, and secondly, when much larger quantities are administered intravenously (5 mL of 10% solution).

In a study of one patient who received an intravenous dose of fluorescein (5 mL of 10% fluorescein = 500 mg), breastmilk levels were monitored for over 76 hours.[1] Concentrations of 372 μg/L at 6 hours and 170 μg/L at 76 hours after the dose were reported. In this patient, the half-life of fluorescein in breastmilk appeared quite long, approximating 62 hours. While the authors conclude that this is a high dose via milk, in another patient who received slightly more (910 mg IV), the patient's plasma levels of fluorescein monoglucuronide were 37,000 μg/L.[2] Using this data, it would appear that an approximation of the milk/plasma ratio would be about 0.018, which suggests that very little of the absolute maternal dose enters milk. Nevertheless, fluorescein-induced phototoxicity remains a possibility in an infant fed breastmilk containing sodium fluorescein. One case of severe fluorescein phototoxicity has been reported in an infant receiving fluorescein intravenously.[3]   If the infant is not undergoing phototherapy, it would appear that there is little risk to a breastfeeding infant.

Pregnancy Risk Category: C

Lactation Risk Category: L3

Adult Concerns: Fluorescein-induced phototoxicity.   Nausea, vomiting, dizziness, syncope, pruritus, seizures, following IV therapy. Severe reactions are rare. Oral fluorescein appears to elicit very few adverse reaction.

Pediatric Concerns: None reported via milk, but avoid phototherapy if used.

Drug Interactions: Interferes with numerous laboratory tests.

Theoretic Infant Dose: 55.8 µg/kg/day

Relative Infant Dose: 0.78%

Adult Dose: 500 mg intravenous

Alternatives:

T½ =	4.4 hours(metab.)	M/P =	
PHL =		PB =	70-85%
T$_{max}$ =	1 hour	Oral =	50%
MW =	376	pKa =	
Vd =	0.5		

References:
1. Maquire AM, Bennett J. Fluorescein elimination in human breastmilk. Arch Ophthalmol 1988; 106(6):718-719.
2. Kearns GL, Williams BJ, Timmons OD. Fluorescein phototoxicity in a premature infant. J Pediatr 1985; 107(5):796-798.
3. Kearns GL, Williams BJ, Timmons OD. Fluorescein phototoxicity in a premature infant. J Pediatr 1985; 107(5):796-798.

FLUORIDE
Trade: Pediaflor, Flura
Can/Aus/UK: Fluor-A-Day, Fluotic, Fluorigard
Uses: Hardening enamel of teeth
LRC: L2
AAP: Reported as having no effect on breastfeeding

Fluoride is an essential element required for bone and teeth development.   It is available as salts of sodium and stannis (tin). Excessive levels are known to stain teeth irreversibly. One study shows breastmilk levels of 0.024 - 0.172 ppm in milk (mean=0.077 ppm) of a population exposed to fluoridated water (0.7ppm).[1]

In another study of breastfeeding women from areas low and rich in fluoride, milk fluoride levels were similar.[2] The mean fluoride concentration was 0.36 μmol/L for colostrum and 0.37 μmol/L for mature milk in the region with 1 ppm fluoride enriched water. In the region with 0.2 ppm fluoride, the mean fluoride concentration of colostrum was 0.28 μmol/L. There was no statistical difference in any of these milk fluoride levels.

Fluoride probably forms calcium fluoride salts in milk which may limit the oral bioavailability of the fluoride provided by human milk. Maternal supplementation is unnecessary and not recommended in areas with high fluoride content (> 0.7 ppm) in water.[3] Allergy to fluoride has been reported in one infant.[4] Younger children (2-6 yrs) should be instructed to use minimal quantities of toothpaste and to not swallow large amounts. The American Academy of Pediatrics no longer recommends supplementing of breastfed infants with oral fluoride.

Fluoride Ion and Dosing Recommendations

Fluoride Content of Drinking Water	Daily Dose, Oral (mg) In Non-Breastfed Infants
<0.3 ppm	
Birth - 2 y	0.25
2-3 y	0.5
3-12 y	1
0.3-0.7 ppm	
Birth - 2 y	0
2-3 y	0.25
3-12 y	0.5

Pregnancy Risk Category: C

Lactation Risk Category: L2

Adult Concerns: Stained enamel, allergic rash

Pediatric Concerns: Allergy to fluoride has been reported in one infant. Do not use maternal doses > 0.7 ppm.

Drug Interactions: Decreased absorption when used with magnesium, aluminum, and calcium containing products.

Theoretic Infant Dose:

Relative Infant Dose:

Adult Dose: 1 mg daily

Alternatives:

T½ =	6 hours	M/P =	
PHL =		PB =	
T$_{max}$ =		Oral =	90% (Na)
MW =	19	pKa =	
Vd =	0.5-0.7		

References:
1. Latifah R, Razak IA. Fluoride levels in mother's milk. J Pedod 1989; 13(2):149-154.
2. Spak CJ, Hardell LI, De Chateau P. Fluoride in human milk. Acta Paediatr Scand 1983; 72(5):699-701.
3. Fluoride supplementation of the breast-fed infant JAMA 1990; 263(16):2179.
4. Shea J. et.al. Allergy to fluoride. Ann Allergy 1967; 25:388.

FLUOROURACIL
Trade: 5FU, Adrucil, Efudex, Fluoroplex
Can/Aus/UK: Adrucil, Fluoroplex, Efudix, Efudex
Uses: Anticancer drug, actinic keratosis
LRC: L5
AAP: Not reviewed

Fluorouracil is a potent antineoplastic agent generally used topically for various skin cancers and IV for various carcinomas. No data are available on its transfer into breastmilk. 5FU is an extremely toxic and dangerous compound and is probably contraindicated in breastfeeding women following IV therapy.[1] It is rapidly cleared by the liver and two long-half-life metabolites (FdUMP, FUTP) are formed. The clinical effect and half-life of these metabolites is unknown.

5FU is commonly used topically as a cream for actinic or solar keratosis. The topical absorption of 5FU is minimal, reported to be less than 6%. Although it is unlikely that significant quantities of 5FU would be transferred to a breastfed infant following topical application to small areas, caution is urged.

Pregnancy Risk Category: D during 1st and 2nd trimesters
X during 3rd trimester

Lactation Risk Category: L5

Adult Concerns: Nausea, vomiting, anorexia, blood dyscrasias, bone marrow suppression, myocardial toxicity, dyspnea, cardiogenic shock, rashes

Pediatric Concerns: None reported but caution is urged.

Drug Interactions: Drug interactions are numerous and include allopurinol, cimetidine, methotrexate, leucovorin and others.

Theoretic Infant Dose:

Relative Infant Dose:

Adult Dose: 6-12 mg/kg injection (IV) daily

Alternatives:

T½ =	8-22 minutes	M/P =	
PHL =		PB =	8-12%
T$_{max}$ =	Immediate(IV)	Oral =	0-80%
MW =	130	pKa =	
Vd =	0.12		

References:
1. McEvoy GE. (ed):AFHS Drug Information. New York, NY: 2003.

FLUOXETINE

Trade: Prozac
Can/Aus/UK: Prozac, Apo-Fluoxetine, Novo-Fluoxetine, Lovan, Zactin
Uses: Antidepressant
LRC: L2 in older infants
L3 if used in neonatal period
AAP: Drugs whose effect on nursing infants is unknown but may be of concern

Fluoxetine is a very popular serotonin reuptake inhibitor (SSRI) currently used for depression and a host of other syndromes. Fluoxetine absorption is rapid and complete and the parent compound is rapidly metabolized to norfluoxetine, which is an active, long half-life metabolite (360 hrs). Both fluoxetine and norfluoxetine appear to permeate breastmilk to levels approximately 1/5 to 1/4 of maternal plasma. In one patient at steady-state (dose=20mg/day), plasma levels of fluoxetine were 100.5 μg/L and levels of norfluoxetine were 194.5 μg/L.[1] Fluoxetine levels in milk were 28.8 μg/L and norfluoxetine levels were 41.6 μg/L. Milk/plasma ratios were 0.286 for fluoxetine and 0.21 for norfluoxetine.

In another patient receiving 20 mg daily at bedtime, the milk concentration of fluoxetine was 67 μg/L and norfluoxetine 52 μg/L at four hours.[2] At 8 hours postdose, the concentration of fluoxetine was 17 μg/L and norfluoxetine was 13 μg/L. Using this data, the authors estimated that the total daily dose was only 15-20 μg/kg per day which represents a low exposure.

In another study of 10 breastfeeding women receiving 0.39 mg/kg/day of fluoxetine, the average breastmilk levels for fluoxetine and norfluoxetine ranged from 24.4-181.1 μg/L and 37.4-199.1 μg/L respectively.[3] Peak milk concentrations occurred within 6 hours. The milk/plasma ratios for fluoxetine and norfluoxetine were 0.88 and 0.72 respectively. Fluoxetine plasma levels in one infant were undetectable (< 1 ng/mL). Using this data, an infant consuming 150 mL/kg/day would consume approximately 9.3-57 μg/kg/day total fluoxetine (and metabolite), which represents 5-9% of the maternal dose. No adverse effects were noted in the infants in this study.

Severe colic, fussiness, and crying have been reported in one case report.[4] The mother was receiving a dose of 20 mg fluoxetine per day. Concentrations of fluoxetine and norfluoxetine in breastmilk were 69 μg/L and 90 μg/L respectively. The plasma levels in the infant for fluoxetine and norfluoxetine were 340 ng/mL and 208 ng/mL respectively which is almost twice that of normal maternal ranges. The author does not report the maternal plasma levels but suggests they were similar to Isenberg's adult levels (100.5 ng/mL and 194.5 ng/mL for fluoxetine and norfluoxetine). In this infant, the plasma levels would approach those of a mother receiving twice the above 20 mg dose per day (40 mg/day). The symptoms resolved upon discontinuation of fluoxetine by the mother.

In a study by Brent [5], an infant exposed in utero and postpartum via milk, had moderate plasma fluoxetine levels that increased in the three weeks postpartum due to breastmilk ingestion. The infant's plasma levels of fluoxetine went from none detectable at day 13 to 61 ng/mL at day 21. The mean adult therapeutic range is 145 ng/mL. The infant in this study exhibited slight seizure activity at 3 weeks, 4 months, and 5 months.

Ilett[6] reports that in a group of 14 women receiving 0.51 mg/kg/day fluoxetine, the mean M/P ratio was 0.67 (range 0.35 to 0.13) and 0.56 for norfluoxetine. Mean total infant dose in fluoxetine equivalents was 6.81% of the weight-adjusted maternal dose. The reported infant fluoxetine and norfluoxetine plasma levels ranged from 20-252 μg/L and 17-187 μg/L respectively.

It is not known if these reported side effects (seizures, colic, fussiness, crying) are common, although this author has received numerous other personal communications similar to this. Indeed in one case, the infant became comatose at 11 days postpartum with high plasma levels of norfluoxetine.[7] At present, fluoxetine is the only antidepressant cleared for use in pregnancy. This may pose an added problem in breastfed infants. Infants born of mothers receiving fluoxetine are born with full steady state plasma levels of the medication, and each time they are breastfed the level in the infant may rise further.

Several methods of reducing the risk to newborns is to reduce or eliminate the use of fluoxetine just prior to delivery or to switch to an alternate antidepressant while breastfeeding (sertraline, paroxetine, etc.). While we do not know the real risk of side effects, they are apparently low for the population. If the patient cannot tolerate switching to another antidepressant, then fluoxetine should be continued.

Age at institution of therapy is of importance. Use in older infants (4-6 months or older) is far less hazardous because they can metabolize and excrete the medication more rapidly. Data published in 1999 also suggest that weight gain in infants breastfed from mothers who were taking fluoxetine demonstrated a growth curve significantly below that of infants who were breastfed by mothers who did not take the drug. The average deficit in measurements taken between 2 and 6 months of age was 392 grams body weight. None of these infants were noted to have unusual behavior.[8]

Another recent report suggests that fluoxetine may induce a state of anesthesia of the vagina and nipples.[9] The author has had another report of a paroxetine-induced reduction of milk ejection reflex. Whether or not a loss of MER is related to an anesthesia of the nipples is purely speculative.

Thus far, neurobehavioral development seems to be normal at least in one small study.[10]

Current data on Sertraline and Paroxetine suggest these medications have difficulty entering milk and, more importantly, the infant. Therefore, they are preferred agents over fluoxetine for therapy of depression in breastfeeding mothers. However, it is important to remember that the risks of not breastfeeding far outweigh the risk of using fluoxetine and women who can only take fluoxetine should be advised to continue breastfeeding and observe the infant for side effects.

The new product Symbyax contains both fluoxetine and olanzapine for treatment of Bipolar Depression.

Pregnancy Risk Category: C

Lactation Risk Category: **L2 in older infants**
L3 if used in neonatal period

Adult Concerns: Nausea, tachycardia, hypotension, headache, anxiety, nervousness, insomnia, dry mouth, anorexia, and visual disturbances

Pediatric Concerns: Severe colic, fussiness, and crying have been reported in one case study.

Drug Interactions: Cimetidine may increase plasma levels 50%. Hallucinations have occurred when used with dextromethorphan. Serious fatal reactions have occurred when used after MAO inhibitors. Phenytoin may reduce plasma levels of fluoxetine by 50%. CNS toxicity may result if used with L-tryptophan. Fluoxetine may increase plasma levels of tricyclic antidepressants. Significant increase in propranolol levels have been reported. Effects of buspirone may be decreased. Serum carbamazepine levels may be increased resulting in toxicity. Bradycardia has been reported when used with diltiazem. Use with digoxin reduces digoxin levels by 15%. Lithium levels may be increased by fluoxetine with possible neurotoxicity. Sertraline did not effect lithium levels. Methadone levels have been significantly increased with SSRIs. Clearance of theophylline may be decreased by three fold. When used with warfarin, a significant increase in bleeding time has been reported.

Theoretic Infant Dose: 57 µg/kg/day

Relative Infant Dose: 6.8%

Adult Dose: 20-40 mg daily

Alternatives: Sertraline, Paroxetine, Citalopram

$T\frac{1}{2}$ =	2-3 days(fluoxetine)	M/P =	0.286-0.67
PHL =		PB =	94.5%
T_{max} =	1.5 - 12 hours	Oral =	100%
MW =	309	pKa =	
Vd =	2.6		

References:
1. Isenberg KE. Excretion of fluoxetine in human breastmilk. J Clin Psychiatry 1990; 51(4):169.
2. Burch KJ, Wells BG. Fluoxetine/norfluoxetine concentrations in human milk. Pediatrics 1992; 89(4 Pt 1):676-677.
3. Taddio A, Ito S, Koren G. Excretion of fluoxetine and its metabolite, norfluoxetine, in human breastmilk. J Clin Pharmacol 1996; 36(1):42-47.
4. Lester BM, Cucca J, Andreozzi L, Flanagan P, Oh W. Possible association between fluoxetine hydrochloride and colic in an infant. J Am Acad Child Adolesc Psychiatry 1993; 32(6):1253-1255.
5. Brent NB, Wisner KL. Fluoxetine and carbamazepine concentrations in a nursing mother/infant pair. Clin Pediatr (Phila) 1998; 37(1):41-44.
6. Kristensen JH, Ilett KF, Hackett LP, Yapp P, Paech M, Begg EJ. Distribution and excretion of fluoxetine and norfluoxetine in human milk. Br J Clin Pharmacol 1999; 48(4):521-527.
7. Hale TW, Shum S, Grossberg M. Fluoxetine toxicity in a breastfed infant. Clin Pediatr (Phila) 2001; 40(12):681-684.
8. Chambers CD, Anderson PO, Thomas RG, Dick LM, Felix RJ, Johnson KA, Jones KL. Weight gain in infants breastfed by mothers who take fluoxetine. Pediatrics 1999; 104(5):e61.
9. Michael A, Mayer C. Fluoxetine-induced anaesthesia of vagina and nipples. Br J Psychiatry 2000; 176:299.
10. Yoshida K, Smith B, Craggs M, Kumar RC. Fluoxetine in breast-milk and developmental outcome of breast-fed infants. Br J Psychiatry 1998; 172:175-178.

FLUPHENAZINE

Trade: Prolixin, Permitil
Can/Aus/UK: Apo-Fluphenazine, Modecate, Anatensol, Moditen
Uses: Psychotherapeutic agent
LRC: L3
AAP: Not reviewed

Fluphenazine is a phenothiazine tranquilizer and presently has the highest milligram potency of this family. Fluphenazine decanoate injections (IM) provide extremely long plasma levels with half-lives approaching 14.3 days at steady state. Members of this family generally have milk/plasma ratios ranging from 0.5 to 0.7.[1] No specific reports on fluphenazine breastmilk levels have been located.

Pregnancy Risk Category: C

Lactation Risk Category: L3

Adult Concerns: Depression, seizures, appetite stimulation, blood dyscrasias, weight gain, hepatic toxicity, sedation

Pediatric Concerns: None reported but observe for sedation.

Drug Interactions: Increased toxicity when administered with ethanol. CNS effects may be increased when used with lithium. May stimulate the effects of narcotics including respiratory depression.

Theoretic Infant Dose:

Relative Infant Dose:

Adult Dose: 1-5 mg daily

Alternatives:

T½ =	10-20 hours	M/P =	
PHL =		PB =	91-99%
T_{max} =	1.5 - 2 hours	Oral =	Complete
MW =	438	pKa =	3.9, 8.1
Vd =	220		

References:
1. Ayd FJ. Excretion of psychotropic drugs in breastmilk. In: International Drug Therapy Newsletter.Ayd Medical Communications 8[November-December]. 1973.

FLURAZEPAM

Trade: Dalmane
Can/Aus/UK: Apo-Flurazepam, Novo-Flupam, Dalmane
Uses: Sedative, hypnotic
LRC: L3
AAP: Not reviewed

Flurazepam is a sedative, hypnotic generally used as an aid for sleep. It belongs to the benzodiazepine (Valium) family. It is rapidly and completely metabolized to several long half-life active metabolites. Because most benzodiazepines are secreted into human milk, flurazepam entry into milk should be expected[1]. However, no specific data on flurazepam breastmilk levels are available. See diazepam.

Pregnancy Risk Category: X

Lactation Risk Category: L3

Adult Concerns: Sedation, tachycardia, jaundice, apnea

Pediatric Concerns: None reported but caution is recommended. Observe for sedation.

Drug Interactions: Decreased effect when used with enzyme inducers such as barbiturates. Increased toxicity when used with other CNS depressants and cimetidine.

Theoretic Infant Dose:

Relative Infant Dose:

Adult Dose: 15-30 mg daily

Alternatives: Lorazepam, Alprazolam

$T\frac{1}{2}$ =	47-100 hours	M/P =	
PHL =		PB =	97%
T_{max} =	0.5-1 hours	Oral =	Complete
MW =	388	pKa =	1.9, 8.2
Vd =	3.4-5.5		

References:
1. Drug Facts and Comparisons 1995 ed. ed. St. Louis: 1995.

FLURBIPROFEN

Trade: Ansaid, Froben, Ocufen
Can/Aus/UK: Ansaid, Froben, Ocufen,
Uses: Analgesic
LRC: L2
AAP: Not reviewed

Flurbiprofen is a nonsteroidal analgesic similar in structure to ibuprofen but used both as an ophthalmic preparation (in eyes) and orally. In one study of 12 women and following nine oral doses (50mg/dose, 3-5 days postpartum) the concentration of flurbiprofen in two women ranged from 0.05 to 0.07 mg/L of milk but was < 0.05 mg/L in 10 of the 12 women[1]. Concentrations in breastmilk and plasma of nursing mothers suggest that a nursing infant would receive less than 0.1 mg flurbiprofen per day, a level considered exceedingly low.

In another study of 10 nursing mothers following a single 100 mg dose, the average peak concentration of flurbiprofen in breastmilk was 0.09 mg/L, or about 0.05% of the maternal dose[2]. Both of these studies suggest that the amount of flurbiprofen transferred in human milk would be clinically insignificant to the infant.

Pregnancy Risk Category: **B during 1st and 2nd trimester**
    C during 3rd trimester

Lactation Risk Category: **L2**

Adult Concerns: GI distress, diarrhea, constipation, cramping, may worsen jaundice

Pediatric Concerns: None reported.

Drug Interactions: May prolong prothrombin time when used with warfarin. Antihypertensive effects of ACEi family may be blunted or completely abolished by NSAIDs. Some NSAIDs may block antihypertensive effect of beta blockers, diuretics. Use with cyclosporin may dramatically increase renal toxicity. May increase digoxin, phenytoin, lithium levels. May increase toxicity of methotrexate. May increase bioavailability of penicillamine. Probenecid may increase NSAID levels.

Theoretic Infant Dose: 13.5 µg/kg/day

Relative Infant Dose:

Adult Dose: 200-300 mg daily

Alternatives: Ibuprofen

T½ =	3.8-5.7 hours	M/P =	0.008 - 0.013
PHL =	2.71 hours(children)	PB =	99%
T_{max} =	1.5 hours	Oral =	Complete
MW =	244	pKa =	4.2
Vd =	0.1		

References:
1. Smith IJ, Hinson JL, Johnson VA, Brown RD, Cook SM, Whitt RT, Wilson JT. Flurbiprofen in post-partum women: plasma and breastmilk disposition. J Clin Pharmacol 1989; 29(2):174-184.
2. Cox SR, Forbes KK. Excretion of flurbiprofen into breastmilk. Pharmacotherapy 1987; 7(6):211-215.

FLUTICASONE

Trade: Flonase, Flovent, Cutivate
Can/Aus/UK: Flovent, Flonase, Flixotide, Flixonase
Uses: Intranasal, inhaled steroid
LRC: L3
AAP: Not reviewed

Fluticasone is a typical steroid primarily used intranasally for allergic rhinitis and intrapulmonary for asthma. Intranasal form is called Flonase, inhaled form is Flovent. When instilled intranasally, the absolute bioavailability is less than 2%, so virtually none of the dose instilled is absorbed systemically.[1] Oral absorption following inhaled fluticasone is approximately 30% although almost instant first-pass absorption virtually eliminates plasma levels of fluticasone.[2] Peak plasma levels following inhalation of 880 µg is only 0.1 to 1.0 nanogram/mL. Adrenocortical suppression following oral or even systemic absorption at normal doses is extremely rare due to limited plasma levels.[3] Plasma levels are not detectable when using suggested doses. Although fluticasone is secreted into milk of rodents, the dose used was many times higher than found under normal conditions. With the above oral and systemic bioavailability and rapid first-pass uptake by the liver, it is not likely that milk levels will be clinically relevant, even with rather high doses.

Pregnancy Risk Category: C

Lactation Risk Category: L3

Adult Concerns: Intranasal: pruritus, headache (1-3%), burning (3-6%), epistaxis. Adverse effects associated with inhaled fluticasone include headache, nasal congestion, and oral candidiasis.

Pediatric Concerns: When used topically on large surface areas, some adrenal suppression has been noted. No effects have been reported in breastfeeding infants. In children receiving up to 5 times the normal inhaled dose (1000 µg/day), some growth suppression was noted.

Drug Interactions:

Theoretic Infant Dose:

Relative Infant Dose:

Adult Dose: 50-110 μg/inhalation daily

Alternatives:

T½ =	7.8 hours	M/P =	
PHL =		PB =	
T$_{max}$ =	15-60 minutes	Oral =	Oral(1%),
			Inhaled(18%)
MW =	500	pKa =	
Vd =	4.2		

References:

1. Pharmaceutical Manufacturer Prescribing Information. 1996.
2. Harding SM. The human pharmacology of fluticasone propionate. Respir Med 1990; 84 Suppl A:25-29.
3. Todd G, Dunlop K, McNaboe J, Ryan MF, Carson D, Shields MD. Growth and adrenal suppression in asthmatic children treated with high-dose fluticasone propionate. Lancet 1996; 348(9019):27-29.

FLUTICASONE AND SALMETEROL

Trade: Advair
Can/Aus/UK:
Uses: Anti-asthmatic
LRC: L3
AAP: Not reviewed

Advair is a combination product containing fluticasone and salmeterol, used for the treatment of asthma. See individual monographs for fluticasone (Flovent) and Salmeterol (Serevent).

Pregnancy Risk Category:

Lactation Risk Category: L3

FLUVASTATIN

Trade: Lescol, Lescol XL
Can/Aus/UK: Lescol,Vastin
Uses: Reduces blood cholesterol levels
LRC: L3
AAP: Not reviewed

Fluvastatin is an inhibitor of cholesterol synthesis in the liver. Fluvastatin levels in human milk are reported to be 2 fold that of serum levels.[1,2]   Effect on infant is unknown but could reduce cholesterol synthesis in infant.   Atherosclerosis is a chronic process and discontinuation of lipid-lowering drugs during pregnancy, and lactation should have little to no impact on the outcome of long-term therapy of primary hypercholesterolemia.   Cholesterol and other products of cholesterol biosynthesis are essential components for fetal and neonatal development and the use of cholesterol-lowering drugs would not be advisable under any circumstances.

Pregnancy Risk Category: X

Lactation Risk Category: L3

Adult Concerns: Headache, insomnia, dyspepsia, diarrhea, gas, elevated liver enzymes

Pediatric Concerns: None reported, but reduced plasma cholesterol levels could occur.

Drug Interactions: Anticoagulant effect of warfarin may be increased.

Theoretic Infant Dose:

Relative Infant Dose:

Adult Dose: 20-40 mg daily

Alternatives:

$T\frac{1}{2}$ =	1.2 hours	M/P =	2.0
PHL =		PB =	> 98%
T_{max} =	< 1 hour	Oral =	20-30%
MW =		pKa =	
Vd =			

References:
1. Drug Facts and Comparisons 1994 ed. ed. St. Louis: 1994.
2. Pharmaceutical Manufacturer Prescribing Information. 1995.

FLUVOXAMINE

Trade: Luvox
Can/Aus/UK: Luvox, Apo-Fluvoxamine, Alti-Fluvoxamine, Faverin, Floxyfral, Myroxim
Uses: Antidepressant
LRC: L2
AAP: Drugs whose effect on nursing infants is unknown but may be of concern

Although structurally dissimilar to the other serotonin reuptake inhibitors, fluvoxamine provides increased synaptic serotonin levels in the brain. It has several hepatic metabolites which are not active. Its primary indications are for the treatment of obsessive-compulsive disorders (OCD) although it also functions as an antidepressant. There are a number of significant drug-drug interactions with this product.

In a case report of one 23 year old mother and following a dose of 100 mg twice daily for 2 weeks, the maternal plasma level of fluvoxamine base was 0.31 mg/Liter and the milk concentration was 0.09 mg/Liter.[1] The authors reported a theoretical dose to infant of 0.0104 mg/kg/day of fluvoxamine, which is only 0.5% of the maternal dose. According to the authors, the infant suffered no unwanted effects as a result of this intake and that this dose poses little risk to a nursing infant.

In a study of one patient receiving 100 mg twice daily, the AUC milk/serum ratio averaged 1.32. The absolute daily dose of fluvoxamine ingested by the newborn was calculated to be 48 μg/kg/d and the relative dose was calculated to be 1.58% of the weight-adjusted maternal dose.[2]

In another study of two breastfeeding women, the AUC average concentration of fluvoxamine in milk was 36 and 256 μg/L respectively.[3] The absolute infant dose was estimated at 5.4 and 38.4 μg/kg/d with a relative infant dose (% of maternal dose) of 0.8% and 1.38%. A Denver assessment on one infant indicated normal development. Fluvoxamine was not detected in the plasma of either infant (limit of detection = 2 μg/L).

In a case report of a single mother receiving 25 mg three times daily, the highest milk concentration was 40 μg/L.[4] Using this data, an infant would ingest approximately 6 μg/kg/day, which is 0.62% of the maternal weight-adjusted dose. Interestingly, the maternal serum concentration at 10 hours was 20 ng/mL while the infant plasma level was 9 ng/mL. Considering the clinical dose to the infant is low, this plasma level in the infant appears high. The authors suggest this may be an atypical case or that this infant's clearance of fluvoxamine is poor. The infant showed no symptoms of adverse effects.

Yoshida reported a case of a mother receiving 100 mg/day and an infant 15 weeks postpartum.[5] In this case the concentration of fluvoxamine in maternal serum and milk was 170 μg/L and 50 μg/L respectively and a milk/plasma ratio of 0.29. The authors estimated the dose to the infant at 7.5 μg/kg/day. Developmental assessments of the infant at 4 months and 21 months suggested normal development.

In a report of 2 breastfeeding women receiving 300 mg/d, Piontek was unable to detect any fluvoxamine in the plasma of two breastfed infants.[6]

In summary, the data from these 8 cases suggests that only miniscule amounts of fluvoxamine are transferred to infants, that plasma levels in infants are too low to be detected, and no adverse effects have been noted.

Pregnancy Risk Category: C

Lactation Risk Category: L2

Adult Concerns: Somnolence, insomnia, nervousness, nausea

Pediatric Concerns: None reported several studies.

Drug Interactions: Increased toxicity may be result when used with terfenadine and astemizole. Sometimes serious fatal reactions have occurred close following the use of MAO inhibitors. Smokers have a 25% increase in the metabolism of fluvoxamine. Enhanced CNS toxicity when used with L-tryptophan. Plasma tricyclic antidepressant levels may be increased when used with fluvoxamine. Plasma levels of propranolol have been increased by five fold when used with fluvoxamine.

Bradycardia has resulted when used with diltiazem. Lithium levels may be increased by fluvoxamine with possible neurotoxicity. Increased bleeding time may result when used with warfarin.

Theoretic Infant Dose: 38.4 μg/kg/day

Relative Infant Dose: 1.3%

Adult Dose: 50-300 mg daily

Alternatives: Sertraline, Paroxetine

T½ =	15.6 hours	M/P =	1.34
PHL =		PB =	80%
T$_{max}$ =	3-8 hours	Oral =	53%
MW =	318	pKa =	
Vd =			

References:
1. Wright S, Dawling S, Ashford JJ. Excretion of fluvoxamine in breastmilk. Br J Clin Pharmacol 1991; 31(2):209.
2. Hagg S, Granberg K, Carleborg L. Excretion of fluvoxamine into breastmilk. Br J Clin Pharmacol 2000; 49(3):286-288.
3. Kristensen JH, Hackett LP, Kohan R, Paech M, Ilett KF. The amount of fluvoxamine in milk is unlikely to be a cause of adverse effects in breastfed infants. J Hum Lact 2002; 18(2):139-143.
4. Arnold LM, Suckow RF, Lichtenstein PK. Fluvoxamine concentrations in breastmilk and in maternal and infant sera. J Clin Psychopharmacol 2000; 20(4):491-493.
5. Yoshida K, Smith B, Kumar RC. Fluvoxamine in breast-milk and infant development. Br J Clin Pharmacol 1997; 44(2):210-211.
6. Piontek CM, Wisner KL, Perel JM, Peindl KS. Serum fluvoxamine levels in breastfed infants. J Clin Psychiatry 2001; 62(2):111-113.

FOLIC ACID

Trade: Folacin, Wellcovorin
Can/Aus/UK: Apo-Folic, Folvite, Novo-Folacid, Accomin, Bioglan Daily, Megafol
Uses: Vitamin
LRC: L1
AAP: Maternal Medication Usually Compatible with Breastfeeding

Folic acid is an essential vitamin. Individuals most susceptible to folic acid deficiency are the pregnant patient, and those receiving anticonvulsants or birth control medications. Folic acid supplementation is now strongly recommended in women prior to becoming pregnant due to a documented reduction of spinal cord malformations. Folic acid is actively secreted into breastmilk even if mother is deficient.[1] If maternal diet is adequate, folic acid is not generally required. The infant receives all required from a normal milk supply. Cooperman determined milk folic acid content to be 15.2 ng/mL in colostrum, 16.3 ng/mL in transitional, and 33.4 ng/mL in mature milk.[2]

In one study of 11 breastfeeding mothers receiving 0.8-1 mg/day of folic acid, the folic acid secreted into human milk averaged 45.6 μg/L.[3] Excessive doses (> 1 mg/day) are not generally recommended.

Pregnancy Risk Category: A during 1st and 2nd trimester
                                C during 3rd trimester

Lactation Risk Category: L1

Adult Concerns: Allergies, rash, nausea, anorexia, bitter taste

Pediatric Concerns: None reported.

Drug Interactions: May increase phenytoin metabolism and reduce levels. Phenytoin, primidone, sulfasalazine, and para-aminosalicylic acid may decrease serum folate concentrations and cause deficiency. Oral contraceptives also impair folate metabolism producing depletion.

Theoretic Infant Dose: 6.84 μg/kg/day

Relative Infant Dose: 47.8%

Adult Dose: 0.4-0.8 mg daily

Alternatives:

T½ =		M/P =		
PHL =		PB =		
T$_{max}$ =	30-60 minutes	Oral =	76-93%	
MW =	441	pKa =		
Vd =				

References:

1. Tamura T, Yoshimura Y, Arakawa T. Human milk folate and folate status in lactating mothers and their infants. Am J Clin Nutr 1980; 33(2):193-197.
2. Cooperman JM, Dweck HS, Newman LJ, Garbarino C, Lopez R. The folate in human milk. Am J Clin Nutr 1982; 36(4):576-580.
3. Smith AM, Picciano MF, Deering RH. Folate supplementation during lactation: maternal folate status, human milk folate content, and their relationship to infant folate status. J Pediatr Gastroenterol Nutr 1983; 2(4):622-628.

FOLLICLE STIMULATING HORMONES

Trade: Metrodin, Fertinex, FSH, Follistim, Follitropin Alpha, Follitropin Beta, GONAL-F
Can/Aus/UK: Fertinorm HP, Metrodin, Metrodin
Uses: FSH, follicle stimulating hormone
LRC: L3
AAP: Not reviewed

Follicle-stimulating hormone (FSH) is a glycoprotein gonadotropin secreted by the anterior pituitary in response to gonadotropin-releasing hormone (GnRH) from the hypothalamus.[1-3] FSH and Lutenizing hormone bind to receptors in the testis and ovary and regulate gonadal function by promoting sex steroid production and gametogenesis. In the female, FSH induces growth of the graafian follicle in the ovary preparatory to the release of the ovum. Approximately 15 µg is secreted daily by the pituitary in normal individuals. Numerous forms of FSH are available and are listed below, but all work similarly. FSH is a large molecular weight peptide (34,000 daltons) and is very unlikely to enter milk or be orally bioavailable to an infant. However, it is not known if the administration of FSH and the subsequent maternal changes in estrogen and progesterone would alter the production of milk. It is likely, since the onset of pregnancy is commonly followed by a decrease in milk production in most mothers.

Urofollitropin (Metrodin, Fertinex)
Urofollitropin is a preparation of gonadotropin (FSH) extracted from the urine of postmenopausal women.

Follitropin Alpha (Gonal-F) and Follitropin Beta (Follistim)
Follitropin alpha and follitropin beta human FSH preparations of recombinant DNA origin.

Menotropins are combination products containing both FSH and lutenizing hormone(LH). See Menotropins.

Pregnancy Risk Category: X

Lactation Risk Category: L3

Adult Concerns: Pulmonary and vascular complications, ovarian hyperstimulation, abdominal pain, fever and chills, abdominal pain, nausea, vomiting, diarrhea, pain at injection site, bruising. Ovarian hyperstimulation.

Pediatric Concerns: None reported via milk. FSH is very unlikely to penetrate milk, and it would not be orally bioavailable. However, observe closely for reduced milk production.

Drug Interactions: Urofollitropin does not effect prolactin levels.

Theoretic Infant Dose:

Relative Infant Dose:

Adult Dose: 75 units daily

Alternatives:

$T\frac{1}{2}$ =	3.9 and 70.4 hours	M/P =	
PHL =		PB =	
T_{max} =	6-18 hours	Oral =	None
MW =	34,000	pKa =	
Vd =	0.06, 1.08		

References:
1. Sharma V, Riddle A, et al: Studies on folliculogenesis and in vitro fertilization outcome after the administration of follicle-stimulating hormone at different times during the menstrual cycle. Fertil Steril 51:298-303, 1989.
2. Kjeld JM, Harsoulis P, et al: Infusions of hFSH and hLH in normal men: kinetics of human follicle stimulating hormone. Acta Endocrinologica 81:225-233, 1976.
3. Yen SSC, Llerena LA, Pearson OH et al: Disappearance rates of endogenous follicle-stimulating hormone in serum following surgical hypophysectomy in man. J Clin Endocrinol 30:325-329, 1970.

FORMALDEHYDE
Trade: Formaldehyde, Formalin, Methyl Aldehyde
Can/Aus/UK:
Uses: Preservative
LRC: L4
AAP: Not reviewed

Formaldehyde exposure in laboratory or embalming environments is strictly controlled by federal regulations to a permissible level of 2 ppm. At room temperature it is a colorless gas with a pungent, irritating odor detectable at 0.5 ppm. At exposure to 1-4 ppm, formaldehyde is a strong mucous membrane irritant, producing burning and lacrimation.[1] Formaldehyde is rapidly destroyed by plasma and tissue enzymes and it is very unlikely than any would enter human milk following environmental exposures. However, acute intoxications following high oral or inhaled doses could lead to significant levels of maternal plasma formic acid which could enter milk. There are no data suggesting untoward side effects in nursing infants as a result of mild to minimal environmental exposure of the mother.

Pregnancy Risk Category: X

Lactation Risk Category: L4

Adult Concerns: Cough, mucous membrane irritation, chest pain, dyspnea, and wheezing occur in individuals exposed to 5-30 ppm.

Pediatric Concerns: None reported via milk.

Drug Interactions:

Theoretic Infant Dose:

Relative Infant Dose:

Adult Dose:

Alternatives:

T½ =		M/P =
PHL =		PB =
T$_{max}$ =		Oral =
MW =	30	pKa =
Vd =		

References:

1. Ellenhorn MJ. Medical toxicology: a primer for the medicolegal age. Clin Toxicol 1978; 13(4):439-462.

FORMOTEROL FUMARATE

Trade: Foradil Aerolizer
Can/Aus/UK:
Uses: Bronchodilator
LRC: L3
AAP: Not reviewed

Formoterol is a long-acting selective beta-2 adrenoceptor agonist used for asthma and COPD. Following inhalation of a 120 μg dose, the maximum plasma concentration of 92 picograms/mL occurred within 5 minutes.[1] No data are available on its transfer into human milk, but the extremely low plasma levels would suggest that milk levels would be incredibly low, if even measurable. Studies of oral absorption in adults suggests that while absorption is good, plasma levels are still below detectable levels and may require large oral doses prior to attaining measurable plasma levels.[2,3] It is not likely the amount present in human milk would be clinically relevant to a breastfed infant.

Pregnancy Risk Category: C

Lactation Risk Category: L3

Adult Concerns: Tremor, headache, dizziness, restlessness, palpitations, nausea, dry mouth, muscle cramps, and cough. Low serum potassium and elevated blood glucose levels can occur with high doses. Blood pressure and heart rate are minimally affected.

Pediatric Concerns: None reported via milk.

Drug Interactions: Concurrent use of xanthing derivatives, steroids, or diuretics may potentiate any hypokalemic effect. Do not use with MAO inhibitors, tricyclic antidepressants, or drugs known to prolong QTc interval. Beta-adrenergic agents may inhibit effect of formoterol.

Theoretic Infant Dose:

Relative Infant Dose:

Adult Dose: 12 μg every 12 hours

Alternatives: Salmeterol, albuterol.

T½ =	10 hours	M/P =	
PHL =		PB =	64%
T$_{max}$ =	5 minutes	Oral =	Good
MW =	840	pKa =	
Vd =			

References:
1. Pharmaceutical Manufacturer Prescribing Information.
2. Tattersfield AE. Long-acting beta 2-agonists. Clin Exp Allergy 1992; 22(6):600-605.
3. Maesen FP, Smeets JJ, Gubbelmans HL, Zweers PG. Bronchodilator effect of inhaled formoterol vs salbutamol over 12 hours. Chest 1990; 97(3):590-594.

FOSCARNET SODIUM

Trade: Foscavir
Can/Aus/UK: Foscavir
Uses: Antiviral for herpes, CMV infections
LRC: L4
AAP: Not reviewed

Foscarnet is an antiviral used to treat mucocutaneous herpes simplex manifestations and cytomegalovirus retinal infections in patients with AIDS. It is not known if foscarnet is secreted into human milk, but studies in animals indicate levels in milk were three times higher than serum levels (suggesting a Milk/plasma ratio of 3.0).[1,2] Foscarnet is a potent and potentially dangerous drug including significant renal toxicity, seizures, and deposition in bone and teeth.

Pregnancy Risk Category: C

Lactation Risk Category: L4

Adult Concerns: Fever, nausea, diarrhea, vomiting, tremor, headache, fatigue, kidney toxicity, anemia due to bone marrow suppression

Pediatric Concerns: None reported but caution is urged.

Drug Interactions: Increased hypocalemia with pentamidine, and increased seizures with ciprofloxacin.

Theoretic Infant Dose:

Relative Infant Dose:

Adult Dose: 34-51 mg/kg injection (IV) daily
Alternatives:

$T\frac{1}{2}$ =	3 hours	M/P =	3.0
PHL =		PB =	14-17%
T_{max} =	Immediate(IV)	Oral =	12-21%
MW =	192	pKa =	
Vd =			

References:
1. Pharmaceutical Manufacturer Prescribing Information. 1995.
2. Sjovall J, Karlsson A, Ogenstad S, Sandstrom E, Saarimaki M. Pharmacokinetics and absorption of foscarnet after intravenous and oral administration to patients with human immunodeficiency virus. Clin Pharmacol Ther 1988; 44(1):65-73.

FOSFOMYCIN TROMETAMOL

Trade: Monuril
Can/Aus/UK: Monuril
Uses: Urinary antibiotic
LRC: L3
AAP: Not reviewed

Fosfomycin is a broad-spectrum antibiotic used primarily for uncomplicated urinary tract infections. It is believed safe for use in pregnancy and has been used in children less than 1 year of age. Fosfomycin absorption is largely dependent on the salt form; trometamol salts are modestly absorbed (34-58%) and calcium salts are poorly absorbed (< 12%). Fosfomycin secreted into human milk would likely be in the calcium form and is unlikely to be absorbed as secreted in human milk. Foods and the acidic milieu of the stomach both significantly reduce oral absorption.[1-3]

Levels secreted into human milk have been reported to be about 10% of the maternal plasma level.[4]   Generally, a single 3 mg oral dose is effective treatment for many urinary tract infections in women. It is not likely that the levels present in breastmilk would produce untoward effects in a breastfeeding infant.

Pregnancy Risk Category: B

Lactation Risk Category: L3

Adult Concerns: GI symptoms include nausea, vomiting, diarrhea, epigastric discomfort, anorexia. Skin rashes and pruritus have been reported.

Pediatric Concerns: None reported via milk.

Drug Interactions: Antacids, calcium salts, and foods will reduce absorption. Metoclopramide reduces serum concentration by reducing oral bioavailability.

Theoretic Infant Dose:

Relative Infant Dose:

Adult Dose: 3 gm/d

Alternatives:

$T\frac{1}{2}$ =	4-8 hours	M/P =	0.1
PHL =	5-7 hours	PB =	< 3%
T_{max} =	1.5-3 hours	Oral =	34-58%
MW =	138	pKa =	
Vd =	0.22		

References:
1. Bergan T. Degree of absorption, pharmacokinetics of fosfomycin trometamol and duration of urinary antibacterial activity. Infection 1990; 18 Suppl 2:S65-S69.
2. Bergan T. Pharmacokinetic comparison between fosfomycin and other phosphonic acid derivatives. Chemotherapy 1990; 36 Suppl 1:10-18.
3. Segre G, Bianchi E, Cataldi A, Zannini G. Pharmacokinetic profile of fosfomycin trometamol (Monuril). Eur Urol 1987; 13 Suppl 1:56-63.
4. Kirby WM. Pharmacokinetics of fosfomycin. Chemotherapy 1977; 23 Suppl 1:141-151.

FOSINOPRIL

Trade: Monopril
Can/Aus/UK: Monopril, Staril
Uses: Antihypertensive, ACE inhibitor
LRC: L3
         L4 if used in neonatal period
AAP: Not reviewed

Fosinopril is a prodrug that is metabolized by the gut and liver upon absorption to fosinoprilat, which is an ACE inhibitor used as an antihypertensive. The manufacturer reports that the ingestion of 20 mg daily for three days resulted in barely detectable levels in human milk although no values are provided.[1,2] See enalapril, benazepril, captopril as alternatives.

Pregnancy Risk Category: D

Lactation Risk Category: L3
         L4 if used in neonatal period

Adult Concerns: Anemia, dry cough, headache, dizziness, diarrhea, fatigue, nausea, vomiting, hypotension

Pediatric Concerns: None reported via milk.

Drug Interactions: Bioavailability of ACEIs may be decreased when used with antacids. Capsaicin may exacerbate coughing associated with ACEi treatment. Pharmacologic effects of ACE inhibitors may be increased. Increased plasma levels of digoxin may result. Increased serum lithium levels may result when used with ACE inhibitors.

Theoretic Infant Dose:

Relative Infant Dose:

Adult Dose: 20-40 mg daily

Alternatives: Enalapril, Benazepril, Captopril

$T\frac{1}{2}$ =	11-35 hours	M/P =	
PHL =		PB =	95 %
T_{max} =	3 hours	Oral =	30-36%
MW =	564	pKa =	
Vd =			

References:
1. Drug Facts and Comparisons 1995 ed. ed. St. Louis: 1995.
2. Pharmaceutical Manufacturer Prescribing Information. 1995.

FOSPHENYTOIN
Trade: Cerebyx
Can/Aus/UK:
Uses: Anticonvulsant
LRC: L2
AAP: Maternal Medication Usually Compatible with Breastfeeding

Fosphenytoin is a prodrug of phenytoin. Following the parenteral injection of fosphenytoin, it is rapidly converted to the anticonvulsant phenytoin with a brief half-life of 15 minutes.[1] Thus the active drug is phenytoin. See phenytoin for breastmilk specifics.

Pregnancy Risk Category: D

Lactation Risk Category: L2

Adult Concerns: Side effects include headache, nausea, ecchymosis, nystagmus, tremor, etc. See phenytoin.

Pediatric Concerns: Only one case of methemoglobinemia, drowsiness, and poor sucking has been reported with phenytoin. Most other studies suggest no problems.

Drug Interactions: See phenytoin.

Theoretic Infant Dose:

Relative Infant Dose:

Adult Dose: 4-6 mg phenytoin equivalents/kg/day

Alternatives: Phenytoin

$T\frac{1}{2}$ =	15 minutes	M/P =	
PHL =		PB =	99%
T_{max} =	0.5 hour	Oral =	
MW =	406	pKa =	
Vd =	4-10.8		

References:
1. Pharmaceutical Manufacturers prescribing information, 2003.

FROVATRIPTAN SUCCINATE
Trade: Frova
Can/Aus/UK:
Uses: Anti-migraine, 5-HT1B/1D receptor agonist
LRC: L3
AAP: Not reviewed

Frovatriptan is believed to act on intracranial arteries to prevent excessive dilation of these vessels commonly found in migraine attacks.[1]

It is from the same family as sumatriptan(Imitrex). No data on its transfer to milk are available. Some studies suggest sumatriptan may be more effective. Sumatriptan is recommended as we have good data suggesting milk levels of sumatriptan are low and its oral bioavailability is low.

Pregnancy Risk Category: C

Lactation Risk Category: L3

Adult Concerns: May increase coronary vasoconstriction. Use cautiously in patients with coronary artery disease. Events reported have included coronary artery vasospasm, transient myocardial ischemia, myocardial infarction, ventricular tachycardia and ventricular fibrillation. Commonly reported complaints include dizziness,headache, paresthesia. GI symptoms include dry mouth, dyspepsia. Fatigue, hot and cold sensations, skeletal pain, and flushing have been reported.

Pediatric Concerns: None reported via milk.

Drug Interactions: Levels of frovatriptan may increase 30% in subjects taking oral contraceptives. Frovatriptan levels may be significantly reduced (25%) by concomitant use of ergotamine. Propranol may increase plasma levels of frovatriptan by 16-23% and half-life as well.

Theoretic Infant Dose:

Relative Infant Dose:

Adult Dose: 2.5 mg initially followed by one after 2 hours if no response.

Alternatives: Sumatriptan

$T\frac{1}{2}$ =	26 hours	M/P =	
PHL =		PB =	15%
T_{max} =	2-4 hours	Oral =	30%
MW =	379	pKa =	
Vd =	4.2		

References:
1. Pharmaceutical Manufacturer Prescribing Information.

FURAZOLIDONE

Trade: Furoxone
Can/Aus/UK: Furoxone
Uses: Gastrointestinal antibiotic.
LRC: L2
 L4 early postpartum
AAP: Not reviewed

Furazolidone belongs to the nitrofurantoin family of antibiotics (see nitrofurantoin). It has a broad spectrum of activity against gram-positive and gram-negative enteric organisms including cholera but is generally used for giardiasis.[1]

Following an oral dose, furazolidone is poorly absorbed (< 5%) and is largely inactivated in the gut. Concentrations transferred to milk are unreported, but the total amounts would be exceedingly low due to the low maternal plasma levels attained by this product. Due to poor oral absorption, systemic absorption in a breastfeeding infant would likely be minimal. Caution should be observed in early postpartum newborns.

Pregnancy Risk Category: C

Lactation Risk Category: L2
 L4 early postpartum

Adult Concerns: Hemolytic anemia in newborns, nausea, vomiting, diarrhea, abdominal pain. Dark yellow to brown discoloration of urine.

Pediatric Concerns: Caution is urged in neonates < 1 month due to possibility of hemolytic anemia.

Drug Interactions: Increased effect when used with sympathomimetic amines, tricyclic antidepressants, MAO inhibitors, meperidine, dextromethorphan, fluoxetine, paroxetine, sertraline, trazodone.

Theoretic Infant Dose:

Relative Infant Dose:

Adult Dose: 100 mg QID

Alternatives:

T½ =		M/P =	
PHL =		PB =	
T$_{max}$ =		Oral =	< 5%
MW =	225	pKa =	
Vd =			

References:
1. Pharmaceutical Manufacturer Prescribing Information.

FUROSEMIDE
Trade: Lasix
Can/Aus/UK: Apo-Furosemide, Novo-Semide, Lasix, Frusemide, Uremide, Frusid
Uses: Loop diuretic
LRC: L3
AAP: Not reviewed

Furosemide is a potent loop diuretic with a rather short duration of action. Furosemide has been found in breastmilk although the levels are unreported. Diuretics, by reducing blood volume, could potentially reduce breastmilk production although this is largely theoretical.[1] Furosemide is frequently used in neonates in pediatric units, so pediatric use is common. The oral bioavailability of furosemide in newborns is exceedingly poor and very high oral doses are required (1-4mg/kg BID).[2] It is very unlikely the amount transferred into human milk would produce any effects in a nursing infant although its maternal use could suppress lactation.

Pregnancy Risk Category: C

Lactation Risk Category: L3

Adult Concerns: Hypotension, fluid loss, potassium loss

Pediatric Concerns: None reported via milk.

Drug Interactions: Furosemide interferes with hypoglycemic effect of antidiabetic agents. NSAIDS may reduce diuretic effect of furosemide. Effects of antihypertensive agents may be increased. Renal clearance of lithium is decreased. Increases ototoxicity of aminoglycosides.

Theoretic Infant Dose:

Relative Infant Dose:

Adult Dose: 40-80 mg BID

Alternatives:

$T\frac{1}{2}$ =	92 minutes	M/P =	
PHL =		PB =	> 98%
T_{max} =	1-2 hours	Oral =	60-70%
MW =	331	pKa =	
Vd =			

References:
1. Healy M. Suppressing lactation with oral diuretics. The Lancet 1961;1353-1354.
2. Pharmaceutical Manufacturer Prescribing Information. 1995.

GABAPENTIN

Trade: Neurontin
Can/Aus/UK: Neurontin
Uses: Anticonvulsant
LRC: L3
AAP: Not reviewed

Gabapentin is a newer anticonvulsant used primarily for partial (focal) seizures with or without secondary generalization. Unlike many anticonvulsants, gabapentin is almost completely renally excreted without metabolism. It does not induce hepatic enzymes and is remarkably well tolerated.[1-3] No published reports are available on its transfer into human milk. However, in preliminary results from a study of one breastfeeding mother who was receiving 1800 mg/d, milk levels were 11.1, 11.3, and 11.0 mg/L at 2, 4, and 8 hours respectively, following a dose of 600 mg.[4] In another patient receiving 2400 mg/d milk levels were 9.8, 9.0, and 7.2 mg/L at 2,4, and 8 hours respectively, after a dose of 800 mg. Using this data an infant would consume approximately 3.7% to 6.5% of the weight-adjusted maternal dose per day. No adverse events were noted in these two infants.

Pregnancy Risk Category: C

Lactation Risk Category: L3

Adult Concerns: Dizziness, somnolence, weight gain, vomiting, tremor, and CNS depression. Abrupt withdrawal may induce severe seizures.

Pediatric Concerns: None reported. Cleared for children > 12 yrs.

Drug Interactions: Antacids reduce gabapentin absorption by 20%. Cimetidine may decrease clearance of gabapentin. No interaction has been reported with other anticonvulsants. Antacids may reduce oral absorption by 20%.

Theoretic Infant Dose: 1.69 mg/kg/day

Relative Infant Dose: 6.5%

Adult Dose: 300-600 mg TID

Alternatives:

$T\frac{1}{2}$ =	5-7 hours	M/P =	
PHL =		PB =	< 3%
T_{max} =	1-3 hours	Oral =	50-60%
MW =		pKa =	
Vd =	0.8		

References:
1. Goa KL, Sorkin EM. Gabapentin. A review of its pharmacological properties and clinical potential in epilepsy. Drugs 1993; 46(3):409-427.

2. Ramsay RE. Clinical efficacy and safety of gabapentin. Neurology 1994; 44(6 Suppl 5):S23-S30.
3. Dichter MA, Brodie MJ. New antiepileptic drugs. N Engl J Med 1996; 334(24):1583-1590.
4. Hale TW, Ilett KF, Hackett P. Personal communication. 2002.

GADODIAMIDE

Trade: Omniscan
Can/Aus/UK: Omniscan
Uses: Radiocontrast agent for MRI scans
LRC: L3
AAP: Not reviewed

Gadodiamide is a gadolinium-containing, non-ionic, non-iodinated water soluble contrast medium commonly used in Magnetic Resonance Imaging scans.[1] It is quite similar to Magnevist, another gadolinium-containing agent. These agents penetrate peripheral compartments poorly, especially the brain. As such they are extremely unlikely to enter milk as well. Data for gadopentetate (Magnevist) support this as its transfer into milk is negligible (< 0.04%). Neither of these compounds are well absorbed orally and neither are metabolized to any degree. It is likely that gadodiamide will penetrate milk only minimally, but without specific data this remains undocumented.

Pregnancy Risk Category: C

Lactation Risk Category: L3

Adult Concerns: The most common reported adverse effects include nausea, headache, dizziness, and urticaria.

Pediatric Concerns: None reported via milk. Cleared for children > 2 years of age.

Drug Interactions: Increased plasma levels with probenecid.

Theoretic Infant Dose:

Relative Infant Dose:

Adult Dose: 0.2 mL/kg administered as a bolus.

Alternatives: Gadopentetate

$T\frac{1}{2}$ =	77 minutes	M/P =	
PHL =		PB =	0%
T_{max} =		Oral =	Nil
MW =	573	pKa =	
Vd =	0.2		

References:

1. Pharmaceutical Manufacturers prescribing information, 2003.

GADOPENTETATE
Trade: Magnevist, Gadolinium
Can/Aus/UK: Magnevist
Uses: Radiocontrast agent (MRI)
LRC: L2
AAP: Maternal Medication Usually Compatible with Breastfeeding

Gadopentetate is a radiopaque agent used in magnetic resonance imaging of the kidney. It is nonionic, non-iodinated and has low osmolarity and contains a gadolinium ion as the radiopaque entity. Following a dose of 7 mmol (6.5 gm), the amount of gadopentetate secreted in breastmilk was 3.09, 2.8, 1.08, and 0.5 μmol/L at 2, 11, 17, and 24 hours respectively.[1] The cumulative amount excreted from both breasts in 24 hours was only 0.023% of the administered dose. Oral absorption is minimal, only 0.8% of gadopentetate is absorbed. These authors suggest that only 0.013 micromole of a gadolinium-containing compound would be absorbed by the infant in 24 hours, which is incredibly low. They further suggest that 24 hours of pumping would eliminate risks although this seems rather extreme in view of the short (1.6 hr) half-life, poor oral bioavailability, and limited milk levels.

In another study of 19 lactating women who received 0.1 mmol/kg and one additional woman who received 0.2 mmol/kg, the cumulative amount of gadolinium excreted in breastmilk during 24 hours was 0.57 μmol.[2] This resulted in an excreted dose of < 0.04% of the IV administered maternal dose. A similar amount was noted in the patient receiving a double dose (0.2 mmol/kg). Thus for any neonate weighing more than 1000 gm, the maximal orally ingested dose would be less than 1% of the permitted intravenous dose of 0.2 mmol/kg. According to the authors, "the very small amount of gadopentetate dimeglumine transferred to a nursing infant does not warrant a potentially traumatic 24-hour suspension of breast feeding for lactating women."

Pregnancy Risk Category: C
Lactation Risk Category: L2
Adult Concerns: Headache, rash, nausea, dry mouth, altered taste
Pediatric Concerns: Virtually none enters milk. No reported side-effects via milk.
Drug Interactions:
Theoretic Infant Dose: 0.42 mg/kg/day
Relative Infant Dose: 0.45%
Adult Dose:

Alternatives:

T½ =	1.6 hours	M/P =	
PHL =		PB =	
T$_{max}$ =	Immediate((V)	Oral =	0.8%
MW =	938	pKa =	
Vd =			

References:
1. Rofsky NM, Weinreb JC, Litt AW. Quantitative analysis of gadopentetate dimeglumine excreted in breastmilk. J Magn Reson Imaging 1993; 3(1):131-132.
2. Kubik-Huch RA, Gottstein-Aalame NM, Frenzel T, Seifert B, Puchert E, Wittek S, Debatin JF. Gadopentetate dimeglumine excretion into human breastmilk during lactation. Radiology 2000; 216(2):555-558.

GADOTERIDOL

Trade: Prohance
Can/Aus/UK: Prohance
Uses: Radiocontrast agent for MRI
LRC: L3
AAP: Not reviewed

Gadoteridol is a nonionic, non-iodinated gadolinium chelate complex used as a radiocontrast agent in MRI scans. The metabolism of gadoteridol is unknown, but a similar gadolinium salt (gadopentetate) is not metabolized at all.[1] The half-life is brief (1.6 hours) and the volume of distribution is very small, suggesting that gadoteridol does not penetrate tissues well and is unlikely to penetrate milk in significant quantities. A similar compound, gadopentetate, is barely detectable in breastmilk. Although not reported, the oral bioavailability is probably similar to gadopentetate, which is minimal to none. No data are available on the transfer of gadoteridol into human milk although it is probably minimal. A brief interruption of breastfeeding for 12-24 hours should remove any risk although it is not necessary.

Pregnancy Risk Category: C

Lactation Risk Category: L3

Adult Concerns: Nausea, bad taste, headache, rash, urticaria, chest pain rarely

Pediatric Concerns: None reported via milk.

Drug Interactions:

Theoretic Infant Dose:

Relative Infant Dose:

Adult Dose: 0.2-0.4 mL/kg X 2

Alternatives: Gadopentetate

T½ =	1.6 hours	M/P =	
PHL =		PB =	
T$_{max}$ =		Oral =	Poor
MW =		pKa =	
Vd =	0.2		

References:
1. Pharmaceutical Manufacturer Prescribing Information. 1997.

GADOVERSETAMIDE
Trade: OptiMARK
Can/Aus/UK: OptiMARK
Uses: Radiocontrast agent used for MRI scans
LRC: L3
AAP: Not reviewed

Gadoversetamide is a paramagnetic agent used as a contrast agent in magnetic resonance imaging (MRI). It does not enter most compartments and is confined to extracellular water with a low volume of distribution. As with gadopentetate, this agent is very unlikely to penetrate milk or be orally bioavailable. However, no human data are available. Rat studies show some penetration of gadoversetamide into rat milk, but rodent lactation studies do not correlate with humans (always high).

Pregnancy Risk Category: C

Lactation Risk Category: L3

Adult Concerns: Adverse symptoms include headache, abdominal pain, asthenia, back pain, flushing, nausea, vomiting, diarrhea, pain at injection site, and allergic reactions.

Pediatric Concerns: None reported via human milk. Some found in rat milk. This agent is unlikely to penetrate into human milk in clinically relevant amounts.

Drug Interactions: None reported.

Theoretic Infant Dose:

Relative Infant Dose:

Adult Dose: 0.2 mL/kg.

Alternatives: Gadopentetate

T½ =	1.7 hours	M/P =	
PHL =		PB =	0%
T$_{max}$ =		Oral =	Nil
MW =	662	pKa =	
Vd =	0.162		

References:
1. Pharmaceutical Manufacturer Prescribing Information. 2003.

GALLIUM-67 CITRATE
Trade: Gallium-67 Citrate
Can/Aus/UK:
Uses: Radioactive isotope
LRC: L4
AAP: Radioactive compound that requires temporary cessation of breastfeeding

Gallium-67 Citrate is a radioactive substance used for bone scanning. In one breastfeeding mother who received 3 mCi, the radioactive content in breastmilk was 0.15, 0.045, and 0.01 uCi/mL at 3, 7, and 14 days respectively.[1] If the infant ingested milk, the whole body exposure would have been very significant, 1.4-2.0 rad/mCi. This is significantly more than the mother's exposure of only 0.26 rad/mCi. Therefore, a significant radioactive hazard exists. Whole body scans showed intense radiation in the breast tissue of the mother. With a 14 day waiting period, the theoretical whole body dose to the infant would be 0.04 rads and 0.07 rads to the skeleton. Radioactive half-life of Gallium-67 is 78.3 hours, while the biological half-life of the gallium ion is 9 days. These approximations suggest that breastfeeding should be interrupted for a minimum of 1 week following a dose of 0.2 mCi, 2 weeks for 1.3 mCi, or 1 month for 4 mCi. Check the NRC guidelines in the appendix.

Pregnancy Risk Category:

Lactation Risk Category: L4

Adult Concerns: Radiation hazard

Pediatric Concerns: Significant radiation exposure. Remove from breast for 14 days.

Drug Interactions:

Theoretic Infant Dose:

Relative Infant Dose:

Adult Dose: 200 mg/sq. meter IV daily

Alternatives:

$T^{1/2}$ =	78.3 hours	M/P =	
PHL =		PB =	
T_{max} =		Oral =	
MW =		pKa =	
Vd =			

References:
1. Tobin RE, Schneider PB. Uptake of 67Ga in the lactating breast and its persistence in milk: case report. J Nucl Med 1976; 17(12):1055-1056.

GANIRELIX ACETATE

Trade: Antagon
Can/Aus/UK:
Uses: Synthetic gonotrophic-releasing hormone antagonist.
LRC: L3
AAP: Not reviewed

Ganirelix acts by competitively inducing a rapid, reversible suppression of gonadotropin secretion.[1] This subsequently inhibits release of leuteinizing hormone. The midcycle LH surge initiates several physiologic actions including ovulation, resumption of meiosis in the oocyte, and luteinization. This product is used to prevent the premature LH surge found in some infertile women. No data are available on the transfer of this decapeptide into human milk, but it is unlikely due to its peptide structure and its larger molecular weight In addition, it is very unlikely this decapeptide would be stable in the infants GI tract or orally bioavailable.

Pregnancy Risk Category: X

Lactation Risk Category: L3

Adult Concerns: Adverse events include abdominal pain, fetal death, headache, ovarian hyperstimulation syndrome, and vaginal bleeding.

Pediatric Concerns: None reported via milk, but no studies are available.

Drug Interactions:

Theoretic Infant Dose:

Relative Infant Dose:

Adult Dose: 250 µg subcutaneously daily

Alternatives:

T½ =	16.2 hours	M/P =	
PHL =		PB =	82
T$_{max}$ =	1.1 hours	Oral =	Nil
MW =	1570	pKa =	
Vd =	0.62		

References:
1. Pharmaceutical Manufacturer Prescribing Information. 2003.

GARLIC

Trade: Allium, Stinkin Rose, Rustic Treacle, Camphor Of The Poor
Can/Aus/UK:
Uses: Herbal antioxidant
LRC: L3
AAP: Not reviewed

Garlic contains a number of sulfur-containing compounds that, when ground, are metabolized to allicin, which is responsible for the pungent odor of garlic and the pharmacologic effects attributed to garlic.[1,2] Garlic has been reported to increase the levels of important plasma antioxidants, glutathione, and catalase probably due to the allicin content. Five sulfur containing compounds have been isolated that produce profound inhibition of lipid peroxidation in liver cells. A number of studies have found hypolipidemic effects of garlic oil, reducing plasma cholesterol, triglyceride levels, and elevating HDL levels significantly. Garlic oil also inhibits platelet aggregation thus reducing risk of thrombosis. Taken together, there is significant evidence to suggest that garlic oil may reduce the risks of cardiovascular disease, reducing plasma lipids and reducing the risk of clot formation. Garlic is known to be modestly antimicrobial, having about 1% of the antimicrobial potency of penicillin. Interestingly, the hypolipidemic and antimicrobial properties appear to reside in the odiferous constituents and may not be present in the "deodorized" oils.

Although garlic oil is commonly used, the safety for long term use is still unresolved. The extract has caused a reduction in liver and kidney protein in animal studies and a potential interaction with other anticoagulants (warfarin) should be expected. Transfer of the odorous components in human milk has been documented.[3,4]

Pregnancy Risk Category:

Lactation Risk Category: L3

Adult Concerns: Few reported but observe for excessive bleeding.

Pediatric Concerns: No studies available.

Drug Interactions: May enhance anticoagulant effects of warfarin.

Theoretic Infant Dose:

Relative Infant Dose:

Adult Dose:

Alternatives:

References:
1. Bissett NG. In: Herbal Drugs and Phytopharmaceuticals. Medpharm Scientific Publishers, CRC Press, Boca Raton, 1994.

2. Review of Natural Products Facts and Comparisons, St Louis, MO 1996.
3. Mennella JA, Beauchamp GK. Maternal diet alters the sensory qualities of human milk and the nursling's behavior. Pediatrics 1991; 88(4):737-744.
4. Mennella JA, Beauchamp GK. The effects of repeated exposure to garlic-flavored milk on the nursling's behavior. Pediatr Res 1993; 34(6):805-808.

GATIFLOXACIN

Trade: Tequin
Can/Aus/UK:
Uses: Fluoroquinolone antibiotic
LRC: L3
AAP: Not reviewed

Gatifloxacin is a fluoroquinolone antibiotic similar to ofloxacin, levofloxacin, and ciprofloxacin. As such, its use in pediatric age patients is not generally recommended although newer data suggest this family is safe in pediatric patients. While the manufacturer reports that gatifloxacin is secreted into animal milk, no data are available on humans. Of the numerous fluoroquinolone antibiotics, ofloxacin[1] and levofloxacin are probably preferred in breastfeeding patients due to lower milk levels. The only major risk to an infant is a change in gut flora and the possibility of overgrowth of C. Difficile (pseudomembranous colitis). If used, observe for bloody diarrhea.

Ophthalmic Product (Gatifloxacin):
No data on its transfer into human milk are available, but the maximum plasma levels reported in users was only 2.7 nanograms/mL. The mean C_{max} and estimated daily exposure values were 1600 and 1000 times lower than the C_{max} and AUC reported after therapeutic 400 mg oral does of moxifloxacin.[1] Thus ophthalmic exposure is extremely unlikely to produce clinically relevant levels in milk. The fluoroquinolones are becoming more popular for use in pediatric patients due to a number of recent studies and reviews.[2]

Pregnancy Risk Category: C

Lactation Risk Category: L3

Adult Concerns: Diarrhea, nausea, vaginitis, headache, dizziness, allergic reaction, chills, fever, palpitations, abdominal pain, and other symptoms have been reported. CNS agitation, nervousness, insomnia, and paranoia have been reported. Hypo and hyperglycemia have been reported in diabetic patients.

Pediatric Concerns: None reported via milk but no studies yet.

Drug Interactions: Probenecid may increase plasma levels of gatifloxacin by 42%. Absorption of gatifloxacin is reduced by concomitant administration with ferrous sulfate or antacids containing aluminum and magnesium salts. A minor increase in digoxin plasma levels has been reported.

Theoretic Infant Dose:

Relative Infant Dose:

Adult Dose:　400 mg daily

Alternatives:　Ofloxacin, Levofloxacin

$T\frac{1}{2}$ =	7.1 hours	M/P =	
PHL =		PB =	20%
T_{max} =	1-2 hours	Oral =	96%
MW =	402	pKa =	
Vd =	1.5		

References:
1. Giamarellou H, Kolokythas E, Petrikkos G, Gazis J, Aravantinos D, Sfikakis P. Pharmacokinetics of three newer quinolones in pregnant and lactating women. Am J Med 1989; 87(5A):49S-51S.

GEMFIBROZIL

Trade: Lopid, Gemcor
Can/Aus/UK: Apo-Gemfibrozil, Lopid, Ausgem, Gemhexal
Uses: Antilipemic agent
LRC: L3
AAP: Not reviewed

Gemfibrozil is a hypolipidemic agent primarily used to lower triglyceride levels by decreasing serum very low density lipoproteins.[1] A slight reduction in serum cholesterol may likewise occur. Following a dose of 800 mg, mean peak plasma levels were 33 μg/mL. There are no data on its transfer into human milk. Reproductive studies in rodents at high doses have not revealed any evidence of harm to the fetus. But the risks of using lipid lowering drugs while pregnant, and probably while breastfeeding, may be higher than the overall risks of hyperlipidemia and, therefore, are not usually justified.

Pregnancy Risk Category:　C

Lactation Risk Category:　L3

Adult Concerns: Epigastric pain, dry mouth, constipation, diarrhea, and flatulence. Changes in blood chemistry including hematocrit, white blood cells, hemoglobin. Elevation of liver enzymes.

Pediatric Concerns: None reported via milk, but risk vs. benefit evaluation is recommended.

Drug Interactions:　Stimulation of anticoagulants including Anisidone, dicoumarol, warfarin. Increased risk of myopathy when coadministered with HMG-CoA reductase inhibitors such as atorvastatin, fluvastatin, and other statins. Increased risk of hypoglycemia when used with glyburide, and perhaps other hypoglycemics.

Theoretic Infant Dose:

Relative Infant Dose:

Adult Dose: 600 mg BID

Alternatives:

T½ =	1.5 hours	M/P =	
PHL =		PB =	99%
T$_{max}$ =	1-2 hours	Oral =	97%
MW =	250	pKa =	
Vd =			

References:
1. McEvoy GE. (ed): AFHS Drug Information. New York, NY: 1999.

GENTAMICIN

Trade: Garamycin
Can/Aus/UK: Alocomicin, Cidomycin, Garamycin, Garatec, Palacos, Septopal
Uses: Aminoglycoside antibiotic
LRC: L2
AAP: Not reviewed

Gentamicin is a narrow spectrum antibiotic generally used for gram negative infections. The oral absorption of gentamicin (< 1%) is generally nil with the exception of premature neonates, where small amounts may be absorbed.[1] In one study of 10 women given 80 mg three times daily IM for 5 days postpartum, milk levels were measured on day 4.[2] Gentamicin levels in milk were 0.42, 0.48, 0.49, and 0.41 mg/L at 1, 3, 5, and 7 hours respectively. The milk/plasma ratios were 0.11 at one hour and 0.44 at 7 hours. Plasma gentamicin levels in neonates were small, were found in only 5 of the 10 neonates, and averaged 0.41 µg/mL. The authors estimate that daily ingestion via breastmilk would be 307 µg for a 3.6 kg neonate (normal neonatal dose = 2.5 mg/kg every 12 hours). These amounts would be clinically irrelevant in most infants.

Pregnancy Risk Category: C

Lactation Risk Category: L2

Adult Concerns: Changes in GI flora, diarrhea, kidney damage, etc.

Pediatric Concerns: None reported.

Drug Interactions: Increased toxicity when used with certain penicillins, cephalosporins, amphotericin B, loop diuretics, and neuromuscular blocking agents.

Theoretic Infant Dose: 73.5 µg/kg/day

Relative Infant Dose: 2.1%

Adult Dose: 1.5-2.5 mg/kg q 8 hours

Alternatives:

T½ =	2-3 hours	M/P =	0.11-0.44
PHL =	3-5.5 hours (neonates)	PB =	< 10-30 %
Tmax =	30-90 minutes (IM)	Oral =	< 1%
MW =		pKa =	8.2
Vd =	0.28(adult)		

References:
1. Nelson JD, McCracken GH, Jr. The current status of gentamicin for tne neonate and young infant. Am J Dis Child 1972; 124(1):13-14.
2. Celiloglu M, Celiker S, Guven H, Tuncok Y, Demir N, Erten O. Gentamicin excretion and uptake from breastmilk by nursing infants. Obstet Gynecol 1994; 84(2):263-265.

GENTIAN VIOLET

Trade: Crystal Violet, Methylrosailine Chloride, Gentian Violet
Can/Aus/UK:
Uses: Antifungal, antimicrobial
LRC: L3
AAP: Not reviewed

Gentian violet is an older product that, when used topically and orally, is an exceptionally effective antifungal and antimicrobial.[1] It is a strong purple dye that is difficult to remove. Gentian violet has been found to be equivalent to ketoconazole and far superior to nystatin in treating oral (not esophageal) candidiasis in patients with advanced AIDS.

Gentian violet (GV) solutions generally come as 1-2% Gentian violet dissolved in a 10% solution of alcohol. For use with infants, the solution should be diluted with distilled water to 0.25 to 0.5% Gentian violet. This reduces the irritant properties of GV and reduces the alcohol content as well. While the alcohol is irritating to the nipple, it is not detrimental to the infant.[2] Higher concentrations of GV are known to be very irritating, leading to oral ulceration and necrotic skin reactions in children. If used, a small swab should be soaked in the solution, and then have the baby suck on the swab, or apply it directly to the affected areas in the mouth no more than once or twice daily for no more than 3-7 days. Direct application to the nipple has been reported and is indicated for candidiasis of the nipple.

Pregnancy Risk Category: C

Lactation Risk Category: L3

Adult Concerns: Oral ulceration, stomatitis, staining of skin and clothing, nausea, vomiting, diarrhea

Pediatric Concerns: Irritation leading to buccal ulcerations and necrotic skin reactions if used excessively and in higher concentrations. Nausea, vomiting, diarrhea.

Drug Interactions:

Theoretic Infant Dose:

Relative Infant Dose:

Adult Dose: N/A

Alternatives:

$T\frac{1}{2}$ =		M/P =	
PHL =		PB =	
T_{max} =		Oral =	
MW =	408	pKa =	
Vd =			

References:
1. McEvoy GE. (ed):AFHS Drug Information. New York, NY: 2003.
2. Newman J. Personal communication. 1997.

GINKGO BILOBA

Trade: Ginko
Can/Aus/UK:
Uses: Herbal antioxidant
LRC: L3
AAP: Not reviewed

Ginkgo Biloba is the world's oldest living tree. Extracts of the leaves (GBE) contain numerous chemical compounds including dimeric flavones and their glycosides, amino acids such as 6-hydroxyknurenic acid, and numerous other compounds. The seeds contain ginkgo toxin, which is particularly toxic, and should not be consumed. Numerous studies reviewing gingko have been reported, including treatments for cerebral insufficiency, asthma, dementia, and circulatory disorders. Gingko appears particularly efficient at increasing cerebral blood flow, with increases varying from 20-70%.[1,2] Older patients were more responsive. This supports the clinical use of GBE to treat cognitive impairment in the elderly. The anxiolytic properties of GBE have been reported to be due to MAO inhibition in animal studies. Ginkgolides inhibit platelet-activating factor and is believed responsible for the anti-allergic and anti-asthmatic properties of this extract. No data are available on the transfer of GBE into human milk. Thus far, with exception of the seeds, GBE appears relatively non-toxic.

Pregnancy Risk Category:

Lactation Risk Category: L3

Adult Concerns: Headache, dizziness, heart palpitations, GI symptoms, dermatologic reactions

Pediatric Concerns: None reported via human milk.

Drug Interactions:

Theoretic Infant Dose:

Relative Infant Dose:

Adult Dose:

Alternatives:

References:
1. Review of Natural Products Facts and Comparisons 1998.
2. Newall C, Anderson LA, Phillipson JD. Chamomile, German. In. Herbal Medicine. A guide for the healthcare professionals. The Pharmaceutical Press, London, 1996.

GINSENG

Trade: Panax
Can/Aus/UK: Minomycin, Red Kooga
Uses: Herbal tonic
LRC: L3
AAP: Not reviewed

Ginseng is perhaps the most popular and widely recognized product in the herbal remedy market. It is available in many forms, but the most common is the American root called Panax quinquefolium L. The root primarily contains steroid-like saponin glycosides (ginsenosides), of which there are at least two dozen and vary as a function of species, age, location, and season when harvested.[1]

Early claims have suggested that ginseng provided "strengthening" effects and included increased mental capacity for work. Animal studies have suggested that ginseng can increase swimming time, prevent stress-induced ulcers, stimulate certain immune cells, etc. A number of studies, mostly small and poorly controlled, have been reported and many suggest beneficial effects of ingesting ginseng with minimal side effects. Reported toxicities have included estrogen-like effects including diffuse mammary nodularity, vaginal bleeding, etc.[2] The most commonly reported event is nervousness, excitation, morning diarrhea, and inability to concentrate. In one case report, germanium, an ingredient in ginseng preparations, produced a significant diuretic resistance.[3]   No data was found concerning transfer into human milk. It is recommended that it not be used for more than 6 weeks.[4]

Pregnancy Risk Category:

Lactation Risk Category: L3

Adult Concerns: Excitement, nervousness, inability to concentrate, diarrhea, skin eruptions, hypertension, hypoglycemia,   mammary nodularity.   Ginseng products sometimes contain germanium,   which can induce a state of severe loop-diuretic resistance.

Pediatric Concerns: None reported, but caution is urged.

Drug Interactions:

Theoretic Infant Dose:

Relative Infant Dose:

Adult Dose:

Alternatives:

References:

1.   Review of Natural Products Facts and Comparisons, St Louis, MO 1996.
2.   Bissett NG. In: Herbal Drugs and Phytopharmaceuticals. Medpharm Scientific Publishers, CRC Press, Boca Raton, 1994.
3.   Becker BN, Greene J, Evanson J, Chidsey G, Stone WJ. Ginseng-induced diuretic resistance. JAMA 1996; 276(8):606-607.
4.   The Complete German Commission E Monographs. Ed. M. Blumenthal Amer Botanical Council 1998.

GLATIRAMER

Trade: Copaxone
Can/Aus/UK:
Uses: Relapsing multiple sclerosis
LRC: L3
AAP: Not reviewed

Glatiramer is a synthetic polypeptide indicated for the treatment of relapsing, remitting multiple sclerosis. It is primarily indicated for those who do not respond to interferons.   Glatiramer is a mixture of random polymers of four amino acids: L-alanine, L-glutamic acid, L-lysine, and L-tyrosine. Its molecular weight ranges from 4,700 to 13,000 daltons, which would reduce its ability to enter milk.[1] It is antigenically similar to myelin basic protein, a natural component of the myelin sheath of neurons. No data are available on its transfer into human milk, but it is very unlikely. If ingested orally, it would likely be depolymerized into individual amino acids, so toxicity is unlikely.

Pregnancy Risk Category: B

Lactation Risk Category: L3

Adult Concerns: Dizziness, chest pain, palpitations, anxiety, hypertonia, sweating, nausea, weakness. Rash, hives, or severe pain where the shot is given.

Pediatric Concerns: None via milk.

Drug Interactions:

Theoretic Infant Dose:

Relative Infant Dose:

Adult Dose: 20 mg subcutaneously once daily

Alternatives:

T½ =		M/P =	
PHL =		PB =	
T$_{max}$ =		Oral =	Minimal
MW =	4700+	pKa =	
Vd =			

References:
1.   Pharmaceutical Manufacturer Prescribing Information.

GLIMEPIRIDE

Trade: Amaryl
Can/Aus/UK:
Uses: Lowers plasma glucose.
LRC: L4
AAP: Not reviewed

Glimepiride is a second-generation sulfonylurea used to lower plasma glucose in patients with non-insulin dependent diabetes mellitus.   No data are available on the transfer of this product into human milk. However, rodent studies demonstrated significant transfer and elevated plasma levels in pups.[1,2]   Caution is urged if used in breastfeeding humans. Observe for hypoglycemia.

Pregnancy Risk Category: B

Lactation Risk Category: L4

Adult Concerns: Hypoglycemia, nausea, hyponatremia, dizziness, headache, elevated liver enzymes, blurred vision

Pediatric Concerns: None reported via milk.   Observe for hypoglycemia.

Drug Interactions: The hypoglycemic effect of sulfonylureas may be increased by non-steroidal analgesics, salicylates, sulfonamides, coumarins, probenecid, and other drugs with high protein binding. Numerous other interactions exist, see product information.

Theoretic Infant Dose:

Relative Infant Dose:

Adult Dose: 1-4 mg daily

Alternatives:

T½ =	6-9 hours	M/P =	
PHL =		PB =	> 99.5%
T$_{max}$ =	2-3 hours	Oral =	100%
MW =	490	pKa =	
Vd =	0.113		

References:
1. Pharmaceutical Manufacturer Prescribing Information.
2. Bressler R, Johnson DG. Pharmacological regulation of blood glucose levels in non-insulin-dependent diabetes mellitus. Arch Intern Med 1997; 157(8):836-848.

GLIPIZIDE

Trade: Glucotrol XL, Glucotrol
Can/Aus/UK: Melizide, Minidiab, Glibenese
Uses: Prolonged release hypoglycemic agent
LRC: L3
AAP: Not reviewed

Glipizide is a potent hypoglycemic agent that belongs to sulfonylurea family. It is formulated in regular and extended release formulations, and it is used only for non insulin-dependent (Type II) diabetes. Thus the half-life and time-to-peak depends on the formulation used. It reduces glucose levels by stimulating insulin secretion from the pancreas.[1] No reports on transfer into human milk were found. Other sulfonylureas (tolbutamide, chlorpropamide) are known to pass into milk in low concentrations. Although hypoglycemia in infants is a potential problem, no reports of such have been published. AHL= 2-5 hrs (Glucotrol), 24 hrs (Glucotrol-XL).

The new product Metaglip contains Glipizide and metformin.

Pregnancy Risk Category: C

Lactation Risk Category: L3

Adult Concerns: Hypoglycemia, jaundice, nausea, vomiting, diarrhea, constipation

Pediatric Concerns: None reported but observe for hypoglycemia.

Drug Interactions: The hypoglycemic effect may be enhanced by : anticoagulants, chloramphenicol, clofibrate, fenfluramine, fluconazole, H2 antagonists, magnesium salts, methyldopa, MAO inhibitors, probenecid, salicylates, TCAs, sulfonamides. The hypoglycemic effect may be reduced by: beta blockers, cholestyramine, diazoxide, phenytoin, rifampin, thiazide diuretics.

Theoretic Infant Dose:

Relative Infant Dose:

Adult Dose: 15-40 mg daily

Alternatives:

T½ =	1.1-3.7 hours	M/P =	
PHL =		PB =	92-99 %
T$_{max}$ =	6-12 hours (XL)	Oral =	80-100%
MW =	446	pKa =	
Vd =			

References:
1.   Pharmaceutical Manufacturer Prescribing Information.

GLUCOSAMINE
Trade: Glucosamine
Can/Aus/UK:
Uses: Antiarthritic
LRC: L3
AAP: Not reviewed

Glucosamine is an endogenous aminomonosaccharide that has been reported effective in resolving symptoms of osteoarthritis. Administered in large doses, most is sequestered in the liver with only minimal amounts reaching other tissues, thus oral bioavailability is low. Most of the oral dose is hepatically metabolized and subsequently incorporated into other plasma proteins.[1]   No data are available on transfer into human milk. Because glucosamine is primarily sequestered and metabolized in the liver, and because the plasma levels are almost undetectable, it is unlikely that much would enter human milk. Further, the fact it is so poorly bioavailable, it is unlikely that an infant would receive clinically relevant amounts.

Pregnancy Risk Category:

Lactation Risk Category: L3

Adult Concerns: Minimal but include nausea, dyspepsia, vomiting, drowsiness, headache, and skin rash. Peripheral edema and tachycardia have been reported.

Pediatric Concerns: None reported via milk.

Drug Interactions:

Theoretic Infant Dose:

Relative Infant Dose:

Adult Dose:

Alternatives:

T½ =	0.3 hours	M/P =	
PHL =		PB =	0%
T$_{max}$ =		Oral =	< 26%
MW =	179	pKa =	
Vd =	0.035		

References:
1. Setnikar I, Palumbo R, Canali S, Zanolo G. Pharmacokinetics of glucosamine in man. Arzneimittelforschung 1993; 43(10):1109-1113.

GLYBURIDE
Trade: Micronase, Diabeta, Glynase, Glucovance
Can/Aus/UK: Diabeta, Euglucon, Gen-Glybe, Diaformin, Daonil
Uses: Hypoglycemic, antidiabetic agent
LRC: L3
AAP: Not reviewed

Glyburide is a "second generation" sulfonylurea agent useful in the treatment of non insulin-dependent (Type II) diabetes mellitus. It belongs to the sulfonylurea family (tolbutamide, glipizide) of hypoglycemic agents of which glyburide is one of the most potent.[1,2] Glyburide apparently stimulates insulin secretion, thus reducing plasma glucose. Although no data exist on the secretion of glyburide into breastmilk, others in this family are secreted in low levels, and it is likely that this product may attain even lower levels than the first generation family. Glyburide apparently does not even cross the placenta. Although we do not have reports of breastmilk levels, it is likely (theoretical) that breastmilk levels will be very low as well. The product Glucovance contains metformin and glyburide.

Pregnancy Risk Category: B

Lactation Risk Category: L3

Adult Concerns: Hypoglycemia, headache, anorexia, nausea, heartburn, allergic skin rashes

Pediatric Concerns: None reported but observe for hypoglycemia, weakness.

Drug Interactions: Thiazide diuretics and beta blockers may decrease efficacy of glyburide. Increased toxicity may result from use with phenylbutazone, oral anticoagulants, hydantoins, salicylates, NSAIDS, sulfonamides. Alcohol increases disulfiram effect.

Theoretic Infant Dose:

Relative Infant Dose:

Adult Dose: 1.25-20 mg daily

Alternatives:

T½ =	4-13.7 hours	M/P =	
PHL =		PB =	99%
T$_{max}$ =	2-3 hours	Oral =	Complete
MW =	494	pKa =	
Vd =	0.73		

References:
1. Pharmaceutical Manufacturer Prescribing Information.
2. McEvoy GE. (ed):AFHS Drug Information. New York, NY: 2003.

GLYCOPYRROLATE
Trade: Robinul
Can/Aus/UK: Robinul
Uses: Anticholinergic
LRC: L3
AAP: Not reviewed

Glycopyrrolate is a quaternary ammonium anticholinergic used prior to surgery to dry secretions.   After administration, its plasma half-life is exceedingly short (< 5 minutes) with most of the product being distribution out of the plasma compartment rapidly.[1,2]   No data are available on its transfer into human milk, but due to its short plasma half-life and its quaternary structure, it is very unlikely that significant quantities would penetrate milk. Further, along with the poor oral bioavailability of this product, it is very remote that glycopyrrolate would pose a significant risk to a breastfeeding infant.

Pregnancy Risk Category: B

Lactation Risk Category: L3

Adult Concerns: Blurred vision, dry mouth, tachycardia

Pediatric Concerns: None reported via milk.

Drug Interactions: May reduce effect of levodopa. Increased toxicity when used with amantadine and cyclopropane.

Theoretic Infant Dose:

Relative Infant Dose:

Adult Dose: 1-2 mg TID

Alternatives:

T½ =	1.7 hours	M/P =		
PHL =		PB =		
T~max~ =	5 hours(oral)	Oral =	10-25%	
MW =	398	pKa =		
Vd =	0.64			

References:
1. Lacy C. Drug information handbook. Lexi-Comp Inc. Cleveland, OH, 1996.
2. Drug Facts and Comparisons 1996 ed. ed. St. Louis: 1996.

GOLD COMPOUNDS

Trade: Ridura, Myochrysine, Solganal
Can/Aus/UK: Myochrysine, Ridaura, Myocrisin
Uses: Antiarthritic
LRC: L5
AAP: Maternal Medication Usually Compatible with Breastfeeding

Gold salts antiinflammatory agents used to treat rheumatoid arthritis. Gold Salts are potent and toxic   Two injectable forms exist--gold sodium thiomalate (Myochrysine) and sodium aurothioglucose (Solganal). One oral form exists, auranofin (Ridura).   The plasma kinetics of the gold salts are highly variable and are difficult to report but in general, their half-lives are very extended and increase as duration of treatment continues. Auranofin is the only orally available salt form and is approximately 20-25% bioavailable.   They are all probably secreted into breastmilk in small quantities.

In a study by Blau [1], milk levels of gold following a cumulative dose of 135 mg ranged from 0.86-0.99 mg/100mL. These are quite high and exceed the data of others.

In one study of a patient receiving Myochrysine, 50 mg/week for 7 weeks, the concentration of gold sodium thiomalate varied from 0.022 to 0.04 mg/L at 66 hours and 7 days post-dose respectively[2]. Although the infant showed no signs or symptoms of toxicity at this time, the authors noted that 3 months after treatment the infant developed transient facial edema of unexplained origin.

Approximately 10% or more of the concentration of gold measured in maternal serum appears in breastmilk. In two patients treated with 50 mg aurothiomalate, levels in milk varied from 27-153 μg/L.[3]   Gold is retained in the human body for long periods of time (months).   For this reason prolonged exposure of a nursing infant may not be justified.

Pregnancy Risk Category: C

Lactation Risk Category: L5

Adult Concerns: GI distress, diarrhea, nausea, vomiting, exfoliative dermatitis, nephrotoxicity, proteinuria, and blood dyscrasias

Pediatric Concerns: Possible facial edema 3 months after therapy. Relationship is questionable.

Drug Interactions: Decreased gold effects with penicillamine and acetylcysteine.

Theoretic Infant Dose: 22.95 µg/kg/day

Relative Infant Dose: 3.2%

Adult Dose: 25-50 mg/week

Alternatives:

T½ =	3-26 days	M/P =	0.02-0.3
PHL =		PB =	95%
T$_{max}$ =	3-6 hours (IM)	Oral =	20-25%(auranofin
MW =		pKa =	
Vd =	0.1		

References:
1. Blau SP. Letter: Metabolism of gold during lactation. Arthritis Rheum 1973; 16(6):777-778.
2. Bell RA, Dale IM. Gold secretion in maternal milk. Arthritis Rheum 1976; 19(6):1374.
3. Ostensen M, Skavdal K, Myklebust G, Tomassen Y, Aarbakke J. Excretion of gold into human breastmilk. Eur J Clin Pharmacol 1986; 31(2):251-252.

GONADORELIN ACETATE

Trade: Lutrepulse
Can/Aus/UK: Lutrepulse, Wyerth-Ayerst HRF, Fertiral
Uses: Gonadotropin-releasing hormone
LRC: L3
AAP: Not reviewed

Gonadorelin is used for the induction of ovulation in anovulatory women with primary hypothalamic amenorrhea. Gonadorelin is a small decapeptide identical to the physiologic GnRH secreted by the hypothalamus which stimulates the pituitary release of luteinizing hormone (LH) and to a lesser degree follicle stimulating hormone (FSH). LH and FSH subsequently stimulate the ovary to produce follicles.

Gonadorelin plasma half-life is very brief (< 2-4 minutes), and it is primarily distributed to the plasma only.[1] Gonadorelin has been detected in human breastmilk at concentrations of 0.1 to 3 nanograms/mL (adult dose = 20-100 micrograms) although its oral bioavailability in the infant would be minimal to none.[2]

Pregnancy Risk Category: B

Lactation Risk Category: L3

Adult Concerns: Ovarian hyperstimulation, bronchospasm, tachycardia, flushing, urticaria, induration at injection site

Pediatric Concerns: None reported via milk.

Drug Interactions:

Theoretic Infant Dose: 0.45 µg/kg/day

Relative Infant Dose: 32.1%

Adult Dose: 1-20 µg daily

Alternatives:

T½ =	2-4 minutes	M/P =	
PHL =		PB =	
T$_{max}$ =		Oral =	None
MW =		pKa =	
Vd =	0.14		

References:
1. Reynolds JEF. (Ed): Martindale: The Extra Pharmacopoeia (electronic version). Denver, CO: Micromedex, Inc., 1990.
2. Drug Facts and Comparisons 1996 ed. ed. St. Louis: 1996.

GOSERELIN ACETATE IMPLANT
Trade: Zoladex
Can/Aus/UK:
Uses: Inhibitor of luteinizing hormone
LRC: L3
AAP: Not reviewed

Goserelin is a synthetic decapeptide analogue of luteinizing hormone releasing factor and it acts as a potent inhibitor of pituitary gonadotropin secretion. Following initial administration in males, goserelin causes an initial increase in serum luteinizing hormone (LH) and follicle stimulating hormone (FSH) levels.[1] Chronic administration of goserelin leads to sustained suppression of pituitary gonadotropins, and serum levels testosterone in males. In females, a down-regulation of the pituitary gland following chronic exposure leads to suppression of gonadotropin secretion, a decrease in serum estradiol to levels consistent with the menopausal state. Serum LH and FSH are suppressed to follicular phase levels within four weeks. No data are available on its transfer into human milk but due to its structure and molecular weight it is very unlikely to enter milk, or to be orally bioavailable in the infant.

Pregnancy Risk Category: X

Lactation Risk Category: L3

Adult Concerns: Adverse events include hot flashes, sexual dysfunction, vaginitis, emotional lability, headache, abdominal pain, pelvic pain, depression, sweating, breast atrophy, edema, etc.

Pediatric Concerns: None reported via milk. While it is unlikely this peptide would enter milk, or be orally bioavailable to an infant, it is not known how it would affect milk production. Some caution is recommended concerning loss of milk supply.

Drug Interactions: None studied.

Theoretic Infant Dose:

Relative Infant Dose:

Adult Dose: 3.6 mg subcutaneously every 28 days

Alternatives:

$T\frac{1}{2}$ =	2.3 hours	M/P =	
PHL =		PB =	Low
T_{max} =	12-15 days	Oral =	Nil
MW =	1269	pKa =	
Vd =	0.28 (females)		

References:
1. Pharmaceutical Manufacturers prescribing information, 2003.

GRANISETRON

Trade: Kytril
Can/Aus/UK:
Uses: Antiemetic
LRC: L3
AAP: Not reviewed

Granisetron is an antinauseant and antiemetic agent commonly used with chemotherapy. Following a 1 mg IV dose, the peak plasma concentration was only 3.63 ng/mL.[1] No data are available on its transfer into human milk but its levels are likely to be low. Further, this family of products (see ondansetron) are not highly toxic and are commonly used in children (2 years +). It is unlikely that this product will be overtly toxic to a breastfed infant. However, when used with chemotherapeutic agents, long waiting periods should be used for elimination of the chemotherapeutic agents anyway.

Pregnancy Risk Category: B

Lactation Risk Category: L3

Adult Concerns: Headache, asthenia, somnolence, diarrhea, dyspepsia, abdominal pain, constipation, and fever. Rarely elevations of liver enzymes been reported.

Pediatric Concerns: None reported via milk.

Drug Interactions: Ketoconazole may inhibit the metabolism of granisetron.

Theoretic Infant Dose:

Relative Infant Dose:

Adult Dose: 2 mg Orally

Alternatives: Ondansetron

$T\frac{1}{2}$ =	3-14 hours	M/P =	
PHL =		PB =	65%
T_{max} =	1 hour	Oral =	60%
MW =	312	pKa =	
Vd =	2-4		

References:
1. Pharmaceutical Manufacturer Prescribing Information. 2002

GREPAFLOXACIN
Trade: Raxar
Can/Aus/UK: Raxar
Uses: Fluoroquinolone antibiotic
LRC: L4
AAP: Not reviewed

Grepafloxacin is a typical fluoroquinolones antibiotic similar to Ciprofloxacin. The manufacturer suggests that grepafloxacin is detectable in human milk after a 400 mg dose but does not provide the exact levels.[1] Studies in rodents suggest a concentrating mechanism of about 16 times that of the plasma compartment. Because this fluoroquinolone has a rather long half-life, high volume of distribution, the ability to enter many body compartments, and is concentrated in rodent milk, it is probably advisable to use this product with extreme caution, if at all, in breastfeeding women.

Pregnancy Risk Category: C

Lactation Risk Category: L4

Adult Concerns: Nausea, taste perversion, dizziness, headache, diarrhea, abdominal pain

Pediatric Concerns: None reported with this product, but diarrhea and pseudomembranous colitis has been reported with ciprofloxacin. Arthropathy has been reported following pediatric use of fluoroquinolones.

Drug Interactions: Decreased absorption with antacids. Quinolones cause increased levels of caffeine, warfarin, cyclosporine, theophylline. Cimetidine, probenecid, azlocillin increase ciprofloxacin levels. Increased risk of seizures when used with foscarnet.

Theoretic Infant Dose:

Relative Infant Dose:

Adult Dose: 400-600 mg daily

Alternatives: Norfloxacin, Ofloxacin, Levofloxacin, Ciprofloxacin

$T^{1/2}$ =	15.7 hours	M/P =		
PHL =		PB =	50%	
T_{max} =	2-3 hours	Oral =	72%	
MW =	422	pKa =		
Vd =	5.07			

References:
1. Pharmaceutical Manufacturer Prescribing Information. 1999.

GRISEOFULVIN

Trade: Fulvicin, Gris-Peg
Can/Aus/UK: Fulvicin, Grisovin-FP, Fulcin, Griseostatin
Uses: Antifungal
LRC: L2
AAP: Not reviewed

Griseofulvin is an older class antifungal. Much better safety profiles with the newer families of antifungals have reduced the use of griseofulvin. The drug is primarily effective against tinea species and not candida albicans.[1,2] There are no data available for humans. In one study in cows following a dose of 10mg/kg/day for 5 days (human dose => 5 mg/kg/day) milk concentrations were 0.16 mg/L. Although these data cannot be directly extrapolated to humans, they indicate transfer to milk in some species. Oral use in adults is associated with low risk of hepatic cancer. Griseofulvin is still commonly used in pediatric tinea capitis (ringworm), where it is a preferred medication.

Pregnancy Risk Category: C

Lactation Risk Category: L2

Adult Concerns: Headache, depression, hepatotoxicity, skin rashes, hallucinations. Symptoms of overdose include lethargy, vertigo, blurred vision, nausea, vomiting, and diarrhea.

Pediatric Concerns: None reported from breastmilk.

Drug Interactions: Barbiturates may reduce plasma levels. May inhibit warfarin activity. May reduce effectiveness of oral contraceptives. May produce increased toxicity and tachycardia when used with alcohol.

Theoretic Infant Dose:

Relative Infant Dose:

Adult Dose: 500-1000 mg daily (micro) or 330-375 mg daily (ultra)

Alternatives: Fluconazole

T½ =	9-24 hours	M/P =	
PHL =		PB =	
T$_{max}$ =	4-8 hours	Oral =	Poor to 50%
MW =	353	pKa =	
Vd =			

References:
1. McEvoy GE. (ed):AFHS Drug Information. New York, NY: 2003.
2. Huddleston WA. Antifungal activity of Penicillium griseofulvin mycelium. Vet Rec 1970; 86(3):75-76.

GUAIFENESIN

Trade: GG, Robitussin
Can/Aus/UK: Balminil, Resyl, Robitussin, Benylin-E, Orthoxicol, Respenyl
Uses: Expectorant, loosens respiratory tract secretions
LRC: L2
AAP: Not reviewed

Guaifenesin is an expectorant used to irritate the gastric mucosa and stimulate respiratory tract secretions in order to reduce phlegm viscosity. It does not suppress coughing and should not be used in persistent cough such as with smokers. No data are available on transfer into human breastmilk. In general, clinical studies documenting the efficacy of guaifenesin are lacking, and the usefulness of this product as an expectorant is highly questionable.[1] Poor efficacy of these drugs (expectorants in general) would suggest that they do not provide enough justification for use in lactating mothers. But untoward effects have not been reported. Pediatric dose: < 2 years = 12 mg/kg/day in 6 divided doses; 2-5 years = 50-100 mg every 4 hours; 6-11 years = 100-200 mg every 4 hours; Children > 12 years and adults = 200-400 mg every 4 hours for a maximum of 2.4 gm/day. Always dose with large volumes of fluids.

Pregnancy Risk Category: C

Lactation Risk Category: L2

Adult Concerns: Vomiting, diarrhea, nausea, sedation, skin rash, GI dyspepsia

Pediatric Concerns: None reported.

Drug Interactions:

Theoretic Infant Dose:

Relative Infant Dose:

Adult Dose: 200-400 mg q 4 hours

Alternatives:

T½ =	< 7 hours	M/P =	
PHL =		PB =	
T$_{max}$ =		Oral =	Complete
MW =	198	pKa =	
Vd =	1.0		

References:
1. Lacy C. Drug information handbook. Lexi-Comp Inc. Cleveland, OH, 1996.

GUANFACINE
Trade: Tenex
Can/Aus/UK:
Uses: Antihypertensive
LRC: L3
AAP: Not reviewed

Guanfacine is a centrally acting antihypertensive that stimulates alpha-2 adrenergic receptors (similar to Clonidine). Studies in animals indicate that guanfacine is secreted into milk (M:P ratio = 0.75), but human studies are lacking.[1,2] Because this product has a low molecular weight (246), a high volume of distribution 6.3 L/kg), and penetrates the CNS at high levels, it is likely to penetrate milk at significant levels. Caution is urged.

Pregnancy Risk Category: B

Lactation Risk Category: L3

Adult Concerns: Bradycardia, hypotension, dry mouth, sedation, weakness, constipation

Pediatric Concerns: None reported but observe for hypotension, sedation, weakness.

Drug Interactions: Decreased hypotensive effect when used with tricyclic antidepressants. Increased effect when used with other antihypertensive agents.

Theoretic Infant Dose:

Relative Infant Dose:

Adult Dose: 1 mg daily

Alternatives:

T½ =	17 hours	M/P =	
PHL =		PB =	20-30%
T_max =	2.6 hours	Oral =	81-100%
MW =	246	pKa =	
Vd =	6.3		

References:
1. Pharmaceutical Manufacturer Prescribing Information. 1995.
2. Lacy C. Drug information handbook. Lexi-Comp Inc. Cleveland, OH, 1996.

HAEMOPHILUS B CONJUGATE VACCINE

Trade: Hibtiter, Haemophilus B Vaccine, Prohibit, Omnihib
Can/Aus/UK: Act-HIB, PedvaxHIB, Hib Titer
Uses: H. influenza Vaccine
LRC: L3
AAP: Not reviewed

Hib Vaccine is a purified capsular polysaccharide vaccine made from haemophilus influenza bacteria. It is non-infective. It is currently recommended for initial immunizations in children at 2 months, and at 2 month intervals, for a total of 3 injections.[1] A booster is recommended at 12-15 months. Although there are no reasons for administering to adult mothers, it would not be contraindicated in breastfeeding mothers.

Pregnancy Risk Category: C

Lactation Risk Category: L3

Adult Concerns: Itching, skin rash, injection site reaction, vomiting, fever. Few anaphylactoid-type reaction.

Pediatric Concerns: Itching, skin rash, injection site reaction, vomiting, fever. Few anaphylactoid-type reaction.

Drug Interactions: Decreased immunogenicity when used with immunosuppressive agents. Immunoglobulins with 1 month may decrease antibody production.

Theoretic Infant Dose:

Relative Infant Dose:

Adult Dose:

Alternatives:

References:
1. Pharmaceutical Manufacturer Prescribing Information. 1996.

HALAZEPAM

Trade: Paxipam
Can/Aus/UK:
Uses: Benzodiazepine antianxiety drug
LRC: L3
AAP: Not reviewed

Halazepam is a benzodiazepine (Valium family) used to treat anxiety disorders. Halazepam is metabolized to desmethyldiazepam, which has an elimination half-life of 50-100 hours.[1] Although no information is available on halazepam levels in human milk, it should be similar to diazepam. See diazepam.

Pregnancy Risk Category: D

Lactation Risk Category: L3

Adult Concerns: Sedation, bradycardia, euphoria, disorientation, confusion, nausea, constipation, hypotension

Pediatric Concerns: None reported but see diazepam.

Drug Interactions:

Theoretic Infant Dose:

Relative Infant Dose:

Adult Dose: 20-40 mg TID-QID

Alternatives: Alprazolam, Lorazepam

$T\frac{1}{2}$ =	14 hours	M/P =	
PHL =		PB =	High
T_{max} =	1-3 hours	Oral =	Complete
MW =	353	pKa =	
Vd =	1.0		

References:
1. Pharmaceutical Manufacturer Prescribing Information. 1995.

HALOPERIDOL

Trade: Haldol
Can/Aus/UK: Apo-Haloperidol, Haldol, Novo-Peridol, Peridol, Serenace
Uses: Antipsychotic
LRC: L2
AAP: Drugs whose effect on nursing infants is unknown but may be of concern

Haloperidol is a potent antipsychotic agent that is reported to increase prolactin levels in some patients. In one study of a woman treated for puerperal hypomania and receiving 5 mg twice daily, the concentration of haloperidol in milk was 0.0, 23.5, 18.0, and 3.25 µg/L on day 1, 6, 7, and 21 respectively.[1] The corresponding maternal plasma levels were 0, 40, 26, and 4 µg/L at day 1, 6, 7, and 21 respectively. The milk/plasma ratios were 0.58, 0.69, and 0.81 on days 6, 7, and 21 respectively. After 4 weeks of therapy the infant showed no symptoms of sedation and was feeding well.

In another study after a mean daily dose of 29.2 mg, the concentration of haloperidol in breastmilk was 5 µg/L at 11 hours post-dose.[2] In a study of 3 women on chronic haloperidol therapy receiving 3, 4, and 6 mg daily, milk levels were reported to be 32, 17, and 4.7 ng/mL.[3] The latter levels(4.7) were taken from a patient believed to be noncompliant.

Bennett calculates the relative infant dose to be 0.2-2.1% to 9.6% of the weight-adjusted maternal daily dose.[4]

Pregnancy Risk Category: C

Lactation Risk Category: L2

Adult Concerns: Extrapyramidal symptoms, sedation, anemia, tachycardia, hypotension

Pediatric Concerns: None reported via milk. Observe for sedation, weakness.

Drug Interactions: Carbamazepine may increase metabolism and decrease effectiveness of haloperidol. CNS depressants may increase adverse effects. Epinephrine may cause hypotension. Concurrent use with lithium has caused acute encephalopathy syndromes.

Theoretic Infant Dose: 3.5 µg/kg/day

Relative Infant Dose: 2.4%

Adult Dose: 0.5-5 mg BID-TID

Alternatives:

T½ =	12-38 hours	M/P =	0.58-0.81
PHL =		PB =	92%
T$_{max}$ =	2-6 hours	Oral =	60%
MW =	376	pKa =	8.3
Vd =	18-30		

References:
1. Whalley LJ, Blain PG, Prime JK. Haloperidol secreted in breastmilk. Br Med J (Clin Res Ed) 1981; 282(6278):1746-1747.
2. Stewart RB, Karas B, Springer PK. Haloperidol excretion in human milk. Am J Psychiatry 1980; 137(7):849-850.
3. Ohkubo T, Shimoyama R, Sugawara K. Measurement of haloperidol in human breastmilk by high-performance liquid chromatography. J Pharm Sci 1992; 81(9):947-949.
4. Bennett PN. Use of the monographs on drugs: In: Drugs and Human Lactation. Amsterdam, Elsevier, 1996.

HALOTHANE

Trade: Fluothane
Can/Aus/UK: Fluothane
Uses: Anesthetic gas
LRC: L2
AAP: Maternal Medication Usually Compatible with Breastfeeding

Halothane is an anesthetic gas similar to enflurane, methoxyflurane, and isoflurane. Approximately 60-80% is rapidly eliminated by exhalation the first 24 hours postoperative, and only 15% is actually metabolized by the liver. Cote (1976) reviewed the secretion of halothane in breastmilk.[1] After a 3 hour surgery, only 2 ppm was detected in milk. At another exposure in one week only 0.83 and 1.9 ppm were found. The authors assessed the exposure to the infant as negligible.

Halothane is probably stored in the adipose tissue and eliminated for several days. There is no available information on the oral bioavailability of halothane. Pumping and dumping milk the first 24 hours postoperatively is generally recommended but is probably unnecessary.

Pregnancy Risk Category: C

Lactation Risk Category: L2

Adult Concerns: Nausea, vomiting, sedation, transient hepatotoxicity

Pediatric Concerns: None reported.

Drug Interactions: When used with rifampin, or phenytoin, may have increased risk of hepatotoxicity.

Theoretic Infant Dose:

Relative Infant Dose:

Adult Dose:

Alternatives:

T½ =		M/P =	
PHL =		PB =	
T$_{max}$ =	10-20 minutes	Oral =	
MW =	197	pKa =	
Vd =	1		

References:
1. Cote CJ, Kenepp NB, Reed SB, Strobel GE. Trace concentrations of halothane in human breastmilk. Br J Anaesth 1976; 48(6):541-543.

HCTZ PLUS TRIAMTERENE
Trade: Dyrenium, Maxzide
Can/Aus/UK: Dyazide, Novo-Triamzide, Dyazide, Hydrene
Uses: Diuretic
LRC: L3
AAP: Not reviewed

Numerous diuretic products contain varying combinations of hydrochlorothiazide (HCTZ) and triamterene. For specifics on HCTZ, see the monograph on hydrochlorothiazide. Triamterene is a potassium sparing diuretic. Following a dose of 100-200 mg, it attains plasma levels in adults of 26-30 μg/L.[1] It is secreted in small amounts in cow's milk but no human data are available. Assuming a high milk/plasma ratio of one, an infant ingesting 125 mL/kg/day would theoretically ingest less than 4 μg/kg/day, an amount unlikely to provide clinical problems.

Pregnancy Risk Category: B

Lactation Risk Category: L3

Adult Concerns: Diarrhea, nausea, vomiting, hepatitis, leukopenia, hyperkalemia

Pediatric Concerns: None reported. Hyperkalemia.

Drug Interactions: Increased risk of hyperkalemia when given with amiloride, spironolactone, and ACE inhibitors. Increased risk of toxicity with amantadine.

Theoretic Infant Dose: 4.5 μg/kg/day

Relative Infant Dose: 0.15%

Adult Dose: 25-50 mg HCTZ (37.5-75 mg Triamterene) daily

Alternatives:

T½ =	1.5-2.5 hours	M/P =	
PHL =		PB =	55%
Tmax =	1.5-3 hours	Oral =	30-70%
MW =	253	pKa =	6.2
Vd =			

References:
1. Pharmaceutical Manufacturer Prescribing Information.

HEPARIN
Trade: Heparin
Can/Aus/UK: Hepalean, Canusal, Heplok, Pularin
Uses: Anticoagulant
LRC: L1
AAP: Not reviewed

Heparin is a large protein molecule.[1] It is used SC, IM, and IV because it is not absorbed orally in mother or infant.   Due to its high molecular weight (40,000 Daltons), it is unlikely any would   transfer into breastmilk. Any that did enter the milk would be rapidly destroyed in the gastric contents of the infant.

Pregnancy Risk Category: C

Lactation Risk Category: L1

Adult Concerns: Hemorrhage

Pediatric Concerns: None reported via milk.

Drug Interactions: Increased toxicity with NSAIDS, aspirin, dipyridamole, hydroxychloroquine.

Theoretic Infant Dose:

Relative Infant Dose:

Adult Dose: 4,000-5,000 units q 4 hours

Alternatives:

T½ =	1-2 hours	M/P =	
PHL =		PB =	
Tmax =	20 minutes	Oral =	None
MW =	30000	pKa =	
Vd =			

References:
1. McEvoy GE. (ed):AFHS Drug Information. New York, NY: 2003.

HEPATITIS B INFECTION

Trade: Hepatitis B Infection
Can/Aus/UK:
Uses: Hepatitis B exposure
LRC:
AAP: Not reviewed

Hepatitis B virus (HBV) causes a wide spectrum of infections, ranging from a mild asymptomatic form to a fulminant fatal hepatitis. Mild asymptomatic illness is most common in pediatric patients although the chronic infectious state occurs in as many as 90% of infants who become infected by perinatal transmission. Chronically infected individuals are at increased risk for chronic liver diseases and liver cancer in later life. HBV is transmitted through blood or body fluids. Hepatitis B antigen has been detected in breastmilk.[1-3]

Infants of mothers who are HBV positive (HBsAg) should be given Hepatitis immune globulin (HBIG) (preferably within 1 hour of birth) and a Hepatitis B vaccination AT BIRTH, which is believed to effectively reduce the risk of post-natal transmission, particularly via breastmilk.[4] Inject in different sites. Thus far, several older studies have indicated that breastfeeding poses no additional risk of transmission, and thus far no cases of horizontal transmission of Hepatitis B via breastmilk have been reported following immunization.

Pregnancy Risk Category:

Lactation Risk Category:

Adult Concerns: Hepatitis, increased risk of liver cancer

Pediatric Concerns: None reported if immunized with HBIG and HB vaccination.

Drug Interactions:

Theoretic Infant Dose:

Relative Infant Dose:

Adult Dose:

Alternatives:

References:

1. Boxall EH, Flewett TH, Dane DS, Cameron CH, MacCallum FO, Lee TW. Letter: Hepatitis-B surface antigen in breastmilk. Lancet 1974; 2(7887):1007-1008.
2. Beasley RP, Stevens CE, Shiao IS, Meng HC. Evidence against breast-feeding as a mechanism for vertical transmission of hepatitis B. Lancet 1975; 2(7938):740-741.

3. Woo D, Cummins M, Davies PA, Harvey DR, Hurley R, Waterson AP. Vertical transmission of hepatitis B surface antigen in carrier mothers in two west London hospitals. Arch Dis Child 1979; 54(9):670-675.
4. American Academy of Pediatrics. Committee on Infectious Diseases. Red Book. 1994.

HEPATITIS A INFECTION

Trade:
Can/Aus/UK:
Uses: Hepatitis A infection
LRC:
AAP: Compatible with Breastfeeding

Hepatitis A is an acute viral infection characterized by jaundice, fever, anorexia, and malaise. In infants, the syndrome is either asymptomatic or causes only mild nonspecific symptoms.[1] Current therapy recommended following exposure to Hepatitis A is an injection of gamma globulin. A majority of the population is immune to Hepatitis A due to prior exposure. Fulminant hepatitis A infection is rare in children and a carrier state is unknown. It is spread through fecal-oral contact and can be spread in day care centers. Viral shedding continues from onset up to 3 weeks. Unless the mother is jaundiced and acutely ill, breastfeeding can continue without interruption.[2] Proper hygiene should be stressed. Protect infant with IM gamma globulin.

Pregnancy Risk Category:

Lactation Risk Category:

Adult Concerns: Jaundice, fever, malaise

Pediatric Concerns: None reported. Protect with gamma globulin injection.

References:
1. American Academy of Pediatrics. Committee on Infectious Diseases. Red Book. 1997.
2. Gartner L. Personal communication. 1997.

HEPATITIS A VACCINE

Trade: Havrix
Can/Aus/UK: Havrix, Vaqta
Uses: Vaccine
LRC: L2
AAP: Not reviewed

Hepatitis A vaccine is an inactivated, noninfectious viral vaccination for Hepatitis A. Although there are no specific data on the use of Hepatitis A vaccine in breastfeeding women, Hepatitis A vaccine can be used in pregnant women after 14 weeks and in children 2 years of age.[1,2] There is little likelihood that Hepatitis A vaccinations in breastfeeding women would cause untoward effects in breastfed infants.

Pregnancy Risk Category: C

Lactation Risk Category: L2

Adult Concerns: Lymphadenopathy. Headache, insomnia, vertigo, fatigue and malaise, fever, anorexia and nausea, photophobia, injection-site soreness.

Pediatric Concerns: None reported via milk.

Drug Interactions:

Theoretic Infant Dose:

Relative Infant Dose:

Adult Dose: 1 mL X 2 over 6-12 months

Alternatives:

References:
1. Drug Facts and Comparisons 1997 ed. ed. St. Louis: 1997.
2. Pharmaceutical Manufacturer Prescribing Information. 1997.

HEPATITIS B IMMUNE GLOBULIN

Trade: H-Big, Hep-B-Gammagee, Hyperhep
Can/Aus/UK:
Uses: Anti-Hepatitis B Immune globulins
LRC: L2
AAP:

HBIG is a sterile solution of immunoglobulin (10-18% protein) containing a high titer of antibody to hepatitis B surface antigen.[1] It is most commonly used as prophylaxis therapy for infants born to hepatitis B surface antigen positive mothers. The carrier state can be prevented in about 75% of such infections in newborns given HBIG immediately after birth. HBIG is generally administered to infants from HBsAg positive mothers who wish to breastfeed. The prophylactic dose for newborns is 0.5 mL IM (thigh) as soon after birth as possible, preferably within 1 hour.[2] The infant should also be immunized with Hepatitis B vaccine (0.5 mL IM) within 12 hours of birth (use separate site), and again at 1 and 6 months.

Pregnancy Risk Category: C

Lactation Risk Category: L2

Adult Concerns: Pain at injection site, erythema, rash, dizziness, malaise

Pediatric Concerns: Pain at injection site, erythema, rash.

Drug Interactions:

Theoretic Infant Dose:

Relative Infant Dose:

Adult Dose: 0.06 mL/kg post-exposure X 3 over 6 weeks

Alternatives:

T½ =		M/P =	
PHL =		PB =	
Tmax =	1-6 days	Oral =	None
MW =		pKa =	
Vd =			

References:
1.   Pharmaceutical Manufacturer Prescribing Information. 1995.
2.   Lawrence RA. Breastfeeding: A guide for the medical profession. St. Louis: Mosby Publishers, 1994.

HEPATITIS B VACCINE
Trade: Heptavax-B, Energix-B, Recombivax Hb
Can/Aus/UK:
Uses: Hepatitis B vaccination
LRC: L2
AAP: Not reviewed

Hepatitis B vaccine is an inactivated non-infectious hepatitis B surface antigen vaccine. It can be used in pediatric patients at birth. No data are available on its use in breastfeeding mothers, but it is unlikely to produce untoward effects on a breastfeeding infant. Hepatitis B vaccination is approximately 80-95% effective in preventing acute hepatitis B infections.[1,2] It requires at least 3 immunizations and the immunity lasts about 5-7 years. In infants born of HB surface antigen positive mothers, the American Academy of Pediatrics recommends hepatitis B vaccine (along with HBIG) should be administered to the infant within 1-12 hours of birth (0.5 mL IM) and again at 1 and 6 months. If so administered, breastfeeding poses no additional risk for acquisition of HBV by the infant.

Pregnancy Risk Category: C

Lactation Risk Category: L2

Adult Concerns: Pain at injection site, swelling, erythema, fever

Pediatric Concerns: Fever, malaise, fatigue when directly injected. None reported via breastmilk.

Drug Interactions: Immunosuppressive agents would decrease effect.

Theoretic Infant Dose:

Relative Infant Dose:

Adult Dose: 20 μg each for three injections over 7 months

Alternatives:

References:
1.   Pharmaceutical Manufacturer Prescribing Information. 1996.
2.   American Academy of Pediatrics. Committee on Infectious Diseases. Red Book. 1997.

HEPATITIS C INFECTION
Trade: Hepatitis C Infection
Can/Aus/UK:
Uses: Hepatitis exposure
LRC: L2
AAP: Not reviewed

Hepatitis C (HCV) is characterized by a mild or asymptomatic infection with jaundice and malaise. On average, 50% of patients develop chronic liver disease, including cirrhosis, and liver cancer in later life.   HCV infection can be spread by blood-blood transmission although most are not associated with blood transfusions and may be transmitted by other unknown methods.

Although perinatal transmission can occur, its incidence is known to be very low[2].   The average incubation period is 7-9 weeks.   Mothers infected with HCV should be advised that transmission of HCV by breastfeeding is possible but has not been documented.   In one study, while transmission of HCV was significantly high (21%) in HIV infected individuals, perinatal transmission was not associated with breastfeeding.[1]

It is not known with certainty if the virus is shed in breastmilk although several studies so suggest. In one study of 17 HCV positive mothers, 11 of the 17 had HCV antibody present in milk, but zero of 17 had HCV-RNA in milk after birth, suggesting that the virus itself was not detected in milk.[3] Although it is possible that during episodes of direct exposure to blood such as from bleeding nipples or following initial infection and viremia that transmission could occur, this does not appear to be certain at this time.

Currently a number of other studies have yet to document vertical transmission of HCV by breastmilk.[4-5] Available data seem to suggest an elevated risk of vertical transmission to the infant occurs in HIV infected women and women with elevated titers of HCV RNA. The risk of transmission of HCV via breastmilk is unknown at this time. HCV-infected women should be counseled that transmission of HCV by breastfeeding is theoretically possible but has not yet been documented.[6,7] The Center for Disease Control (CDC) does not consider chronic hepatitis C infection in the mother as a contraindication to breastfeeding. The decision to breastfeed should be based largely on informed discussion between the mother and her health care provider.

Pregnancy Risk Category:

Lactation Risk Category: L2

References:

1. Paccagnini S, Principi N, Massironi E, Tanzi E, Romano L, Muggiasca ML, Ragni MC, Salvaggio L. Perinatal transmission and manifestation of hepatitis C virus infection in a high risk population. Pediatr Infect Dis J 1995; 14(3):195-199.
2. Nagata I, Shiraki K. et.al. Mother to infant transmission of hepatitis C virus. J Pediatrics 1992; 120:432-434.
3. Grayson ML, Braniff KM, Bowden DS, Turnidge JD. Breastfeeding and the risk of vertical transmission of hepatitis C virus. Med J Aust 1995; 163(2):107.
4. Lin HH, Kao JH, Hsu HY, Ni YH, Chang MH, Huang SC, Hwang LH, Chen PJ, Chen DS. Absence of infection in breast-fed infants born to hepatitis C virus-infected mothers. J Pediatr 1995; 126(4):589-591.
5. Zanetti. et.al. Mother to infant transmission of hepatitis C virus. Lancet 1995; 345(8945):289-291.
6. American Academy of Pediatrics. Committee on Infectious Diseases. Red Book. 1997.
7. Lawrence RA. Breastfeeding: A guide for the medical profession. St. Louis: Mosby Publishers, 1994.

HERBAL TEAS

Trade: Herbal Teas
Can/Aus/UK:
Uses: Herbal teas, tablets, powders, antioxidants.
LRC:
AAP: Not reviewed

Herbal teas should be used with great caution, if at all. A number of reports in the literature indicate potential toxicity in pregnant women from some herbal teas which contain pyrrolizidine alkaloids (PA).[1,2] Such alkaloids have been associated with feticide, birth defects, and liver toxicity.

Other reports of severe hepatotoxicity requiring liver transplant have occurred with an herbal antioxidant called "Chaparral".[3] A Chinese herbal product called "Jin Bu Huan" has been implicated in clinically recognized hepatitis in 7 patients.[3] Other hepatotoxic remedies include germander, comfrey, mistletoe and skullcap, margosa oil, mate tea, Gordolobo yerba tea, and pennyroyal (squawmint) oil.[4-5] A recent report of seven poisonings with anticholinergic symptoms following ingestion of "Paraguay Tea" was published and was an apparent adulteration.[6] A recent report on Blue Cohosh suggests it may be cardiotoxic when used late in pregnancy (see blue cohosh).[7,8]

Because exact ingredients are seldom listed on many teas, this author strongly suggests that lactating mothers limit exposure to these substances as much as possible. Never consume herbal remedies of unknown composition. Remember, breastfeeding infants are much more susceptible to such toxicants than are adults.

Pregnancy Risk Category:

Lactation Risk Category:

Adult Concerns: Severe toxicity including hepatotoxicity, anticholinergic poisoning, etc.

Pediatric Concerns: None reported via breastmilk but caution is recommended. Agents listed above would be contraindicated.

References:
1. Anonymous. Drug Therapy. J 1993; 16:64.
2. Ellenhorn MJ. Medical toxicology: a primer for the medicolegal age. Clin Toxicol 1978; 13(4):439-462.
3. Gordon DW, Rosenthal G, Hart J, Sirota R, Baker AL. Chaparral ingestion. The broadening spectrum of liver injury caused by herbal medications. JAMA 1995; 273(6):489-490.
4. Hsu CK, Leo P, Shastry D, Meggs W, Weisman R, Hoffman RS. Anticholinergic poisoning associated with herbal tea. Arch Intern Med 1995; 155(20):2245-2248.
5. Siegel RK. Herbal Intoxication. JAMA 1976; 236:473-477.

6. Rosti L, Nardini A, Bettinelli ME, Rosti D. Toxic effects of a herbal tea mixture in two newborns. Acta Paediatr 1994; 83(6):683.
7. Jones TK, Lawson BM. Profound neonatal congestive heart failure caused by maternal consumption of blue cohosh herbal medication. J Pediatr 1998;132:550-2.
8. Gunn TR, Wright IMR. The use of blue and black cohosh in labour. NZ Med J 1996;109:410-1.

HEROIN

Trade: Heroin
Can/Aus/UK:
Uses: Narcotic analgesic
LRC: L5
AAP: Contraindicated by the American Academy of Pediatrics in Breastfeeding Mothers

Heroin is diacetyl-morphine (diamorphine), a prodrug that is rapidly converted by plasma cholinesterases to 6-acetylmorphine and more slowly to morphine. With oral use, rapid and complete first-pass metabolism occurs in the liver. The half-life of diamorphine is only 3 minutes, with the large majority of the prodrug converted to morphine. Peak levels of morphine occur in about 30 minutes following oral doses. As an analgesic, morphine is generally considered to be an ideal choice for breastfeeding mothers when used postoperatively or for other forms of pain "in normal dosage ranges". Unfortunately, addicts and recreational users may use extraordinarily large doses of heroin, and at such doses, it is likely to be very dangerous for a breastfed infant. Heavily dependent users should probably be advised against breastfeeding and their infants converted to formula. While it could be argued that recreational users could continue to breastfeed if they avoid doing so while under the influence of the heroin or prior to its use, this still may not be advisable as it requires some understanding of the kinetics of morphine and its elimination. Heroin, as is morphine, is known to transfer into breastmilk.[1,2] See morphine for kinetics.

Pregnancy Risk Category: B

Lactation Risk Category: L5

Adult Concerns: Sedation, hypotension, euphoria, nausea, vomiting, dry mouth, respiratory depression, constipation

Pediatric Concerns: Caution, observe for sedation. Tremors, restlessness, vomiting, poor feeding.

Drug Interactions:

Theoretic Infant Dose:

Relative Infant Dose:

Adult Dose:

Alternatives:

T½ =	1.5-2 hours	M/P =	2.45
PHL =		PB =	35%
T$_{max}$ =	0.5-1 hours	Oral =	Poor
MW =	369	pKa =	7.6
Vd =	25		

References:
1. Feilberg VL, Rosenborg D, Broen CC, Mogensen JV. Excretion of morphine in human breastmilk. Acta Anaesthesiol Scand 1989; 33(5):426-428.
2. Wittels B, Scott DT, Sinatra RS. Exogenous opioids in human breastmilk and acute neonatal neurobehavior: a preliminary study. Anesthesiology 1990; 73(5):864-869.

HERPES SIMPLEX INFECTIONS
Trade:
Can/Aus/UK:
Uses: Herpes simplex type I, II
LRC:
AAP: Breastfeeding is acceptable if no lesions are on the breast or are adequately covered

HSV-1 and HSV-2 have been isolated from human milk, even in the absence of vesicular lesions or drainage.[1,2] Transmission after birth can occur and herpetic infections during the neonatal period are often severe and fatal.[3] Exposure to the virus from skin lesions of caregivers, including lesions of the breast, have been described. On average, however, perinatal infection is generally believed to occur during delivery rather than through breastmilk. Breastmilk does not appear to be a common mode of transmission although women with active lesions around the breast and nipple should refrain from breastfeeding until the lesions are adequately covered. Lesions directly on the nipple generally preclude breastfeeding. A number of cases of herpes simplex transmission via breastmilk have been reported.[4-5] Women with active lesions should be extremely meticulous in hand washing to prevent spread of the disease from other active lesions.

Pregnancy Risk Category:

Lactation Risk Category:

Adult Concerns: Skin eruptions, CNS changes, gingivostomatitis, skin lesions, fever

Pediatric Concerns: Transfer of virus to infants has been reported but may be from exposure to lesions. Cover lesions on breast.

Drug Interactions:

Theoretic Infant Dose:

Relative Infant Dose:

Adult Dose: N/A

References:
1. Light IJ. Postnatal acquisition of herpes simplex virus by the newborn infant: a review of the literature. Pediatrics 1979; 63(3):480-482.
2. Sullivan-Bolyai JZ, Fife KH, Jacobs RF, Miller Z, Corey L. Disseminated neonatal herpes simplex virus type 1 from a maternal breast lesion. Pediatrics 1983; 71(3):455-457.
3. Whitley RJ, Nahmias AJ, Visintine AM, Fleming CL, Alford CA. The natural history of herpes simplex virus infection of mother and newborn. Pediatrics 1980; 66(4):489-494.
4. Dunkle LM, Schmidt RR, O'Connor DM. Neonatal herpes simplex infection possibly acquired via maternal breastmilk. Pediatrics 1979; 63(2):250-251.
5. Quinn PT, Lofberg JV. Maternal herpetic breast infection: another hazard of neonatal herpes simplex. Med J Aust 1978; 2(9):411-412.

HEXACHLOROPHENE

Trade: Septisol, Phisohex, Septi-Soft
Can/Aus/UK: pHisoHex, Sapoderm, Dermalex
Uses: Antiseptic scrub
LRC: L4
AAP: Not reviewed

Hexachlorophene is an antibacterial that is an effective inhibitor of gram positive organisms.[1] It is generally used topically as a surgical scrub and sometimes vaginally in mothers. Due to its lipophilic structure, it is well absorbed through intact and denuded skin producing significant levels in plasma, brain, fat, and other tissues in both adults and infants. It has been implicated in causing brain lesions (spongiform myelinopathy), blindness, and respiratory failure in both animals and humans.[2] Although there are no studies reporting concentrations of this compound in breastmilk, it is probably transferred to some degree. Transfer into breastmilk is known to occur in rodents. Topical use in infants is absolutely discouraged due to the high absorption of hexachlorophene through an infant's skin and proven toxicity.

Pregnancy Risk Category: C

Lactation Risk Category: L4

Adult Concerns: Seizures, respiratory failure, hypotension, brain lesions, blindness in overdose

Pediatric Concerns: Following direct application, CNS injury, seizures, irritability have been reported in neonates. Toxicity via breastmilk has not been reported.

Drug Interactions:

Theoretic Infant Dose:

Relative Infant Dose:

Adult Dose:

Alternatives:

T½ =		M/P =	
PHL =	6.1-44.2 hours	PB =	
T$_{max}$ =		Oral =	Complete
MW =	407	pKa =	
Vd =			

References:
1. Pharmaceutical Manufacturer Prescribing Information. 1996.
2. Tyrala EE, Hillman LS, Hillman RE, Dodson WE. Clinical pharmacology of hexachlorophene in newborn infants. J Pediatr 1977; 91(3):481-486.

HIV INFECTION
Trade: Aids
Can/Aus/UK:
Uses: Aids, HIV infections
LRC: L5 in developed countries
AAP: Advise not to breastfeed

The AIDS (HIV) virus has been isolated from human milk. In addition, recent reports from throughout the world have documented the transmission of HIV through human milk.[1-3] At least 9 or more cases in the literature currently suggest that HIV-1 is secreted and can be transmitted horizontally to the infant via breastmilk. Although these studies clearly indicate a risk, currently no studies clearly show the exact risk associated with breastfeeding in HIV infected women. However, women who develop a primary HIV infection while breastfeeding may shed especially high concentrations of HIV viruses and pose a high risk of transmission to their infants. In some studies, the risk of transmission during primary infection was 29%. In various African populations, recent reports suggest the incremental risk of transmitting HIV via breastfeeding ranges from 3-12%.[6] Because the risk is now well documented, HIV infected mothers in the USA and others countries with safe alternative sources of feeding should be advised to not breastfeed their infants.[7] Mothers at-risk for HIV should be screened and counseled prior to initiating breastfeeding.

Pregnancy Risk Category:

Lactation Risk Category: L5 in developed countries

Adult Concerns:

Pediatric Concerns: HIV transmission has been documented.   HIV infected women are advised not to breastfeed.

References:

1. Commitee on Pediatric AIDS. Human milk, breastfeeding, and transmission of human immunodeficiency virus in the United States. Pediatrics 1995; 96:977-979.
2. Oxtoby MJ. Human immunodeficiency virus and other viruses in human milk: placing the issues in broader perspective. Pediatr Infect Dis J 1988; 7(12):825-835.
3. Goldfarb J. Breastfeeding. AIDS and other infectious diseases. Clin Perinatol 1993; 20(1):225-243.
4. Van de PP, Simonon A, Hitimana DG, Dabis F, Msellati P, Mukamabano B, Butera JB, Van Goethem C, Karita E, Lepage P. Infective and anti-infective properties of breastmilk from HIV-1-infected women. Lancet 1993; 341(8850):914-918.
5. Dunn DT, Newell ML, Ades AE, Peckham CS. Risk of human immunodeficiency virus type 1 transmission through breastfeeding. Lancet 1992; 340(8819):585-588.
6. St. Louis ME. et.al. The timing of HIV-1 transmission in an African setting. Presented at the First National Conference on Human Retroviruses and Related Infections. December 12-16; Washington DC. 1993.
7. Report of the committee on Infectious Diseases. American Academy of Pediatrics. 1994.

HYDRALAZINE

Trade: Apresoline
Can/Aus/UK: Apresoline, Novo-Hylazin, Apo-Hydralazine, Alphapress
Uses: Antihypertensive
LRC: L2
AAP: Maternal Medication Usually Compatible with Breastfeeding

Hydralazine is a popular antihypertensive used for severe pre-eclampsia and gestational and postpartum hypertension. In a study of one breastfeeding mother receiving 50 mg three times daily, the concentrations of hydralazine in breastmilk at 0.5 and 2 hours after administration was 762, and 792 nmol/L respectively.[1] The respective maternal serum levels were 1525 and 580 nmol/L at the aforementioned times. From these data, an infant consuming 1000 cc of milk would consume only 0.17 mg of hydralazine, an amount too small to be clinically relevant. The published pediatric dose for hydralazine is 0.75 to 1 mg/kg/day.

Pregnancy Risk Category: C

Lactation Risk Category: L2

Adult Concerns: Hypotension, tachycardia, renal failure, liver toxicity, paresthesias

Pediatric Concerns: None reported but observe for hypotension, sedation, weakness.

Drug Interactions: Increased effect with other antihypertensives, MAO inhibitors. Decreased effect when used with indomethacin.

Theoretic Infant Dose: 25.5 μg/kg/day

Relative Infant Dose: 1.19%

Adult Dose: 10-25 mg QID

Alternatives:

T½ =	1.5-8 hours	M/P =	0.49-1.36
PHL =		PB =	87%
T_{max} =	2 hours	Oral =	30-50%
MW =	160	pKa =	7.1
Vd =	1.6		

References:
1. Liedholm H, Wahlin-Boll E, Hanson A, Ingemarsson I, Melander A. Transplacental passage and breastmilk concentrations of hydralazine. Eur J Clin Pharmacol 1982; 21(5):417-419.

HYDROCHLOROTHIAZIDE

Trade: Hydrodiuril, Esidrix, Oretic
Can/Aus/UK: Apo-Hydro, Diuchlor H, Hydrodiuril, Novo-Hydrazide, Amizide, Dyazide, Modizide, Direma, Esidrex
Uses: Thiazide diuretic.
LRC: L2
AAP: Maternal Medication Usually Compatible with Breastfeeding

Hydrochlorothiazide (HCTZ) is a typical thiazide diuretic. In one study of a mother receiving a 50 mg dose each morning, milk levels were almost 25% of maternal plasma levels.[1] The dose ingested (assuming milk intake of 600 mL) would be approximately 50 μg/day, a clinically insignificant amount. The concentration of HCTZ in the infant's serum was undetectable(< 20 ng/mL). Some authors suggest that HCTZ can produce thrombocytopenia in nursing infant although this is remote and unsubstantiated. Thiazide diuretics could potentially reduce milk production by depleting maternal blood volume although it is seldom observed. Most thiazide diuretics are considered compatible with breastfeeding if doses are kept low.

Pregnancy Risk Category: D

Lactation Risk Category: **L2**

Adult Concerns: Fluid loss, hypotension. May reduce milk supply.

Pediatric Concerns: None reported via milk but may reduce milk supply in mother.

Drug Interactions: May increase hypoglycemia with antidiabetic drugs. May increase hypotension associated with other antihypertensives. May increase digoxin associated arrhythmias. May increase lithium levels.

Theoretic Infant Dose:

Relative Infant Dose:

Adult Dose: 25-100 mg daily

Alternatives:

T½ =	5.6-14.8 hours	M/P =	0.25
PHL =		PB =	58%
Tmax =	2 hours	Oral =	72%
MW =	297	pKa =	7.9, 9.2
Vd =	3		

References:
1. Miller ME, Cohn RD, Burghart PH. Hydrochlorothiazide disposition in a mother and her breast-fed infant. J Pediatr 1982; 101(5):789-791.

HYDROCODONE
Trade: Lortab, Vicodin
Can/Aus/UK: Hycodan, Robidone, Hycomine, Actron
Uses: Analgesic for pain
LRC: L3
AAP: Not reviewed

Hydrocodone is a narcotic analgesic and antitussive structurally related to codeine although somewhat more potent. It is commonly used in breastfeeding mothers throughout the USA. Most authors suggest that doses of 5 mg every 4 hours or more has a minimal effect on nursing infants, particularly older infants.[1-3] However, no data on hydrocodone levels in milk are available. To reduce exposure of the infant, attempt to feed infant prior to taking the medication. Neonates may be more sensitive to this product: observe for sedation or constipation. Lortab and Vicodin also contain acetaminophen.

Pregnancy Risk Category: **B**

Lactation Risk Category: **L3**

Adult Concerns: Sedation, dizziness, apnea, bradycardia, nausea, or constipation

Pediatric Concerns: None reported via milk but observe closely for sedation, apnea, constipation.

Drug Interactions: May reduce analgesia when used with phenothiazines. May increase toxicity associated with CNS depressants and tricyclic antidepressants.

Theoretic Infant Dose:

Relative Infant Dose:

Adult Dose: 5-10 mg q 4-6 hours

Alternatives: Codeine

$T\frac{1}{2}$ =	3.8 hours	M/P =	
PHL =		PB =	
T_{max} =	1.3 hours	Oral =	Complete
MW =	299	pKa =	8.9
Vd =	3.3-4.7		

References:
1. Horning MG. Identification and quantification of drugs and drug metabolites in human milk using GC-MS-COM methods. Mod Probl Pediatr 1975; 15:73-79.
2. Kwit NT, Hatcher RA. Excretion of drugs in milk. Am J Dis Child 1935; 49:900-904.
3. Anderson PO. Medication use while breast feeding a neonate. Neonatal Pharmacology Quarterly 1993; 2:3-12.

HYDROCORTISONE TOPICAL
Trade: Westcort
Can/Aus/UK: Cortate, Cortone, Emo-Cort, Aquacort, Dermaid, Egocort, Hycor, Cortef, Dermacort
Uses: Corticosteroid
LRC: L2
AAP: Not reviewed

Hydrocortisone is a typical corticosteroid with glucocorticoid and mineralocorticoid activity. When applied topically it suppresses inflammation and enhances healing. Initial onset of activity when applied topically is slow and may require several days for response. Absorption topically is dependent on placement; percutaneous absorption is 1% from the forearm, 2% from rectum, 4% from the scalp, 7% from the forehead, and 36% from the scrotal area.[1] The amount transferred into human milk has not been reported, but as with most steroids, is believed minimal. Topical application to the nipple is generally approved by most authorities if amounts applied and duration of use are minimized. Only small amounts should be applied and then only after feeding; larger quantities should be removed prior to breastfeeding. 0.5 to 1 % ointments, rather than creams, are generally preferred.

Pregnancy Risk Category: C

Lactation Risk Category: L2

Adult Concerns: Local irritation

Pediatric Concerns: None reported via milk.

Drug Interactions:

Theoretic Infant Dose:

Relative Infant Dose:

Adult Dose: Apply topical QID

Alternatives:

T½ =	1-2 hours	M/P =	
PHL =		PB =	90%
T$_{max}$ =		Oral =	96%
MW =	362	pKa =	
Vd =	0.48		

References:
1. Derendorf H, Mollmann H, Barth J, Mollmann C, Tunn S, Krieg M. Pharmacokinetics and oral bioavailability of hydrocortisone. J Clin Pharmacol 1991; 31(5):473-476.

HYDROMORPHONE

Trade: Dilaudid
Can/Aus/UK: Dilaudid, Hydromorph Contin, Palladone
Uses: Opiate analgesic
LRC: L3
AAP: Not reviewed

Hydromorphone is a potent semisynthetic narcotic analgesic used to alleviate moderate to severe pain. It is approximately 7-10 times more potent that morphine but is used in equivalently lower doses.[1] No data are available on its transfer into human milk, but it is likely quite low and similar to that of morphine.

Pregnancy Risk Category: C

Lactation Risk Category: L3

Adult Concerns: Dihydromorphone is highly addictive. Adverse effects include dizziness, sedation, agitation, hypotension, respiratory depression, nausea, and vomiting.

Pediatric Concerns: None reported via milk, but sedation is possible in infants whose mothers ingest higher doses at frequent intervals.

Drug Interactions:

Theoretic Infant Dose:

Relative Infant Dose:

Adult Dose: 2-10 mg q 3-6 hours PRN

Alternatives: Codeine, Hydrocodone

T½ =	2.5 hours	M/P =	
PHL =		PB =	
T$_{max}$ =		Oral =	51%
MW =		pKa =	
Vd =	2.9		

References:

1. Baselt RC. Disposition of toxic drugs and chemicals in man. Foster City, CA: Chemical Toxicology Institute, 2000: 426-427.

HYDROQUINONE

Trade: Esoterica, Eldoquin, Melpaque, Melanex, Solaquin, Nuquin, Viquin

Can/Aus/UK:

Uses: Depigmenting agent for topical applications

LRC: L3

AAP: Not reviewed

Hydroquinone is used for depigmentation of skin due to conditions such as freckles, melasma, senile lentigo, and inactive chloasma.[1] Hydroquinone is rapidly and extensively absorbed from the gut of animals. Absorption via the skin is slower but may be more rapid with vehicles such as alcohols. The transcutaneous absorption is reported to be about 35% which is relatively high for topical preparations. Hydroquinone distributes rapidly and widely and is metabolized to p-benzoquinone and other products. It is metabolized in the liver by conjugation to monoglucuronide, monosulfate, and mercapturic derivatives. The excretion of hydroquinone and its metabolites is rapid and occurs primarily via the urine. No data are available on its transfer into human milk. Although it is quite polar and water soluble, it also has a rather high pKa (9.96) which could lead to some trapping in human milk. While it does not seem to be very toxic, its chronic use in breastfeeding mothers is probably not warranted for such benign syndromes that could wait until the mother has weaned.

Pregnancy Risk Category: C

Lactation Risk Category: L3

Adult Concerns: Adverse effects include mild skin irritation and sensitivity, dryness, and fissuring of paranasal and infraorbital areas. Cases of intoxication and death have been reported from the oral ingestion of photographic developing agents. Dermal applications of hydroquinone at concentration levels below 3% in different bases caused negligible effects in male volunteers. However, there are case reports suggesting that skin lightening creams containing 2% hydroquinone have produced leucoderma as well as ochronosis.

Pediatric Concerns: No reports of its use in breastfeeding mothers. While not highly risky, its use in breastfeeding mothers may not be justified.

Drug Interactions: Combinations with corticosteroids may reduce skin irriatation.

Theoretic Infant Dose:

Relative Infant Dose:

Adult Dose: Apply 2-4% solutions twice daily. Limit areas treated.

Alternatives: Azelaic acid

References:
1. Pharmaceutical Manufacturers Package Insert, 2003.

HYDROXYCHLOROQUINE
Trade: Plaquenil
Can/Aus/UK: Plaquenil
Uses: Antimalarial, Antirheumatic, Lupus
LRC: L2
AAP: Maternal Medication Usually Compatible with Breastfeeding

Hydroxychloroquine (HCQ) is effective in the treatment of malaria but is also used in immune syndromes such as rheumatoid arthritis and Lupus erythematosus. HCQ is known to produce significant retinal damage and blindness if used over a prolonged period, and this could occur (theoretically) in breastfed infants. Patients on this product should see an ophthalmologist routinely. In one study of a mother receiving 400 mg HCQ daily, the concentrations of HCQ in breastmilk were 1.46, 1.09, and 1.09 mg/L at 2.0, 9.5, and 14 hours after the dose.[1] The average milk concentration was 1.1 mg/L. The milk/plasma ratio was approximately 5.5. On a body-weight basis, the infant's dose would be 2.9% of the maternal dose.

In a second study of one mother receiving 200 mg twice daily milk levels were much lower and than previous study. Only a total of 3.2 micrograms of HCQ was detected in her milk over 48 hours.[2] HCQ is mostly metabolized to chloroquine and has an incredibly long half-life. The pediatric dose for malaria prophylaxis is 5 mg/kg/week. See chloroquine.

Pregnancy Risk Category: C

Lactation Risk Category: L2

Adult Concerns: Blood dyscrasias, nausea, vomiting, diarrhea, retinopathy, rash, aplastic anemia, psychosis, porphyries, psoriasis, corneal deposits

Pediatric Concerns: None reported, but observe for retinal damage, blood dyscrasias.

Drug Interactions: Increased risk of blood dyscrasias when used with aurothioglucose. May increase serum digoxin levels.

Theoretic Infant Dose: 0.165

Relative Infant Dose: 2.89%

Adult Dose: 400 mg q week X 10 weeks

Alternatives:

T½ =	> 40 days	M/P =	5.5
PHL =		PB =	63%
T$_{max}$ =	1-2 hours	Oral =	74%
MW =	336	pKa =	
Vd =	580-815		

References:

1. Nation RL, Hackett LP, Dusci LJ, Ilett KF. Excretion of hydroxychloroquine in human milk. Br J Clin Pharmacol 1984; 17(3):368-369.
2. Ostensen M, Brown ND, Chiang PK, Aarbakke J. Hydroxychloroquine in human breastmilk. Eur J Clin Pharmacol 1985; 28(3):357.

HYDROXYUREA

Trade: Hydrea
Can/Aus/UK: Hydrea
Uses: Antineoplastic agent
LRC: L2
AAP: Not reviewed

Hydroxyurea is an antineoplastic agent used to treat melanoma, leukemias, and other neoplasms. It is well absorbed orally and rapidly metabolized to urea by the liver. In one study following a dose of 500 mg three times daily for 7 days, milk samples were collected two hours after the last dose.[1] The concentration of hydroxyurea in breastmilk averaged 6.1 mg/L (range 3.8 to 8.4 mg/L). Hydroxyurea is rapidly cleared from the plasma compartment and appears to leave no residuals or metabolites. Approximately 80% of the dose is excreted renally within 12 hours.

Pregnancy Risk Category: D

Lactation Risk Category: L2

Adult Concerns: Bone marrow suppression, drowsiness, convulsion, hallucinations, fever, nausea, vomiting, diarrhea, constipation.

Pediatric Concerns: None reported via milk, but extreme caution is recommended due to overt toxicity of this product.

Drug Interactions: May have increased toxicity and neurotoxicity when used with fluorouracil.

Theoretic Infant Dose: 0.915 mg/kg/day

Relative Infant Dose: 4.27%

Adult Dose: 80 mg/kg q 3 days

Alternatives:

T½ =	2-3 hours	M/P =	
PHL =		PB =	
T$_{max}$ =	2 hours	Oral =	Complete
MW =	76	pKa =	
Vd =			

References:
1. Sylvester RK, Lobell M, Teresi ME, Brundage D, Dubowy R. Excretion of hydroxyurea into milk. Cancer 1987; 60(9):2177-2178.

HYDROXYZINE

Trade: Atarax, Vistaril
Can/Aus/UK: Apo-Hydroxyzine, Atarax, Novo-Hydroxyzin
Uses: Antihistamine, antiemetic
LRC: L1
AAP: Not reviewed

Hydroxyzine is an antihistamine structurally similar to cyclizine and meclizine. It produces significant CNS depression, anticholinergic side effects (drying), and antiemetic side effects.[1] Hydroxyzine is largely metabolized to cetirizine (Zyrtec). No data are available on secretion into breastmilk.

Pregnancy Risk Category: C

Lactation Risk Category: L1

Adult Concerns: Sedation, hypotension, dry mouth

Pediatric Concerns: None reported via milk but observe for sedation, tachycardia, dry mouth.

Drug Interactions: May reduce epinephrine vasopressor response. Increased sedation when used with CNS depressants. Increased anticholinergic side effects when admixed with other anticholinergics.

Theoretic Infant Dose:

Relative Infant Dose:

Adult Dose: 50-100 mg QID

Alternatives: Cetirizine, Loratadine

T½ =	3-7 hours	M/P =	
PHL =	7.1 hours	PB =	
T$_{max}$ =	2 hours	Oral =	Complete
MW =	375	pKa =	2.1, 7.1
Vd =	13-31		

References:
1. Paton DM, Webster DR. Clinical pharmacokinetics of H1-receptor antagonists (the antihistamines). Clin Pharmacokinet 1985; 10(6):477-497.

HYLAN G-F 20

Trade: Synvisc
Can/Aus/UK:
Uses: Joint lubricant for arthritic pain.
LRC: L2
AAP: Not reviewed

Hylan G-F 20 (Synvisc) is a elastoviscous fluid containing hylan polymers produced from chicken combs. Hylans are a natural complex sugar of the glycosaminoglycan family.[1] Hylans are large molecular weight polymers and would not be expected to enter milk. Average molecular weight is 6 million daltons.

Pregnancy Risk Category:

Lactation Risk Category: L2

Adult Concerns: Knee pain or swelling, rash, itching, nausea, vomiting

Pediatric Concerns: None reported via milk. Probably too large to enter milk in clinically relevant amounts.

Drug Interactions:

Theoretic Infant Dose:

Relative Infant Dose:

Adult Dose:

Alternatives:

T½ =		M/P =	
PHL =		PB =	
T$_{max}$ =		Oral =	None
MW =	6 mil	pKa =	
Vd =			

References:
1. Pharmaceutical Manufacturer Prescribing Information. 1999.

HYOSCYAMINE

Trade: Anaspaz, Levsin, Nulev
Can/Aus/UK: Buscopan, Levsin, Hyoscine
Uses: Anticholinergic, antisecretory agent
LRC: L3
AAP: Not reviewed

Hyoscyamine is an anticholinergic, antisecretory agent that belongs to the belladonna alkaloid family. Its typical effects are to dry secretions, produce constipation, dilate pupils, blur vision, and may produce urinary retention.[1,2]   Although no exact amounts are listed, hyoscyamine is known to be secreted into breastmilk in trace amounts.[3] Thus far, no untoward effects from breastfeeding while using hyoscyamine have been found. Levsin (hyoscyamine) drops have in the past been used directly in infants for colic although it is no longer recommended for this use. As with atropine, infants and children are especially sensitive to anticholinergics and their use is discouraged. Atropine is composed of two isomers of hyoscyamine. See atropine. Use with caution.

Pregnancy Risk Category: C

Lactation Risk Category: L3

Adult Concerns: Tachycardia, dry mouth, blurred vision, constipation, urinary retention

Pediatric Concerns: Decreased heart rate, anticholinergic effects from direct use but none reported from breastmilk ingestion.   Never use directly in infants with projectile vomiting or in infants with bilious (green) vomitus.

Drug Interactions: Decreased effect with antacids.   Increased toxicity with amantadine, antimuscarinics, haloperidol, phenothiazines, tricyclic antidepressants, MAO inhibitors.

Theoretic Infant Dose:

Relative Infant Dose:

Adult Dose: 0.125-0.25 mg QID

Alternatives:

$T\frac{1}{2}$ =	3.5 hours	M/P =	
PHL =		PB =	50%
T_{max} =	40-90 minutes (oral)	Oral =	81%
MW =	289	pKa =	
Vd =			

References:
1. Drug Facts and Comparisons 1995 ed. ed. St. Louis: 1995.
2. Pharmaceutical Manufacturer Prescribing Information. 1995.
3. Wilson J. Drugs in Breastmilk. New York: ADIS Press 1981.

I-125 I-131 I-123
Trade: Radioactive Iodine, Iodine-125, Iodine-131, Iodine-123, Iodotope, I-125, I-131, I-123
Can/Aus/UK:
Uses: Radioactive iodine
LRC: L4
AAP: Radioactive compound that requires temporary cessation of breastfeeding

Radioactive iodine concentrates in the thyroid gland as well as in breastmilk, and if ingested by an infant, it may suppress its thyroid function or increase the risk of future thyroid carcinomas, and produce thyroid destruction in the infant. Radioactive iodine is clinically used to ablate or destroy the thyroid (dose= 355 MBq), or in much smaller doses (7.4 MBq), to scan the thyroid for malignancies. Following ingestion, radioactive iodine concentrates in the thyroid and lactating tissues, and it is estimated 27.9% of total radioactivity is secreted via breast milk.[1]

Two potential half-lives exist for radioactive iodine. One is the radioactive half-life which is solely dependent on radioactive decay of the molecule. And two, the biological half-life, which is often briefer, and is the half-life of the iodine molecule itself in the human being. The latter half-life is influenced most by elimination via the kidneys and other routes.

Previously published data have suggested that Iodine-125 is present in milk for at least 12 days and Iodine-131 is present for 2-14 days, but these studies may be in error as they ignored the second component of the biexponential breastmilk disappearance curve.[2] The radioactive half-life of ^{131}I is 8.1 days. The half-life of ^{125}I is 60.2 days and the half-life of ^{123}I is 13.2 hours. The biological half-life may be shorter due to excretion in urine, feces, and milk.

A well done study by Dydek reviewed the transfer of both tracer and ablation doses of ^{131}I into human milk.[3] If the tracer doses are kept minimal (0.1 uCi or 3.7 kBq), breastfeeding could resume as early as the eighth day. However, if larger tracer doses (8.6 uCi or 0.317 MBq) are used, nursing could not resume until 46 days following therapy. Doses used for ablation of the maternal thyroid (111 MBq) would require an interruption of breastfeeding for a minimum of 106 days or more.

However, an acceptable dose to an infant, as a result of ingestion of radioiodine, is a matter for debate although an effective dose of < 1 mSv has been suggested.

In another study of ^{131}I use in a mother, breastmilk levels were followed for 32 days. These authors recommend discontinuing breastfeeding for up to 50-52 days to ensure safety of the infant thyroid. Thyroid scans use either radioactive iodine or technetium-99m pertechnetate. Technetium has a very short half-life and should be preferred in breastfeeding mothers for thyroid scanning.[3]

Due to the fact that significant concentrations of ^{131}I are concentrated in breastmilk, women should discontinue breastfeeding prior to treatment, as the cumulative exposure to breast tissues could be excessively high. It is sometimes recommended that women discontinue breastfeeding several days to weeks before undergoing therapy or that they pump and discard milk for several weeks after exposure to iodine to reduce the overall radioactive exposure to breast tissues. The estimated dose of radioactivity to the breasts would give a "theoretical" probability of induction of breast cancer of 0.32%.[1] In addition, holding the infant close to the breast or thyroid gland for long periods may expose the infant to gamma irradiation and is not recommended. Patients should consult with the radiologist concerning exposure of the infant.

One case of significant exposure was reported in a breastfed infant.[4] The mother received a 3.02 millicurie dose of ^{131}I and continued to breastfeed for the next 7 days before the mother admitted breastfeeding. During this 7 day period, the infant's thyroid contained 2.7 microcuries of iodine-131 which is an effective dose equivalent of 5.5 rads. Had the mother continued to breastfeed, the dose would have been much larger and potentially dangerous.

In another case report of a patient who received 14 microcuries of oral [131]Iodine, and then 5 millicuries of [99]technetium, the mother's milk was withdrawn and screened for radiation with a gamma counter.[5] On day 8 the measured radioactivity was 94 counts per minute(cpm). On day 13, the measured radioactivity was 30 cpm, and by day 20, the radioactivity was measured at background levels (20 cpm). This data suggests that if the [131]I
levels administered are equal to or less than 14 microcuries, then the mother could potentially return to breastfeeding after 20 days.

Another alternative is ^{123}I, a newer isotope that is increasing in popularity. [123]I has a short half-life of only 13.2 hours and is radiologically ideal for thyroid and other scans. If radioactive iodine compounds are mandatory for various "scanning" procedures, ^{123}I should be preferred, followed by pumping and dumping for 12-24 hours depending on the dose. However, the return to breastfeeding following 123I therapy is dependent on the purity of this product. During manufacture of 123I, 124I and 125I are created. If using 123I, breastfeeding should be temporarily interrupted (see table in appendices). 123I is not used for ablation of the thyroid.

In a study by Morita of the transfer of 123I-sodium iodide, 123I was excreted exponentially with an effective half-life of 5.5 hours.[6] A total of 2.5% of the total radioactivity administered was excreted in the breast milk over the 93 h, 95% of which was excreted within the first 24 h, and 98.2% within 36 h. The first milk sample collected at 7 hours after administration contained 48.5% of the total radioactivity excreted. The authors estimated the potential absorption of radioactivity to an infant's thyroid in uninterrupted breast-feeding to be 30.3 mGy. With a 24-hour interruption, the absorbed radioactivity would be 1.25 mGy; with a 36-hour interruption, it would be 0.24 mGy. They recommend that breastfeeding should be curtailed for 36 h to reduce the infant's exposure to 123I radioactivity.

The Nuclear Regulatory Commission has released a table of instructions to mothers concerning the use of radioisotopes (see appendix). These instructions conclude that patients should not breastfeed following the use of 131I. In a study by Hammami, radioactive 131I was found to transfer into breasts weeks following cessation of lactation.[7] They suggest the breast is a "radioiodine reservoir".

Pregnancy Risk Category:

Lactation Risk Category: L4

Adult Concerns: Ablation of thyroid function. Theoretical risk of breast cancer if used in lactating women.

Pediatric Concerns: None reported, but damage to thyroid is probable if the infant is breastfed while I-131 levels are high.

Drug Interactions:

Theoretic Infant Dose:

Relative Infant Dose:

Adult Dose:

Alternatives: Technetium-99M

References:
1.   Robinson PS, Barker P, Campbell A, Henson P, Surveyor I, Young PR. Iodine-131 in breast milk following therapy for thyroid carcinoma. J Nucl Med 1994; 35(11):1797-1801.
2.   Palmer KE. Excretion of 125I in breast milk following administration of labelled fibrinogen. Br J Radiol 1979; 52(620):672-673.
3.   Dydek GJ, Blue PW. Human breast milk excretion of iodine-131 following diagnostic and therapeutic administration to a lactating patient with Graves' disease. J Nucl Med 1988; 29(3):407-410.

4. Iodine-131 dose for whole body scan administered to a breast-feeding patient. Preliminary notification of event or unusual occurrence PNO-198-038. NRC. http://www.nrc.gov/OPA/pn/pn19838.htm. 2004.
5. Saenz RB. Iodine-131 elimination from breast milk: a case report. J. Hum. Lact. 2000:; 16(1):44-46
6. Morita S, Umezaki N, Ishibashi M, Kawamura S, Inada C, Hayabuchi N. Determining the breast-feeding interruption schedule after administration of 123I-iodide. Ann Nucl Med 1998; 12(5):303-306.
7. Bakheet SM, Hammami MM. Patterns of radioiodine uptake by the lactating breast. Eur J Nucl Med 1994; 21(7):604-608.

IBUPROFEN

Trade: Advil, Nuprin, Motrin, Pediaprofen
Can/Aus/UK: Actiprofen, Advil, Amersol, Motrin, ACT-3, Brufen, Nurofen, Rafen
Uses: Analgesic, antipyretic
LRC: L1
AAP: Maternal Medication Usually Compatible with Breastfeeding

Ibuprofen is a nonsteroidal antiinflammatory analgesic. It is frequently used for fever in infants. Ibuprofen enters milk only in very low levels (less than 0.6% of maternal dose). Even large doses produce very small milk levels. In one patient receiving 400 mg twice daily, milk levels were less than 0.5 mg/L.[1]

In another study of twelve women who received 400 mg doses every 6 hours for a total of 5 doses, all breastmilk levels of ibuprofen were less than 1.0 mg/L, the lower limit of the assay.[2] Data in these studies document that no measurable concentrations of ibuprofen are detected in breastmilk following the above doses. Ibuprofen is presently popular for therapy of fever in infants. The current recommended dose for children is 5-10 mg/kg every 6 hours.

Pregnancy Risk Category: B in 1st and 2nd trimester.
                                D in 3rd trimester.

Lactation Risk Category: L1

Adult Concerns: Nausea, epigastric pain, dizziness, edema, GI bleeding

Pediatric Concerns: None reported from breastfeeding.

Drug Interactions: Aspirin may decrease serum ibuprofen levels. May prolong prothrombin time when used with warfarin. Antihypertensive effects of ACEi family may be blunted or completely abolished by NSAIDs. Some NSAIDs may block antihypertensive effect of beta blockers, diuretics. Used with cyclosporin, may dramatically increase renal toxicity. May increase digoxin, phenytoin, lithium levels. May increase toxicity of methotrexate. May increase bioavailability of penicillamine. Probenecid may increase NSAID levels.

Theoretic Infant Dose: 75 µg/kg/day

Relative Infant Dose: < 0.65%

Adult Dose: 400 mg q 4-6 hours

Alternatives: Acetaminophen

T½ =	1.8-2.5 hours	M/P =	
PHL =		PB =	> 99%
T$_{max}$ =	1-2 hours	Oral =	80%
MW =	206	pKa =	4.4
Vd =	0.14		

References:
1. Weibert RT, Townsend RJ, Kaiser DG, Naylor AJ. Lack of ibuprofen secretion into human milk. Clin Pharm 1982; 1(5):457-458.
2. Townsend RJ, Benedetti TJ, Erickson SH, Cengiz C, Gillespie WR, Gschwend J, Albert KS. Excretion of ibuprofen into breastmilk. Am J Obstet Gynecol 1984; 149(2):184-186.

IMIPENEM-CILASTATIN

Trade: Primaxin
Can/Aus/UK: Primaxin
Uses: Antibiotic
LRC: L2
AAP: Not reviewed

Imipenem is structurally similar to penicillins and acts similarly. Cilastatin is added to extend the half-life of imipenem. Both imipenem and cilastatin are poorly absorbed orally and must be administered IM or IV.[1,2] Imipenem is destroyed by gastric acidity. Transfer into breastmilk is probably minimal, but no data are available. Changes in GI flora could occur but is probably remote.

Pregnancy Risk Category: C

Lactation Risk Category: L2

Adult Concerns: Nausea, diarrhea, vomiting, abdominal pain, decreased white blood cells, decreased hemoglobin, seizures

Pediatric Concerns: No studies available. Probably similar to other penicillins.

Drug Interactions: May have increased toxicity when used with other beta lactam antibiotics. Probenecid may increase toxic potential.

Theoretic Infant Dose:

Relative Infant Dose:

Adult Dose: 500-750 mg BID

Alternatives:

T½ =	0.85-1.3 hours	M/P =	
PHL =	1.5-2.6 hours (neonate)	PB =	20-35%
T$_{max}$ =	Immediate(IV)	Oral =	Poor
MW =	317	pKa =	
Vd =			

References:

1. Pharmaceutical Manufacturer Prescribing Information. 1995.
2. McEvoy GE. (ed):AFHS Drug Information. New York, NY: 2003.

IMIPRAMINE

Trade: Tofranil, Janimine

Can/Aus/UK: Apo-Imipramine, Impril, Novo-Pramine, Melipramine, Tofranil

Uses: Tricyclic antidepressant

LRC: L2

AAP: Drugs whose effect on nursing infants is unknown but may be of concern

Imipramine is a classic tricyclic antidepressant.   Imipramine is metabolized to desipramine, the active metabolite.   Milk levels approximate those of maternal serum.   In a patient receiving 200 mg daily at bedtime, the milk levels at 1, 9, 10, and 23 hours were 29, 24, 12, and 18 µg/L respectively.[1] However, in this previous study the mother was not in a therapeutic range.[2]   In a mother with full therapeutic levels, it is suggested that an infant would ingest approximately 0.2 mg/Liter of milk. This represents a dose of only 30 µg/kg/day, far less than the 1.5 mg/kg dose recommended for older children. The long half-life of this medication in infants could, under certain conditions, lead to high plasma levels although they have not been reported. Although no untoward effects have been reported, the infant should be monitored closely.   Therapeutic plasma levels in children 6-12 yrs. are 200-225 ng/mL.   Two good reviews of psychotropic drugs in breastfeeding patients are available. [3,4]

Pregnancy Risk Category: D

Lactation Risk Category: L2

Adult Concerns: Dry mouth, sedation, hypotension, arrhythmias, confusion, agitation, seizures

Pediatric Concerns: None reported, but observe for sedation, dry mouth.

Drug Interactions: Barbiturates may lower serum levels of TCAs. Central and respiratory depressant effects may be additive. Cimetidine has increased serum TCA concentrations. Anticholinergic symptoms may be exacerbated. Use with clonidine may produce dangerous elevation in blood pressure and hypertensive crisis. Dicumarol anticoagulant capacity may be increased when used with TCAs. Co-use with fluoxetine may increase the toxic levels and effects of TCAs. Symptoms may persist for several weeks after discontinuation of fluoxetine. Haloperidol may increase serum concentrations of TCAs. MAO inhibitors should never be given immediately after or with tricyclic antidepressants. Oral contraceptives may inhibit the metabolism of tricyclic antidepressants and may increase their plasma levels.

Theoretic Infant Dose: 4.35 µg/kg/day

Relative Infant Dose: 0.15%

Adult Dose: 75-100 mg daily

Alternatives: Amoxapine

T½ =	8-16 hours	M/P =	0.5-1.5
PHL =		PB =	90%
T$_{max}$ =	1-2 hours	Oral =	90%
MW =	280	pKa =	9.5
Vd =	20-40		

References:
1. Sovner R, Orsulak PJ. Excretion of imipramine and desipramine in human breastmilk. Am J Psychiatry 1979; 136(4A):451-452.
2. Erickson SH, Smith GH, Heidrich F. Tricyclics and breast feeding. Am J Psychiatry 1979; 136(11):1483-1484.
3. Buist A, Norman TR, Dennerstein L. Breastfeeding and the use of psychotropic medication: a review. J Affect Disord 1990; 19(3):197-206.
4. Wisner KL, Perel JM, Findling RL. Antidepressant treatment during breast-feeding. Am J Psychiatry 1996; 153(9):1132-1137.

INDAPAMIDE
Trade: Lozol
Can/Aus/UK: Lozide, Gen-Indapamide, Apo-Indapamide, Dapa-Tabs, Nadide, Napamide, Natrilix
Uses: Antihypertensive diuretic
LRC: L3
AAP: Not reviewed

Indapamide is the first of a new class of indoline diuretics used to treat hypertension. No data exists on transfer into human milk.[1] Some diuretics may reduce the production of breastmilk. See hydrochlorothiazide as alternative.

Pregnancy Risk Category: D

Lactation Risk Category: L3

Adult Concerns: Sodium and potassium loss, hypotension, dizziness, nausea, vomiting, constipation

Pediatric Concerns: None reported but observe for reduction in milk supply and volume depletion.

Drug Interactions: May reduce effect of oral hypoglycemics. Cholestyramine may reduce absorption of indapamide. May increase the effect of furosemide and other diuretics. May increased toxicity and levels of lithium.

Theoretic Infant Dose:

Relative Infant Dose:

Adult Dose: 2.5-5 mg daily

Alternatives:

$T\frac{1}{2}$ =	14 hours	M/P =	
PHL =		PB =	71%
T_{max} =	0.5-2 hours	Oral =	Complete
MW =	366	pKa =	
Vd =			

References:

1. Pharmaceutical Manufacturer Prescribing Information. 1996.

INDIUM - 111M

Trade: 111-Indium
Can/Aus/UK:
Uses: Radioactive diagnostic agent
LRC: L4
AAP: Radioactive compound that requires temporary cessation of breastfeeding

Indium-111 is a radioactive material used for imaging neuroendocrine tumors. While the plasma half-life is extremely short (< 10 minutes), with the majority of this product leaving the plasma compartment and distributing to tissue sites, the radioactive half-life is 2.8 days. In one patient receiving 12 MBq (0.32 mCi), the concentration in milk at 6 and 20 hours was 0.09 Bq/mL and 0.20 Bq/mL per MBq injected.[1] These data indicate that breastfeeding may be safe if this radiopharmaceutical is used. Assuming an ingestion of 500 cc daily, the infant would receive approximately 100 Bq per MBq given to the mother (approximately 0.1 uCi). The NRC recommends a waiting period of 1 week with doses of 20 Mbq (0.5 mCi). See appendix.

Pregnancy Risk Category:

Lactation Risk Category: **L4**

Adult Concerns: Nausea, dizziness, headache, flushing, hypotension

Pediatric Concerns: None reported but slight risk of radiation exposure.

Drug Interactions:

Theoretic Infant Dose:

Relative Infant Dose:

Adult Dose:

Alternatives:

T½ =	2.8 days	M/P =
PHL =		PB =
T~max~ =	Immediate (IV)	Oral =
MW =	358	pKa =
Vd =		

References:
1. Pullar M, Hartkamp A. Excretion of radioactivity in breastmilk following administration of an 113-Indium labeled chelate complex. Br J Radial 1977; 50:846.

INDOMETHACIN

Trade: Indocin
Can/Aus/UK: Apo-Indomethacin, Indocid, Novo-Methacin, Arthrexin, Hicin, Indoptol
Uses: Non-steroidal antiinflammatory
LRC: L3
AAP: Maternal Medication Usually Compatible with Breastfeeding

Indomethacin is a potent, nonsteroidal antiinflammatory agent frequently used in arthritis. It is also used in newborns in neonatal units to close a patent ductus arteriosus. There is one reported case of convulsions in an infant of a breastfeeding mother early postpartum (day 7).[1]

In another report of 16 women, of 20 milk samples analyzed 12 were less than 20 µg/L(limit of detection), and the median milk/plasma ratio was 0.37.[2] The eight measurable samples ranged from 23 to 115 µg/L. The authors suggest the total infant dose, assuming daily milk intake of 150 mL/kg, would range from 0.07% to 0.98% of the weight adjusted maternal dose. Plasma samples derived from 6 of the 7 infants were below the sensitivity of the assay (< 20 µg/L) and 47 µg/L in only one infant. Dose calculations for all 16 infants showed that absolute dose ranged from < 0.003 to 0.017 mg/kg/day. In six of seven infants, indomethacin levels were below detection. In one infant the plasma level was 47 μg/L. No adverse effects were noted in this study.

Pregnancy Risk Category: **B in 1st and 2nd trimester**
D in 3rd trimester

Lactation Risk Category: **L3**

Adult Concerns: Renal dysfunction, GI distress, gastric bleeding, diarrhea, clotting dysfunction

Pediatric Concerns: One case of seizures in neonate. Additional report suggests no untoward effects. Frequently used in neonatal nurseries for patent ductus.

Drug Interactions: May prolong prothrombin time when used with warfarin. Antihypertensive effects of ACEi family may be blunted or completely abolished by NSAIDs. Some NSAIDs may block antihypertensive effect of beta blockers, diuretics. Used with cyclosporin, may dramatically increase renal toxicity. May increase digoxin, phenytoin, lithium levels. May increase toxicity of methotrexate. May increase bioavailability of penicillamine. Probenecid may increase NSAID levels.

Theoretic Infant Dose: 16.95 μg/kg/day

Relative Infant Dose: < 1.18%

Adult Dose: 25-50 mg BID-TID

Alternatives: Ibuprofen

T½ =	4.5 hours	M/P =	0.37
PHL =	30 hours (prematures)	PB =	> 90%
T$_{max}$ =	1-2 :2-4(SR) hours	Oral =	90%
MW =	357	pKa =	4.5
Vd =	0.33-0.40		

References:
1. Eeg-Olofsson O, Malmros I, Elwin CE, Steen B. Convulsions in a breast-fed infant after maternal indomethacin. Lancet 1978; 2(8082):215.
2. Lebedevs TH, Wojnar-Horton RE, Yapp P, Roberts MJ, Dusci LJ, Hackett LP, Ilett KF. Excretion of indomethacin in breastmilk. Br J Clin Pharmacol 1991; 32(6):751-754.

INFLIXIMAB

Trade: Remicade
Can/Aus/UK: Remicade
Uses: Treatment of Crohn's, Rheumatoid arthritis
LRC: L2
AAP: Not reviewed

Infliximab is a monoclonal antibody to tumor necrosis factor-alpha (TNF-alpha) used to treat Crohn's disease and rheumatoid arthritis. Infliximab is a very large molecular weight antibody and is largely retained in the vascular system. In a study of one breastfeeding patient who received 5 mg/kg IV, infliximab levels were determined in milk at 0, 2, 4, 8, 24, 48, 72 hours, and 4, 5, and 7 days.[1] None was detected in milk at any time (detection limit < 0.1 µg/mL). While these are preliminary study results that are continuing, infliximab is probably too large to enter milk in clinically measurable amounts. It would not be orally bioavailable.

Pregnancy Risk Category: C

Lactation Risk Category: L2

Adult Concerns: Infusion-related reactions include fever, chills, pruritus, urticaria, chest pain, hypotension. A state of immunosuppression is induced thus serious infection including sepsis, disseminated tuberculosis and other infections have been reported.

Pediatric Concerns: None reported in three patients.

Drug Interactions:

Theoretic Infant Dose:

Relative Infant Dose:

Adult Dose: 5 mg/kg (Crohn's)

Alternatives:

T½ =	8-9.5 days	M/P =	
PHL =		PB =	
T$_{max}$ =		Oral =	Nil
MW =	149100	pKa =	
Vd =	3		

References:
1. Hale TW, Fasanmade A. Personal communication. 2002.

INFLUENZA VIRUS VACCINE
Trade: Vaccine- Influenza, Flu-Imune, Fluogen, Fluzone
Can/Aus/UK: Fluviral, Fluzone
Uses: Vaccine
LRC: L1
AAP: Not reviewed

Influenza vaccine is prepared from inactivated, non-viable influenza viruses and infection of the neonate via milk would not be expected. There are no reported side effects nor published contraindications for using influenza virus vaccine during lactation.[1,2] Influenza vaccine is now indicated for infants by the American Academy of Pediatrics.

Pregnancy Risk Category: C

Lactation Risk Category: L1

Adult Concerns: Fever, myalgia

Pediatric Concerns: None reported in breastfeeding mothers.

Drug Interactions: Decreased effect with immunosuppressants. Influenza vaccine may be administered simultaneously (but at a separate site and with a different syringe) with other routine immunizations in children.

Theoretic Infant Dose:

Relative Infant Dose:

Adult Dose: 0.5 mL injection once

Alternatives:

References:
1. Kilbourne ED. Questions and answers. Artificial influenza immunization of nursing mothers not harmful. JAMA 1973; 226:87.
2. Pharmaceutical Manufacturer Prescribing Information. 1996.

INSECT STINGS
Trade: Insect Stings, Spider Stings, Bee Stings
Can/Aus/UK:
Uses: Insect stings, envenomations
LRC:
AAP: Not reviewed

Insect stings are primarily composed of small peptides, enzymes such as hyaluronidase, and other factors such as histamine. Because the total injectant is so small, most reactions are local. In cases of systemic reactions, the secondary release of maternal reactants produces the allergic response in the injected individual. Nevertheless, the amount of injection is exceedingly small. In the case of black widow spiders, the venom is so large in molecular weight, it would not likely penetrate milk. In addition, most of the venoms and allergens would be destroyed in the acidic milieu of the infant's stomach. The sting of the Loxosceles spider (brown recluse, fiddleback) is primarily a local necrosis without systemic effects. No reports of toxicity to nursing infants have been reported from insect stings.

Pregnancy Risk Category:

Lactation Risk Category:

Adult Concerns: Nausea, vomiting

Pediatric Concerns: None reported via milk.

References:

INSULIN
Trade: Humulin
Can/Aus/UK: Novolin, Humulin, Humalog, Iletin, Mixtard, Protaphane, Monotard
Uses: Human insulin
LRC: L1
AAP: Not reviewed

Insulin is a large peptide that is not secreted into milk. Even if secreted, it would be destroyed in the infant's GI tract leading to minimal or no absorption.

Pregnancy Risk Category: B

Lactation Risk Category: L1

Adult Concerns: Hypoglycemia

Pediatric Concerns: None reported via milk.

Drug Interactions: A decreased hypoglycemic effect may result when used with oral contraceptives, corticosteroids, diltiazem, epinephrine, thiazide diuretics, thyroid hormones, and niacin. Increased hypoglycemic effects may result when used with alcohol, beta blockers, fenfluramine, MAO inhibitors, salicylates, tetracyclines.

Theoretic Infant Dose:

Relative Infant Dose:

Adult Dose:

Alternatives:

T½ =		M/P =	
PHL =		PB =	
Tmax =		Oral =	0%
MW =	> 6000	pKa =	
Vd =	0.37		

References:

INTERFERON ALPHA-N3
Trade: Alferon N, Interferon Alpha, Peg-Intron
Can/Aus/UK:
Uses: Immune modulator, antiviral.
LRC: L2
AAP: Not reviewed

Interferon alpha is a pure clone of a single interferon subspecies with antiviral, antiproliferative, and immunomodulatory activity. The alpha-interferons are active against various malignancies and viral syndromes such as hairy cell leukemia, melanoma, AIDS-related Kaposi's sarcoma, condyloma acuminata, and chronic hepatitis B and C infection.[1] Other forms of interferons such as the Alfa-2b (Peg-Intron) are also available.

Very little is known about the secretion of interferons in human milk although some interferons are known to be secreted normally and may contribute to the antiviral properties of human milk. However, interferons are large in molecular weight (16-28,000 daltons) which would limit their transfer into human milk. Following treatment with a massive dose of 30 million units IV in one breastfeeding patient, the amount of interferon alpha transferred into human milk was 894, 1004, 1551, 1507, 788, 721 units at 0 (baseline), 2, 4, 8, 12, and 24 hours respectively.[2] Hence, even following a massive dose, no change in breastmilk levels were noted from baseline. One thousand international units is roughly equivalent to 500 nanograms of interferon.

The oral absorption of interferons is controversial and is believed to be minimal. Interferons are relatively nontoxic unless extraordinarily large doses are administered parenterally. Interferons are sometimes used in infants and children to treat idiopathic thromboplastinemia (ITP) in huge doses.

Pregnancy Risk Category: C

Lactation Risk Category: L2

Adult Concerns: Thrombocytopenia and neutropenia. Flu-like syndrome which occurs 30 minutes after administration and persists for several hours. Fatigue, hyperglycemia, nausea and vomiting.

Pediatric Concerns: None reported via milk.

Drug Interactions: Hematologic abnormalities (granulocytopenia, thrombocytopenia) may occur when used with ACE inhibitors.

Theoretic Infant Dose:

Relative Infant Dose:

Adult Dose: 0.05-0.5 mL per wart twice weekly

Alternatives:

$T\frac{1}{2}$ =	5-7 hours		M/P =	
PHL =			PB =	
T_{max} =	Immediate		Oral =	Low
MW =	28,000		pKa =	
Vd =	0.44			

References:
1. Pharmaceutical Manufacturer Prescribing Information. 1997.
2. Kumar AR, Hale TW, Mock RE. Transfer of interferon alfa into human breastmilk. J Hum Lact 2000; 16(3):226-228.

INTERFERON BETA - 1A
Trade: Avonex, Rebif
Can/Aus/UK: Avonex, Rebif
Uses: Immune modulator
LRC: L3
AAP: Not reviewed

Interferon Beta-1A is a glycoprotein with antiviral, antiproliferative, and immunomodulator activity presently used for reducing the severity and frequency of exacerbations of relapsing-remitting multiple sclerosis.[1] Very little is known about the secretion of interferons in human milk although some interferons are known to be secreted normally and may contribute to the antiviral properties of human milk. However, interferons are large in molecular weight, generally containing 166 amino acids, which would limit their transfer into human milk. Their oral absorption is controversial but is believed to be minimal. However, interferons are relatively nontoxic unless extraordinarily large doses are administered parenterally. Interferons are sometimes used in infants and children to treat idiopathic thromboplastinemia (ITP) in huge doses. See Interferon Alpha, Interferon 1B.

Pregnancy Risk Category: C

Lactation Risk Category: L3

Adult Concerns: Headache, myalgia, nausea, diarrhea, dyspepsia, fever, chills, malaise, sweating, depression, flu-like symptoms. These effects generally follow huge doses.

Pediatric Concerns: None reported via milk.

Drug Interactions: Do not use with live viral vaccines.

Theoretic Infant Dose:

Relative Infant Dose:

Adult Dose: 30 μg weekly I.M.

Alternatives:

T½ =	10 Hours	M/P =	
PHL =		PB =	
T$_{max}$ =	3-15 hours	Oral =	Minimal
MW =	22,500	pKa =	
Vd =	61.6 L		

References:

1. Chofflon M. Recombinant human interferon beta in relapsing-remitting multiple sclerosis: a review of the major clinical trials. Eur J Neurol 2000; 7(4):369-380.

INTERFERON BETA-1B

Trade: Betaseron
Can/Aus/UK: Betaseron, Betaferon
Uses: Antiviral, immunomodulator
LRC: L3
AAP: Not reviewed

Interferon Beta-1B is a glycoprotein with antiviral, antiproliferative, and immunomodulatory activity presently used for treatment of multiple sclerosis.[1,2] Very little is known about the secretion of interferons in human milk although some interferons are known to be secreted normally and may contribute to the antiviral properties of human milk. However, interferons are large in molecular weight, generally containing 165 amino acids, which would limit their transfer into human milk. Their oral absorption is controversial but is believed to be minimal. However, interferons are relatively nontoxic unless extraordinarily large doses are administered parenterally. Interferons are sometimes used in infants and children to treat idiopathic thromboplastinemia (ITP) in huge doses. See Interferon Alpha.

Pregnancy Risk Category: C

Lactation Risk Category: L3

Adult Concerns: Headache, myalgia, nausea, diarrhea, dyspepsia, fever, chills, malaise, sweating, depression, flu-like symptoms. These effects generally follow huge doses.

Pediatric Concerns: None reported via milk.

Drug Interactions: Hematologic abnormalities (granulocytopenia, thrombocytopenia) may occur when added to ACE inhibitors.

Theoretic Infant Dose:

Relative Infant Dose:

Adult Dose: 0.25 mg every other day

Alternatives:

$T\frac{1}{2}$ =	4.3 hours	M/P =		
PHL =		PB =		
T_{max} =	3-15 hours (IM)	Oral =	Poor	
MW =		pKa =		
Vd =	2.9			

References:

1. Chiang J, Gloff CA, Yoshizawa CN, Williams GJ. Pharmacokinetics of recombinant human interferon-beta ser in healthy volunteers and its effect on serum neopterin. Pharm Res 1993; 10(4):567-572.
2. Wills RJ. Clinical pharmacokinetics of interferons. Clin Pharmacokinet 1990; 19(5):390-399.

IODINATED GLYCEROL

Trade: Organidin, Iophen, R-Gen
Can/Aus/UK: Organidin
Uses: Expectorant
LRC: L4
AAP: Not reviewed

This product contains 50% organically bound iodine. High levels of iodine are known to be secreted in milk.[1] Milk/plasma ratios as high as 26 have been reported. Following absorption by the infant, high levels of iodine could lead to severe thyroid depression in infants. Normal iodine levels in breastmilk are already four times higher than RDA for infant. Expectorants, including iodine, work very poorly. Recently, many iodine containing products have been replaced with guaifenesin, which is considered safer. High levels of iodine-containing drugs should not be used in lactating mothers.

Pregnancy Risk Category: X

Lactation Risk Category: L4

Adult Concerns: Depressed thyroid function. Diarrhea, nausea, vomiting. Acne, dermatitis. Metallic taste.

Pediatric Concerns: Iodine concentrates in milk and should not be administered to breastfeeding mothers. Infantile thyroid suppression is likely.

Drug Interactions: Increased toxicity with disulfiram, metronidazole, procarbazine, MAO inhibitors, CNS depressants, lithium.

Theoretic Infant Dose:

Relative Infant Dose:

Adult Dose:

Alternatives:

$T\frac{1}{2}$ =		M/P =	
PHL =		PB =	
T_{max} =		Oral =	Complete
MW =	258	pKa =	
Vd =			

References:
1.   Postellon DC, Aronow R. Iodine in mother's milk. JAMA 1982; 247(4):463.

IOHEXOL
Trade: Omnipaque
Can/Aus/UK: Omnipaque
Uses: Radiopaque agent
LRC: L2
AAP: Maternal Medication Usually Compatible with Breastfeeding

Iohexol is a nonionic, radiocontrast agent.   Radiopaque agents (except barium) are iodinated compounds used to visualize various organs during X-ray, CAT scans, and other radiological procedures.   These compounds are highly-iodinated, benzoic acid derivatives.   Although under usual circumstances iodine products are contraindicated in nursing mothers (due to ion trapping in milk),   these products are unique in that they are extremely inert and are largely cleared without metabolism.   The iodine is organically bound to the structure and is not biologically active.

In a study of 4 women who received 0.755 g/kg (350 mg iodine/mL) of iohexol IV, the mean peak level of iohexol in milk was 35 mg/L at 3 hours post-injection.[1]   The average concentration in milk was only 11.4 mg/L over 24 hours.   Assuming a daily milk intake of 150 mL/kg body weight, the amount of iohexol transferred to an infant during the first 24 hours would be 1.7 mg/kg which corresponds to 0.23% of the maternal dose.

As a group, these radiocontrast agents are virtually unabsorbed after oral administration (< 0.1%).   Iohexol has a brief half-life of just 2 hours and the estimated dose ingested by the infant is only 0.2 % of the radiocontrast dose used clinically for various scanning procedures in infants. Although most company package inserts suggest that an infant be removed from the breast for 24 hours, no untoward effects have been reported with these products in breastfed infants. Because the amount of iohexol transferred into milk is so small, the authors conclude that breastfeeding is acceptable after intravenously administered iohexol.

Pregnancy Risk Category: B

Lactation Risk Category: L2

Adult Concerns: Hypersensitivity to iodine. Arrhythmias, renal failure. Volume expansion.

Pediatric Concerns: None reported via milk in one study.

Drug Interactions: Lower seizure threshold when used with amitriptyline, other tricyclics, CNS stimulants, MAO inhibitors. Should not be used in patients on metformin therapy.

Theoretic Infant Dose: 1.71 mg/kg/day

Relative Infant Dose: 0.23%

Adult Dose: 10-75 mL X 1

Alternatives:

T½ =	2 hours	M/P =	
PHL =		PB =	
T$_{max}$ =	3-10 minutes	Oral =	Nil
MW =		pKa =	
Vd =	0.55		

References:
1. Nielsen ST, Matheson I, Rasmussen JN, Skinnemoen K, Andrew E, Hafsahl G. Excretion of iohexol and metrizoate in human breastmilk. Acta Radiol 1987; 28(5):523-526.

IOPAMIDOL

Trade: Isovue-128
Can/Aus/UK: Ascorbef, Gastromiro
Uses: Radiocontrast agent
LRC: L3
AAP: Not reviewed

Iopamidol is a nonionic radiocontrast agent used for numerous radiological procedures. Although it contains significant iodine content, the iodine is covalently bound to the parent molecule and the bioavailability of the iodine molecule is miniscule.[1] As with other ionic and nonionic radiocontrast agents, it is primarily extracellular and intravascular, its does not pass the blood-brain barrier, and it would be extremely unlikely that it would penetrate into human milk. However, no data are available on its transfer into human milk. As with most of these products, it is poorly absorbed from the GI tract and rapidly excreted from the maternal circulation due to a extremely short half-live.

Pregnancy Risk Category:

Lactation Risk Category: L3

Adult Concerns: Infrequently seizures, deformed and dehydrated red blood cells. Hot flashes, angina, flushing.

Pediatric Concerns: None reported.

Drug Interactions:

Theoretic Infant Dose:

Relative Infant Dose:

Adult Dose: 10-60 mL X 1

Alternatives:

$T\frac{1}{2}$ =	< 2 hours	M/P =	
PHL =		PB =	< 2 hours
T_{max} =	Immediate	Oral =	None
MW =	777	pKa =	
Vd =	0.35		

References:
1.   Pharmaceutical Manufacturer Prescribing Information. 1997.

IOPANOIC ACID
Trade: Telepaque
Can/Aus/UK: Telepaque
Uses: Radiocontrast agent
LRC: L2
AAP: Maternal Medication Usually Compatible with Breastfeeding

Iopanoic acid is a radiopaque organic iodine compound similar to dozens of other radiocontrast agents. It contains 66.7% by weight of iodine. As with all of these compounds, the iodine is organically bound to the parent molecule, and only minimal amounts are free in solution or metabolized by the body. In a group of 5 breastfeeding mothers who received an average of 2.77 gm of iodine (as Iopanoic acid), the amount of iopanoic acid excreted into human milk during the following 19-29 hours was 20.8 mg or about 0.08% of the maternal dose.[1] No untoward effects were noted in the infants.

Pregnancy Risk Category: D

Lactation Risk Category: **L2**

Adult Concerns: Nausea, vomiting, diarrhea, cramps

Pediatric Concerns: None reported via milk. Levels are low.

Drug Interactions:

Theoretic Infant Dose: 3.12 mg/kg/day

Relative Infant Dose: 7.8%

Adult Dose: 3 g X 1-2

Alternatives:

T½ =	24 hours		M/P =	
PHL =			PB =	97%
T$_{max}$ =			Oral =	Poor
MW =	571		pKa =	4.8
Vd =				

References:
1. Holmdahl KH. Cholecystography during lactation. Acta Radiol 1956; 45(4):305-307.

IOVERSOL 160-350
Trade: Optiray 160-350
Can/Aus/UK: Optiray
Uses: Radiocontrast/Radiopaque media
LRC: L3
AAP: Not reviewed

Ioversol is a typical iodinated radiocontrast agent used in computed tomographic imaging (CT scans). The concentration of iodine varies from 16% organically bound iodine(160) to 35% iodine (350). Ioversol is not metabolized, but is excreted largely unchanged. Iodine is only minimally released; therefore, thyroid function tests remain unchanged with exception of iodine uptake studies (PBI, radioactive iodine uptake). The vascular half-life is brief, only 20 minutes. No data are available on its transfer to milk, but many others in this family have been studied (see appendix) and transfer to milk at extraordinarily low levels. Further none of these agents are orally bioavailable.

Pregnancy Risk Category: B

Lactation Risk Category: L3

Adult Concerns: Adverse reactions include angina pectoris, hypotension, shock, vomiting, dry mouth, allergic reactions, etc.

Pediatric Concerns: None reported via milk. It is extremely unlikely to penetrate milk.

Drug Interactions: Alterations in thyroid iodine uptake studies have been reported. Lactic acidosis can occur with admixed with metformin.

Theoretic Infant Dose:

Relative Infant Dose:

Adult Dose: Variable

Alternatives:

$T^{1/2}$ =	1.5 hours	M/P =		
PHL =		PB =	0%	
T_{max} =	30 seconds	Oral =	Nil	
MW =	807	pKa =		
Vd =				

References:
1. Pharmaceutical Manufacturers prescribing information, 2003.

IPRATROPIUM BROMIDE

Trade: Atrovent
Can/Aus/UK: Atrovent, Apo-Ipravent
Uses: Bronchodilator in asthmatics
LRC: L2
AAP: Not reviewed

Ipratropium is an anticholinergic drug that is used via inhalation for dilating the bronchi of asthmatics.[1] Ipratropium is a quaternary ammonium compound, and although no data exists, it probably penetrates into breastmilk in exceedingly small levels due to its structure. It is unlikely that the infant would absorb any due to the poor tissue distribution and oral absorption of this family of drugs.

Pregnancy Risk Category: B

Lactation Risk Category: L2

Adult Concerns: Nervousness, dizziness, nausea, GI distress, drug mouth, bitter taste

Pediatric Concerns: None reported. Commonly used in pediatric patients.

Drug Interactions: Albuterol may increase effect of ipratropium. May have increased toxicity when used with other anticholinergics.

Theoretic Infant Dose:

Relative Infant Dose:

Adult Dose: 36 μg QID

Alternatives:

T½ =	2 hours	M/P =	
PHL =		PB =	
T$_{max}$ =	1-2 hours	Oral =	0-2%
MW =	412	pKa =	
Vd =			

References:
1. Pharmaceutical Manufacturer Prescribing Information. 1996.

IRBESARTAN

Trade: Avapro
Can/Aus/UK: Avalide, Avapro, Accuretic, Adizem, Amizide
Uses: Antihypertensive
LRC: L3
AAP: Not reviewed

Irbesartan is an angiotensin-II receptor antagonist used as an antihypertensive. Low concentrations are known to be secreted into rodent milk, but human studies are lacking.[1] Both the ACE inhibitor family and the specific AT1 inhibitors such as irbesartan are contraindicated in the 2nd and 3rd trimesters of pregnancy due to severe hypotension, neonatal skull hypoplasia, irreversible renal failure, and death in the newborn infant. However, some of ACE inhibitors can be used in breastfeeding mothers postpartum. Extreme caution is recommended.

Pregnancy Risk Category: C in 1 st trimester
                          D in 2nd or 3rd trimester

Lactation Risk Category: L3

Adult Concerns: Headache, back pain, pharyngitis, and dizziness have been reported. The use of ACE inhibitors and angiotensin receptor blockers during pregnancy or the neonatal period is extremely dangerous and has resulted in hypotension, neonatal skull hypoplasia, anuria, renal failure, and death.

Pediatric Concerns: None reported via milk, but caution is recommended.

Drug Interactions: None reported thus far.

Theoretic Infant Dose:

Relative Infant Dose:

Adult Dose: 150-300 mg daily

Alternatives: Captopril, enalapril

T½ =	11-15 hours	M/P =	
PHL =		PB =	90%
T$_{max}$ =	1.5-2 hours	Oral =	60-80%
MW =	428	pKa =	
Vd =	1.3		

References:
1. Pharmaceutical Manufacturer Prescribing Information. 1999.

IRON
Trade: Fer-In-Sol
Can/Aus/UK: Infufer, Jectofer, Slow-Fe, Feospan
Uses: Metal supplement
LRC: L1
AAP: Not reviewed

The secretion of iron salts into breastmilk appears to be very low although the bioavailability of that present in milk is high. One recent study suggests that supplementation is not generally required until the 4th month postpartum when some breastfed infants may become iron deficient although these assumptions are controversial.[1] Premature infants are more susceptible to iron deficiencies because they do not have the same hepatic stores available as full term infants. These authors recommend iron supplementation, particularly in exclusively breastfed infants, beginning at 4th month.[1] Supplementation in pre-term infants should probably be initiated earlier. However, oral supplemental iron may block some of the antibacterial properties of human milk. Again, avoid excessively high doses.

Pregnancy Risk Category:

Lactation Risk Category: L1

Adult Concerns: Constipation, GI distress

Pediatric Concerns: None reported via milk.

Drug Interactions: Decreased iron absorption when used with antacids, cimetidine, levodopa, penicillamine, quinolones, tetracyclines. Slightly increased absorption with ascorbic acid.

Theoretic Infant Dose:

Relative Infant Dose:

Adult Dose: 50-100 mg TID

Alternatives:

T½ =		M/P =	
PHL =		PB =	
T$_{max}$ =		Oral =	< 30%
MW =	56	pKa =	
Vd =			

References:
1. Calvo EB, Galindo AC, Aspres NB. Iron status in exclusively breast-fed infants. Pediatrics 1992; 90(3):375-379.

IRON DEXTRAN
Trade: Infed
Can/Aus/UK:
Uses: Iron supplement
LRC: L2
AAP: Not reviewed

Iron dextran is a colloidal solution of ferric hydroxide in a complex with partially hydrolyzed low molecular weight dextran. It is used for severe iron deficiency anemia. Its molecular weight is approximately 180,000 daltons. Approximately 99% of the iron in iron dextran is present as a stable ferric-dextran complex. Following IM injection, iron dextran is absorbed from the site principally through the lymphatic system and subsequently transferred to the reticuloendothelial system in the liver for metabolism. The initial phase of absorption lasts 3 days, which accounts for 60% of an IM dose. The other 40% requires up to 1-3 weeks to several months for complete absorption. While there are no data available on the transfer of iron dextran into human milk, it is extremely unlikely due to its massive molecular weight. Further, iron is transferred into human milk by a tightly controlled pumping system that first chelates the iron to a high molecular weight protein and then transfers it into the milk compartment. It is generally well known that dietary supplements of iron do not change milk levels of iron.[1] Please note: While the pregnancy risk category is only C, it has been shown to be teratogenic in other species. Great care should be used in pregnant women.

Pregnancy Risk Category: C

Lactation Risk Category: L2

Adult Concerns: Local reactions at the site of injection. Abdominal pain, dyspepsia, nausea, vomiting, and diarrhea. Headache, paresthesias, weakness, changes in taste perception, faintness, syncope, folic acid deficiency, and leukocytosis. Please note: while the pregnancy risk category is only C, it has been shown to be teratogenic in other species, and great care should be used in pregnant women.

Pediatric Concerns: None via breastmilk.

Drug Interactions:

Theoretic Infant Dose:

Relative Infant Dose:

Adult Dose:

Alternatives:

References:
1. Lawrence RA. Breastfeeding: A guide for the medical profession. St. Louis: Mosby Publishers, 1994.

ISOETHARINE
Trade: Bronkosol, Bronkometer
Can/Aus/UK: Numotac
Uses: Bronchodilator
LRC: L2
AAP: Not reviewed

Isoetharine is a selective beta-2 adrenergic bronchodilator for asthmatics. There are no reports on its secretion into human milk.[1] However, plasma levels following inhalation are exceedingly low, and breastmilk levels would similarly be low. Isoetharine is rapidly metabolized in the GI tract, so oral absorption by the infant would likely be minimal.

Pregnancy Risk Category: C

Lactation Risk Category: L2

Adult Concerns: Tremors and excitement, hypertension, anxiety, insomnia

Pediatric Concerns: None reported via milk.

Drug Interactions: May have decreased effect with beta blockers and increased toxicity with other adrenergic stimulants such as epinephrine.

Theoretic Infant Dose:

Relative Infant Dose:

Adult Dose:

Alternatives:

$T\frac{1}{2}$ =	1-3 hours	M/P =	
PHL =		PB =	
T_{max} =	5-15 minutes (inhaled)	Oral =	
MW =	239	pKa =	
Vd =			

References:
1. Pharmaceutical Manufacturer Prescribing Information. 1995.

ISOMETHEPTENE MUCATE
Trade: Midrin
Can/Aus/UK: Midrin
Uses: For tension and migraine headache.
LRC: L3
AAP: Not reviewed

Isometheptene is a mild stimulate (sympathomimetic) that apparently acts by constricting dilated cranial and cerebral arterioles, thus reducing vascular headaches. It is listed as "possibly" effective by the FDA and is probably only marginally effective.[1] Midrin also contains acetaminophen and a mild sedative dichloralphenazone, of which little is known.

No data are available on transfer into human milk. Due to its size and molecular composition, it is likely to attain low to moderate levels in breastmilk. Because better drugs exist for migraine therapy, this product is probably not a good choice for breastfeeding mothers. See sumatriptan, amitriptyline, or propranolol as alternatives.

Pregnancy Risk Category:

Lactation Risk Category: L3

Adult Concerns: Dizziness, skin rash, hypertension, sedation

Pediatric Concerns: None reported. Observe for stimulation.

Drug Interactions:

Theoretic Infant Dose:

Relative Infant Dose:

Adult Dose:

Alternatives: Sumatriptan, amitriptyline, propranolol

References:
1.   Pharmaceutical Manufacturer Prescribing Information. 1995.

ISONIAZID
Trade: Inh, Laniazid
Can/Aus/UK: Isotamine, PMS Isoniazid, Pycazide, Rimifon
Uses: Antituberculosis agent
LRC: L3
AAP: Maternal Medication Usually Compatible with Breastfeeding

Isoniazid (INH) is an antimicrobial agent primarily used to treat tuberculosis. It is secreted into milk in quantities ranging from 0.75 to

2.3% of the maternal dose. Following doses of 5 and 10 mg/kg, one report measured peak milk levels at 6 mg/L and 9 mg/L respectively.[1] Isoniazid was not measurable in the infant's serum but was detected in the urine of several infants.

In another study, following a maternal dose of 300 mg of isoniazid, the concentration of isoniazid in milk peaked at 3 hours at 16.6 mg/L while the acetyl derivative (AcINH) was 3.76 mg/L.[2] The 24 hour excretion of INH in milk was estimated at 7 mg. The authors felt this dose was potentially hazardous to a breastfed infant.

Caution and close monitoring of infant for liver toxicity and neuritis are recommended. Peripheral neuropathies, common in INH therapy, can be treated with 10-50 mg/day pyroxidine in adults. PHL= 8-20 hrs (neonate), 2-5 hrs (1.5-15 yrs).

Pregnancy Risk Category: C

Lactation Risk Category: L3

Adult Concerns: Mild hepatic dysfunction, peripheral neuritis, nausea, vomiting, dizziness

Pediatric Concerns: None reported, but the infant should be closely monitored for toxicity including hepatitis, vision changes. Observe for fatigue, weakness, malaise, anorexia, nausea, vomiting.

Drug Interactions: Decreased effect/plasma levels of isoniazide with aluminum products. Increased toxicity/levels of oral anticoagulants, carbamazepine, cycloserine, phenytoin, certain benzodiazepines. Disulfiram reactions.

Theoretic Infant Dose: 1.35 mg/kg/day

Relative Infant Dose: 13.5%

Adult Dose: 5 mg/kg daily

Alternatives:

$T\frac{1}{2}$ =	1.1 - 3.1 hours	M/P =	
PHL =	8-20 hours (neonate)	PB =	10-15%
T_{max} =	1-2 hours (oral)	Oral =	Complete
MW =	137	pKa =	1.9, 3.5,
Vd =	0.6		

References:
1. Snider DE, Jr., Powell KE. Should women taking antituberculosis drugs breast-feed? Arch Intern Med 1984; 144(3):589-590.
2. Berlin CM, Lee C. Isoniazid and acetylisoniazid disposition in human milk, saliva and plasma. Fed Proc 1979; 38:426.

ISOPROTERENOL
Trade: Medihaler-Iso, Isuprel
Can/Aus/UK: Isuprel, Medihaler-Iso, Isoprenaline, Saventrine
Uses: Bronchodilator
LRC: L2
AAP: Not reviewed

Isoproterenol is an old adrenergic bronchodilator.[1] Currently it is seldom used for this purpose. There are no data available on breastmilk levels. It is probably secreted into milk in extremely small levels. Isoproterenol is rapidly metabolized in the gut, and it is unlikely a breastfeeding infant would absorb clinically significant levels.

Pregnancy Risk Category: C

Lactation Risk Category: L2

Adult Concerns: Insomnia, excitement, agitation, tachycardia

Pediatric Concerns: None reported.

Drug Interactions: Increased toxicity when used with other adrenergic stimulants and elevation of blood pressure. When used with isoproterenol, general anesthetics may cause arrhythmias.

Theoretic Infant Dose:

Relative Infant Dose:

Adult Dose: 10-30 mg QID

Alternatives: Albuterol

$T\frac{1}{2}$ =	1-2 hours	M/P =	
PHL =		PB =	
T_{max} =	10 minutes (Inhaled)	Oral =	Poor
MW =	211	pKa =	8.6
Vd =	0.5		

References:
1. Drug Facts and Comparisons 1995 ed. ed. St. Louis: 1995.

ISOTRETINOIN
Trade: Accutane
Can/Aus/UK: Accutane, Isotrex, Accure, Roaccutane
Uses: Vitamin A derivative used for acne
LRC: L5
AAP: Not reviewed

Isotretinoin is a synthetic derivative of the Vitamin A family called retinoids. Isotretinoin is known to be incredibly teratogenic producing profound birth defects in exposed fetuses.[1]   It is primarily used for cystic acne where it is extremely effective if used by skilled physicians. While only 25% reaches the plasma, the remaining is either metabolized in the GI tract or removed first-pass by the liver. It is distributed to the liver, adrenals, ovaries, and lacrimal glands.   Unlike vitamin A, isotretinoin is not stored in the liver. Secretion into milk is unknown but is likely as with other retinoids.   Isotretinoin is extremely lipid soluble,   and   concentrations   in   milk   may   be   significant.   The manufacturer strongly recommends against using isotretinoin in a breastfeeding mother.

Pregnancy Risk Category: X

Lactation Risk Category: L5

Adult Concerns: Cheilitis (inflammation of the lips), dry nose, pruritus, elevated serum triglycerides, arthralgia, altered CBC, fatigue, headache, anorexia, nausea, vomiting, abnormal liver function tests, birth defects.

Pediatric Concerns: None reported, but this product poses too many risks to use in a lactating woman.

Drug Interactions: May increased clearance of carbamazepine. Avoid use of other vitamin A products.

Theoretic Infant Dose:

Relative Infant Dose:

Adult Dose: 0.5-2 mg/kg daily
Alternatives:

$T\frac{1}{2}$ =	>20 hours	M/P =	
PHL =		PB =	99.9%
T_{max} =	3.2 hours	Oral =	25%
MW =	300	pKa =	
Vd =			

References:
1. Zbinden G. Investigation on the toxicity of tretinoin administered systemically to animals. Acta Derm Verereol Suppl(Stockh) 1975; 74:36-40.

ISRADIPINE

Trade: Dynacirc
Can/Aus/UK: Prescal
Uses: Calcium channel blocker, antihypertensive
LRC: L3
AAP: Not reviewed

It is not known if isradipine is secreted into milk. However, other calcium channel blockers are transferred only minimally (see verapamil, nifedipine).[1]   Observe for lethargy, low blood pressure, and headache. See verapamil or nifedipine as alternatives.

Pregnancy Risk Category: C

Lactation Risk Category: L3

Adult Concerns: Hypotension, headache, dizziness, fatigue, bradycardia, nausea, dyspnea

Pediatric Concerns: None reported but observe for hypotension, fatigue, bradycardia, apnea.

Drug Interactions: H2 blockers may increased oral absorption of isradipine. Carbamazepine levels may be increased. Cyclosporine levels may be increased. May increase hypotension associated with fentanyl use. Digitalis levels may be increased. May increase quinidine levels including bradycardia, arrhythmias, and hypotension.

Theoretic Infant Dose:

Relative Infant Dose:

Adult Dose: 2.5-10 mg BID

Alternatives: Nifedipine, Verapamil, Nimodipine

$T\frac{1}{2}$ =	8 hours	M/P =	
PHL =		PB =	95%
T_{max} =	1.5 hours	Oral =	17%
MW =	371	pKa =	
Vd =			

References:
1.   Pharmaceutical Manufacturer Prescribing Information. 1996.

ITRACONAZOLE
Trade: Sporanox
Can/Aus/UK: Sporanox
Uses: Antifungal
LRC: L2
AAP: Not reviewed

Itraconazole is an antifungal agent active against a variety of fungal strains. It is extensively metabolized to hydroxyitraconazole, an active metabolite.[1,2]   Itraconazole has an enormous volume of distribution, and large quantities (20 fold compared to plasma) concentrate in fatty tissues, liver, kidney, and skin. In a study of two women who received two oral doses of 200 mg itraconazole 12 hours apart, the average milk concentrations at 4, 24, and 48 hours after the second dose were 70, 28, and 16 µg/L respectively.[3]   After 72 hours, itraconazole levels in one mother were 20   µg/L and undetectable in the other. Reported milk/plasma ratios at 4, 24, and 48 hours were 0.51, 1.61, and 1.77 respectively.   However, itraconazole oral absorption in an infant is somewhat unlikely as it requires an acidic milieu for absorption, which may be unlikely in a diet high in milk.

Never use with terfenadine or astemizole. Itraconazole has also been reported to induce significant bone defects in newborn animals, and it is not cleared for pediatric use. Until further studies are done, fluconazole is probably a preferred choice in breastfeeding mothers.

Pregnancy Risk Category: C

Lactation Risk Category: L2

Adult Concerns: Nausea, vomiting, diarrhea, epigastric pain, dizziness, rash, hypertension, abnormal liver enzymes

Pediatric Concerns: None reported via breastmilk. Absorption via milk is unlikely.

Drug Interactions: Decreased serum levels with isoniazid, rifampin, and phenytoin.   Decreased absorption under alkaline conditions. Agents which increase stomach pH such as H-2 blockers (cimetidine, famotidine, nizatidine, ranitidine),   omeprazole, sucralfate, and milk significantly reduce absorption. Cyclosporin levels are significantly increased by 50%.   May increase phenytoin levels, inhibit warfarin metabolism, and increase digoxin levels.   Significantly increases terfenadine, astemizole plasma levels.

Theoretic Infant Dose: 10.5 μg/kg/day

Relative Infant Dose: 0.187%

Adult Dose: 200-400 mg daily

Alternatives: Fluconazole

T½ =	64 hours	M/P =	0.51-1.77
PHL =		PB =	99.8%
T$_{max}$ =	4 hours	Oral =	55%
MW =	706	pKa =	
Vd =	10		

References:
1.   Drug Facts and Comparisons 1994 ed. ed. St. Louis: 1994.
2.   Pharmaceutical Manufacturer Prescribing Information. 1996.
3.   Janssen Pharmaceuticals, personal communication. 1996.

IVERMECTIN

Trade: Mectizan
Can/Aus/UK: Stromectol
Uses: Antiparasitic
LRC: L3
AAP: Maternal Medication Usually Compatible with Breastfeeding

Ivermectin is now widely used to treat human onchocerciasis, lymphatic filariasis, and other worms and parasites such as head lice. In a study of 4 women given 150 µg/kg orally, the maximum breastmilk concentration averaged 14.13 µg/L.[1] Milk/plasma ratios ranged from 0.39 to 0.57 with a mean of 0.51. Highest breastmilk concentration was at 4-6 hours. Average daily ingestion of ivermectin was calculated at 2.1 µg/kg which is 10 fold less than the adult dose. No adverse effects were reported.

Pregnancy Risk Category: C

Lactation Risk Category: L3

Adult Concerns: Headaches, pruritus, transient hypotension

Pediatric Concerns: None reported.

Drug Interactions:

Theoretic Infant Dose: 2.1 µg/kg/day

Relative Infant Dose: 1.4%

Adult Dose: 150-200 µg/kg once

Alternatives:

$T\frac{1}{2}$ =	28 hours	M/P =	0.39-0.57
PHL =		PB =	
T_{max} =	4 hours	Oral =	Variable
MW =		pKa =	
Vd =			

References:
1. Ogbuokiri JE, Ozumba BC, Okonkwo PO. Ivermectin levels in human breastmilk. Eur J Clin Pharmacol 1994; 46(1):89-90.

KANAMYCIN
Trade: Kebecil, Kantrex
Can/Aus/UK: Kannasyn
Uses: Antibiotic
LRC: L2
AAP: Maternal Medication Usually Compatible with Breastfeeding

Kanamycin is an aminoglycoside antibiotic primarily used for gram negative infections. In a study of 3 patients who received 1000 mg IV, milk levels at 1, 2, 4, and 6 hours were zero, 0.1 mg/L, 0.3 mg/L, 0.5 and 0.8 mg/L respectively.[1] The average milk level in this study was 0.25 mg/L although the highest milk level occurred at 1 hour following the IV infusion. The milk/plasma ratio at 6 hours was 0.045. It is probably advisable to refrain from breastfeeding for several hours following placement of the IV. This will drastically reduce the infant's exposure to kanamycin. However, poor oral absorption (only 1%) in the infant would limit amount absorbed although changes in GI flora are possible.

Pregnancy Risk Category: D

Lactation Risk Category: L2

Adult Concerns: Diarrhea, ototoxicity, nephrotoxicity

Pediatric Concerns: None reported but observe for diarrhea.

Drug Interactions: May have increased toxicity when used with penicillins, cephalosporins, amphotericin B, and diuretics. May increase neuromuscular blockade when used with neuromuscular blocking agents.

Theoretic Infant Dose: 0.0375 mg/kg/day

Relative Infant Dose: 0.26%

Adult Dose: 5-7.5 mg/kg q 8-12 hours

Alternatives:

$T^{1/2}$ =	2.4 hours	M/P =	0.045
PHL =	4-18 hours	PB =	0%
T_{max} =	1 hour	Oral =	1%
MW =		pKa =	7.2
Vd =	0.2-0.3		

References:
1. Matsuda S. Transfer of antibiotics into maternal milk. Biol Res Pregnancy Perinatol 1984; 5(2):57-60.

KAOLIN - PECTIN

Trade: Kaolin, Kaopectate
Can/Aus/UK: Donnagel-MB, Kao-Con, Kaopectate
Uses: Antidiarrhea
LRC: L1
AAP: Not reviewed

Kaolin and pectin (attapulgite) are used as antidiarrhea agents. Kaolin is a natural hydrated aluminum silicate. Pectin is a purified polymerized carbohydrate obtained from citrus fruits. Kaolin and pectin are not absorbed following oral use. Some preparations may contain opiate compounds and atropine-like substances. Observe bottle for ingredients. Never use in children less than 3 years of age.

Pregnancy Risk Category: C

Lactation Risk Category: L1

Adult Concerns: Constipation, fecal impaction, reduce drug absorption

Pediatric Concerns: None reported via milk.

Drug Interactions: Decreases oral absorption of clindamycin, tetracyclines, penicillamine, digoxin.

Theoretic Infant Dose:

Relative Infant Dose:

Adult Dose: 60-120 mL PRN

Alternatives:

$T\frac{1}{2}$ =		M/P =
PHL =		PB =
T_{max} =		Oral = 0%
MW =		pKa =
Vd =		

References:

KAVA-KAVA
Trade: Awa, Kew, Tonga
Can/Aus/UK:
Uses: Sedative and sleep enhancement
LRC: L5
AAP: Not reviewed

Kava is the dried rhizome and roots of Piper methysticum. While more than 20 varieties are know, the black and white grades are most popular. Kava drink is prepared from the rhizome by steeping the pulverized root in hot water. It is then filtered and drunk. It is indigenous to the islands of the South Pacific where it is used similar to alcohol to induce relaxation.[1] The activity of kava appears to be related to several dihydropyrones that possess CNS activity including methysticine, kawain, dihydromethysticin, and yangonin. Studies of these agents suggest that they may induce mephenesin-like muscle relaxation in animals, similar in effect to the local anesthetics. Masticated kava induces a local anesthetic effect in the mouth. It is not known with certainty how these agents work, but it is apparently not at the opiate receptors. However, they do induce sleep and reduce anxiety. The CNS activity of kava is due to the lipid components, not the more polar water soluble components. In humans, kava produces mild euphoria, happiness, fluent and lively speech. High doses may lead to muscle weakness, visual and auditory changes. Heavy users are underweight, have reduced plasma protein levels, facial edema, scaly rashes, elevated HDL cholesterol, blood in the urine, and abnormal CBS (elevated RBCs, reduced platelets, and lymphocytes). Discolored, flaky skin, and reddened eyes is common. Ethanol dramatically increases the toxicity of kava and should not be co-mixed. No data are available on its use in breastfeeding mothers, but care should be exercised. The German Commission E monographs state that it is contraindicated in pregnant and lactating women.[2]

Pregnancy Risk Category:

Lactation Risk Category: L5

Adult Concerns: High doses may lead to muscle weakness, visual and auditory changes. Heavy users are underweight, have reduced plasma protein levels, facial edema, scaly rashes, elevated HDL cholesterol, blood in the urine, and abnormal CBS (elevated RBCs, reduced platelets, and lymphocytes). Discolored, flaky skin and reddened eyes is common. Ethanol dramatically increases the toxicity of kava and should not be co-mixed.

Pediatric Concerns: None reported but caution is recommended.

Drug Interactions: Admixing with alcohol dramatically increases toxicity of kava.

455

Theoretic Infant Dose:

Relative Infant Dose:

Adult Dose:

Alternatives:

References:
1. Review of Natural Products Facts and Comparisons, St Louis, MO 1996.
2. The Complete German Commission E Monographs. Ed. M. Blumenthal Amer Botanical Council 1998.

KETOCONAZOLE

Trade: Nizoral Shampoo, Nizoral
Can/Aus/UK: Nizoral
Uses: Antifungal, anti-dandruff
LRC: L2
AAP: Maternal Medication Usually Compatible with Breastfeeding

Ketoconazole is an antifungal similar in structure to miconazole and clotrimazole. It is used orally, topically, and via shampoo.[1] Ketoconazole is not detected in plasma after chronic shampooing. In a study of one patient (82 kg) receiving 200 mg daily for 10 days, milk samples were taken at 1.75, 3.25, 6.0, 8.0, and 24 hours after the tenth dose.[2] The average concentration of ketoconazole over the 24 hours was 68 μg/L while the C_{max} at 3.25 hours was 0.22 mg/L. The absorption of ketoconazole is highly variable and could be reduced in infants due to the alkaline condition induced by milk ingestion.[3] Ketoconazole requires acidic conditions to be absorbed, and its absorption and distribution in children is not known. Regardless, ketoconazole is probably safe in breastfeeding infants.

Pregnancy Risk Category: C

Lactation Risk Category: L2

Adult Concerns: Nausea, vomiting, itching, dizziness, fever, chills, hypertension, hepatotoxicity

Pediatric Concerns: None reported in one case.

Drug Interactions: Decreased ketoconazole levels occur with rifampin, isoniazid and phenytoin use. Theophylline levels may be reduced. Absorption requires acid pH, so anything increasing gastric pH will significantly reduce absorption. This includes cimetidine, ranitidine, famotidine, omeprazole, sucralfate, antacids, etc. Do not coadminister with cisapride or terfenadine (very dangerous). May increase cyclosporin levels by 50%, inhibits warfarin metabolism and prolongs coagulation.

Theoretic Infant Dose: 10.2 μg/kg/day

Relative Infant Dose: 0.4%

Adult Dose: 200-400 mg daily

Alternatives: Fluconazole

T½ =	2-8 hours	M/P =	
PHL =		PB =	99%
T$_{max}$ =	1-2 hours	Oral =	Variable (75%)
MW =	531	pKa =	
Vd =			

References:
1. Pharmaceutical Manufacturer Prescribing Information. 1996.
2. Moretti ME, Ito S, Koren G. Disposition of maternal ketoconazole in breastmilk. Am J Obstet Gynecol 1995; 173(5):1625-1626.
3. Force RW, Nahata MC. Salivary concentrations of ketoconazole and fluconazole: implications for drug efficacy in oropharyngeal and esophageal candidiasis. Ann Pharmacother 1995; 29(1):10-15.

KETOPROFEN

Trade: Orudis, Oruvail
Can/Aus/UK: Apo-Keto, Orudis, Rhodis, Oruvail, Rhovail
Uses: NSAID analgesic
LRC: L3
AAP: Not reviewed

Ketoprofen is a typical nonsteroidal analgesic. It is structurally similar to ibuprofen. Due to tablet formulation (Oruvail), maternal absorption is prolonged during the day requiring 6-7 hours to peak levels.[1] Studies in animals indicate the milk concentration to be 4-5% of maternal plasma levels. There is no information available on levels produced in human breastmilk. See ibuprofen as alternative.

Pregnancy Risk Category: B

Lactation Risk Category: L3

Adult Concerns: GI distress, diarrhea, vomiting, gastric bleeding

Pediatric Concerns: None reported but observe for GI symptoms including diarrhea, cramping.

Drug Interactions: May prolong prothrombin time when used with warfarin. Antihypertensive effects of ACEi family may be blunted or completely abolished by NSAIDs. Some NSAIDs may block antihypertensive effect of beta blockers, diuretics. Used with cyclosporin, may dramatically increase renal toxicity. May increase digoxin, phenytoin, lithium levels. May increase toxicity of methotrexate. May increase bioavailability of penicillamine. Probenecid may increase NSAID levels.

Theoretic Infant Dose:

Relative Infant Dose:

Adult Dose: 50-75 mg TID-QID

Alternatives: Ibuprofen

$T\frac{1}{2}$ =	2-4 hours	M/P =	
PHL =		PB =	> 99%
T_{max} =	1.2	Oral =	90%
MW =	254	pKa =	4.0
Vd =	0.1-0.5		

References:
1. Pharmaceutical Manufacturer Prescribing Information. 1996.

KETOROLAC
Trade: Toradol, Acular
Can/Aus/UK: Acular, Toradol
Uses: Non-steroidal antiinflammatory, analgesic
LRC: L2
AAP: Maternal Medication Usually Compatible with Breastfeeding

Ketorolac is a popular, nonsteroidal analgesic. Although previously used in labor and delivery, its use has subsequently been contraindicated because it is believed to adversely effect fetal circulation and inhibit uterine contractions, thus increasing the risk of hemorrhage.

In a study of 10 lactating women who received 10 mg orally four times daily, milk levels of ketorolac were not detectable in 4 of the subjects.[1] In the 6 remaining, the concentration of ketorolac in milk 2 hours after a dose ranged from 5.2 to 7.3 µg/L on day 1 and 5.9 to 7.9 µg/L on day 2. In most patients, the breastmilk level was never above 5 µg/L. The maximum daily dose an infant could absorb (maternal dose = 40 mg/day) would range from 3.16 to 7.9 µg/day assuming a milk volume of 400 mL or 1000 mL. An infant would therefore receive less than 0.2% of the daily maternal dose (Please note, the original paper contained a misprint on the daily intake of ketorolac (mg instead of µg).

Pregnancy Risk Category: B in 1st and 2nd trimester
                                            D in 3rd trimester

Lactation Risk Category: L2

Adult Concerns: GI irritability, dry mouth, nausea, vomiting, edema, or rash

Pediatric Concerns: None reported in one study.

Drug Interactions: May prolong prothrombin time when used with warfarin. Antihypertensive effects of ACEi family may be blunted or completely abolished by NSAIDs. Some NSAIDs may block antihypertensive effect of beta blockers, diuretics. Used with cyclosporin, may dramatically increase renal toxicity. May increase digoxin, phenytoin, lithium levels. May increase toxicity of methotrexate. May increase bioavailability of penicillamine. Probenecid may increase NSAID levels.

Theoretic Infant Dose: 1.18 μg/kg/day

Relative Infant Dose: < 0.2%

Adult Dose: 30 mg q 6 hours

Alternatives: Ibuprofen

T½ =	2.4-8.6 hours	M/P =	0.015-0.037
PHL =		PB =	99%
T$_{max}$ =	0.5 - 1 hours	Oral =	> 81%
MW =	255	pKa =	3.5
Vd =	0.15-0.33		

References:

1. Wischnik A, Manth SM, Lloyd J, Bullingham R, Thompson JS. The excretion of ketorolac tromethamine into breastmilk after multiple oral dosing. Eur J Clin Pharmacol 1989; 36(5):521-524.

KOMBUCHA TEA
Trade:
Can/Aus/UK:
Uses: Herbal tea
LRC: L5
AAP: Not reviewed

Kombucha tea is a popular health beverage made by incubating the Kombucha mushroom in sweet black tea. During 1995, several reported cases of toxicity and one fatality were reported to the CDC.[1] Based on these reports, the Iowa Department of Health has recommended that persons refrain from drinking Kombucha tea until the role of the tea in these cases has been resolved.

Pregnancy Risk Category:

Lactation Risk Category: L5

Adult Concerns: Shortness of breath, respiratory distress, fatigue, metabolic acidosis, disseminated intravascular coagulopathy

Pediatric Concerns: Caution is recommended.

Drug Interactions:

Theoretic Infant Dose:

Relative Infant Dose:

Adult Dose: N/A

Alternatives:

References:

1.   Unexplained severe illness possibly associated with consumption of Kombucha tea--Iowa, 1995 MMWR Morb Mortal Wkly Rep 1995; 44(48):892-900.

LABETALOL
Trade: Trandate, Normodyne
Can/Aus/UK: Trandate, Presolol, Labrocol
Uses: Antihypertensive, beta blocker
LRC: L2
AAP: Maternal Medication Usually Compatible with Breastfeeding

Labetalol is a selective beta blocker with moderate lipid solubility that is used as an antihypertensive and for treating angina.   In one study of 3 women receiving   600 mg, 600 mg, or 1200 mg/day,   the peak concentration of labetalol in breastmilk was 129, 223, and 662 µg/L respectively.[1]   In only one infant were measurable plasma levels found, 18 µg/L following a maternal dose of 600 mg.   Therefore, only small amounts are secreted into human milk.

Pregnancy Risk Category: C

Lactation Risk Category: L2

Adult Concerns: Bradycardia, hypotension, dizziness, nausea, aggravation of asthma, lethargy

Pediatric Concerns: None reported but observe for hypotension, apnea.

Drug Interactions: Decreased effect when used with aluminum salts, barbiturates, calcium salts, cholestyramine, NSAIDs, ampicillin, rifampin, and salicylates. Beta blockers may reduce the effect of oral sulfonylureas (hypoglycemic agents).   Increased toxicity/effect when used with other antihypertensives, contraceptives, MAO inhibitors, cimetidine, and numerous other products.   See   drug interaction reference for complete listing.

Theoretic Infant Dose: 99.3 µg/kg/day

Relative Infant Dose: 0.57%

Adult Dose: 200-400 mg BID

Alternatives: Propranolol, Metoprolol

T½	=	6-8 hours	M/P	=	0.8-2.6
PHL	=		PB	=	50%
Tmax	=	1-2 hours (oral)	Oral	=	30-40%
MW	=	328	pKa	=	A7.4, B8.7
Vd	=	10			

References:
1. Lunell NO, Kulas J, Rane A. Transfer of labetalol into amniotic fluid and breastmilk in lactating women. Eur J Clin Pharmacol 1985; 28(5):597-599.

LAMIVUDINE
Trade: Epivir-Hbv, 3TC
Can/Aus/UK: 3TC, 3TC
Uses: Antiviral
LRC: L2
AAP: Not reviewed

Lamivudine is a synthetic nucleoside analogue antiviral used for the treatment of Hepatitis B or HIV infections. It is presently in numerous other combination products(Combivir, Ziagen, etc.). In a study of 20 women receiving either 300 mg once daily or 150 mg twice daily one week postpartum, the mean breastmilk concentration was 1.22 mg/L (range= 0.5-6.09) or 0.183 mg/kg/day. This is significantly less than the clinical dose normally administered to infants (4-8 mg/kg/d). The authors suggested that the amount ingested via breastmilk was negligible relative to therapeutic dosing and would not provide adequate antiretroviral drug concentrations for a neonate.

Pregnancy Risk Category: C

Lactation Risk Category: L2

Adult Concerns: Adverse events include lactic acidosis, severe hepatomegaly, pancreatitis, malaise, fatigue, upper respiratory infections, nausea, vomiting, headache, and mylagia.

Pediatric Concerns: None reported in one study. Dose via milk is apparently too low to produce adverse effects.

Drug Interactions: Use with cotrimoxazole (trimethoprim and sulfamethoxazole) could potentially elevate levels of lamivudine. Plasma levels of loviride were reduced by lamivudine. Do not use with ribavirin due to risk of fatal lactic acidosis.

Theoretic Infant Dose: 0.183 mg/kg/day

Relative Infant Dose: 4.2%

Adult Dose: 100 mg daily for hepatitis B infections.

Alternatives:

T½ =	5-7 hours	M/P =	
PHL =	13.95 hours	PB =	< 36%
T_{max} =	1-1.5 hours	Oral =	82%
MW =	229	pKa =	
Vd =	1.0		

References:

1   Moodley J, Moodley D, Pillay K, Coovadia H, Saba J, van Leeuwen R,
     Goodwin C, Harrigan PR, Moore KH, Stone C, Plumb R, Johnson MA.
     Pharmacokinetics and antiretroviral activity of lamivudine alone or when
     coadministered with zidovudine in human immunodeficiency virus type 1-
     infected pregnant women and their offspring. J Infect Dis 1998;
     178(5):1327-1333.

LAMOTRIGINE

Trade: Lamictal
Can/Aus/UK: Lamictal
Uses: Anticonvulsant
LRC: L3
AAP: Drugs whose effect on nursing infants is unknown but may
be of concern

Lamotrigine is a new anticonvulsant primarily indicated for treatment of
simple and complex partial seizures. In a study of a 24 year old female
receiving 300 mg/day lamotrigine during pregnancy, maternal serum
levels and cord levels of lamotrigine at birth were 3.88 µg/mL in the
mother and 3.26 µg/mL in the cord blood.[1] By day 22, the maternal
serum levels were 9.61 µg/mL, the milk concentration was 6.51 mg/L,
and the infant's serum level was 2.25 µg/mL. Following a reduction in
dose, the prior levels decreased significantly over the next weeks. The
milk/plasma ratio at the highest maternal serum level was 0.562. The
estimated dose to infant would be approximately 2-5 mg per day
assuming a maternal dose of 200-300mg per day. The infant developed
normally in every way.

In another study of a single mother receiving 200 mg/day lamotrigine,
milk levels of lamotrigine immediately prior to the next dose (trough) at
steady state were 3.48 mg/L (13.6 uM).[2] They estimated the daily dose
to infant to be 0.5 mg/kg/day. The above authors suggest that infants,
while developing normally, should probably be monitored periodically
for plasma levels of lamotrigine.

The manufacturer reports that in a group of 5 women (no dose listed),
breastmilk concentrations of lamotrigine ranged from 0.07-5.03 mg/L.[3]
Breastmilk levels averaged 40-45% of maternal plasma levels. No ill
effects were noted in the infants.

In a study by Ohman of 9 breastfeeding women at 3 weeks postpartum, the median milk/plasma ratio was 0.61, and the nursed infants maintained lamotrigine concentrations of approximately 30% of the mother's plasma levels.[4] The authors estimated the dose to the infant at >= 0.2-1 mg/kg/d. No adverse effects were noted in the infants.

Pregnancy Risk Category: C

Lactation Risk Category: L3

Adult Concerns: Rash, fatigue, ataxia, dizziness, ataxia, somnolence, tremor, nausea, vomiting, and headache.   Breast pain has been infrequently reported.

Pediatric Concerns: Breastmilk levels are relatively high and RID is high as well.   Reported infant plasma levels are about 30% of maternal plasma levels. However, no untoward effects have been noted in any of these studies.

Drug Interactions: Acetaminophen reduces lamotrigine half-life by 15-20% and may require increased doses.   Carbamazepine, phenytoin, phenobarbital, and other anticonvulsants may reduce plasma levels of lamotrigine by increasing clearance, but this is highly variable.

Theoretic Infant Dose: 0.97 mg/kg/day

Relative Infant Dose: 22.7%

Adult Dose: 150-250 mg BID

Alternatives:

T½ =	29 hours	M/P =	0.562
PHL =		PB =	55%
T$_{max}$ =	1-4 hours	Oral =	98%
MW =	256	pKa =	5.7
Vd =	0.9-1.3 L/kg		

References:

1. Rambeck B, Kurlemann G, Stodieck SR, May TW, Jurgens U. Concentrations of lamotrigine in a mother on lamotrigine treatment and her newborn child. Eur J Clin Pharmacol 1997; 51(6):481-484.
2. Tomson T, Ohman I, Vitols S. Lamotrigine in pregnancy and lactation: a case report. Epilepsia 1997; 38(9):1039-1041.
3. Biddlecombe RA. Analysis of breastmilk samples for lamotrigine. Internal document BDCR/93/0011. Glaxo-Wellcome 2004.
4. Ohman I, Vitols S, Tomson T. Lamotrigine in pregnancy: pharmacokinetics during delivery, in the neonate, and during lactation. Epilepsia 2000; 41(6):709-713.

LANSOPRAZOLE

Trade: Prevacid, Prevpac, Prevacid Naprapak
Can/Aus/UK: Prevacid, Zoton
Uses: Reduces stomach acid secretion.
LRC: L3
AAP: Not reviewed

Lansoprazole is a new proton pump inhibitor that suppresses the release of acid protons from the parietal cells in the stomach, effectively raising the pH of the stomach. Structurally similar to omeprazole, it is very unstable in stomach acid and to a large degree is denatured by acidity of the infant's stomach.[1] A new study shows milk levels of omeprazole are minimal (see omeprazole) and it is likely milk levels of lansoprazole are small as well. Although there are no studies of lansoprazole in breastfeeding mothers, transfer to milk and its oral absorption (via milk) is likely to be minimal in a breastfed infant.

Lansoprazole is secreted in animal milk although no data are available on the amount secreted in human milk. The only likely untoward effects would be a reduced stomach acidity. This product has no current pediatric indications although it is occasionally used in severe cases of erosive gastritis.

Prevpac contains Lansoprazole, Amoxicillin, and Clarithromycin. It is primarily indicated for treatment of H.Pylori infections which cause stomach ulcers.

Prevacid NapraPAC contains 15 mg lansoprazole and 500 mg naproxen for use in reducing the risk of NSAID-associated gastric ulcers in patients with a history of documented gastric ulcer who require the use of an NSAID for treatment of the signs and symptoms of rheumatoid arthritis, osteoarthritis, and ankylosing spondylitis.

Pregnancy Risk Category: B

Lactation Risk Category: L3

Adult Concerns: Reduced stomach acidity. Diarrhea, nausea, elevated liver enzymes.

Pediatric Concerns: None reported via milk. It is unlikely to be absorbed while dissolved in milk due to instability in acid.

Drug Interactions: Decreased absorption of ketoconazole, itraconazole, and other drugs dependent on acid for absorption. Theophylline clearance is increased slightly. Reduced lansoprazole absorption when used with sucralfate (30%).

Theoretic Infant Dose:

Relative Infant Dose:

Adult Dose: 15-30 mg TID

Alternatives: Omeprazole, famotidine

T½ =	1.5 hours	M/P =	
PHL =		PB =	97%
T$_{max}$ =	1.7 hours	Oral =	80%
			(Enteric only)
MW =	369	pKa =	
Vd =			

References:
1. Pharmaceutical Manufacturer Prescribing Information.

LATANOPROST

Trade: Xalatan
Can/Aus/UK: Optimol, Xalatan, Betim
Uses: Prostaglandin for glaucoma
LRC: L3
AAP: Not reviewed

Latanoprost is a prostaglandin F2-alpha analogue used for the treatment of ocular hypertension and glaucoma. One drop used daily is usually effective.[1] No data are available on the transfer of this product into human milk, but it is unlikely. Prostaglandins are by nature, rapidly metabolized. Plasma levels are barely detectable and then only for 1 hour after use. Combined with the short half-life, minimal plasma levels, and poor oral bioavailability, untoward effects via milk are unlikely.

Pregnancy Risk Category: C

Lactation Risk Category: L3

Adult Concerns: Ocular irritation, headache, rash, muscle aches, joint pain

Pediatric Concerns: None reported via milk.

Drug Interactions:

Theoretic Infant Dose:

Relative Infant Dose:

Adult Dose: 1 drop in affected eye daily

Alternatives:

T½ =	< 30 minutes	M/P =	
PHL =		PB =	
T$_{max}$ =	< 1 hour	Oral =	Nil
MW =		pKa =	
Vd =	0.16		

References:
1. Pharmaceutical Manufacturer Prescribing Information.

LEAD
Trade:
Can/Aus/UK:
Uses: Environmental pollutant
LRC: L5
AAP: Not reviewed

Lead is an environmental pollutant. It serves no useful purpose in the body and tends to accumulate in the body's bony structures based on their exposure. Due to the rapid development of the nervous system, children are particularly sensitive to elevated levels.

Lead apparently transfers into human milk at a rate proportional to maternal blood levels, but the absolute degree of transfer is controversial. Studies of milk lead levels vary enormously and probably reflect the enormous difficulty in accurately measuring lead in milk.

One study evaluated lead transfer into human milk in population of women with an average blood lead of 45 µg/dL (considered very high).[1] The average lead level in milk was 2.47 µg/dL. Using these parameters, the average intake in an infant would be 8.1 µg/kg/d. The daily permissible level by WHO is 5.0 µg/kg/d. Using these parameters, mothers contaminated with lead should not breastfeed their infants.

However, in another study of two lactating women whose blood lead levels were 29 and 33 µg/dl, the breastmilk levels were < 0.005 µg/mL and < 0.010 µg/mL respectively.[2] Although both infants had high lead levels (38 µg/dl and 44 µg/dl), it was probably derived from the environment or in-utero. Using these data, breastfeeding would appear to be safe.

In a larger study of Shanghai mothers (n=165), the transfer of lead to the fetus was highly correlated with maternal blood lead levels (maternal blood vs. cord = 13.2 µg/dL and 6.9 µg/dL).[3] Lead levels in the cord blood and breastmilk increased with the lead level in the maternal blood, with coefficient of correlation of 0.714 and 0.353 respectively. The average concentration of lead in breastmilk for 12 occupationally exposed women (lead-exposed jobs) was 52.7 µg/L, which was almost 12 times higher than that for the occupationally non-exposed population(4.43 mg/dL). These results suggest that lead levels in milk could pose a potential health hazard to the breastfed infant but only in those moms with high plasma lead levels.

In another rather elegant study of milk lead levels, Gulson et.al. collected samples from 21 mothers and 24 infants over a 6 month period.[4] They reported lead concentrations in milk ranging from 0.09-3.1 µg Pb/kg or ppb (mean 0.73 µg/kg) while the blood lead levels were all less than 5 µg/dL with exception of one mother. The major source of lead to the infant during this period was from maternal bone and diet.

Nashashibi reports on the transfer of lead from the mother to fetus and into her breastmilk.[5] In a group of 47 women, the mean maternal blood lead concentration was 14.9 µg/dL, while in milk the mean lead level was 2.0 µg/dL. Mean lead level in cord blood was 13.1 µg/dL. These data suggest a close correlation between maternal blood and cord blood lead levels, and maternal blood and milk levels.

In the last decade, the permissible blood level (according to CDC) in children has dropped from 25 to less than 10 µg/dL. Lead poisoning is known to significantly alter IQ and neuropsychologic development, particularly in infants. Therefore, infants receiving breastmilk from mothers with high lead levels should be closely monitored, and both mother and infant may require chelation and the infant transferred to formula. Depending on the choice of chelator, mothers undergoing chelation therapy to remove lead may mobilize significant quantities of lead and should not breastfeed during the treatment period unless the chelator is Succimer.

Pregnancy Risk Category:

Lactation Risk Category: **L5**

Adult Concerns: Constipation, abdominal pain, anemia, anorexia, vomiting, lethargy

Pediatric Concerns: Pediatric lead poisoning but appears unlikely via milk. More likely environmental.

Drug Interactions:

Theoretic Infant Dose:

Relative Infant Dose:

Adult Dose:

Alternatives:

T½ =	20-30 years (bone)	M/P =	
PHL =		PB =	
T$_{max}$ =		Oral =	5-10%
MW =	207	pKa =	
Vd =			

References:

1. Namihira D, Saldivar L, Pustilnik N, Carreon GJ, Salinas ME. Lead in human blood and milk from nursing women living near a smelter in Mexico City. J Toxicol Environ Health 1993; 38(3):225-232.
2. Baum C, Shannon M. Lead-Poisoned lactating women have insignificant lead in breastmilk. J Clin Toxicol 1995; 33(5):540-541.
3. Li PJ, Sheng YZ, Wang QY, Gu LY, Wang YL. Transfer of lead via placenta and breastmilk in human. Biomed Environ Sci 2000; 13(2):85-89.
4. Gulson BL, Jameson CW, Mahaffey KR, Mizon KJ, Patison N, Law AJ, Korsch MJ, Salter MA. Relationships of lead in breastmilk to lead in blood, urine, and diet of the infant and mother. Environ Health Perspect 1998; 106(10):667-674.
5. Nashashibi N, Cardamakis E, Bolbos G, Tzingounis V. Investigation of kinetic of lead during pregnancy and lactation. Gynecol Obstet Invest 1999; 48(3):158-162.

LEFLUNOMIDE

Trade: Arava
Can/Aus/UK: Arava
Uses: Antimetabolite anti-inflammatory
LRC: L4
AAP: Not reviewed

Leflunomide is a new anti-inflammatory agent used for arthritis. It is an immunosuppressant that reduces pyrimidine synthesis.[1] Leflunomide is metabolized to the active metabolite referred to as M1, which has a long half-life and slow elimination. This product is a potent immunosuppressant with a potential elevated risk of malignancy and teratogenicity in pregnant women. It is not known if it transfers into human milk, but use of this product while breastfeeding would be a highly risky.

Pregnancy Risk Category: X

Lactation Risk Category: L4

Adult Concerns: Hypertension, diarrhea, respiratory infection, alopecia, and rash are the most common adult side effects.

Pediatric Concerns: No reports via milk, but due to the danger of this product, breastfeeding is not recommended.

Drug Interactions: Cholestyramine produces a rapid reduction of plasma levels of the active metabolite. A significant increase in hepatotoxicity when admixed with other hepatotoxic drugs. Increased plasma drug levels (M1) when used with NSAIDs and rifampin May increase plasma free drug levels of tolbutamide.

Theoretic Infant Dose:

Relative Infant Dose:

Adult Dose: 20 mg daily

Alternatives:

T½ =	> 15-18 hours	M/P =	
PHL =		PB =	
Tmax =	6-12 hours	Oral =	80%
MW =	270	pKa =	
Vd =			

References:
1.   Pharmaceutical Manufacturer Prescribing Information. 1999.

LEPIRUDIN
Trade: Refludan
Can/Aus/UK: Refludan
Uses: Thrombin inhibitor, anticoagulant
LRC: L3
AAP: Not reviewed

Lepirudin is a large molecular weight polypeptide that is a direct inhibitor of thrombin. It is a polypeptide that consists of 65 amino acids and has a molecular weight of 6979 daltons. It is very unlikely this large peptide would be transported into human milk after 48 hours postnatally. Most risk would be the first 24-48 hours postnatally when many proteins can be transported into human milk. However, it is unlikely this agent would be stable or absorbed in the GI tract of an infant. No data on human milk levels are available.

Pregnancy Risk Category: B

Lactation Risk Category: L3

Adult Concerns: Hemorrrhagic events, bleeding.   Bronchospasm, cough, stridor, dyspnea have been reported as common.

Pediatric Concerns: None reported via milk.

Drug Interactions: Additive with other anticoagulants such as coumarin or antithrombotic agents, etc.

Theoretic Infant Dose:

Relative Infant Dose:

Adult Dose: 0.15 mg/kg/hour administered continuously.

Alternatives:

T½ =	1.3 hours	M/P =	
PHL =		PB =	
T$_{max}$ =	3-4 hours sc	Oral =	Nil
MW =	6979	pKa =	
Vd =			

References:
1. Pharmaceutical Manufacturers Prescribing Information, 2003.

LETROZOLE

Trade: Femara
Can/Aus/UK: Femara
Uses: Aromatase inhibitor of estrogen synthesis.
LRC: L4
AAP: Not reviewed

Letrozole is an aromatase inhibitor of estrogen synthesis and is used to treat estrogen-receptor positive breast cancer and other syndromes.[1] No data are available on its transfer to human milk, but I would suspect the levels are low. However, it has a very long half-life which is concerning in a breastfed infant and could lead to higher plasma levels over time. Therefore, the transfer of small amounts of this agent to an infant could seriously impair bone growth and sexual development of an infant, and for this reason it is probably somewhat hazardous to use in a breastfeeding mother.

Pregnancy Risk Category: D

Lactation Risk Category: L4

Adult Concerns: Adverse reactions include fatigue, chest pain, edema, hot flushes, hypertension, nausea, constipation, diarrhea, vomiting, bone pain, back pain, arthralgia, limb pain, dyspnea, cough, and chest wall pain.

Pediatric Concerns: None reported via milk, but this agent is probably too hazardous to use in a breastfeeding woman.

Drug Interactions: Tamoxifen may reduce letrozole plasma levels by 38%.

Theoretic Infant Dose:

Relative Infant Dose:

Adult Dose: 2.5 mg/day.

Alternatives:

T½ =	48 hours	M/P =	
PHL =		PB =	Weak
T$_{max}$ =		Oral =	90%
MW =	285	pKa =	
Vd =	1.9		

References:
1. Pharmaceutical Manufacturers prescribing information, 2003.

LEUPROLIDE ACETATE

Trade: Lupron, Viadur
Can/Aus/UK: Lupron, Prostap
Uses: Gonadotropin-Releasing Hormone Analog
LRC: L5
AAP: Not reviewed

Leuprolide is a synthetic nonapeptide analog of naturally occurring gonadotropin-releasing hormone with greater potency than the naturally occurring hormone. After initial stimulation, it inhibits gonadotropin release from the pituitary and, after sustained use, suppresses ovarian and testicular hormone synthesis(2-4 weeks).[1] Almost complete suppression of estrogen, progesterone, and testosterone result.[2] Although Lupron is contraindicated in pregnant women, no reported birth defects have been reported in humans. It is commonly used prior to fertilization but should never be used during pregnancy.

It is not known whether leuprolide transfers into human milk, but due to its nonapeptide structure, it is not likely that its transfer would be extensive. In addition, animal studies have found that it has zero oral bioavailability; therefore, it is unlikely it would be orally bioavailable in the human infant if ingested via milk. Its effect on lactation is unknown, but it could suppress lactation particularly early postpartum.[3] Lupron would reduce estrogen and progestin levels to menopausal ranges, which may or may not suppress lactation, depending on the duration of lactation. Interestingly, several studies show no change in prolactin levels although these were not in lactating women. One study of a hyperprolactinemic patient showed significant suppression of prolactin which is the reason for my L5 risk categorization. It is of no risk to the breastfed infant, only to milk production.

Pregnancy Risk Category: X

Lactation Risk Category: L5

Adult Concerns: Vasomotor hot flashes, gynecomastia, edema, bone pain, thrombosis, and GI disturbances. Body odor, fever, headache.

Pediatric Concerns: May suppress lactation, particularly early in lactation.

Drug Interactions:

Theoretic Infant Dose:

Relative Infant Dose:

Adult Dose: 3.75 mg q month

Alternatives:

T½ =	3.6 hours	M/P =	
PHL =		PB =	43-49%
T$_{max}$ =	4-6 hours	Oral =	None
MW =	1400	pKa =	
Vd =	0.52		

References:
1. Sennello LT, Finley RA, Chu SY, Jagst C, Max D, Rollins DE, Tolman KG. Single-dose pharmacokinetics of leuprolide in humans following intravenous and subcutaneous administration. J Pharm Sci 1986; 75(2):158-160.
2. Chantilis SJ, Barnett-Hamm C, Byrd WE, Carr BR. The effect of gonadotropin-releasing hormone agonist on thyroid-stimulating hormone and prolactin secretion in adult premenopausal women. Fertil Steril 1995; 64(4):698-702.
3. Frazier SH. Personnal communication. 1997.

LEVALBUTEROL

Trade: Xopenex
Can/Aus/UK:
Uses: Bronchodilator
LRC: L2
AAP: Not reviewed

Levalbuterol is the active (R)-enantiomer of the drug substance racemic albuterol. It is a popular and new bronchodilator used in asthmatics.[1] No data are available on breastmilk levels. After inhalation, plasma levels are incredibly low, averaging 1.1 nanogram/mL. It is very unlikely that enough would enter milk to produce clinical effects in an infant. This product is commonly used in infancy for asthma and other bronchoconstrictive illnesses.

Pregnancy Risk Category: C

Lactation Risk Category: L2

Adult Concerns: Tachycardia, tremors, dizziness, dyspepsia

Pediatric Concerns: None reported via milk.

Drug Interactions: Levalbuterol effects are reduce when used with beta blockers. Cardiovascular effects are potentiated when used with MAO inhibitors, tricyclic antidepressants, amphetamines, and inhaled anesthetics (enflurane).

Theoretic Infant Dose:

Relative Infant Dose:

Adult Dose: 0.63 mg every 6-8 hours by nebulization

Alternatives:

T½ =	3.3 hours	M/P =	
PHL =		PB =	
T$_{max}$ =	0.2 (inhalation)	Oral =	100%
MW =	275	pKa =	
Vd =			

References:
1.   Pharmaceutical Manufacturer Prescribing Information.

LEVETIRACETAM
Trade: Keppra
Can/Aus/UK: Keppra
Uses: Anticonvulsant
LRC: L3
AAP: Not reviewed

Levetiracetam is an new broad-spectrum antiepileptic agent.[1] It is structurally and pharmacologically dissimilar to all the other known anticonvulsants. No data are available on its transfer into human milk. The physicochemistry of this product would suggest that milk levels will be moderate, as it is not bound by protein, it is low in molecular weight, it is 100% orally bioavailable, it is lipophilic, and it is neuroactive. Although this product is popular for it limited side effect profile, some caution is recommended until data are available.

Pregnancy Risk Category: C

Lactation Risk Category: L3

Adult Concerns: Somnolence, weakness, infection, headache, and dizziness

Pediatric Concerns: None reported but caution is recommended.

Drug Interactions: Levetiracetam may significantly increase phenytoin plasma levels by as much as 52%.

Theoretic Infant Dose:

Relative Infant Dose:

Adult Dose: 1000 - 3000 mg daily

Alternatives:

T½ =	6-8 hours	M/P =	
PHL =		PB =	< 10%
T$_{max}$ =	1 hour	Oral =	100%
MW =	170	pKa =	
Vd =	0.7		

References:
1. Pharmaceutical Manufacturer Prescribing Information.

LEVOBUNOLOL

Trade: Bunolol
Can/Aus/UK: Betagan, Ophtho-Bunolol
Uses: Beta blocker for glaucoma
LRC: L3
AAP: Not reviewed

Levobunolol is a typical beta blocker used intraophthalmic for treatment of glaucoma.[1] Some absorption has been reported with resultant bradycardia in patients. No data on transfer to human milk are available.

Pregnancy Risk Category: C

Lactation Risk Category: L3

Adult Concerns: Bradycardia, hypotension, headache, dizziness, fatigue, lethargy

Pediatric Concerns: None reported via milk, but transfer of some beta blockers is reported. Observe for lethargy, hypotension, bradycardia, apnea.

Drug Interactions: May have increased toxicity when used with other systemic beta adrenergic blocking agents. May produce bradycardia following use with quinidine and verapamil.

Theoretic Infant Dose:

Relative Infant Dose:

Adult Dose: 1-2 drops BID

Alternatives:

T½ =	6.1 hours	M/P =	
PHL =		PB =	
T$_{max}$ =	3 hours	Oral =	Complete
MW =	291	pKa =	
Vd =	5.5		

References:
1. Pharmaceutical Manufacturer Prescribing Information. 1997.

LEVOCABASTINE
Trade: Livostin
Can/Aus/UK: Livostin
Uses: Ophthalmic antihistamine for itching
LRC: L2
AAP: Not reviewed

Levocabastine is an antihistamine primarily used via nasal spray and eye drops.[1] It is used for allergic rhinitis and ophthalmic allergies.[1] After application to eye or nose, very low levels are attained in the systemic circulation (< 1 ng/mL). In one nursing mother, it was calculated that the daily dose of levocabastine in the infant was about 0.5 µg, far too low to be clinically relevant.

Pregnancy Risk Category: C

Lactation Risk Category: L2

Adult Concerns: Sedation, dry mouth, fatigue, eye and nasal irritation

Pediatric Concerns: None reported via milk.

Drug Interactions:

Theoretic Infant Dose:

Relative Infant Dose:

Adult Dose: 1 drop QID

Alternatives:

$T\frac{1}{2}$ =	33-40 hours	M/P =	
PHL =		PB =	
T_{max} =	1-2 hours	Oral =	100%
MW =		pKa =	
Vd =			

References:
1. Pharmaceutical Manufacturer Prescribing Information. 1996.

LEVODOPA

Trade: Dopar, Larodopa
Can/Aus/UK: Sinemet, Prolopa, Endo Levodopa/Carbidopa, Kinson, Madopar, Brocadopa, Eldopa, Weldopa
Uses: Antiparkinsonian
LRC: L4
AAP: Not reviewed

Levodopa is a prodrug of dopamine used primarily for parkinsonian symptoms. Its use during pregnancy is extremely dangerous. In one group of 30 patients, levodopa significantly reduced prolactin plasma levels.[1] It could under certain circumstances reduce milk production as well.

Pregnancy Risk Category: C

Lactation Risk Category: L4

Adult Concerns: Nausea, vomiting, anorexia, orthostatic hypotension. Reduces prolactin levels and may reduce milk production. Do not use in glaucoma patients with MAO inhibitors, asthmatics, peptic ulcer disease, or parkinsonian disease.

Pediatric Concerns: None reported via milk, but reduced milk supply is a possible adverse effect.

Drug Interactions: MAO inhibitors may predispose to hypertensive reactions. Decreased effect when administered with phenytoin, pyridoxine, phenothiazines.

Theoretic Infant Dose:

Relative Infant Dose:

Adult Dose: 1-2 g TID

Alternatives:

$T^{1/2}$ =	1-3 hours	M/P =	
PHL =		PB =	< 36%
T_{max} =	1-2 hours	Oral =	41%-70%
MW =	197	pKa =	
Vd =			

References:
1. Barbieri C, Ferrari C, Caldara R, Curtarelli G. Growth hormone secretion in hypertensive patients: evidence for a derangement in central adrenergic function. Clin Sci (Lond) 1980; 58(2):135-138.

LEVOFLOXACIN

Trade: Levaquin, Quixin
Can/Aus/UK: Levaquin
Uses: Antibiotic
LRC: L3
AAP: Not reviewed

Levofloxacin is a pure (S) enantiomer of the racemic fluoroquinolone Ofloxacin. Its kinetics including milk levels should be identical.[1,2] See ofloxacin for specifics. The use of fluoroquinolones is increasing in pediatrics due to minimal toxicity.[3]

Pregnancy Risk Category: C

Lactation Risk Category: L3

Adult Concerns: Nausea, vomiting, diarrhea, abdominal cramps, GI bleeding

Pediatric Concerns: None reported, see ofloxacin.

Drug Interactions: Decreased absorption with antacids. Quinolones cause increased levels of caffeine, warfarin, cyclosporine, theophylline. Cimetidine, probenecid, azlocillin may increase ofloxacin levels. Increased risk of seizures when used with foscarnet.

Theoretic Infant Dose:

Relative Infant Dose:

Adult Dose: 500 mg daily

Alternatives: Norfloxacin, Ofloxacin, Trovafloxacin

$T\frac{1}{2}$ =	6-8 hours	M/P =	
PHL =		PB =	24-38%
T_{max} =	1-1.8 hours	Oral =	99%
MW =	370	pKa =	
Vd =	1.27		

References:
1. Pharmaceutical Manufacturer Prescribing Information.
2. McEvoy GE. (ed): AFHS Drug Information. New York, NY: 1997.
3. Ghaffar F, McCracken GH. Quinolones in Pediatrics. In: Hooper DC, Rubinstein E, editors. Quinolone Antimicrobial Agents. Washington, D.C.: ASM Press, 2003: 343-354.

LEVONORGESTREL

Trade: Norplant, Seasonale, Mirena
Can/Aus/UK: Norplant, Triquilar, Levelen, Microlut, Microval, Norgeston
Uses: Implantable, oral, and intrauterine contraceptives
LRC: L2
L3 for Seasonale
AAP: Maternal Medication Usually Compatible with Breastfeeding

Levonorgestrel (LNG) is the active progestin in Norplant and Mirena. Norplant is a contraceptive method that involves placing six match-size, flexible capsules under the skin of a woman's upper arm. These release a low dose of synthetic progestin continuously for up to five years. Mirena is a levonorgestrel-releasing intrauterine (IUD) contraceptive that delivers 20 μg/day of levonorgestrel directly into the uterus and protects against pregnancy for up to 5 full years. The contraceptive effect of Mirena is mainly based on the local effects of levonorgestrel in the uterine cavity.

From several studies, levonorgestrel appears to produce limited if any effect on milk volume or quality.[1] One report of 120 women with implants at 5-6 weeks postpartum showed no change in lactation.[2] The level of progestin in the infant is approximately 10% that of maternal circulation. In a study of 9 women who were taking levonorgestrel oral minipills (30 μg daily) and 10 women who were using the subdermal implants from 4-15 weeks postpartum, no significant differences in infant follicle stimulating hormone (FSH), luteinizing hormone (LH), or testosterone levels in urine were noted when compared to controls.[3] These results suggest that the sexual development of children exposed via milk to trace levels of LNG is normal.

The plasma concentration of levonorgestrel produced by Mirena are even lower than those produced by LNG contraceptive implants and with oral contraceptives. Because Mirena produces even lower plasma levels of this progestin, it is probably less likely to affect milk production than oral or implantable forms of progestins.

The new oral contraceptive Seasonale is extended-cycle oral contraceptive and contains both levonorgestrel and ethinyl estradiol. It is used continuously for a three month period followed by withdrawal and menstruation. Due to its estrogen content, caution is recommended in breastfeeding mothers due to potential reduced milk supply.

Pregnancy Risk Category: X

Lactation Risk Category: **L2**
L3 for Seasonale

Adult Concerns: Interruption of the menstrual cycle and spotting with headache, weight gain, and occasional depression

Pediatric Concerns: None reported via milk. However, Seasonale should be used with caution due to estrogen content. Some mothers have reported reduced milk supply with some oral and injectable progestin-only contraceptives.

Drug Interactions: Reduced effect of carbamazepine and phenytoin.

Theoretic Infant Dose:

Relative Infant Dose:

Adult Dose: Six 36 mg capsules subcutaneously

Alternatives:

T½ =	11-45 hours	M/P =	
PHL =		PB =	
Tmax =		Oral =	Complete
MW =	312	pKa =	
Vd =			

References:

1. Shaaban MM, Salem HT, Abdullah KA. Influence of levonorgestrel contraceptive implants, NORPLANT, initiated early postpartum upon lactation and infant growth. Contraception 1985; 32(6):623-635.
2. Shaaban MM. Contraception with progestogens and progesterone during lactation. J Steroid Biochem Mol Biol 1991; 40(4-6):705-710.
3. Shikary ZK, Betrabet SS, Toddywala WS, Patel DM, Datey S, Saxena BN. Pharmacodynamic effects of levonorgestrel (LNG) administered either orally or subdermally to early postpartum lactating mothers on the urinary levels of follicle stimulating hormone (FSH), luteinizing hormone (LH) and testosterone (T) in their breast-fed male infants. Contraception 1986; 34(4):403-412.

LEVONORGESTREL (Plan B)

Trade: Plan B
Can/Aus/UK:
Uses: Emergency contraceptive
LRC: L2
AAP: Not reviewed

Levonorgestrel is a progestin that can be used as an emergency contraceptive. It is believed to act by preventing ovulation or fertilization by altering tubal transport of sperm and/or ova.[1] It may as well partially inhibit implantation by altering the endometrium. For more details on detailed monograph on levonorgestrel.

Plan B is an emergency contraceptive that can be used to prevent pregnancy following unprotected intercourse or a known or suspected contraceptive failure. It is not effective if the woman is already pregnant or once the process of implantation has begun. To obtain maximal efficacy, the first tablet should be taken as soon as possible within 72 hours of intercourse. The second tablet should be taken 12 hour later.

Pregnancy Risk Category:

Lactation Risk Category: **L2**

Adult Concerns: Adverse effects include nausea(23%), vomiting(6%), abdominal pain, fatigue, headache, heavier menstrual bleeding, dizziness, breast tenderness.

Pediatric Concerns: None reported via milk, but this progestin is unlikely to bother a breastfed infant or alter milk production in general.

Drug Interactions:

Theoretic Infant Dose:

Relative Infant Dose:

Adult Dose: 0.75 mg (one tablet) initially following in 12 hours by second tablet.

Alternatives:

$T\frac{1}{2}$ =	11-45	M/P =	
PHL =		PB =	
T_{max} =	1.6 hours	Oral =	Complete
MW =	312	pKa =	
Vd =			

References:
1. Pharmaceutical Manufacturers prescribing information, 2003.

LEVONORGESTREL + ETHINYL ESTRADIOL (Preven)

Trade: Preven
Can/Aus/UK:
Uses: Emergency contraceptive
LRC: L3
AAP: Not reviewed

Levonorgestrel and ethinyl estradiol (Preven) can be used as an emergency contraceptive.[1] It is believed to act by preventing ovulation or fertilization by altering tubal transport of sperm and/or ova. It may as well partially inhibit implantation by altering the endometrium. For more details on each ingredient see their individual monographs.

Preven is an emergency contraceptive that can be used to prevent pregnancy following unprotected intercourse or a known or suspected contraceptive failure. It is not effective if the woman is already pregnant or once the process of implantation has begun. Each tablet contains 0.25 mg levonorgestrel and 0.05 mg ethinyl estradiol. They should not be used in known or suspected pregnancy, in patients with pulmonary edema, ischemic heart disease, deep vein thrombosis, etc. The initial treatment of 2 tablets should be administered as soon as possible but within 72 hours of unprotected intercourse. This is followed by the second dose of 2 tablets 12 hours later.

Pregnancy Risk Category:

Lactation Risk Category: L3

Adult Concerns: Adverse events include nausea, vomiting, menstrual cycle disturbances, breast tenderness, headaches, abdominal pain, and dizziness.

Pediatric Concerns: None reported in infants via milk. However estrogens and even progestins may in some patients suppress milk production. Caution is recommended.

Drug Interactions:

Theoretic Infant Dose:

Relative Infant Dose:

Adult Dose: 2 tablets followed in 12 hours by 2 additional tablets.

Alternatives: Plan B

References:
1. Pharmaceutical Manufacturers prescribing information, 2003.

LEVOTHYROXINE
Trade: Synthroid, Levothroid, Unithyroid, Eltroxin, Levoxyl, Thyroid
Can/Aus/UK: Eltroxin, Synthroid, Thyroxine, Oroxine,
Uses: Thyroid supplements
LRC: L1
AAP: Maternal Medication Usually Compatible with Breastfeeding.

Levothyroxine is also called T4. Most studies indicate that minimal levels of maternal thyroid are transferred into human milk, and further, that the amount secreted is extremely low and insufficient to protect a hypothyroid infant even while nursing.[1-3] The amount secreted after supplementing a breastfeeding mother is highly controversial and numerous reports conflict. Anderson indicates that levothyroxine is not detectable in breastmilk although others using sophisticated assay methods have shown extremely low levels (4 ng/mL).[4] It is generally recognized that some thyroxine will transfer but the amount will be extremely low. It is important to remember that supplementation with levothyroxine is designed to bring the mother into a euthyroid state, which is equivalent to the normal breastfeeding female. Hence, the risk of using exogenous thyroxine is no different than in a normal euthyroid mother. Liothyronine (T3) appears to transfer into milk in higher concentrations than levothyroxine (T4), but liothyronine is seldom used in clinical medicine due to its short half-life (< 1 day).[4]

Pregnancy Risk Category: A

Lactation Risk Category: L1

Adult Concerns: Nervousness, tremor, agitation, weight loss

Pediatric Concerns: None reported via milk.

Drug Interactions: Phenytoin may decrease levothyroxine levels. Cholestyramine may decreased absorption of levothyroxine. May increase oral hypoglycemic requirements and doses. May increase effects of oral
anticoagulants. Use with tricyclic antidepressants may increase toxicity.

Theoretic Infant Dose: 0.6 ng/kg/day

Relative Infant Dose:

Adult Dose: 75-125 µg daily

Alternatives:

$T\frac{1}{2}$ =	6-7 days	M/P =	
PHL =		PB =	99%
T_{max} =	2-4 hours	Oral =	50-80%
MW =	798	pKa =	
Vd =			

References:

1. Mizuta H, Amino N, Ichihara K, Harada T, Nose O, Tanizawa O, Miyai K. Thyroid hormones in human milk and their influence on thyroid function of breast-fed babies. Pediatr Res 1983; 17(6):468-471.
2. Oberkotter LV. Thyroid function and human breastmilk. Am J Dis Child 1983; 137(11):1131.
3. Sack J, Amado O, Lunenfeld B. Thyroxine concentration in human milk. J Clin Endocrinol Metab 1977; 45(1):171-173.
4. Anderson PO. Drugs and breast feeding. Semin Perinatol 1979; 3(3):271-278.

LIDOCAINE

Trade: Xylocaine
Can/Aus/UK: Xylocard, Xylocaine, Lignocaine, EMLA
Uses: Local anesthetic
LRC: L2
AAP: Maternal Medication Usually Compatible with Breastfeeding

Lidocaine is an antiarrhymic and a local anesthetic. In one study of a breastfeeding mother who received IV lidocaine for ventricular arrhythmias, the mother received approximately 965 mg over 7 hours including the bolus starting doses.[1] At seven hours, breastmilk samples were drawn and the concentration of lidocaine was 0.8 mg/L or 40% of the maternal plasma level (2.0 mg/L). Assuming that the mother's plasma was maintained at 5 μg/mL (therapeutic = 1.5-5 μg/mL), an infant consuming 1 L per day of milk would ingest approximately 2 mg/day. This amount is exceedingly low in view of the fact that the oral bioavailability of lidocaine is very poor (35%). The lidocaine dose recommended for pediatric arrhythmias is 1 mg/kg given as a bolus. Once absorbed by the liver, lidocaine is rapidly metabolized. These authors suggest that a mother could continue to breastfeed while on parenteral lidocaine.

Dryden and Lo have reported the transfer of lidocaine following tumescent liposuction in a 80 kg patient.[2] The areas undergoing liposuction were infiltrated with a 52 .5 mg/kg dose of lidocaine dissolved in 8400 cc of solution (total=4200 mg). Milk samples were drawn 17 hours, and plasma levels were drawn 18 hours following the procedure because other studies show lidocaine peaks in the plasma compartment at this time postoperatively. Milk levels of lidocaine were 0.55 mg/L while plasma levels were 1.2 mg/L. Breastmilk levels were 46% of the serum level. The authors conclude that it is unlikely toxic levels would be reached in a nursing infant.

In a study of 27 parturients who received an average of 82.1 mg bupivacaine and 183.3 mg lidocaine via an epidural catheter, lidocaine milk levels at 2, 6 , and 12 hours post administration were 0.86, 0.46, and 0.22 mg/L respectively.[3] Levels of bupivacaine in milk at 2, 6, and 12 hours were 0.09, 0.06, 0.04 mg/L respectively. The milk/serum ratio bases upon area under the curve values (AUC) were 1.07 and 0.34 for lidocaine and bupivacaine respectively. Based on AUC data of lidocaine and bupivacaine milk levels, the average milk concentration of these agents over 12 hours was 0.5 and 0.07 mg/L. Most of the infants had a maximal APGAR score.

In a study of 7 nursing mothers who received 3.6-7.2 mL of 2% lidocaine without adrenaline, the concentration of lidocaine in milk 3 and 6 hours after injection averaged 97.5 μg/L and 52.7 μg/L respectively.[4] These authors suggest that mothers who receive local injections of lidocaine can safely breastfeed.

Recommended doses are as follows: Caudal blockade, < 300 mg; Epidural blockade, < 300 mg; Dental nerve block, < 100 mg; tumescent liposuction, 4200 mg. When administered as a local anesthetic for dental and other surgical procedures, only small quantities are used, generally less than 40 mg. However, following liposuction, the amount used via instillation in the tissues is quite high. Nevertheless, maternal plasma and milk levels do not seem to approach high concentrations, and the oral bioavailability in the infant would be quite low (< 35%).

Pregnancy Risk Category: C

Lactation Risk Category: L2

Adult Concerns: Bradycardia, confusion, cardiac arrest, drowsiness, seizures, bronchospasm

Pediatric Concerns: None reported via milk.

Drug Interactions: Use of local anesthetics with sulfonamides may reduce antibacterial efficacy.

Theoretic Infant Dose: 0.075 mg/kg/day

Relative Infant Dose: 2.8%

Adult Dose: 50-100 mg PRN

Alternatives:

$T\frac{1}{2}$ =	1.8 hours	M/P =	0.4
PHL =	3 hours (neonate)	PB =	70%
T_{max} =	Immediate (IM, IV)	Oral =	< 35%
MW =	234	pKa =	7.9
Vd =	1.3		

References:
1. Zeisler JA, Gaarder TD, De Mesquita SA. Lidocaine excretion in breastmilk. Drug Intell Clin Pharm 1986; 20(9):691-693.
2. Dryden RM, Lo MW. Breastmilk lidocaine levels in tumescent liposuction. Plast Reconstr Surg 2000; 105(6):2267-2268.
3. Ortega D, Viviand X, Lorec AM, Gamerre M, Martin C, Bruguerolle B. Excretion of lidocaine and bupivacaine in breastmilk following epidural anesthesia for cesarean delivery. Acta Anaesthesiol Scand 1999; 43(4):394-397.
4. Giuliani M, Grossi GB, Pileri M, Lajolo C, Casparrini G. Could local anesthesia while breast-feeding be harmful to infants? J Pediatr Gastroenterol Nutr 2001; 32(2):142-144.

LINCOMYCIN
Trade: Lincocin
Can/Aus/UK: Lincocin
Uses: Antibiotic
LRC: L2
AAP: Not reviewed

Lincomycin is an effective antimicrobial used for gram positive and anaerobic infections. It is secreted into breastmilk in small but detectable levels. In a group of 9 mothers who received 500 mg every 6 hrs for 3 days, breastmilk concentrations ranged from 0.5 to 2.4 mg/L (mean = 1.28). In this same group, the maternal plasma levels averaged 1.37 mg/L.[1] Although effects on infant are unlikely, some modification of gut flora or diarrhea is possible.

Pregnancy Risk Category: B

Lactation Risk Category: L2

Adult Concerns: Diarrhea, changes in GI flora, colitis, blood dyscrasias, jaundice

Pediatric Concerns: None reported via milk but observe for GI symptoms such as diarrhea.

Drug Interactions: GI absorption of lincomycin is decreased when used with kaolin-pectin antidiarrheals. The actions of neuromuscular blockers may be enhanced when used with lincomycin.

Theoretic Infant Dose: 0.192 mg/kg/day

Relative Infant Dose: 0.67%

Adult Dose: 500 mg q 6-8 hours

Alternatives: Clindamycin

T½ =	4.4-6.4 hours	M/P =	0.9
PHL =		PB =	72%
T$_{max}$ =	2-4 hours	Oral =	< 30%
MW =	407	pKa =	
Vd =			

References:
1. Medina A, Fiske N, Hjelt-Harvey I, Brown CD, Prigot A. Absorption, diffusion, and excretion of a new antibiotic lincomycin. Antimicrob Agents Chemother 1963; 161:189-196.

LINDANE

Trade: Kwell, G-Well, Scabene
Can/Aus/UK: Hexit, Kwellada, PMS-Lindane, Quellada, Desitan
Uses: Pediculicide, scabicide
LRC: L4
AAP: Not reviewed

Lindane is an older pesticide also called gamma benzene hexachloride. It is primarily indicated for treatment of pediculus capitis (head lice) and less so for scabies (crab lice).[1,2] Because of its lipophilic nature, it is significantly absorbed through the skin of neonates (up to 13%) and has produced elevated liver enzymes, seizures disorders, and hypersensitivity. It is not recommended for use in neonates or young children. Lindane is transferred into human milk although the exact amounts are unpublished. Estimates by the manufacturer indicate a total daily dose of an infant ingesting 1 Liter of milk daily (30 ng/mL) would be approximately 30 µg/day, an amount that would probably be clinically insignificant.

If used in children, lindane should not be left on the skin for more than 6 hours before being washed off as peak plasma levels occur in children at about 6 hours after application. Although there are reports of some resistance, head lice and scabies should generally be treated with permethrin products (NIX, Elimite) which are much safer in pediatric patients. See permethrin.

Pregnancy Risk Category: B

Lactation Risk Category: L4

Adult Concerns: Dermatitis, seizures (excess dose), nervousness, irritability, anxiety, insomnia, dizziness, aplastic anemia, thrombocytopenia, neutropenia

Pediatric Concerns: Lindane is not recommended for children. Potential CNS toxicity includes lethargy, disorientation, restlessness, and tonic-clonic seizures.

Drug Interactions: Oil based hair dressings may enhance skin absorption.

Theoretic Infant Dose:

Relative Infant Dose:

Adult Dose: Topical

Alternatives:

T½ =	18-21 hours	M/P =	
PHL =	17-22 hours	PB =	
T$_{max}$ =	6 hours	Oral =	
MW =	290	pKa =	
Vd =			

References:
1. Pharmaceutical Manufacturer Prescribing Information. 1996.
2. Drug Facts and Comparisons 1996 ed. ed. St. Louis: 1996.

LINEZOLID
Trade: Zyvox
Can/Aus/UK:
Uses: Antibiotic
LRC: L3
AAP: Not reviewed

Linezolid is a new oxazolidinone family of antibiotics primarily used for gram positive infections but has some spectrum for gram negative and anaerobic bacteria. It is active against many strains including resistant staph aureus, streptococcus pneumonia, streptococcus pyogenes, and others. It is indicated for use in patients with vancomycin resistant enterococcus faceulum infections, staph aureus pneumonias, resistant streptococcus pneumonia infections, etc. Linezolid was found in the milk of lactating rats at concentrations similar to plasma levels although the dose was not indicated (rat milk levels are always higher than humans). Using these data, with an average maternal plasma concentration of 11.5 µg/mL and a theoretical milk/plasma ratio of 1.0, an infant would ingest approximately 1.7 mg/kg/day following a maternal dose of 1200 mg/day. This amount is likely a high estimate as doses given animals are extraordinarily high. Observe for changes in gut flora and diarrhea.

Pregnancy Risk Category: C

Lactation Risk Category: L3

Adult Concerns: Thrombocytopenia has been reported in one patient. Observe for diarrhea, sometimes induced by overgrowth of C. Difficle (pseudomembranous colitis). Side effects include headache, nausea, tongue discoloration, taste perversion, and vomiting. Note numerous drug-drug interactions.

Pediatric Concerns: None via milk but observe for diarrhea.

Drug Interactions: Linezolid is a reversible, nonselective inhibitor of monoamine oxidase. Therefore , it has the potential for interaction with adrenergic and serotonergic agents. This includes phenylephrine, phenylpropanolamine, pseudoephedrine, dopamine, and epinephrine.

Thus far coadministration with SSRIs has not posed a problem but caution is recommended.

Theoretic Infant Dose:

Relative Infant Dose:

Adult Dose: 400-600 mg every 12 hours

Alternatives:

T½ =	5.2 hours	M/P =		
PHL =		PB =	31%	
Tmax =	1.5-2.2 hours	Oral =	100%	
MW =	337	pKa =		
Vd =	0.71			

References:
1. Pharmaceutical Manufacturer Prescribing Information.

LIOTHYRONINE
Trade: Cytomel
Can/Aus/UK: Cytomel, Tertroxin
Uses: Thyroid supplement
LRC: L2
AAP: Not reviewed

Liothyronine is also called T3. It is seldom used for thyroid replacement therapy due to its short half-life. It is generally recognized that only minimal levels of thyroid hormones are secreted in human milk although several studies have shown that hypothyroid conditions only became apparent when breastfeeding was discontinued.[1,2] Although some studies indicate that breastfeeding may briefly protect hypothyroid infants, it is apparent that the levels of T4 and T3 are too low to provide long-term protection from hypothyroid disease.[3,4,5] Levels of T3 reported in milk vary but, in general, are around 238 ng/dl and considerably higher than T4 levels. The maximum amount of T3 ingested daily by an infant would be 357 ng/kg/day or approximately 1/10 the minimum requirement. From these studies, it is apparent that only exceedingly low levels of T3 are secreted into human milk and are insufficient to protect an infant from hypothyroidism.

Pregnancy Risk Category: A

Lactation Risk Category: L2

Adult Concerns: Tachycardia, tremor, agitation, hyperthyroidism

Pediatric Concerns: None reported via milk.

Drug Interactions: Cholestyramine and colestipol may reduce absorption of thyroid hormones. Estrogens may decrease effectiveness of thyroid hormones. The anticoagulant effect of certain medications is increased. Serum digitalis levels are reduced in hyperthyroidism or when the hyperthyroid patient is converted to the euthyroid state. Therapeutic effects of digitalis glycosides may be reduced. A decrease in theophylline clearance can be expected.

Theoretic Infant Dose: 357 ng/kg/day

Relative Infant Dose:

Adult Dose: 25-75 µg daily

Alternatives:

T½ =	25 hours	M/P =	
PHL =		PB =	Low
T$_{max}$ =	1-2 hours	Oral =	95 %
MW =	651	pKa =	
Vd =			

References:
1. Bode HH, Vanjonack WJ, Crawford JD. Mitigation of cretinism by breast-feeding. Pediatrics 1978; 62(1):13-16.
2. Rovet JF. Does breast-feeding protect the hypothyroid infant whose condition is diagnosed by newborn screening? Am J Dis Child 1990; 144(3):319-323.
3. Varma SK, Collins M, Row A, Haller WS, Varma K. Thyroxine, tri-iodothyronine, and reverse tri-iodothyronine concentrations in human milk. J Pediatr 1978; 93(5):803-806.
4. Hahn HB, Jr., Spiekerman AM, Otto WR, Hossalla DE. Thyroid function tests in neonates fed human milk. Am J Dis Child 1983; 137(3):220-222.
5. Letarte J, Guyda H, Dussault JH, Glorieux J. Lack of protective effect of breast-feeding in congenital hypothyroidism: report of 12 cases. Pediatrics 1980; 65(4):703-705.
6. Franklin R, O'Grady C, Carpenter L. Neonatal thyroid function: comparison between breast-fed and bottle-fed infants. J Pediatr 1985; 106(1):124-126.

LISINOPRIL

Trade: Prinivil, Zestril
Can/Aus/UK: Prinivil, Zestril, Apo-Lisinopril, Carace
Uses: Antihypertensive, ACE inhibitor
LRC: L3
AAP: Not reviewed

Lisinopril is a typical long-acting ACE inhibitor used as an antihypertensive.[1] No breastfeeding data are available on this product. See enalapril, benazepril, captopril as alternatives.

Pregnancy Risk Category: D

Lactation Risk Category: L3

Adult Concerns: Hypotension, headache, cough, GI upset, diarrhea, nausea

Pediatric Concerns: None reported but observe for hypotension, weakness.

Drug Interactions: Probenecid increases plasma levels of ACEi. ACEi and diuretics have additive hypotensive effects. Antacids reduce bioavailability of ACE inhibitors. NSAIDS reduce hypotension of ACE inhibitors. Phenothiazines increase effects of ACEi. ACEi increase digoxin and lithium plasma levels. May elevate potassium levels when potassium supplementation is added.

Theoretic Infant Dose:

Relative Infant Dose:

Adult Dose: 20-40 mg daily

Alternatives: Captopril, Enalapril

T½ =	12 hours	M/P =	
PHL =		PB =	Low
T$_{max}$ =	7 hours	Oral =	29%
MW =	442	pKa =	
Vd =			

References:
1.   McEvoy GE. (ed):AFHS Drug Information. New York, NY: 2003.

LITHIUM CARBONATE
Trade: Lithobid, Eskalith
Can/Aus/UK: Carbolith, Duralith, Lithane, Lithicarb, Camcolit, Liskonum, Phasal
Uses: Antimanic drug in bipolar disorders
LRC: L4
AAP: Drugs associated with significant side effects and should be given with caution

Lithium is a potent antimanic drug used in bipolar disorder. Its use in the first trimester of pregnancy may be associated with a number of birth anomalies, particularly cardiovascular.[1] If used during pregnancy, the dose required is generally elevated due to the increased renal clearance during pregnancy. Soon after delivery, maternal lithium levels should be closely monitored as the mother's renal clearance drops to normal in the next several days. Several cases have been reported of lithium toxicity in newborns.

In a study of a 36 year old mother who received lithium during and after pregnancy, the infant's serum lithium level was similar to the mothers at birth (maternal dose =400 mg) but dropped to 0.03 mmol/L by the sixth day.[2] While the mother's dose increased to 800 mg/day postpartum, the infant's serum level did not rise above 10% of the maternal serum levels. At 42 days postpartum, the maternal and infant serum levels were 1.1 and 0.1 mmol/L respectively.

Some toxic effects have been reported. In a mother receiving 600-1200 mg lithium daily during pregnancy, the concentration of lithium in breastmilk at 3 days was 0.6 mEq/L.[3] The maternal and infant plasma levels were 1.5 mEq/L and 0.6 mEq/L respectively at 3 days. In this case the infant was floppy, unresponsive and exhibited inverted T waves which are indicative of lithium toxicity. In another study done 7 days postpartum, the milk and infant plasma levels were 0.3 mEq/L each, while the mother's plasma lithium levels were 0.9 mEq/L.[4] In a case report of a mother receiving 300 mg three times daily and breastfeeding her infant at two weeks postpartum, the mother and infant's lithium levels were 0.62 and 0.31 mmol/L respectively. The infant's neurobehavioral development and thyroid function were reported normal.[5]

From these studies it is apparent that lithium can permeate milk and is absorbed by the breastfed infant. If the infant continues to breastfeed, it is strongly suggested that the infant be closely monitored for serum lithium levels. Lithium does not reach steady state levels for approximately 10 days. Clinicians may wish to wait at least this long prior to evaluating the infant's serum lithium level, or sooner if symptoms occur. In addition, lithium is known to reduce thyroxine production, and periodic thyroid evaluation should be considered. Because hydration status of the infant can alter lithium levels dramatically, the clinician should observe changes in hydration carefully. A number of studies of lithium suggest that lithium administration is not an absolute contraindication to breastfeeding, if the physician monitors the infant closely for elevated plasma lithium. Current studies, as well as unpublished experience, suggest that the infant's plasma levels rise to about 30-40% of the maternal level, most often without untoward effects in the infant. Recent evidence suggests that certain anticonvulsants such as carbamazepine, valproic acid, and others may be equally effective as lithium in treating mania. Because these medications are probably safer to use in breastfeeding mothers, the clinician may wish to explore the use of these medications in certain manic breastfeeding mothers.[6]

Pregnancy Risk Category: D

Lactation Risk Category: L4

Adult Concerns: Nausea, vomiting, diarrhea, frequent urination, tremor, drowsiness

Pediatric Concerns: In one study cyanosis, T-wave abnormalities, and decreased muscle tone were reported. Other studies report no side effects. Evaluate infant lithium levels along with mothers.

Drug Interactions: Decreased lithium effect with theophylline and caffeine. Increased toxicity with alfentanil. Thiazide diuretics reduce clearance and increase toxicity. NSAIDS, haloperidol, phenothiazines, fluoxetine and ACE inhibitors may increase toxicity.

Theoretic Infant Dose:

Relative Infant Dose:

Adult Dose: 600 mg TID

Alternatives: Valproic acid, carbamazepine

T½ =	17-24 hours	M/P =	0.24-0.66
PHL =	17.9 hours	PB =	0%
T$_{max}$ =	2-4 hours	Oral =	Complete
MW =	74	pKa =	
Vd =	0.7-1.0		

References:

1. Schou M. Lithium treatment during pregnancy, delivery, and lactation: an update. J Clin Psychiatry 1990; 51(10):410-413.
2. Sykes PA, Quarrie J, Alexander FW. Lithium carbonate and breast-feeding. Br Med J 1976; 2(6047):1299.
3. Tunnessen WW, Jr., Hertz CG. Toxic effects of lithium in newborn infants: a commentary. J Pediatr 1972; 81(4):804-807.
4. Fries H. Lithium in pregnancy. Lancet 1970; 1(7658):1233.
5. Montgomery A. Use of lithium for treatment of bipolar disorder during pregnancy and lactation. Academy of breastfeeding Medicine News and Views 1997; 3(1):4-5.
6. Llewellyn A, Stowe ZN, Strader JR, Jr. The use of lithium and management of women with bipolar disorder during pregnancy and lactation. J Clin Psychiatry 1998; 59 Suppl 6:57-64.

LOMEFLOXACIN

Trade: Maxaquin
Can/Aus/UK: Okacyn
Uses: Fluoroquinolone antibiotic
LRC: L3
AAP: Not reviewed

Lomefloxacin belongs the fluoroquinolone family of antimicrobials.[1] The use of fluoroquinolone antibiotics in adolescent children has been associated with arthropathy or swollen joints although these studies are now suspect and were in patients receiving several weeks of normal oral doses, not breastmilk. The fluoroquinoles in general are becoming more popular in pediatric-aged patients due to the introduction of recent studies.[2] In addition, the FDA is reviewing several pediatric indications for this group. At least one case of bloody colitis (pseudomembranous colitis) has been reported in a breastfeeding infant whose mother ingested ciprofloxacin. It is reported that lomefloxacin is excreted in the milk of lactating animals although levels are low.

Pregnancy Risk Category: C

Lactation Risk Category: L3

Adult Concerns: GI distress,   diarrhea,   colitis,   headaches, phototoxicity

Pediatric Concerns: None reported with this drug. Pseudomembranous colitis has been reported with another member of this family. Observe closely for bloody diarrhea.

Drug Interactions: Antacids, iron salts, sucralfate, and zinc salts may interfere with the GI absorption of the fluoroquinolones resulting in decreased serum levels. Cimetidine may interfere with the elimination of the fluoroquinolones. Nitrofurantoin may interfere with the antibacterial properties of the fluoroquinolone family. Probenecid may reduce renal clearance as much as 50%. Nephrotoxic side effects of cyclosporine may be significantly increased when used with fluoroquinolones. Phenytoin serum levels may be reduced producing a decrease in therapeutic effects. Anticoagulant effects may be increased when used with fluoroquinolones. Decreased clearance and increased plasma levels and toxicity of theophylline have been reported with the use of the fluoroquinolones.

Theoretic Infant Dose:

Relative Infant Dose:

Adult Dose: 400 mg daily

Alternatives: Norfloxacin, Ofloxacin, Trovafloxacin

$T\frac{1}{2}$ =	8 hours	M/P =	
PHL =		PB =	20.6 %
T_{max} =	0.7-2.0 hours	Oral =	92%
MW =	351	pKa =	
Vd =	2		

References:
1.   Pharmaceutical Manufacturer Prescribing Information. 1996.
2.   Ghaffar F, McCracken GH. Quinolones in Pediatrics. In: Hooper DC, Rubinstein E, editors. Quinolone Antimicrobial Agents. Washington, D.C.: ASM Press, 2003: 343-354.

LOPERAMIDE

Trade: Imodium, Pepto Diarrhea Control, Maalox Anti-Diarrheal Caplets, Kaopectate Ii Caplets, Imodium Advanced
Can/Aus/UK: Imodium, Novo-Loperamide, Gastro-Stop
Uses: Antidiarrheal drug
LRC: L2
AAP: Maternal Medication Usually Compatible with Breastfeeding

Loperamide is an antidiarrheal drug. Because it is only minimally absorbed orally (0.3%), only extremely small amounts are secreted into breastmilk. Following a 4 mg oral dose twice daily in 6 women (early postpartum), milk levels at 12 hours after the following dose averaged 0.18 µg/L, and 6 hours after the second dose were 0.27 µg/L.[1] A breastfeeding infant consuming 165 mL/kg/day of milk would ingest 2000 times less than the recommended daily dose. It is very unlikely these reported levels in milk (Relative infant dose = 0.03%) would ever produce clinical effects in a breastfed infant.

Pregnancy Risk Category: B

Lactation Risk Category: L2

Adult Concerns: Fatigue, dry mouth, respiratory depression, dry mouth, and constipation

Pediatric Concerns: One case of mild delirium has been reported in a 4 year old infant.

Drug Interactions: CNS depressants, phenothiazines, and TCA antidepressants may potentiate adverse effects.

Theoretic Infant Dose: 0.0405 µg/kg/day

Relative Infant Dose: 0.03%

Adult Dose: 4 mg PRN

Alternatives:

$T\frac{1}{2}$ =	10.8 hours	M/P =	0.5-0.36
PHL =		PB =	
T_{max} =	4-5 hours (capsules)	Oral =	0.3%
MW =	477	pKa =	
Vd =			

References:
1. Nikodem VC, Hofmeyr GJ. Secretion of the antidiarrhoeal agent loperamide oxide in breastmilk. Eur J Clin Pharmacol 1992; 42(6):695-696.

LORACARBEF

Trade: Lorabid
Can/Aus/UK:
Uses: Synthetic penicillin-like antibiotic
LRC: L2
AAP: Not reviewed

Loracarbef is a synthetic beta-lactam antibiotic. It is structurally similar to the cephalosporin family.[1] It is used for gram negative and gram positive infections. Pediatric indications are available for infants 6 months and children to 12 years of age. No data are available on levels in breastmilk.

Pregnancy Risk Category: B

Lactation Risk Category: L2

Adult Concerns: Nausea, vomiting, diarrhea, allergic rashes

Pediatric Concerns: None reported. Observe for GI changes such as diarrhea.

Drug Interactions: Probenecid may increase levels of cephalosporins by reducing renal clearance.

Theoretic Infant Dose:

Relative Infant Dose:

Adult Dose: 200-400 mg BID

Alternatives:

T½ =	1 hour	M/P =	
PHL =		PB =	25%
T$_{max}$ =	1.2 hours	Oral =	90%
MW =		pKa =	
Vd =			

References:
1. Pharmaceutical Manufacturer Prescribing Information. 1995.

LORATADINE

Trade: Claritin
Can/Aus/UK: Claritin, Claratyne, Clarityn
Uses: Long-acting antihistamine
LRC: L1
AAP: Maternal Medication Usually Compatible with Breastfeeding

Loratadine is a long-acting antihistamine with minimal sedative properties. During 48 hours following administration, the amount of loratadine transferred via milk was 4.2 μg, which was 0.01% of the administered dose.[1] Through 48 hours, only 6.0 μg of descarboethoxyloratadine (metabolite) (7.5 μg loratadine equivalents) were excreted into breastmilk, or 0.029% of the administered dose of loratadine or its active metabolite were transferred via milk to the infant. A 4 kg infant would receive only 0.46% of the loratadine dose received by the mother on a mg/kg basis (2.9 μg/kg/day). It is very unlikely this dose would present a hazard to infants. Loratadine does not transfer into the CNS of adults, so it is unlikely to induce sedation even in infants. The half-life in neonates is not known although it is likely quite long. Pediatric formulations are available.

Pregnancy Risk Category: B

Lactation Risk Category: L1

Adult Concerns: Sedation, dry mouth, fatigue, nausea, tachycardia, palpitations

Pediatric Concerns: None reported, but observe for sedation, dry mouth, tachycardia.

Drug Interactions: Increased plasma levels of loratadine may result when used with ketoconazole, the macrolide antibiotics, and other products.

Theoretic Infant Dose: 0.9 μg/kg/day

Relative Infant Dose: 0.62%

Adult Dose: 10 mg daily

Alternatives: Cetirizine

$T\frac{1}{2}$ =	8.4-28 hours	M/P =	1.17
PHL =		PB =	97%
T_{max} =	1.5 hours	Oral =	Complete
MW =	383	pKa =	
Vd =			

References:
1. Hilbert J, Radwanski E, Affrime MB, Perentesis G, Symchowicz S, Zampaglione N. Excretion of loratadine in human breastmilk. J Clin Pharmacol 1988; 28(3):234-239.

LORAZEPAM

Trade: Ativan
Can/Aus/UK: Apo-Lorazepam, Ativan, Novo-Lorazepam, Almazine
Uses: Antianxiety, sedative drug
LRC: L3
AAP: Drugs whose effect on nursing infants is unknown but may be of concern

Lorazepam is a typical benzodiazepine from the Valium family of drugs. It is frequently used prenatally and presurgically as a sedative agent. In one prenatal study, it has been found to produce a high rate of depressed respiration, hypothermia, and feeding problems in newborns.[1] Newborns were found to secrete lorazepam for up to 11 days postpartum. In McBrides's study, the infants were unaffected following the prenatal use of 2.5 mg IV prior to delivery.[2] Plasma levels of lorazepam in infants were equivalent to those of the mothers. The rate of metabolism in mother and infant appears slow but equal following delivery. In this study there were no untoward effects noted in any of the infants.

In one patient receiving 2.5 mg twice daily for 5 days postpartum, the breastmilk levels were 12 μg/L.[3] In another patient four hours after an oral dose of 3.5 mg, milk levels averaged 8.5 μg/L.[4] Summerfield reports an average concentration in milk of 9 μg/L and an average milk/plasma ratio of 0.22.[4] It would appear from these studies that the amount of lorazepam secreted into milk would be clinically insignificant under most conditions.

The benzodiazepine family as a rule are not ideal for breastfeeding mothers due to relatively long half-lives and the development of dependence. However, it is apparent that the shorter-acting benzodiazepines are safest during lactation provided their use is short-term or intermittent, low dose, and after the first week of life.[5]

Pregnancy Risk Category: D

Lactation Risk Category: L3

Adult Concerns: Sedation, agitation, respiratory depression, withdrawal syndrome

Pediatric Concerns: None reported via milk but observe for sedation.

Drug Interactions: Increased sedation when used with morphine, alcohol, CNS depressants, MAO inhibitors, loxapine, and tricyclic antidepressants.

Theoretic Infant Dose: 1.8 µg/kg/day

Relative Infant Dose: 2.5%

Adult Dose: 1-3 mg BID-TID

Alternatives: Midazolam

$T^{1/2}$ =	12 hours	M/P =	0.15-0.26
PHL =		PB =	85%
T_{max} =	2 hours	Oral =	90%
MW =	321	pKa =	1.3, 11.5
Vd =	0.9-1.3		

References:

1. Johnstone M. Effect of maternal lorazepam on the neonate. Br Med J (Clin Res Ed) 1981; 282(6280):1973-1974.
2. McBride RJ, Dundee JW, Moore J, Toner W, Howard PJ. A study of the plasma concentrations of lorazepam in mother and neonate. Br J Anaesth 1979; 51(10):971-978.
3. Whitelaw AG, Cummings AJ, McFadyen IR. Effect of maternal lorazepam on the neonate. Br Med J (Clin Res Ed) 1981; 282(6270):1106-1108.
4. Summerfield RJ, Nielsen MS. Excretion of lorazepam into breastmilk. Br J Anaesth 1985; 57(10):1042-1043.
5. Maitra R, Menkes DB. Psychotropic drugs and lactation. N Z Med J 1996; 109(1024):217-218.

LOSARTAN

Trade: Cozaar, Hyzaar
Can/Aus/UK: Cozaar
Uses: ACE-like antihypertensive
LRC: L3
AAP: Not reviewed

Losartan is a new ACE-like antihypertensive. Rather than inhibiting the enzyme that makes angiotensin such as the ACE inhibitor family, this medication selectively blocks the ACE receptor site preventing attachment of angiotensin II.[1,2] No data are available on its transfer to human milk. Although it penetrates the CNS significantly, its rather high protein binding would probably reduce its ability to enter milk. This product is only intended for those few individuals who cannot take ACE inhibitors. No data on transfer into human milk are available. The trade name Hyzaar contains losartan plus hydrochlorothiazide.

Pregnancy Risk Category: C in 1st trimester
D in 2nd and 3rd trimester

Lactation Risk Category: L3

Adult Concerns: Dizziness, insomnia, hypotension, anxiety, ataxia, confusion, depression. Cough, nor angioedema, commonly associated with ACE inhibitors does not apparently occur with losartan.

Pediatric Concerns: None reported.

Drug Interactions: Decreased effect when used with phenobarbital, ketoconazole, troleandomycin, sulfaphenazole. Increased effect when used with cimetidine, moxonidine.

Theoretic Infant Dose:

Relative Infant Dose:

Adult Dose: 25-50 mg daily-BID

Alternatives: Captopril, Enalapril

T½ =	4-9 hours (metabolite)	M/P =	
PHL =		PB =	99.8%
T$_{max}$ =	1 hour	Oral =	25-33%
MW =		pKa =	
Vd =	12		

References:
1. Lacy C. Drug information handbook. Lexi-Comp Inc. Cleveland, OH, 1996.
2. Pharmaceutical Manufacturer Prescribing Information. 1997.

LOVASTATIN
Trade: Mevacor
Can/Aus/UK: Mevacor, Apo-Lovastatin
Uses: Hypocholesterolemic
LRC: L3
AAP: Not reviewed

Lovastatin is an effective inhibitor of hepatic cholesterol synthesis. It is primarily used for hypercholesterolemia. Pregnancy normally elevates maternal cholesterol and triglyceride levels. Following delivery, lipid levels gradually decline to pre-pregnancy levels within about 9 months.

Small but unpublished levels are known to be secreted into human breastmilk.[1] Less then 5% of a dose reaches the maternal circulation due to extensive first-pass removal by the liver. The effect on the infant is unknown, but it could reduce hepatic cholesterol synthesis. There is little justification for using such a drug during lactation, but due to the extremely small maternal plasma levels, it is unlikely that the amount in breastmilk would be clinically active. Others in this same family of drugs include simvastatin, Pravachol, atorvastatin, and fluvastatin. Atherosclerosis is a chronic process, and discontinuation of lipid-lowering drugs during pregnancy and lactation should have little to no impact on the outcome of long-term therapy of primary hypercholesterolemia. Cholesterol and other products of cholesterol biosynthesis are essential components for fetal and neonatal development, and the use of cholesterol-lowering drugs would not be advisable under any circumstances.

Pregnancy Risk Category: X

Lactation Risk Category: L3

Adult Concerns: Diarrhea, dyspepsia, flatulence, constipation, headache

Pediatric Concerns: None reported, but its use is not recommended.

Drug Interactions: Increased toxicity when added to gemfibrozil (myopathy, myalgia, etc), clofibrate, niacin (myopathy), erythromycin, cyclosporine, oral anticoagulants (elevated bleeding time).

Theoretic Infant Dose:

Relative Infant Dose:

Adult Dose: 20-80 mg daily
Alternatives:

T½ =	1.1-1.7	M/P =	
PHL =		PB =	> 95%
T$_{max}$ =	2-4 hours	Oral =	5-30%
MW =	405	pKa =	
Vd =			

References:
1.   Pharmaceutical Manufacturer Prescribing Information. 1999.

LOXAPINE

Trade: Loxitane
Can/Aus/UK: Loxapac, PMS-Loxapine
Uses: CNS tranquilizer
LRC: L4
AAP: Not reviewed

Loxapine produces pharmacologic effects similar to the phenothiazines and haloperidol family.[1]   The drug does not appear to have antidepressant effects and may lower the seizure threshold. It is a powerful tranquilizer and has been found to be secreted into the milk of animals, but no human data are available. This is a potent tranquilizer than could produce significant sequelae in breastfeeding infants. Caution is urged.

Pregnancy Risk Category: C

Lactation Risk Category: L4

Adult Concerns: Drowsiness, tremor, rigidity, extrapyramidal symptoms

Pediatric Concerns: None reported but extreme caution is recommended.

Drug Interactions: Increased toxicity when used with CNS depressants, metrizamide, and MAO inhibitors.

Theoretic Infant Dose:

Relative Infant Dose:

Adult Dose: 10-50 mg BID-QID

Alternatives: Haloperidol

T½ =	19 hours	M/P =	
PHL =		PB =	
T$_{max}$ =	1-2 hours	Oral =	33%
MW =	328	pKa =	6.6
Vd =			

References:
1. McEvoy GE. (ed):AFHS Drug Information. New York, NY: 2003.

LSD
Trade:
Can/Aus/UK:
Uses: Hallucinogen
LRC: L5
AAP: Not reviewed

LSD is a power hallucinogenic drug.[1] No data are available on transfer into breastmilk. However, due to its extreme potency and its ability to pass the blood-brain-barrier, LSD is likely to penetrate milk and produce hallucinogenic effects in the infant. This drug is definitely CONTRAINDICATED. Maternal urine may be positive for LSD for 34-120 hours post ingestion.

Pregnancy Risk Category:

Lactation Risk Category: L5

Adult Concerns: Hallucinations, dilated pupil, salivation, nausea

Pediatric Concerns: None reported via milk, but due to potency, hallucinations are likely. Contraindicated.

Drug Interactions:

Theoretic Infant Dose:

Relative Infant Dose:

Adult Dose:

Alternatives:

T½ =	3 hours	M/P =	
PHL =		PB =	
T$_{max}$ =	30-60 minutes (oral)	Oral =	Complete
MW =	268	pKa =	
Vd =			

References:
1. Ellenhorn MJ, Barceloux DG. In: Medical Toxicology. New York, NY: Elsevier, 1988.

LYME DISEASE

Trade: Lyme Disease, Borrelia
Can/Aus/UK:
Uses: Borrelia Burgdorferi infections.
LRC:
AAP: Not reviewed

Lyme disease is caused by infection with the spirochete, borrelia burgdorferi. This spirochete is transferred in-utero to the fetus and is secreted into human milk[1] and can cause infection in breastfed infants.[2] If diagnosed postpartum or in a breastfeeding mother, the mother and infant should be treated immediately. In children (> 7 yrs) and adults, preferred therapy is doxycycline (100 mg PO twice daily for 14-21 days) or Amoxicillin (500 mg three times daily for 21 days). In breastfeeding patients, amoxicillin therapy is probably preferred. In the infant, amoxicillin (40 mg/kg/day (max 3 gm) with probenecid (25 mg/kg/day) divided in three doses/day for a duration of 21 days.[3]

Alternative therapy for adults includes clarithromycin (500 mg PO twice daily for 21 days), azithromycin (500 mg PO daily for 14-21 days), or cefuroxime axetil (500 mg PO twice daily for 21 days).[4] Although doxycycline therapy is not definitely contraindicated in breastfeeding mothers, alternates such as amoxicillin, cefuroxime, clarithromycin, or azithromycin should be preferred.

Pregnancy Risk Category:

Lactation Risk Category:

References:
1. Schmidt BL, Aberer E, Stockenhuber C, Klade H, Breier F, Luger A. Detection of Borrelia burgdorferi DNA by polymerase chain reaction in the urine and breastmilk of patients with Lyme borreliosis. Diagn Microbiol Infect Dis 1995; 21(3):121-128.

2. Stiernstedt G. Lyme borreliosis during pregnancy. Scand J Infect Dis Suppl 1990; 71:99-100.
3. Bartlett JG. In: Pocket Book of Infectious Disease Therapy. Baltimore, USA: Williams and Wilkins, 1996.
4. Nelson JD. In: Pocket Book of Pediatric Antimicrobial Therapy. Baltimore, USA: Williams and Wilkins, 1995.

LYME DISEASE VACCINE
Trade: LYMErix
Can/Aus/UK:
Uses: Lyme Disease Vaccine
LRC: L2
AAP: Not reviewed

LYMErix is a noninfectious recombinant vaccine containing a lipoprotein from the outer surface of Borrelia burgdorferi. The lipoprotein from this causative agent is a single polypeptide chain of 257 amino acids with lipids covalently bonded to the N terminus.[1] No substance of animal origin is used in the manufacturing process. It is primarily indicated for individuals 15-70 years of age. It is very unlikely to enter milk. Officials from the CDC suggest that it is not contraindicated for use in breastfeeding patients.[2]

Pregnancy Risk Category: C

Lactation Risk Category: L2

Adult Concerns: Pain at injection site, headache, fatigue, arthralgia, myalgia

Pediatric Concerns: None reported via milk. Unlikely to enter milk compartment.

Drug Interactions: No known interactions have been published. Avoid use in patients taking anticoagulants.

Theoretic Infant Dose:

Relative Infant Dose:

Adult Dose:

Alternatives:

References:
1. Pharmaceutical Manufacturer Prescribing Information.
2. Hayes N. Center for Disease Control, Personal communication. 2000.

LYSINE
Trade: Lysine, L-Lysine
Can/Aus/UK:
Uses: Amino acid food supplement
LRC: L2
AAP: Not reviewed

Lysine is a naturally occurring amino acid; the average American ingests from 6-10 grams daily. Aside from its use as a supplement in patients with poor nutrition, it is most often used for the treatment of recurrent herpes simplex infections. The clinical efficacy of lysine in herpes infections is highly controversial with some advocates[1,2] and many detractors.[3] Upon absorption, most is sequestered in the liver, but blood levels do rise transiently. However, the risk of toxicity is considered quite low in both adults and infants. Rather high doses have been studied in infants as young as 4 months, with doses from 60 to 1080 mg L-lysine per 8 ounces of milk.[4] At the higher level, 5.18 grams of L-lysine was consumed. Plasma lysine levels varied only with normal limits, while urinary lysine levels were roughly proportional to the amount of supplementation.

Thomas et.al. has reported an elegant study of the transfer of radiolabeled L-lysine into numerous compartments, including milk.[5-6] In a group of 5 lactating women who received L-lysine (15N-lysine and 13C-lysine (5 mg/kg/each)), milk levels of labeled lysine reached a peak at approximately 150 minutes. Labeled lysine levels in milk were slightly higher with M/P ratios ranging from 1.29 to 1.43. However, the total amount of radiolabeled lysine present in milk was low. Only 0.54% of the administered dose of lysine was secreted into milk proteins. Further, the lysine present in milk was present as protein, not free amino acid.

Therefore supplementation of breastfeeding mothers with L-lysine will probably not result in significantly elevated levels of free lysine in milk.

Pregnancy Risk Category:

Lactation Risk Category: **L2**

Adult Concerns: GI distress. Lysine may cause cholesterol and triglyceride levels in the blood to rise.

Pediatric Concerns: None reported.

Drug Interactions:

Theoretic Infant Dose:

Relative Infant Dose:

Adult Dose:

Alternatives:

T½ =	3.66 hours	M/P =	
PHL =		PB =	
T$_{max}$ =		Oral =	83%
MW =	146	pKa =	
Vd =			

References:
1. Griffith RS, Walsh DE, Myrmel KH, Thompson RW, Behforooz A. Success of L-lysine therapy in frequently recurrent herpes simplex infection. Treatment and prophylaxis. Dermatologica 1987; 175(4):183-190.
2. Walsh DE, Griffith RS, Behforooz A. Subjective response to lysine in the therapy of herpes simplex. J Antimicrob Chemother 1983; 12(5):489-496.
3. DiGiovanna JJ, Blank H. Failure of lysine in frequently recurrent herpes simplex infection. Treatment and prophylaxis. Arch Dermatol 1984; 120(1):48-51.
4. Anderson SA, Raiten DJ. (eds): "Safety of Amino Acids in Dietary Supplements.". Life Sciences Research Office, Bethesda, MD: FASEB Special Publications Office, 1999.
5. Thomas MR, Irving CS, Reeds PJ, Malphus EW, Wong WW, Boutton TW, Klein PD. Lysine and protein metabolism in the young lactating woman. Eur J Clin Nutr 1991; 45(5):227-242.
6. Irving CS, Malphus EW, Thomas MR, Marks L, Klein PD. Infused and ingested labeled lysines: appearance in human-milk proteins. Am J Clin Nutr 1988; 47(1):49-52.

MAGNESIUM HYDROXIDE
Trade: Milk Of Magnesia
Can/Aus/UK: Citro-Mag, Phillip's Milk of Magnesia, Mylanta, Gastrobrom
Uses: Laxative, antacid
LRC: L1
AAP: Not reviewed

Poorly absorbed from maternal GI tract. Only about 15-30 % of an orally ingested magnesium product is absorbed. Magnesium rapidly deposits in bone (> 50%) and is significantly distributed to tissue sites. See magnesium sulfate.

Pregnancy Risk Category: B

Lactation Risk Category: L1

Adult Concerns: Hypotension, diarrhea, nausea

Pediatric Concerns: None reported.

Drug Interactions: Decreased absorption of tetracyclines, digoxin, indomethacin, and iron salts.

Theoretic Infant Dose:

Relative Infant Dose: 0.17%

Adult Dose: 5-30 mL PRN

Alternatives:

T½ =		M/P =	
PHL =		PB =	33%
T$_{max}$ =		Oral =	15-30%
MW =	58	pKa =	
Vd =			

References:

MAGNESIUM SULFATE

Trade: Epsom Salt
Can/Aus/UK: Magnoplasm, Salvital, Zinvit, Epsom Salts
Uses: Saline laxative and anticonvulsant (IV,IM)
LRC: L1
AAP: Maternal Medication Usually Compatible with Breastfeeding

Magnesium is a normal plasma electrolyte. It is used pre and postnatally as an effective anticonvulsant in preeclamptic patients. In one study of 10 preeclamptic patients who received a 4 gm IV loading dose followed by 1 gm per hour IV for more than 24 hours, the average milk magnesium levels in treated subjects were 6.4 mg/dl, only slightly higher than controls (untreated) which were 4.77 mg/dl[1]. On day 2, the average milk magnesium levels in treated groups were 3.83 mg/dl, which was not significantly different from untreated controls, 3.19 mg/dl. By day 3, the treated and control groups breastmilk levels were identical (3.54 vs. 3.52 mg/dl). The mean maternal serum magnesium level on day 1 in treated groups was 3.55 mg/dl, which was significantly higher than control untreated, 1.82 mg/dl. In both treated and control subjects, levels of milk magnesium were approximately twice those of maternal serum magnesium levels, with the milk-to-serum ratio being 1.9 in treated subjects and 2.1 in control subjects.

This study clearly indicates a normal concentrating mechanism for magnesium in human milk. It is well known that oral magnesium absorption is very poor, averaging only 4-30%. Further, this study indicates that in treated groups, infants would only receive about 1.5 mg of oral magnesium more than the untreated controls. It is very unlikely that the amount of magnesium in breastmilk would be clinically relevant.

Pregnancy Risk Category: B

Lactation Risk Category: L1

Adult Concerns: IV-hypotension, sedation, muscle weakness

Pediatric Concerns: None reported via milk. Sedation, hypotonia following in-utero exposure.

Drug Interactions: May decrease the hypertensive effect of nifedipine. May increase the depression associated with other CNS depressants, neuromuscular blocking agents, and the cardiotoxicity associated with ritodrine.

Theoretic Infant Dose: 0.5745 mg/kg/day

Relative Infant Dose:

Adult Dose: 1-2 g q 4-6 hours PRN

Alternatives:

T½ =	< 3 hours	M/P =	1.9
PHL =		PB =	0%
T_max =	Immediate (IV)	Oral =	4-30%
MW =	120	pKa =	
Vd =			

References:
1. Cruikshank DP, Varner MW, Pitkin RM. Breastmilk magnesium and calcium concentrations following magnesium sulfate treatment. Am J Obstet Gynecol 1982; 143(6):685-688.

MANGAFODIPIR TRISODIUM

Trade: Teslascan
Can/Aus/UK: Teslascan
Uses: Radiocontrast agent for MRI scans
LRC: L3
AAP: Not reviewed

Mangafodipir is a manganese-containing radiocontrast agent used in Magnetic Resonance Imaging. It is rapidly redistributed to liver and less so to other tissues. The release of manganese is significant, and whole-body stores are approximately doubled with infusion of this product. Elevated plasma manganese levels drop rapidly with a redistribution half-life of about 25 minutes, while the terminal elimination half-life of manganese in more on the order of 10.1 hours. Manganese is effectively transported into human milk, and milk levels are apparently a function of oral intake in the mother.[1] Hence manganese levels in milk could temporarily be elevated. Infants are somewhat deficient in manganese and have higher oral bioavailability of manganese due to the relative state of deficiency.[2] Thus it is reasonable to assume that the use of this product in a breastfeeding woman could conceivably elevate the levels of her milk significantly although briefly. A brief interruption of breastfeeding for a few hours (4 or more) followed by pumping and discarding would significantly reduce any risk to the infant.

Pregnancy Risk Category: C

Lactation Risk Category: L3

Adult Concerns: Adverse events include nausea, vomiting, chest pain, palpitation, pruritus, heat, flushing, pressure, pain, headache, and gastric distress.

Pediatric Concerns: None reported via milk. A short interruption of 4 hours would probably eliminate most risk.

Drug Interactions: None

Theoretic Infant Dose:

Relative Infant Dose:

Adult Dose: 5 μmol/kg IV

Alternatives:

$T\frac{1}{2}$ =	10 hours (Mn)	M/P =	
PHL =		PB =	Nil
T_{max} =	Immediate	Oral =	Low
MW =	757	pKa =	
Vd =			

References:

1 Vuori E, Makinen SM, Kara R, Kuitunen P. The effects of the dietary intakes of copper, iron, manganese, and zinc on the trace element content of human milk. Am J Clin Nutr 1980; 33(2):227-231.
2. Pharmaceutical Manufacturers prescribing information, 2003.

MANNITOL

Trade: Osmitrol
Can/Aus/UK:
Uses: Osmotic diuretic
LRC: L3
AAP: Not reviewed

Mannitol is a hexahydroxy alcohol chemically related to mannose and is used as an osmotic diuretic.[1] As such, it does not readily enter the cellular compartment and remains in the extracellular compartment. Hepatic metabolism is minimal, and the drug is primarily excreted unchanged in the urine by glomerular filtration. The elimination half-life is 71-100 minutes. Mannitol does not normally enter the CNS or the eye. It is freely filtered by the kidneys with less than 10% tubular reabsorption which is the basis for its use as a diuretic. It is not known if it enters the milk compartment, but it is likely only during the first few days postpartum when the tight-junctions in the alveolar system are immature. After 48-72 hours, the entry of mannitol into human milk is probably minimal. Oral absorption in infants would be minimal except early postpartum when their GI tract is relative porous.

Pregnancy Risk Category: C

Lactation Risk Category: L3

Adult Concerns: Hypernatremia, hyponatremia, elevated potassium, diarrhea, kidney failure, pulmonary edema, and congestive heart failure

Pediatric Concerns: None reported via milk, but watery diarrhea is remotely possible. Due to its osmotic diuresis, it is possible that it could briefly reduce the production of milk.

Drug Interactions: May enhance diuresis with added with loop and other diuretics. May increase elimination of lithium.

Theoretic Infant Dose:

Relative Infant Dose:

Adult Dose: High variable, check other references.

Alternatives:

T½ =	71-100 minutes	M/P =	
PHL =		PB =	0%
T$_{max}$ =		Oral =	17%
MW =	182	pKa =	
Vd =	Low		

References:
1.   Pharmaceutical Manufacturers prescribing information, 2003.

MAPROTILENE

Trade: Ludiomil
Can/Aus/UK: Novo-Maprotilene, Ludiomil
Uses: Antidepressant
LRC: L3
AAP: Not reviewed

Maprotiline is a unique structured (tetracyclic) antidepressant dissimilar to others but has clinical effects similar to the tricyclic antidepressants. While it has fewer anticholinergic side effects than the tricyclics, it is more sedating and has similar toxicities in overdose. In one study following an oral dose of 50 mg three times daily, milk and maternal blood levels were greater than 200 μg/L.[1] Milk/plasma ratios varied from 1.3 to 1.5. While these levels are quite low, it is not known if they are hazardous to a breastfed infant but caution is recommended.

Pregnancy Risk Category: B

Lactation Risk Category: L3

Adult Concerns: Side effects include drowsiness, sedation, vertigo, blurred vision, dry mouth, and urinary retention. Skin rashes, seizures, myoclonus, mania and hallucinations have been reported.

Pediatric Concerns: None reported via milk but caution is recommended.

Drug Interactions: Maprotilene levels may be decreased by barbiturates, phenytoin, and carbamazepine. Increased toxicity may result when used with CNS depressants, quinidine, MAO inhibitors, anticholinergics, sympathomimetics, phenothiazines (seizures), benzodiazepines. Due to hazard of increased QT intervals, do not admix with cisapride.

Theoretic Infant Dose: 30 µg/kg/day

Relative Infant Dose: 1.4%

Adult Dose: 25-75 mg daily

Alternatives: Sertraline, venlafaxine, paroxetine

T½ =	27-58 hours	M/P =	1.5
PHL =		PB =	88%
T$_{max}$ =	12 hours	Oral =	100%
MW =	277	pKa =	
Vd =	22.6		

References:

1. Riess W. The relevance of blood level determinations during the evaluation of maprotiline in man. In:Murphy (ed): Research and Clinical Investigations in Depression. Northhampton: Cambridge Medical Publications, 1976.

MEBENDAZOLE

Trade: Vermox
Can/Aus/UK: Vermox, Sqworm
Uses: Anthelmintic
LRC: L3
AAP: Not reviewed

Mebendazole is an anthelmintic used primarily for pin worms although it is active against round worms, hookworms, and a number of other nematodes. Mebendazole is poorly absorbed orally. In one patient who received 100 mg twice daily for three days, milk production was drastically reduced.[1] However in another report of four postpartum breastfeeding mothers who received 100 mg twice daily for 3 days, milk levels of mebendazole were undetectable in one patient sample. No change in milk production was noted in the latter study.[2] Considering the poor oral absorption and high protein binding, it is unlikely that mebendazole would be transmitted to the infant in clinically relevant concentrations.

Pregnancy Risk Category: C

Lactation Risk Category: L3

Adult Concerns: Diarrhea, abdominal pain,   nausea, vomiting, headache. Observe mother for reduced production of breastmilk.

Pediatric Concerns: None reported via milk.   May inhibit milk production.

Drug Interactions: Carbamazepine and phenytoin may increase metabolism of mebendazole.

Theoretic Infant Dose:

Relative Infant Dose:

Adult Dose: 100 mg BID

Alternatives: Pyrantel

$T\frac{1}{2}$ =	2.8-9 hours	M/P =	
PHL =		PB =	High
T_{max} =	0.5-7.0 hours	Oral =	2-10%
MW =	295	pKa =	
Vd =			

References:
1.   Rao TS. Does mebendazole inhibit lactation? N Z Med J 1983; 96(736):589-590.
2.   Kurzel RB, Toot PJ, Lambert LV, Mihelcic AS. Mebendazole and postpartum lactation. N Z Med J 1994; 107(988):439.

MECLIZINE
Trade: Antivert, Bonine
Can/Aus/UK: Bonamine, Ancolan, Sea-legs
Uses: Antiemetic, antivertigo, motion sickness
LRC: L3
AAP: Not reviewed

Meclizine is an antihistamine frequently used for nausea, vertigo, and motion sickness although it is inferior to scopolamine.   Meclizine was previously used for nausea and vomiting of pregnancy.[1] No data are available on its secretion into breastmilk.   There are no pediatric indications for this product.

Pregnancy Risk Category: B

Lactation Risk Category: L3

Adult Concerns: Drowsiness, sedation, dry mouth, blurred vision

Pediatric Concerns: None reported.

Drug Interactions: May have increased sedation when used with CNS depressants and other neuroleptics and anticholinergics.

Theoretic Infant Dose:

Relative Infant Dose:

Adult Dose: 25-100 mg daily

Alternatives: Hydroxyzine, Cetirizine

T½ =	6 hours	**M/P** =	
PHL =		**PB** =	
T$_{max}$ =	1-2 hours	**Oral** =	Complete
MW =	391	**pKa** =	
Vd =			

References:

1.   Vorherr H. Drug excretion in breastmilk. Postgrad Med 1974; 56(4):97-104.

MEDROXYPROGESTERONE
Trade: Provera, Depo-Provera, Cycrin
Can/Aus/UK: Depo-Provera, Provera, Alti-MPA, Gen-Medroxy, Farlutal, Provelle, Divina, Ralovera
Uses: Injectable progestational agent
LRC: L1
        L4 if used first 3 days postpartum
AAP: Maternal Medication Usually Compatible with Breastfeeding

Depo Medroxyprogesterone (DMPA) is a synthetic progestin compound. It is used orally for amenorrhea, dysmenorrhea, uterine bleeding, and infertility. It is used intramuscularly for contraception. Due to its poor oral bioavailability, it is seldom used orally.

Saxena has reported that the average concentration in milk is 1.03 µg/L.[1] Koetswang reported average milk levels of 0.97 µg/L.[2] In a series of huge studies, the World Health Organization reviewed the developmental skills of children and their weight gain following exposure to progestin-only contraceptives during lactation.[3,4] These studies documented that no adverse effects on overall development, or rate of growth, were notable. Further, they suggested there is no apparent reason to deny lactating women the use of progestin-only contraceptives, preferably after 6 weeks postpartum.

There have been consistent and controversial studies suggesting that males exposed to early postnatal progestins have higher feminine scores.

However, Ehrhardt's studies have provided convincing data that males exposed to early progestins were no different than controls.[5] A number of other short and long-term studies available on development of children have found no differences with control groups.[6,7]

Interestingly, an excellent study of the transfer of DMPA into breastfed infants has been published.[8] In this study of 13 breastfeeding women who received 150 mg injections of DMPA on day 43 and again on day 127 postpartum, urine and plasma collections in infants (n=22) from day 38 to day 137 were collected. Urinary follicle stimulating hormone (FSH), luteinizing hormone (LH), unconjugated testosterone, unconjugated cortisol, medroxyprogesterone, and metabolites were measured. No differences (from untreated controls) were found in LH, FSH, or unconjugated testosterone urine levels in the infants. Urine cortisol levels were not altered from those of control infants. Medroxyprogesterone or its metabolites were at no time detected in any of the infant urine samples. These data conclude that only small trace amounts of MPA are transferred to breastfeeding infants and that these amounts are not expected to have any influence on breastfeeding infants. In support of this, using calculations based on MPA levels in the blood of DMPA users and a plasma to milk MPA ratio, Benagiano and Fraser suggest that the actual amounts of MPA in the infant's system is probably at or below trace levels.[9] Koetsewant states that the small amount of MPA present in milk is unlikely to have any significant clinical adverse effects on the infant.[2] A long-term follow-up study by Jimenez found no changes in growth, development, or health status in 128 breast-fed infants at 4.5 years of age.[10] DMPA mothers lactated significantly longer than controls in this study.

The use of Depo-Provera in breastfeeding women is common but will probably always be somewhat controversial. Depo Provera has been documented to significantly elevate prolactin levels in breastfeeding mothers and increase milk production.[11, 12]

It is well known that estrogens suppress milk production. With progestins, it has been suggested that some women may experience a decline in milk production or arrested early production following an injection of DMPA, particularly when the progestin is used early postpartum (12-48 hrs).[13] At present there are no published data to support this, nor is the relative incidence of this untoward effect known. Therefore, in some instances, it might be advisable to recommend treatment with oral progestin-only contraceptives postpartum, so that women who experience reduced milk supply could easily withdraw from the medication without significant loss of breastmilk supply. No progestin should be used before at least 3 days postpartum and perhaps longer.[13]

Pregnancy Risk Category: D

Lactation Risk Category: **L1**
                                L4 if used first 3 days postpartum

Adult Concerns: Fluid retention, GI distress, menstrual disorders, breakthrough bleeding, weight gain

Pediatric Concerns: None reported via milk although unsubstantiated reports of reduced milk supply have been made.

Drug Interactions: Aminoglutethimide may increase the hepatic clearance of medroxyprogesterone, reducing its efficacy.

Theoretic Infant Dose:

Relative Infant Dose:

Adult Dose: 5-10 mg daily

Alternatives:

$T\frac{1}{2}$ =	14.5 hours		M/P =	
PHL =			PB =	
T_{max} =			Oral =	0.6-10%
MW =	344		pKa =	
Vd =				

References:

1. Saxena NB. et.al. Level of contraceptive steroids in breastmilk and plasma of lactating women. Contraception 1977; 16:605-613.

2. Koetsawang S, Nukulkarn P, Fotherby K, Shrimanker K, Mangalam M, Towobola K. Transfer of contraceptive steroids in milk of women using long-acting gestagens. Contraception 1982; 25(4):321-331.

3. Progestogen-only contraceptives during lactation: I. Infant growth. World Health Organization Task force for Epidemiological Research on Reproductive Health; Special Programme of Research, Development and Research Training in Human Reproduction Contraception 1994; 50(1):35-53.

4. Progestogen-only contraceptives during lactation: II. Infant development. World Health Organization, Task Force for Epidemiological Research on Reproductive Health; Special Programme of Research, Development, and Research Training in Human Reproduction Contraception 1994; 50(1):55-68.

5. Ehrhardt AA, Grisanti GC, Meyer-Bahlburg HF. Prenatal exposure to medroxyprogesterone acetate (MPA) in girls. Psychoneuroendocrinology 1977; 2(4):391-398.

6. Schwallie PC. The effect of depot-medroxyprogesterone acetate on the fetus and nursing infant: a review. Contraception 1981; 23(4):375-386.

7. Pardthaisong T, Yenchit C, Gray R. The long-term growth and development of children exposed to Depo-Provera during pregnancy or lactation. Contraception 1992; 45(4):313-324.3. Benagiano G, Fraser I. The Depo-Provera debate. Commentary on the article "Depo-Provera, a critical analysis". Contraception 1981; 24(5):493-528.

8. Virutamasen P, Leepipatpaiboon S, Kriengsinyot R, Vichaidith P, Muia PN, Sekadde-Kigondu CB, Mati JK, Forest MG, Dikkeschei LD, Wolthers BG, d'Arcangues C. Pharmacodynamic effects of depot-medroxyprogesterone acetate (DMPA) administered to lactating women on their male infants. Contraception 1996; 54(3):153-157.

9. Benagiano G, Fraser I. The Depo-Provera debate. Commentary on the article "Depo-Provera, a critical analysis". Contraception 1981; 24(5):493-528.
10. Jimenez J, Ochoa M, Soler MP, Portales P. Long-term follow-up of children breast-fed by mothers receiving depot-medroxyprogesterone acetate. Contraception 1984; 30(6):523-533.
11. Ratchanon S, Taneepanichskul S. Depot medroxyprogesterone acetate and basal serum prolactin levels in lactating women. Obstet Gynecol 2000; 96(6):926-928.
12. Fraser IS. Long acting injectable hormonal contraceptives. Clin Reprod Fertil 1982; 1(1):67-88.
13. Kennedy KI, Short RV, Tully MR. Premature introduction of progestin-only contraceptive methods during lactation. Contraception 1997; 55(6):347-350.

MEDROXYPROGESTERONE AND ESTRADIOL CYPIONATE

Trade: Lunelle
Can/Aus/UK:
Uses: Once-a-month birth control injection.
LRC: L3
AAP: Not reviewed

Lunelle is a new, once-a-month injectable birth control product. It contains medroxyprogesterone acetate (25 mg), which is the active ingredient in Depo-Provera and also contains 5 mg estradiol cypionate, which is a repository form of estrogen that is slowly released from the injection site over 30 days.

The amount of medroxyprogesterone for this one month injection is 25 mg. The amount of Depo-Provera providing 3 months coverage is 150 mg. Because this injection contains estrogen, it may potentially reduce the production of milk and caution is recommended.[1] Although small amounts of estrogens and progestins may pass into breastmilk, the effects of these hormones on an infant appear minimal. Use of estrogen containing products, particularly early postpartum, may dramatically reduce the volume of milk produced. Mothers should attempt to delay use of these products for as long as possible postpartum (at least 6-8 weeks), if at all. Because of the estrogen content and the prolonged release formula, caution is recommended in breastfeeding mothers.

Pregnancy Risk Category: X

Lactation Risk Category: L3

Adult Concerns: Side effects are typical of oral contraceptives and include thromboembolism, cerebral hemorrhage, hypertension, infarction, cerebral ischemia, gallbladder disease, pulmonary embolism, thrombophlebitis. Abdominal pain, acne, etc. See package insert for numerous others.

Pediatric Concerns: Possibility of reduce milk supply. Long term followup of infants has shown no untoward effects.

Drug Interactions: Aminoglutethimide may decrease effectiveness and serum concentration of MPA. Rifamin may increase metabolism of estrogens/progestins. Anticonvulsans such as phenobarbital, phenytoin, and carbamazepine have been shown to increase metabolism of some estrogens and progestins and could reduce contraceptive effectiveness. Some antibiotics (ampicillin, tetracycline and griseofulvin) may reduce contraceptive effectiveness. St. Johns wort may also reduce contraceptive effectiveness by enhancing metabolism of numerous drugs.

Theoretic Infant Dose:

Relative Infant Dose:

Adult Dose: 25 mg MPA, 5 mg estradiol cypionate monthly

Alternatives: Micronor, Ovrette

References:
1. Booker DE, Pahl IR. Control of postpartum breast engorgement with oral contraceptives. Am J Obstet Gynecol 1967; 98(8):1099-1101.

MEFLOQUINE
Trade: Lariam
Can/Aus/UK: Lariam
Uses: Antimalarial
LRC: L2
AAP: Not reviewed

Mefloquine is an antimalarial and a structural analog of quinine. It is concentrated in red cells and therefore has a long half-life.[1] Following a single 250 mg dose in two women, the milk/plasma ratio was only 0.13 to 0.16 the first 4 days of therapy.[2] The concentration of mefloquine in milk ranged from 32 to 53 μg/L. Unfortunately, these studies were not carried out after steady state conditions, which would probably increase to some degree the amount transferred to the infant. According to the manufacturer, mefloquine is secreted in small concentrations approximating 3% of the maternal dose. Assuming a milk level of 53 μg/L and a daily milk intake of 150 mL/kg/day, an infant would ingest approximately 8 μg/kg/day of mefloquine, which is not sufficient to protect the infant from malaria. The therapeutic dose for malaria prophylaxis is 62 mg in a 15-19 kg infant. Thus far, no untoward effects have been reported.

Pregnancy Risk Category: C

Lactation Risk Category: **L2**

Adult Concerns: GI upset, dizziness, elevated liver enzymes, possible retinopathy

Pediatric Concerns: None reported but discontinue lactation if neuropsychiatric disturbances occur.

Drug Interactions: Decreases effect of valproic acid. Increased toxicity of beta blockers, chloroquine, quinine, quinidine.

Theoretic Infant Dose: 7.95 µg/kg/day

Relative Infant Dose: 0.22 %

Adult Dose: 1.25 g once OR 250 mg q week

Alternatives:

$T\frac{1}{2}$ =	10-21 days	M/P =	0.13-0.27
PHL =		PB =	98%
T_{max} =	1-2 hours	Oral =	85%
MW =	414	pKa =	
Vd =	19		

References:
1. Pharmaceutical Manufacturer Prescribing Information. 1995.
2. Edstein MD, Veenendaal JR, Hyslop R. Excretion of mefloquine in human breastmilk. Chemotherapy 1988; 34(3):165-169.

MELATONIN
Trade:
Can/Aus/UK:
Uses: Hormone
LRC: L3
AAP: Not reviewed

Melatonin (N-acetyl-5-methoxytryptamine) is a normal hormone secreted by the pineal gland in the human brain. It is circadian in rhythm, with nighttime values considerably higher than daytime levels. It is postulated to induce a sleep-like pattern in humans. It is known to be passed into human milk and is believed responsible for entraining the newborn brain to phase shift its circadian clock to that of the mother by communicating the time of day information to the newborn.

On the average, the amount of melatonin in human milk is about 35% of the maternal plasma level but can range to as high as 80%.[1] Post feeding milk levels appear to more closely reflect the maternal plasma level than prefeeding values, suggesting that melatonin may be transported into milk at night during the feeding, rather than being stored in foremilk. In neonates, melatonin levels are low and progressively increase up to the age of 3 months when the characteristic diurnal rhythm is detectible.[2]   Night-time melatonin levels reach a maximum at the age of 1-3 years and thereafter decline to adult values.[3,4,5]   While night-time maternal serum levels average 280 pmol/L, milk levels averaged 99 pmol/L in a group of ten breastfeeding mothers.[1] The effect of orally administered melatonin on newborns is unknown, but melatonin has thus far not been associated with significant untoward effects.

Pregnancy Risk Category:

Lactation Risk Category: L3

Adult Concerns: Headache and confusion, drowsiness, fatigue, hypothermia, and dysphoria in depressed patients.

Pediatric Concerns: None reported.

Drug Interactions:

Theoretic Infant Dose:

Relative Infant Dose:

Adult Dose:

Alternatives:

$T\frac{1}{2}$ =	30-50 minutes	M/P =	0.35-0.8
PHL =		PB =	
T_{max} =	0.5-2 hours	Oral =	Complete
MW =	232	pKa =	
Vd =			

References:
1. Illnerova H, Buresova M, Presl J. Melatonin rhythm in human milk. J Clin Endocrinol Metab 1993; 77(3):838-841.
2. Hartmann L, Roger M, Lemaitre BJ, Massias JF, Chaussain JL. Plasma and urinary melatonin in male infants during the first 12 months of life. Clin Chim Acta 1982; 121(1):37-42.
3. Aldhous M, Franey C, Wright J, Arendt J. Plasma concentrations of melatonin in man following oral absorption of different preparations. Br J Clin Pharmacol 1985; 19(4):517-521.
4. Attanasio A, Rager K, Gupta D. Ontogeny of circadian rhythmicity for melatonin, serotonin, and N-acetylserotonin in humans. J Pineal Res 1986; 3(3):251-256.
5. Dollins AB, Lynch HJ, Wurtman RJ, Deng MH, Kischka KU, Gleason RE, Lieberman HR. Effect of pharmacological daytime doses of melatonin on human mood and performance. Psychopharmacology (Berl) 1993; 112(4):490-496.

MELOXICAM

Trade: Mobic
Can/Aus/UK: Mobic
Uses: Nonsteroidal anti-inflammatory agent
LRC: L3
AAP: Not reviewed

Meloxicam is a nonsteroidal anti-inflammatory drug that appears more selective for the COX-2 receptor.[1] No data are available for transfer into human milk although it does transfer into rodent milk. Due to its long half-life and good bioavailability, another NSAID would probably be preferred.

Pregnancy Risk Category: C

Lactation Risk Category: L3

Adult Concerns: Leukopenia, elevated liver enzymes, headache, abdominal pain, constipation, diarrhea, angina, anaphylaxis in aspirin sensitive patients.

Pediatric Concerns: None reported via milk.

Drug Interactions: May reduce coagulation in patients using anticoagulants and other platelet inhibitory drugs. NSAIDs may decrease the antihypertensive effect of ACE inhibitors. May increase blood pressure in hypertensive patients using beta blockers and other antihypertensives. May increase risk of gastric hemorrhage with calcium channel blockers. Numerous other drug-drug interactions listed, consult another text.

Theoretic Infant Dose:

Relative Infant Dose:

Adult Dose: 7.5 mg/d

Alternatives: Ibuprofen, celecoxib

$T\frac{1}{2}$ =	20.1 hours	M/P =	
PHL =		PB =	99.4
T_{max} =	4.9 hours	Oral =	89%
MW =	351	pKa =	4.2
Vd =	0.14		

References:
1. Pharmaceutical Manufacturer Prescribing Information. 2002

MENINGOCOCCAL VACCINE
Trade: Menomune
Can/Aus/UK:
Uses: Vaccine
LRC: L1
AAP: Not reviewed

Meningococcal polysaccharide vaccine is a freeze-dried preparation of group-specific antigens from Neisseria meningitidis. This vaccine is not infectious. This vaccine is useful to prevent endemic and epidemic meningitis and meningococcemia in children and young adults. There are no contraindications for using this in breastfeeding mothers other than allergic hypersensitivity to some of the ingredients.

Pregnancy Risk Category: C

Lactation Risk Category: L1

Adult Concerns: Pain , erythema, induration at injection site. Headaches, malaise, chills and elevated temperature have been reported.

Pediatric Concerns: None via milk.

Drug Interactions:

Theoretic Infant Dose:

Relative Infant Dose:

Adult Dose: 0.5 mL subcutaneously

Alternatives:

References:
1. Pharmaceutical Manufacturers Prescribing Information, 2003.

MENOTROPINS
Trade: Pergonal, Humegon, Repronex
Can/Aus/UK: Pergonal, Humegon
Uses: Produces follicle growth
LRC: L3
AAP: Not reviewed

Menotropins is a purified preparation of gonadotropins hormones extracted from the urine of postmenopausal women. It is a biologically standardized form containing equal activity of follicle stimulating hormone (FSH) and luteinizing hormone (LH).[1-3] Menotropins and human chorionic gonadotropins (see chorionic gonadotropins) are given sequentially to induce ovulation in the anovulatory female. FSH and LH are large molecular weight peptides and would not likely penetrate into human milk. Further, they are unstable in the GI tract, and their oral bioavailability would be minimal to zero even in an infant.

Pregnancy Risk Category: X

Lactation Risk Category: L3

Adult Concerns: Ovarian enlargement, cysts, hemoperitoneum, fever, chills, aches, join patins, nausea, vomiting, abdominal pain, diarrhea, bloating, rash, dizziness.

Pediatric Concerns: None reported via milk. These agents are very unlikely to enter milk. But observe closely for changes in milk production which could occur.

Drug Interactions:

Theoretic Infant Dose:

Relative Infant Dose:

Adult Dose: 75-150 units each FSH & LH daily

Alternatives:

$T\frac{1}{2}$ =	3.9 and 70.4 hours	M/P =		
PHL =		PB =		
T_{max} =	6 hours	Oral =	0%	
MW =	34,000	pKa =		
Vd =	1.08			

References:
1.   Sharma V, Riddle A, Mason B, Whitehead M, Collins W. Studies on folliculogenesis and in vitro fertilization outcome after the administration of follicle-stimulating hormone at different times during the menstrual cycle. Fertil Steril 1989; 51(2):298-303.
2.   Kjeld JM, Harsoulis P, Kuku SF, Marshall JC, Kaufman B, Fraser TR. Infusions of hFSH and hLH in normal men. I. Kinetics of human follicle stimulating hormone. Acta Endocrinol (Copenh) 1976; 81(2):225-233.
3.   Yen SC, Llerena LA, Pearson OH, Littell AS. Disappearance rates of endogenous follicle-stimulating hormone in serum following surgical hypophysectomy in man. J Clin Endocrinol Metab 1970; 30(3):325-329.

MEPERIDINE

Trade: Demerol
Can/Aus/UK: Demerol, Pethidine
Uses: Narcotic analgesic
LRC: L2
            L3 if used early postpartum
    AAP: Maternal Medication Usually Compatible with Breastfeeding

Meperidine is a potent opiate analgesic. It is rapidly and completely metabolized by the adult and neonatal liver to an active form, normeperidine. Significant but small amounts of meperidine are secreted into breastmilk. In a study of 9 nursing mothers two hours after a 50 mg IM injection, the average concentration of meperidine in milk was 82 μg/L and a milk/plasma ratio of 1.12.[1] The highest concentration of meperidine in breastmilk at 2 hours after dose was 0.13 mg/L.

In another study, the maximum concentration of meperidine in milk ranged from 134 to 244 μg/L in 5 patients at 1-2 hours after administration and 76 to 318 μg/L at 2-4 hours after administration of 25 mg intravenously (in 3 patients).[2] According to these authors, the maximum dose to an infant would be approximately 9.5 μg/kg or 1.2% to 3.5% of the weight-adjusted maternal dose.

In a study of two nursing mothers who received varying amounts of meperidine following delivery (up to 1275 mg within 72 hours), the concentration of meperidine ranged from 36.2 to 314 μg/L with an average of 225 μg/L. Breastmilk levels of normeperidine ranged from zero to 333 μg/L with an average of 142 μg/L.[3] This study clearly shows a much longer half-life for the active metabolite, normeperidine. Normeperidine levels were detected after 56 hours post-administration in human milk (8.1 ng/mL) following a single 50 mg dose. The milk/plasma ratios varied from 0.82 to 1.59 depending on dose and timing of sampling.

Published half-lives for meperidine in neonates (13 hours) and normeperidine (63 hours) are long and with time could concentrate in the plasma of a neonate. Wittels studies clearly indicate that infants from mothers treated with meperidine (PCA post-cesarian) were neurobehaviorally depressed after three days. Infants from similar groups treated with morphine were not affected.

Pregnancy Risk Category: B

Lactation Risk Category: L2
     L3 if used early postpartum

Adult Concerns: Sedation, respiratory depression

Pediatric Concerns: Sedation, poor suckling reflex, neurobehavioral delay.

Drug Interactions: Phenytoin may decrease analgesic effect. Meperidine may aggravate adverse effects of isoniazid. MAO inhibitors, Fluoxetine and other SSRIs, and tricyclic antidepressants may greatly potentiate the effects of meperidine.

Theoretic Infant Dose: 12.3 μg/kg/day

Relative Infant Dose: 1.7%

Adult Dose: 50-100 mg q 3-4 hours PRN

Alternatives: Morphine, Fentanyl, Hydrocodone

T½ =	3.2 hours	M/P =	0.84-1.59
PHL =	6-32 hours (neonates)	PB =	65-80 %
T_{max} =	30-50 minutes (IM)	Oral =	< 50%
MW =	247	pKa =	8.6
Vd =	3.7-4.2		

References:

1. Peiker G, Muller B, Ihn W, Noschel H. [Excretion of pethidine in mother's milk (author's transl)]. Zentralbl Gynakol 1980; 102(10):537-541.
2. Borgatta L, Jenny RW, Gruss L, Ong C, Barad D. Clinical significance of methohexital, meperidine, and diazepam in breastmilk. J Clin Pharmacol 1997; 37(3):186-192.
3. Quinn PG, Kuhnert BR, Kaine CJ, Syracuse CD. Measurement of meperidine and normeperidine in human breastmilk by selected ion monitoring. Biomed Environ Mass Spectrom 1986; 13(3):133-135.
4. Wittels B, Scott DT, Sinatra RS. Exogenous opioids in human breastmilk and acute neonatal neurobehavior: a preliminary study. Anesthesiology 1990; 73(5):864-869.

MEPINDOLOL SULFATE

Trade:
Can/Aus/UK: Corindolan
Uses: Non-specific beta blocker
LRC: L2
AAP: Not reviewed

Mepindolol is a non-selective beta receptor blocking agent. In a study of 5 women (on day 3 postpartum) who received 20 mg daily for 5 days, the concentrations of mepindolol in plasma and milk of five breastfeeding mothers were determined one day one and after 5 daily doses of mepindolol sulphate 20 mg.[1] In the newborns plasma levels were measured once on the first and fifth days of the study. The mean maternal plasma concentration of mepindolol 2 hours after administration was 52 µg/L both after 1 and 5 doses. Average milk concentrations of mepindolol were 18 µg/L after one dose, and 22 µg/L after 5 daily doses. The average milk/plasma ratio was 0.4. Plasma levels in the newborn were below the detection limit of 1 µg/L, except for one baby in whom 2 and 5 µg/L were measured. The "relative" infant dose would be 1.1% of the maternal dose. No drug-related side effects were noted in these 5 infants.

Pregnancy Risk Category: **C in first trimester**
                                D in second and third trimester

Lactation Risk Category: **L2**

Adult Concerns: Bradycardia, asthmatic symptoms, hypotension, sedation, weakness, hypoglycemia

Pediatric Concerns: None reported in one study of 5 breastfed infants.

Drug Interactions: Beta blockers may reduce the effect of oral sulfonylureas (hypoglycemic agents). Increased toxicity/effect when used with other antihypertensives, contraceptives, MAO inhibitors, cimetidine, and numerous other products. See drug interaction reference for complete listing.

Theoretic Infant Dose: 3.3 µg/kg/day

Relative Infant Dose: 1.1%

Adult Dose: 20 mg daily

Alternatives: Propranolol, metoprolol

T½ =	3-4 hours	M/P =	< 0.4
PHL =		PB =	50%
T$_{max}$ =	1-3 hours	Oral =	> 95%
MW =		pKa =	
Vd =	5.7		

References:
1 Krause W, Stoppelli I, Milia S, Rainer E. Transfer of mepindolol to newborns by breast-feeding mothers after single and repeated daily doses. Eur J Clin Pharmacol 1982; 22(1):53-55.

MEPIVACAINE
Trade: Carbocaine, Polocaine
Can/Aus/UK: Carbocaine, Polocaine
Uses: Local anesthetic
LRC: L3
AAP: Not reviewed

Mepivacaine is a long acting local anesthetic similar to bupivacaine.[1-3] Mepivacaine is used for infiltration, peripheral nerve blocks, and central nerve blocks (epidural or caudal anesthesia). No data are available on the transfer of mepivacaine into human milk; however, its structure is practically identical to bupivacaine and one would expect its entry into human milk is similar and low. Bupivacaine enters milk in exceedingly low levels (see bupivacaine). Due to higher fetal levels and reported toxicities, mepivacaine is never used antenatally. For use in breastfeeding patients, bupivacaine is preferred.

Pregnancy Risk Category: C

Lactation Risk Category: L3

Adult Concerns: Sedation, bradycardia, respiratory sedation, transient burning, anaphylaxis

Pediatric Concerns: None reported via milk. Neonatal depression and convulsive seizures occurred in 7 neonates 6 hours after delivery.

Drug Interactions: Increases effect of hyaluronidase, beta blockers, MAO inhibitors, tricyclic antidepressants, phenothiazines, and vasopressors.

Theoretic Infant Dose:

Relative Infant Dose:

Adult Dose: 50-300 mg X 1

Alternatives:

T½ =	1.9-3.2 hours	M/P =	
PHL =	8.7-9 hours	PB =	60-85%
Tmax =	30 minutes	Oral =	
MW =		pKa =	7.6
Vd =			

References:
1. Pharmaceutical Manufacturer Prescribing Information. 1997.
2. Hillman LS, Hillman RE, Dodson WE. Diagnosis, treatment, and follow-up of neonatal mepivacaine intoxication secondary to paracervical and pudendal blocks during labor. J Pediatr 1979; 95(3):472-477.
3. Teramo K, Rajamaki A. Foetal and maternal plasma levels of mepivacaine and foetal acid-base balance and heart rate after paracervical block during labour. Br J Anaesth 1971; 43(4):300-312.

MEPROBAMATE

Trade: Equanil, Miltown
Can/Aus/UK: Equanil, Novo-Mepro, Apo-Meprobamate, Meprate
Uses: Antianxiety drug
LRC: L3
AAP: Not reviewed

Meprobamate is an older antianxiety drug.[1] It is secreted into milk at levels 2-4 times that of the maternal plasma level.[2] It could produce some sedation in a breastfeeding infant.

Pregnancy Risk Category: D

Lactation Risk Category: L3

Adult Concerns: Blood dyscrasias, sedation, hypotension, withdrawal reactions

Pediatric Concerns: None reported, but observe for sedation.

Drug Interactions: May have increased CNS depression when used with other neuroleptic depressants.

Theoretic Infant Dose:

Relative Infant Dose:

Adult Dose: 300-400 mg TID-QID

Alternatives: Lorazepam, Alprazolam

T½ =	6-17 hours	M/P =	2-4
PHL =		PB =	15%
T$_{max}$ =	1-3 hours	Oral =	Complete
MW =	218	pKa =	
Vd =	0.7		

References:
1. Pharmaceutical Manufacturer Prescribing Information. 1993.
2. Wilson JT, Brown RD, Cherek DR, Dailey JW, Hilman B, Jobe PC, Manno BR, Manno JE, Redetzki HM, Stewart JJ. Drug excretion in human breastmilk: principles, pharmacokinetics and projected consequences. Clin Pharmacokinet 1980; 5(1):1-66.

MERCAPTOPURINE
Trade: Purinthol, 6-Mp
Can/Aus/UK: Purinethol, Puri-Nethol
Uses: Antimetabolite, immunosuppressant
LRC: L5
AAP: Not reviewed

Mercaptopurine is an anticancer drug that acts intracellularly as an purine antagonist, ultimately inhibiting DNA and RNA synthesis.[1] It is an extremely toxic drug producing significant bone marrow suppression. Because it has a pKa of 7.6, it would likely penetrate milk although no data are available. Mercaptopurine is probably too dangerous and toxic to use in a breastfeeding mother although it is occasionally used during pregnancy.

Pregnancy Risk Category: D

Lactation Risk Category: L5

Adult Concerns: Bone marrow suppression, liver toxicity, nausea, vomiting, diarrhea

Pediatric Concerns: None reported, but this product is probably too dangerous to continue breastfeeding.

Drug Interactions: When used with allopurinol, reduced mercaptopurine to 1/3 to 1/4 the usual dose. When used with trimethoprim sulfamethoxazole, may enhance bone marrow suppression.

Theoretic Infant Dose:

Relative Infant Dose:

Adult Dose: 1.5-2.5 mg/kg daily

Alternatives: Infliximab

T½ =	0.9 hour	M/P =	
PHL =		PB =	19%
T$_{max}$ =	2 hours	Oral =	50%
MW =	152	pKa =	7.6
Vd =			

References:
1. Pharmaceutical Manufacturer Prescribing Information. 1995.

MERCURY
Trade: Mercury
Can/Aus/UK:
Uses: Environmental contaminate
LRC: L5
AAP: Not reviewed

Mercury is an environmental contaminate that is available in multiple salt forms. Elemental mercury, the form found in thermometers, is poorly absorbed orally (0.01%) but completely absorbed via inhalation (> 80%).[1] Inorganic mercury causes most forms of mercury poisoning and is available in mercury disk batteries (7-15% orally bioavailable). Organic mercury (methyl mercury fungicides, phenyl mercury) is readily absorbed (90% orally). Mercury poisoning produces encephalopathy, acute renal failure, severe GI necrosis, and numerous other systemic toxicities. Mercury transfers into human milk with a milk/plasma ratio that varies according to the mercury form. Pitkin reports that in the USA that 100 nonexposed women had 0.9 µg/L total mercury in their milk.[2] Concentrations of mercury in human milk are generally much higher in populations that ingest large quantities of fish. Mothers known to be contaminated with mercury should not breastfeed.

The transfer of mercury from dental amalgams has been studied to some degree. In mothers with mercury-containing amalgams, the transfer of mercury during gestation to the fetus is generally much higher than from human milk.[3,4] Mercury levels in milk are highest immediately after birth, and these are significantly correlated with the number and size of amalgam fillings present in the mother although others disagree.[5,6,7] In this study breastmilk levels of mercury dropped significantly after 2 months and are more positivitely associated with the amount of fish ingested, rather than the number of amalgam fillings. At birth mercury levels in milk averaged 0.9 µg/L (0.25 to 20.3 µg/L) and after two months mercury levels averaged 0.25 μg/L(0.25-11.7 μg/L). The authors suggest that the exposure to mercury of breastfed infants from maternal amalgam fillings is of minor importance compared to maternal fish consumption.

Oskarsson suggests in a study of Swedish women that the exposure of the infant to mercury from breastmilk was less than 0.3 μg/kg/d. This exposure is only approximately one-half the tolerable daily intake for adults recommended by the World Health Organization.[6]

These studies generally conclude that while mercury fillings may increase the transfer of mercury to the infant, most occurs in utero. Secondly, the transfer of mercury into human milk is transiently high at birth and then drops significantly at 2 months. Apparently the diet provides the greatest source of maternal mercury to human milk, much less is provided by older amalgam fillings. Further, the replacement of amalgam fillings should if possible be postponed until after pregnancy, and breastfeeding as the removal of amalgam fillings while breastfeeding could potentially increase the transfer of mercury to the breastfed infant and largely (this largely depends on the precautions taken by the dentist).

There are several routine precautions that the dentist could use when removing the old amalgam. Because heat during the grinding process can vaporize the mercury and enhance absorption by the mother, suggest that the dentist use copious amounts of cold water irrigation to minimize heat; use a rubber dam to isolate her mouth from the particles, and use an alternate source of air (oxygen) to minimize mercury vapor inhalation during removal of the amalgam.

Pregnancy Risk Category:

Lactation Risk Category: L5

Adult Concerns: Brain damage, acute renal failure, severe GI necrosis, and numerous other systemic toxicities.

Pediatric Concerns: Mercury transfer into milk is significant. Transfer to the infant is a function of levels in the mother. Dental amalgams provide some but not significant levels of transfer. Most mercury transfers in utero, not in milk. Mercury levels in milk drop significantly after 2 months. Caution is recommended in removing amalgams while pregnant or breastfeeding.

Drug Interactions:

Theoretic Infant Dose:

Relative Infant Dose:

Adult Dose:

Alternatives:

T½ =	70 days	M/P =	0.27 -1.0
PHL =		PB =	
T$_{max}$ =		Oral =	Variable
MW =	201	pKa =	
Vd =			

References:

1. Wolff MS. Occupationally derived chemicals in breastmilk. Am J Ind Med. 4:259-281, 1983.
2. Pitkin RM, Bahns JA, Filer LJ, Jr., Reynolds WA. Mercury in human maternal and cord blood, placenta, and milk. Proc Soc Exp Biol Med. 151(3):565-567, 1976.
3. Ramirez G, Cruz MC, Pagulayan O, Ostrea E, Dalisay C. The Tagum study I: analysis and clinical correlates of mercury in maternal and cord blood, breast milk, meconium, and infants' hair. Pediatrics 2000; 106(4):774-781.
4. Yang J, Jiang Z, Wang Y, Qureshi IA, Wu XD. Maternal-fetal transfer of metallic mercury via the placenta and milk. Ann Clin Lab Sci 1997; 27(2):135-141.
5. Drexler H, Schaller KH. The mercury concentration in breast milk resulting from amalgam fillings and dietary habits. Environ Res 1998; 77(2):124-129.
6. Oskarsson A, Schultz A, Skerfving S, Hallen IP, Ohlin B, Lagerkvist BJ. Total and inorganic mercury in breast milk in relation to fish consumption and amalgam in lactating women. Arch Environ Health 1996; 51(3):234-241.
7. Klemann D, Weinhold J, Strubelt O, Pentz R, Jungblut JR, Klink F. [Effects of amalgam fillings on the mercury concentrations in amniotic fluid and breast milk]. Dtsch Zahnarztl Z 1990; 45(3):142-145.

MEROPENEM

Trade: Merrem
Can/Aus/UK: Merrem, Meronem
Uses: Semisynthetic carbapenem antibiotic
LRC: L3
AAP: Not reviewed

Meropenem is a new antibiotic similar to the older imipenem although it has greater activity against gram-negative species, but has slightly less activity against gram-positive species.[1] No data are available on its transfer into human milk but like others in this family, it is likely low. Further this agent is not orally bioavailable to any degree. Changes in gut flora could be expected in breastfed infants.

Pregnancy Risk Category: B

Lactation Risk Category: L3

Adult Concerns: Headache, seizures (0.5%), nausea, abdominal pain, diarrhea, and elevated liver function tests have been reported.

Pediatric Concerns: None reported via milk. Unlikely to enter milk significantly. Changes in gut flora could occur.

Drug Interactions: Increased plasma levels with probenecid.

Theoretic Infant Dose:

Relative Infant Dose:

Adult Dose: 1 gm IV every 8 hours

Alternatives: Imipenem-Cilistatin

T½ =	1 hour	M/P =	
PHL =	1.5 hours	PB =	2%
T$_{max}$ =	Immediate	Oral =	Nil
MW =	437	pKa =	
Vd =	0.28		

References:
1.   Pharmaceutical Manufacturers prescribing information, 2003.

MESALAMINE
Trade: Asacol, Pentasa, Rowasa, Canasa, Colazal
Can/Aus/UK: Salofalk, Mesasal, Quintasa, Mesalazine, Asacol
Uses: Anti-inflammatory in ulcerative colitis
LRC: L3
AAP: Should be given to nursing mothers with caution

Mesalamine is an anti-inflammatory agent used in ulcerative colitis. Although it contains 5-aminosalicylic acid, the mechanism of action is unknown. Some 5-aminosalicylic acid (5-ASA) can be converted into salicylic acid and absorbed, but the amount is very small. Acetyl-5-aminosalicylic (Acetyl-5-ASA) acid is the common metabolite and has been found in breastmilk. The effect of mesalamine is primarily local on the mucosa of the colon itself. Mesalamine is poorly absorbed from the GI tract. Only 5-35% of a dose is absorbed. Oral tablets are enteric coated for delayed absorption.

In one patient receiving 500 mg mesalamine orally three times daily, the concentration of 5-ASA in breastmilk was 0.11 mg/L, and the Acetyl-5-ASA metabolite was 12.4 mg/L of milk. The milk/plasma ratio for 5-ASA was 0.27 and for Acetyl-5-ASA was 5.1.[1] Using these data, the weight-adjusted relative infant dose would be 8.7%.

In another patient receiving 1000 mg PO three times daily, milk levels of 5-ASA following 7 and 11 days of treatment and 5 hours following the dose were both 0.1 mg/L, and the milk/plasma ratios were 0.07 and 0.09.[2]

Mesalamine is useful in patients allergic to sulfasalazine or salicylazosulfapyridine.   At least one report of a watery diarrhea in an infant whose mother was using rectal 5-ASA has been reported.[3]   Each time treatment was reinstated diarrhea recurred. A new product, Colazal (Balsalazide), is a prodrug of mesalamine (5-aminosalicylic acid; 5-ASA).

Pregnancy Risk Category: B

Lactation Risk Category: L3

Adult Concerns: Watery diarrhea, abdominal pain, cramps, flatulence, nausea, headache

Pediatric Concerns: Watery diarrhea in one breastfed patient although this appears rare.

Drug Interactions: May significantly reduce bioavailability of digoxin.

Theoretic Infant Dose: 1.8 mg/kg/day

Relative Infant Dose: 8.7%

Adult Dose: 800 mg TID

Alternatives:

T½ =	5-10 hours (metabolite)	M/P =	0.27, 5.1
PHL =		PB =	55%
Tmax =	4-12 hours	Oral =	15-35%
MW =	153	pKa =	
Vd =			

References:
1. Jenss H, Weber P, Hartmann F. 5-Aminosalicylic acid and its metabolite in breastmilk during lactation. Am J Gastroenterol 1990; 85(3):331.
2. Klotz U, Harings-Kaim A. Negligible excretion of 5-aminosalicylic acid in breastmilk. Lancet 1993; 342(8871):618-619.
3. Nelis GF. Diarrhoea due to 5-aminosalicylic acid in breastmilk. Lancet 1989; 1(8634):383.

MESORIDAZINE

Trade: Serentil
Can/Aus/UK: Serentil
Uses: Phenothiazine antipsychotic
LRC: L4
AAP: Drugs whose effect on nursing infants is unknown but may be of concern

Mesoridazine is a typical phenothiazine antipsychotic used for treatment of schizophrenia. No data on transfer into human milk are available.[1] However, the use of the phenothiazine family in breastfeeding mothers is risky and may increase the risk of SIDS.

Pregnancy Risk Category: C

Lactation Risk Category: L4

Adult Concerns: Adverse effects include leukopenia, eosinophilia, thrombocytopenia, anemia, aplastic anemia, hypotension, drowsiness, agitation, dystonic reactions, seizures, galactorrhea, gynecomastia, dry mouth, nausea, vomiting, constipation, priapism, incontinence, and phototoxicity.

Pediatric Concerns: None reported via milk, but use in breastfeeding mothers is discouraged due to possible sedation in infant and elevated risk of SIDS.

Drug Interactions: Decreased effect with anticonvulsants, anticholinergics. Increased toxicity when used with CNS depressants, metrizamide (increased seizures), and propranolol.

Theoretic Infant Dose:

Relative Infant Dose:

Adult Dose: 25-50 mg TID

Alternatives:

T½ =	24-48 hours	M/P =	
PHL =		PB =	91%
T$_{max}$ =	4 hours	Oral =	Erratic
MW =		pKa =	
Vd =			

References:
1.   Ayd FJ. Excretion of psychotropic drugs in breastmilk. In: International Drug Therapy Newsletter.Ayd Medical Communications 8[November-December]. 1973.

METAXALONE

Trade: Skelaxin
Can/Aus/UK:
Uses: Sedative, skeletal muscle relaxant
LRC: L3
AAP: Not reviewed

Metaxalone is a centrally acting sedative used primarily as a muscle relaxant.[1]   Its ability to relax skeletal muscle is weak and is probably due to its sedative properties.   Hypersensitivity reactions in adults (allergic) have occurred as well as liver toxicity.   No data are available on its transfer into breastmilk.

Pregnancy Risk Category:

Lactation Risk Category: L3

Adult Concerns: Sedation, nausea, vomiting, GI upset, hemolytic anemia, abnormal liver function

Pediatric Concerns: None reported. No data available.

Drug Interactions:

Theoretic Infant Dose:

Relative Infant Dose:

Adult Dose: 800 mg TID-QID

Alternatives:

T½ =	2-3 hours	M/P =
PHL =		PB =
T_{max} =	2 hours	Oral =
MW =	221	pKa =
Vd =		

References:
1. Pharmaceutical Manufacturer Prescribing Information. 1995.

METFORMIN

Trade: Glucophage, Glucovance
Can/Aus/UK: Glucophage, Gen-Metformin, Glycon, Diabex, Diaformin, Diguanil
Uses: Oral hypoglycemic agent for diabetes
LRC: L1
AAP: Not reviewed

Metformin belongs to the biguanide family and is used to reduce glucose levels in non-insulin dependent diabetics. Oral bioavailability is only 50%. In a study of 7 women taking metformin (median dose 1500 mg/d), the mean milk-to-plasma ratio for metformin was 0.35.[1] The mean of its average concentrations in milk over the dose interval was 0.27 mg/L. The absolute infant dose averaged 0.04 mg/kg/d and the mean relative infant dose was 0.28%. Metformin was present in very low or undetectable concentrations in the plasma of four of the infants who were studied. No health problems were found in the six infants who were evaluated.

In another study of five subjects, the median milk/plasma ratio (AUC) for metformin was 0.47. The median calculated infant dose was 0.2% of the weight-adjusted maternal dose. None of the infants exposed to their mothers milk had detectable levels of metformin in their plasma, nor were any side effects noted.

The new product Glucovance contains metformin and glyburide. The new product Metaglip contains Glipizide and metformin.

Pregnancy Risk Category: B

Lactation Risk Category: L1

Adult Concerns: Diarrhea, nausea, vomiting, bloating, lactic acidosis, hypoglycemia

Pediatric Concerns: No side effects noted in two studies. Plasma levels undetectable.

Drug Interactions: Alcohol potentiates the effect of metformin on lactic metabolism. Cimetidine produces a 60% increase in peak metformin plasma levels. Furosemide may increase metformin plasma levels by 22%. Use of iodinated contrast material in patients receiving metformin has produced acute renal failure and been associated with lactic acidosis. Use of nifedipine increases oral bioavailability of metformin by 20%.

Theoretic Infant Dose: 0.04 mg/kg/day

Relative Infant Dose: 0.28%

Adult Dose: 500 mg BID

Alternatives:

T½ =	6.2 hours (plasma)	M/P =	1.0
PHL =		PB =	Minimal
T$_{max}$ =	2.75 hours	Oral =	50%
MW =	129	pKa =	11.5
Vd =	3.7		

References:
1. Hale TW, Kristensen JH, Hackett LP, Kohan R, Ilett KF. Transfer of metformin into human milk. Diabetologia 2002; 45(11):1509-1514.
2. Gardiner SJ, Kirkpatrick CM, Begg EJ, Zhang M, Moore MP, Saville DJ. Transfer of metformin into human milk. Clin Pharmacol Ther 2003; 73(1):71-77.

METHADONE
Trade: Dolophine
Can/Aus/UK: Physeptone, Biodone forte, Physeptone, Methex
Uses: Narcotic analgesic
LRC: L3
AAP: Maternal Medication Usually Compatible with Breastfeeding

Methadone is a potent and very long-acting opiate analgesic. It is primarily used to prevent withdrawal in opiate addiction. In one study of 10 women receiving methadone 10-80 mg/day, the average milk/plasma ratio was 0.83.[1] Due to the variable doses used, the milk concentrations ranged from 0.05 mg/L in one patient receiving 10 mg/day to 0.57 mg/L in a patient receiving 80 mg/day. One infant death has been reported in a breastfeeding mother receiving maintenance methadone therapy.[2] Although it is not clear that the only source of methadone to this infant was from breastmilk.

In a more recent study of 12 breastfeeding women on methadone maintenance doses ranging from 20-80 mg/day, the mean concentration of methadone in plasma and milk was 311 (207-416) μg/L and 116 (72-160) μg/L respectively yielding a mean M/P ratio of 0.44 (0.24-0.64).[3] The mean absolute oral dose to infant was 17.4 (10.8-24) μg/kg/day. This equates to a mean of 2.79% of the maternal dose per day. In this study, 64% of the infants exhibited neonatal abstinence syndrome requiring treatment.

In two women receiving 30 mg twice daily and another who received 73 mg of methadone once daily, the average breastmilk methadone concentrations was 0.169 mg/L and 0.132 mg/L respectively.[4] The milk/plasma ratios were 1.215 and 0.661 respectively. While the infant of the second mother died at 3 1/2 months of SIDS, it was apparently not due to methadone, as none was present in the infant's plasma and the infant was significantly supplemented with formula.

In an excellent study, 8 mother/infant pairs ingesting from 40 to 105 mg/day methadone, the average (AUC) concentration of R-methadone and S-methadone enantiomers varied from 42-259 μg/L and 26-126 μg/L respectively.[5] The relative infant dose was estimated to be 2.8% of the maternal dose. Interestingly, there was little difference in methadone milk levels in immature and mature milk.

Most studies thus far show that only small amounts of methadone pass into breastmilk despite doses as high as 105 mg/day. In fact, neonatal abstinence syndromes are well known to occur in breastfeeding infants following delivery. In one study, 58% of infants developed neonatal abstinence syndrome while still breastfeeding.[6] However, some methadone is undoubtedly transferred via milk, and abrupt cessation of breastfeeding during high dose therapy has resulted in neonatal abstinence in some infants.[7]

In summary, the dose of R plus S methadone transferred via milk is largely dose dependent but generally averages less than 2.8% of the maternal dose.[5] This is significantly less than the conventional cut-off value of 10% of the maternal dose corrected for weight. However, the amount in milk is insufficient to prevent neonatal withdrawal syndrome. The Academy of Pediatrics recently placed methadone in the "approved" category for breastfeeding women.

Pregnancy Risk Category: B

Lactation Risk Category: L3

Adult Concerns: Nausea, vomiting, constipation, respiratory depression, sedation, withdrawal syndrome

Pediatric Concerns: Observe for sedation, respiratory depression, addiction, withdrawal syndrome. Neonatal abstinence syndrome.

Drug Interactions: Phenytoin, pentazocine, and rifampin may increase metabolism of methadone and produce withdrawal syndrome. CNS depressants, phenothiazines, tricyclic antidepressants, and MAO inhibitors may increase adverse effects of methadone.

Theoretic Infant Dose: 38.85 µg/kg/day

Relative Infant Dose: 2.8%

Adult Dose: 2.5-10 mg q 3-4 hours PRN

Alternatives:

T½ =	13-55 hours	M/P =	0.68 (R)
PHL =		PB =	89%
T$_{max}$ =	0.5-1 hours	Oral =	50%
MW =	309	pKa =	8.6
Vd =	4-5		

References:

1. Blinick G, Inturrisi CE, Jerez E, Wallach RC. Methadone assays in pregnant women and progeny. Am J Obstet Gynecol 1975; 121(5):617-621.
2. Smialek JE, Monforte JR, Aronow R, Spitz WU. Methadone deaths in children. A continuing problem. JAMA 1977; 238(23):2516-2517.
3. Wojnar-Horton RE, Kristensen JH, Yapp P, Ilett KF, Dusci LJ, Hackett LP. Methadone distribution and excretion into breastmilk of clients in a methadone maintenance programme. Br J Clin Pharmacol 1997; 44(6):543-547.
4. Geraghty B, Graham EA, Logan B, Weiss EL. Methadone levels in breastmilk. J Hum Lact 1997; 13(3):227-230.
5. Begg EJ, Malpas TJ, Hackett LP, Ilett KF. Distribution of R- and S-methadone into human milk during multiple, medium to high oral dosing. Br J Clin Pharmacol 2001; 52(6):681-685.
6. Wojnar-Horton RE, Kristensen JH, Yapp P, Ilett KF, Dusci LJ, Hackett LP. Methadone distribution and excretion into breastmilk of clients in a methadone maintenance programme. Br J Clin Pharmacol 1997; 44(6):543-547.
7. Malpas TJ, Darlow BA. Neonatal abstinence syndrome following abrupt cessation of breastfeeding. N Z Med J 1999; 112(1080):12-13.

METHICILLIN

Trade: Staphcillin, Celebenin
Can/Aus/UK: Metin, Celbenin
Uses: Penicillin antibiotic
LRC: L3
AAP: Not reviewed

Methicillin is a penicillin antibiotic only available by IM and IV formulations.[1] It is extremely unstable at acid pH (stomach); hence, it would have only limited oral absorption. No data available on transfer into breastmilk although it would appear to be similar to other penicillins.

Pregnancy Risk Category: B

Lactation Risk Category: L3

Adult Concerns: Allergic rash, thrush, diarrhea, drug fever, changes in GI flora, renal toxicity, pseudomembranous colitis

Pediatric Concerns: None reported via milk.

Drug Interactions: The effect of oral contraceptives may be reduced.   Disulfiram and probenecid may significantly increase penicillin levels. Methicillin may increase the effect of anticoagulants.

Theoretic Infant Dose:

Relative Infant Dose:

Adult Dose: 1 g q 6 hours

Alternatives:

T½ =	1-2 hours	M/P =	
PHL =	1.4-2.4 hours (neonates)	PB =	40%
T$_{max}$ =	30-60 minutes	Oral =	Poor
MW =	402	pKa =	
Vd =			

References:
1.   Drug Facts and Comparisons 1994 ed. ed. St. Louis: 1994.

METHIMAZOLE

Trade: Tapazole
Can/Aus/UK: Tapazole
Uses: Antithyroid agent
LRC: L3
AAP: Maternal Medication Usually Compatible with Breastfeeding

Methimazole, carbimazole, and propylthiouracil are used to inhibit the secretion of thyroxine.   Carbimazole is metabolized to the active metabolite, methimazole. Levels depend on maternal dose but appear too low to produce clinical effect. In one study of a patient receiving 2.5 mg methimazole every 12 hours, the milk/serum ratio was 1.16, and the dose per day was calculated at 16-39 μg methimazole.[1] This was equivalent to 7-16% of the maternal dose. In a study of 35 lactating women receiving 5 to 20 mg/day of methimazole, no changes in the infant thyroid function were noted in any infant, even those at higher doses.[2]

Further, studies by Lamberg in 11 women, who were treated with the methimazole derivative carbimazole (5-15 mg daily, equal to 3.3 -10 mg methimazole), found all 11 infants had normal thyroid function following maternal treatments.[3]   Thus, in small maternal doses, methimazole may also be safe for the nursing mother. In a study of a woman with twins who was receiving up to 30 mg carbimazole daily, the average methimazole concentration in milk was 43 µg/L.[4]   The average plasma concentrations in the twin infants were 45 and 52 ng/mL, which is below therapeutic range.   Methimazole milk concentrations peaked at 2-4 hours after a carbimazole dose.   No changes in thyroid function in these infants were noted.

In a large study of over 139 thyrotoxic lactating mothers and their infants, even at methimazole doses of 20 mg/day, no changes in infant TSH, T4, or T3 were noted in over 12 months of study.[5]   The authors conclude that both PTU and methimazole can safely be administered during lactation.   However, during the first few months of therapy, monitoring of infant thyroid functioning is recommended.

Pregnancy Risk Category: D

Lactation Risk Category: L3

Adult Concerns: Hypothyroidism,   hepatic dysfunction, bleeding, drowsiness, skin rash, nausea, vomiting, fever

Pediatric Concerns: None reported in several studies,   but propylthiouracil may be a preferred choice in breastfeeding women.

Drug Interactions: Use with iodinated glycerol, lithium, and potassium iodide may increase toxicity.

Theoretic Infant Dose: 6.45 µg/kg/day

Relative Infant Dose: 1.5%

Adult Dose: 5-30 mg daily

Alternatives: Propylthiouracil

T½ =	6-13 hours	M/P =	1.0
PHL =		PB =	0%
T$_{max}$ =	1 hour	Oral =	80-95%
MW =	114	pKa =	
Vd =			

References:

1. Tegler L, Lindstrom B. Antithyroid drugs in milk. Lancet 1980; 2(8194):591.
2. Azizi F. Effect of methimazole treatment of maternal thyrotoxicosis on thyroid function in breast-feeding infants. J Pediatr 1996; 128(6):855-858.
3. Lamberg BA, Ikonen E, Osterlund K, Teramo K, Pekonen F, Peltola J, Valimaki M. Antithyroid treatment of maternal hyperthyroidism during lactation. Clin Endocrinol (Oxf) 1984; 21(1):81-87.
4. Rylance GW, Woods CG, Donnelly MC, Oliver JS, Alexander WD. Carbimazole and breastfeeding. Lancet 1987; 1(8538):928.

5. Azizi F, Khoshniat M, Bahrainian M, Hedayati M. Thyroid function and intellectual development of infants nursed by mothers taking methimazole. J Clin Endocrinol Metab 2000; 85(9):3233-3238.

METHOCARBAMOL

Trade: Robaxisal, Robaxin
Can/Aus/UK: Robaxin
Uses: Muscle relaxant
LRC: L3
AAP: Not reviewed

Methocarbamol is a centrally acting sedative and skeletal muscle relaxant. Only minimal amounts have been found in milk.[1] Observe for sedation.

Pregnancy Risk Category: C

Lactation Risk Category: L3

Adult Concerns: Drowsiness, nausea, metallic taste, vertigo, blurred vision, fever, headache

Pediatric Concerns: None reported, but studies are limited.

Drug Interactions: May see increased toxicity when used with CNS depressants.

Theoretic Infant Dose:

Relative Infant Dose:

Adult Dose: 4-4.5 g q 4-6 hours

Alternatives:

$T\frac{1}{2}$ =	0.9-1.8 hours	M/P =	
PHL =		PB =	
T_{max} =	1-2 hours	Oral =	Complete
MW =	241	pKa =	
Vd =			

References:
1. Pharmaceutical Manufacturer Prescribing Information. 1995.

METHOHEXITAL

Trade: Brevital
Can/Aus/UK: Brietal
Uses: Anesthetic agent
LRC: L3
AAP: Maternal Medication Usually Compatible with Breastfeeding

Methohexital is an ultra short-acting barbiturate used for induction in anesthesia. The duration of action is approximately 1/2 that of thiopental sodium or less than 8 minutes depending on dose. Within 30 minutes there is complete redistribution of methohexital to tissues other than the brain, primarily the liver.[1,2] While it is not known if methohexital enters milk, it is very unlikely that milk levels will be significant because the drug is so rapidly cleared from the plasma compartment and redistributed to other compartments. A brief interval of a few hours (2-4) following administration will significantly reduce any risk.

Pregnancy Risk Category: B

Lactation Risk Category: L3

Adult Concerns: Hypotension, lethargy, restlessness, confusion, headache, delirium, and excitation

Pediatric Concerns: None reported via milk.

Drug Interactions: CNS depressants such as barbiturates, benzodiazepines, etc, may potentiate sedation with methohexital.

Theoretic Infant Dose:

Relative Infant Dose:

Adult Dose: 20-40 mg q 4-7 minutes during surgery

Alternatives:

T½ =	3.9 hours	M/P =
PHL =		PB =
T$_{max}$ =	Instant	Oral =
MW =	284	pKa =
Vd =		

References:
1. Drug Facts and Comparisons 1999 ed. ed. St. Louis: 1999.
2. McEvoy GE. (ed): AFHS Drug Information. New York, NY: 1999.

METHOTREXATE

Trade: Folex, Rhedumatrex

Can/Aus/UK: Rheumatrex, Ledertrexate, Methoblastin, Arthitrex

Uses: Antimetabolite, anticancer, antirheumatic

LRC: L3 for acute use
L5 for chronic use

AAP: Contraindicated by the American Academy of Pediatrics in Breastfeeding Mothers

Methotrexate is a potent and potentially dangerous folic acid antimetabolite used in arthritic and other immunologic syndromes. It is also used as an abortifacient in tubal pregnancies. Methotrexate is secreted into breastmilk in small levels. Following a dose of 22.5 mg to one patient two hours post-dose, the methotrexate concentration in breastmilk was 2.6 µg/L of milk with a milk/plasma ratio of 0.08.[1] The cumulative excretion of methotrexate in the first 12 hours after oral administration was only 0.32 µg in milk. These authors conclude that methotrexate therapy in breastfeeding mothers would not pose a contraindication to breastfeeding. However, methotrexate is believed to be retained in human tissues (particularly neonatal GI cells and ovarian cells) for long periods (months).[2] One study has indicated a higher risk of fetal malformation in mothers who received methotrexate months prior to becoming pregnant.[3] Therefore, pregnancy should be delayed if either partner is receiving methotrexate for at least 3 months following therapy. It is apparent that the concentration of methotrexate in human milk is minimal although due to the toxicity of this agent, it is probably wise to pump and discard the mother's milk (2-4 half-lives depending on dose) after taking this product.

Pregnancy Risk Category: D

Lactation Risk Category: L3 for acute use
L5 for chronic use

Adult Concerns: Bone marrow suppression, anemia, vasculitis, vomiting, diarrhea, GI bleeding, stomatitis, bloody diarrhea, kidney damage, seizures, etc.

Pediatric Concerns: None reported via milk, but caution is recommended.

Drug Interactions: Aminoglycosides may significantly decrease absorption of methotrexate. Etretinate has produced hepatotoxicity in several patients receiving methotrexate. The use of folic acid or its derivatives may reduce the response to MTX. The use of NSAIDs with methotrexate is contraindicated. Several deaths have occurred due to elevated MTX levels. Phenytoin serum levels may be decreased. Procarbazine may increase nephrotoxicity of MTX.

Theoretic Infant Dose: 0.39 µg/kg/day

Relative Infant Dose: 0.12%

Adult Dose: 10-30 mg

Alternatives:

T½ =	7.2 hours	M/P =	> 0.08
PHL =	1.7 hours	PB =	34-50 %
T$_{max}$ =	1-2 hours	Oral =	33-90%
MW =	454	pKa =	4.3, 5.5
Vd =	2.6		

References:
1. Johns DG, Rutherford LD, Leighton PC, Vogel CL. Secretion of methotrexate into human milk. Am J Obstet Gynecol 1972; 112(7):978-980.
2. Fountain JR, Hutchison DJ, Waring GB, Burchenal JH. Persistence of amethopterin in normal mouse tissues. Proc Soc Exp Biol Med 1953; 83(2):369-373.
3. Walden PA, Bagshawe KD. Pregnancies after chemotherapy for gestational trophoblastic tumours. Lancet 1979; 2(8154):1241.

METHYLDOPA

Trade: Aldomet

Can/Aus/UK: Aldomet, Apo-Methyldopa, Dopamet, Nova-Medopa, Aldopren, Hydopa, Nudopa

Uses: Antihypertensive

LRC: L2

AAP: Maternal Medication Usually Compatible with Breastfeeding

Alpha-methyldopa is a centrally acting antihypertensive. It is frequently used to treat hypertension during pregnancy. In a study of 2 lactating women who received a dose of 500 mg, the maximum breastmilk concentration of methyldopa ranged from 0.2 to 0.66 mg/L.[1] In another patient who received 1000 mg dose, the maximum concentration in milk was 1.14 mg/L.[1] The milk/plasma ratios varied from 0.19 to 0.34. The authors indicated that if the infant were to ingest 750 mL of milk daily (with a maternal dose= 1000mg), the maximum daily ingestion would be less than 855 µg or approximately 0.02 % of the maternal dose.

In another study of 7 women who received 0.750-2.0 gm/day of methyldopa, the free methyldopa concentrations in breastmilk ranged from zero to 0.2 mg/L while the conjugated metabolite had concentrations of 0.1 to 0.9 mg/L.[2] These studies generally indicate that the levels of methyldopa transferred to a breastfeeding infant would be too low to be clinically relevant.

However, gynecomastia and galactorrhea have been reported in one full-term two week old female neonate following seven days of maternal therapy with methyldopa, 250 mg three times daily.[3]

Pregnancy Risk Category: C

Lactation Risk Category: L2

Adult Concerns: Hemolytic anemia, hepatitis, fever, rashes, dizziness, hypotension, sleep disturbances, dry mouth, depression, colitis

Pediatric Concerns: None reported in several studies. Gynecomastia and galactorrhea in one personal communication.

Drug Interactions: Iron supplements can interact and cause a significant increase in blood pressure. Increased toxicity with lithium has been reported.

Theoretic Infant Dose: 0.03 mg/kg/day

Relative Infant Dose: 0.11%

Adult Dose: 250-500 mg BID-QID

Alternatives:

T½ =	105 minutes	M/P =	0.19-0.34
PHL =		PB =	Low
T$_{max}$ =	3-6 hours	Oral =	25-50%
MW =	211	pKa =	
Vd =	0.3		

References:
1. White WB, Andreoli JW, Cohn RD. Alpha-methyldopa disposition in mothers with hypertension and in their breast-fed infants. Clin Pharmacol Ther 1985; 37(4):387-390.
2. Jones HM, Cummings AJ. A study of the transfer of alpha-methyldopa to the human foetus and newborn infant. Br J Clin Pharmacol 1978; 6(5):432-434.
3. E.D.M. Personal Communication. 1997.

METHYLERGONOVINE

Trade: Methergine
Can/Aus/UK: Methergine, Ergometrine, Methylerometrine
Uses: Vasoconstrictor, uterine stimulant
LRC: L2
        L4 for chronic use
AAP: Not reviewed

Methylergonovine is an amine ergot alkaloid used to control postpartum uterine bleeding. The ergots are powerful vasoconstrictors.   In a group of 8 postpartum women receiving 0.125 mg three times daily for 5 days, the concentration of methylergonovine ranged from < 0.5 in 4 patients to 1.3 μg/L in one patient at one hour postdose.[1]   In this study only 5 of 16 milk samples had detectable methylergonovine levels.

Using a dose of 1.3 μg/L of milk, an infant would only consume approximately 0.2 μg/kg/day, which is incredibly low compared to the usual 0.375 mg daily dose. The milk/plasma ratio averaged about 0.3. Short-term (1 week), low-dose regimens of these agents do not apparently pose problems in nursing infants/mothers.[2]   In those situations with longer therapy, a benefit to risk assessment is required, but it is not likely to be overly hazardous to the infant. Methylergonovine is preferred over ergonovine because it does not inhibit lactation to the same degree, and levels in milk are minimal.

Pregnancy Risk Category: C

Lactation Risk Category: L2
                                        L4 for chronic use

Adult Concerns: Nausea, vomiting, diarrhea, dizziness, rapid pulse

Pediatric Concerns: None reported, but long term exposure is not recommended. Methylergonovine is commonly recommended early postpartum for breastfeeding mothers with bleeding.

Drug Interactions: Use caution when using with other vasoconstrictors or pressor agents.

Theoretic Infant Dose: 0.195 μg/kg/day

Relative Infant Dose: 3.6%

Adult Dose: 0.2-0.4 mg q 6-12 hours PRN

Alternatives:

$T\frac{1}{2}$ =	20-30 minutes	M/P =	0.3
PHL =		PB =	36%
T_{max} =	0.5-3 hours	Oral =	60%
MW =	339	pKa =	
Vd =			

References:
1. Erkkola R, Kanto J, Allonen H, Kleimola T, Mantyla R. Excretion of methylergometrine (methylergonovine) into the human breastmilk. Int J Clin Pharmacol Biopharm 1978; 16(12):579-580.
2. Del Pozo E, Brun DR, Hinselmann M. Lack of effect of methyl-ergonovine on postpartum lactation. Am J Obstet Gynecol 1975; 123(8):845-846.

METHYLPHENIDATE

Trade: Ritalin, Concerta, Metadate Cd, Metadate Er, Methylin
Can/Aus/UK: Ritalin, Riphenidate, PMS-Methylphenidate
Uses: CNS stimulant, treatment of ADHD
LRC: L3
AAP: Not reviewed

The pharmacologic effects of methylphenidate are similar to those of amphetamines and include CNS stimulation.[1] It is presently used for narcolepsy and attention deficit hyperactivity syndrome. In one mother who ingested 35 mg, the highest milk concentration was 62 µg/L (Cav=13.3 µg/L). In another mother who ingested 20 mg at 0900 and 20 mg at 1330, the highest concentration was 57 µg/L at 2087 (Cav=28.3).[2] Using this preliminary data, an infant would possibly receive 1.99 to 4.2 µg/kg/day respectively. While these doses seem low, the risk of toxicity must be weighed against the need of mother and infant.

Pregnancy Risk Category: C

Lactation Risk Category: L3

Adult Concerns: Nervousness, hyperactivity, insomnia, agitation, and lack of appetite

Pediatric Concerns: None reported, but observe for stimulation, insomnia, anorexia.

Drug Interactions: Methylphenidate may reduce the effects of guanethidine and bretylium. May increased serum levels of tricyclic antidepressants, phenytoin, warfarin, phenobarbital, and primidone. Use with MAOI may produce significant increased effects of methylphenidate.

Theoretic Infant Dose: 9.3 µg/kg/day (preliminary data)

Relative Infant Dose: 1.8%

Adult Dose: 10 mg BID-TID. Highly variable.

Alternatives:

$T\frac{1}{2}$ =	1-3 hours	M/P =		
PHL =		PB =		
T_{max} =	1 - 3 hours	Oral =	95%	
MW =	233	pKa =	8.8	
Vd =	11-33			

References:

1. Pharmaceutical Manufacturer Prescribing Information. 1996.
2. Ilett KF. Hale TW, Hackett LP. Unpublished data, 2003.

METHYLPREDNISOLONE

Trade: Solu-Medrol, Depo-Medrol, Medrol
Can/Aus/UK: Medrol, Depo-Medrol, Solu-Medrol, Neo-Medrol, Advantan
Uses: Corticosteroid
LRC: L2
AAP: Maternal Medication Usually Compatible with Breastfeeding

Methylprednisolone (MP) is the methyl derivative of prednisolone. Four milligrams of methylprednisolone is roughly equivalent to 5 mg of prednisone. Multiple dosage forms exist and include the succinate salt which is rapidly active, the methylprednisolone base which is the tablet formulation for oral use, and the methylprednisolone acetate suspension (Depo-Medrol) which is slowly absorbed over many days to weeks. Depo-Medrol is generally used intrasynovially, IM, or epidurally and is slowly absorbed from these sites. They would be very unlikely to affect a breastfed infant, but this depends on dose and duration of exposure. For a complete description of corticosteroid use in breastfeeding mothers see the prednisone monograph. In general, the amount of methylprednisolone and other steroids transferred into human milk is minimal as long as the dose does not exceed 80 mg per day.[1] However, relating side effects of steroids administered via breastmilk and their maternal doses is rather difficult and each situation should be evaluated individually. Extended use of high doses could predispose the infant to steroid side effects including decreased linear growth rate, but these require rather high doses. Low to moderate doses are believed to have minimal effect on breastfed infants. See prednisone.

High dose pulsed intravenous or oral administrations of methylprednisolone (MP) have become increasingly important as a treatment for acute relapses or progressively worsening of multiple sclerosis (MS).[2-6] Even though prednisolone is approved by the American Academy of Pediatrics for use in breastfeeding women, when MP is used in such high doses in patients with MS, questions concerning when mothers can return to breastfeeding have arisen. While there are extensive kinetic data on the plasma levels, metabolism, and clearance of methylprednisolone from normal and MS patients, no data are available on the transfer of MP into human milk subsequent to using such high pulse IV doses in breastfeeding mothers.[7,8] Simulation of MP elimination curves by the author shows a rapid and complete elimination from the maternal plasma compartment.[9] From this simulation, it would appear a brief pumping and discarding of milk for a period of 8-24 hours following the IV administration of MP (at doses up to 1 gm) would significantly reduce an infant's exposure to this corticosteroid. This simulation estimates the infant dose at 12 hours post-administration of MP to be approximately 1.24 µg/kg/day. These are only theoretical predictions as no one yet has published milk levels following IV administration of 1 gram doses.

Pregnancy Risk Category: **C**

Lactation Risk Category: **L2**

Adult Concerns: GI bleeding, GI ulceration, edema, osteoporosis

Pediatric Concerns: None reported via breastmilk. Limit dose and length of exposure if possible. High doses and prolonged durations may inhibit epiphyseal bone growth, induce gastric ulcerations, glaucoma, etc.

Drug Interactions: Barbiturates may significantly reduce the effects of corticosteroids. Cholestyramine may reduce absorption of methylprednisone. Oral contraceptives may reduce half-life and concentration of steroids. Ephedrine may reduce the half-life and increase clearance of certain steroids. Phenytoin may increase clearance. Corticosteroid clearance may be decreased by ketoconazole. Certain macrolide antibiotics may significantly decrease clearance of steroids. Isoniazid serum concentrations may be decreased.

Theoretic Infant Dose:

Relative Infant Dose:

Adult Dose: 2-60 mg daily

Alternatives: Prednisone

$T\frac{1}{2}$ =	2.8 hours	M/P =	
PHL =		PB =	
T_{max} =		Oral =	Complete
MW =	374	pKa =	
Vd =	1.5		

References:

1. Anderson PO. Corticosteroid use by breast-feeding mothers. Clin Pharm 1987; 6(6):445.
2. Miller DM, Weinstock-Guttman B, Bethoux F, Lee JC, Beck G, Block V, Durelli L, LaMantia L, Barnes D, Sellebjerg F, Rudick RA. A meta-analysis of methylprednisolone in recovery from multiple sclerosis exacerbations. Mult Scler 2000; 6(4):267-273.
3. Hommes OR, Barkhof F, Jongen PJ, Frequin ST. Methylprednisolone treatment in multiple sclerosis: effect of treatment, pharmacokinetics, future. Mult Scler 1996; 1(6):327-328.
4. Goas JY, Marion JL, Missoum A. High dose intravenous methyl prednisolone in acute exacerbations of multiple sclerosis. J Neurol Neurosurg Psychiatry 1983; 46(1):99.
5. Sellebjerg F, Frederiksen JL, Nielsen PM, Olesen J. Double-blind, randomized, placebo-controlled study of oral, high-dose methylprednisolone in attacks of MS. Neurology 1998; 51(2):529-534.
6. Barnes D, Hughes RA, Morris RW, Wade-Jones O, Brown P, Britton T, Francis DA, Perkin GD, Rudge P, Swash M, Katifi H, Farmer S, Frankel J. Randomised trial of oral and intravenous methylprednisolone in acute relapses of multiple sclerosis. Lancet 1997; 349(9056):902-906.

7. Vree TB, Verwey-van Wissen CP, Lagerwerf AJ, Swolfs A, Maes RA, van Ooijen RD, Eikema Hommes OR, Jongen PJ. Isolation and identification of the C6-hydroxy and C20-hydroxy metabolites and glucuronide conjugate of methylprednisolone by preparative high-performance liquid chromatography from urine of patients receiving high-dose pulse therapy. J Chromatogr B Biomed Sci Appl 1999; 726(1-2):157-168.

8. Vree TB, Lagerwerf AJ, Verwey-van Wissen CP, Jongen PJ. High-performance liquid chromatography analysis, preliminary pharmacokinetics, metabolism and renal excretion of methylprednisolone with its C6 and C20 hydroxy metabolites in multiple sclerosis patients receiving high-dose pulse therapy. J Chromatogr B Biomed Sci Appl 1999; 732(2):337-348.

9. Hale TW, Ilett K. Unpublished data. 2000.

METOCLOPRAMIDE

Trade: Reglan
Can/Aus/UK: Apo-Metoclop, Emex, Maxeran, Reglan, Maxolon, Pramin, Gastromax, Paramid
Uses: GI stimulant, prolactin stimulant
LRC: L2
AAP: Drugs whose effect on nursing infants is unknown but may be of concern

Metoclopramide has multiple functions but is primarily used for increasing the lower esophageal sphincter tone in gastroesophageal reflux in patients with reduced gastric tone. In breastfeeding, it is sometimes used in lactating women to stimulate prolactin release from the pituitary and enhance breastmilk production. Since 1981, a number of publications have documented major increases in breastmilk production following the use of metoclopramide, domperidone, or sulpiride. With metoclopramide, the increase in serum prolactin and breastmilk production appears dose-related up to a dose of 15 mg three times daily.[1] Many studies show 66 to 100 % increases in milk production depending on the degree breastmilk supply in the mother prior to therapy and maybe her initial prolactin levels. Doses of 15 mg/day were found ineffective, whereas doses of 30-45 mg/day were most effective. In most studies, major increases in prolactin were observed such as from 125 ng/mL to 172 ng/mL in one patient.[2]

In Kauppila's study of 37 women, the concentration of metoclopramide in milk was consistently higher than the maternal serum levels.[3] The peak occurred at 2-3 hours after administration of the medication. During the late puerperium, the concentration of metoclopramide in the milk varied from 20 to 125 μg/L, which was less than the 28 to 157 μg/L noted during the early puerperium. The authors estimated the daily dose to infant to vary from 6 to 24 μg/kg/day during the early puerperium and from 1 to 13 μg/kg/day during the late phase. These doses are minimal compared to those used for therapy of reflux in pediatric patients (0.1 to 0.5 mg/kg/day). In these studies, only 1 of 5 infants studied had detectable blood levels of metoclopramide; hence, no accumulation or side effects were observed. While plasma prolactin levels in the newborns were comparable to those in the mothers prior to treatment, Kaupilla found slight increases in prolactin levels in 4 of 7 newborns following treatment with metoclopramide although a more recent study did not find such changes.[6] However, prolactin levels are highly variable and subject to diurnal rhythm, thus timing is essential in measuring prolactin levels and could account for this inconsistency.

In another study[4] of 23 women with premature infants, milk production increased from 93 mL/day to 197 mL/day between the first and 7th day of therapy with 30 mg/day. Prolactin levels although varied, increased from 18.1 to 121.8 ng/mL. While basal prolactin levels were elevated significantly, metoclopramide seems to blunt the rapid rise of prolactin when milk was expressed. Nevertheless, milk production was still elevated. Gupta studied 32 mothers with inadequate milk supply.[5] Following a dose of 10 mg three times daily, a 66-100% increase in milk supply was noted. Of twelve cases of complete lactation failure, 8 responded to treatment in an average of 3-4 days after starting therapy. In this study, 87.5% of the total 32 cases responded to metoclopramide therapy with greater milk production. No untoward effects were noted in the infants.

In a study of 5 breastfeeding women who were receiving 30 mg/day, daily milk production increased significantly from 150.9 mL/day to 276.4 mL/day in this group.[6] However, the plasma prolactin levels in breastfed infants were determined as well on the 5th postnatal day and no changes were noted; thus, the amount of metoclopramide transferred in milk was not enough to change the infant's prolactin levels.

In a study by Lewis in ten patients who received a single oral dose of 10 mg, the mean maternal plasma and milk levels at 2 hours was 68.5 ng/mL and 125.7 μg/L respectively.[7]

It is well recognized that metoclopramide increases a mothers' milk supply, but it is exceedingly dose dependent, and yet some mothers simply do not respond. In those mothers who do not respond, Kaupila's work suggests that such patients may already have elevated prolactin levels. In his study, 3 of the 5 mothers who did not respond with increased milk production had the highest basal prolactin levels (300-400 ng/mL).[3] Thus it may be advisable to do plasma prolactin levels on under-producing mothers prior to instituting metoclopramide therapy to assess the response prior to treating.

Side effects such as gastric cramping and diarrhea limit the compliance of some patients but are rare. Further, it is often found that upon rapid discontinuation of the medication, the supply of milk may in some instances reduce significantly. Tapering of the dose is generally recommended and one possible regimen is to decrease the dose by 10 mg per week. Long-term use of this medication (> 4 weeks) may be accompanied by increased side effects such as depression in the mother although some patients have used it successfully for months. Another dopamine antagonist, Domperidone, due to minimal side effects, is a preferred choice but is unfortunately not available in the USA other than in compounding pharmacies.

Two recent cases of serotonin-like reactions (agitation, dysarthria, diaphoresis, and extrapyramidal movement disorder) have been reported when metoclopramide was used in patients receiving sertraline or venlafaxine.

Pregnancy Risk Category: B

Lactation Risk Category: L2

Adult Concerns: Diarrhea, sedation, gastric upset, nausea, extrapyramidal symptoms, severe depression

Pediatric Concerns: None reported in infants via milk.   Commonly used in pediatrics.

Drug Interactions: Anticholinergic drugs may reduce the effects of metoclopramide.   Opiate analgesics may increased CNS depression. Two cases of serotonin-like syndrome have been reported when used the metoclopramide(Reglan).   Two recent cases of serotonin-like reactions (agitation, dysarthria, diapyhoresis, and extrapyramidal movement disorder) have been reported when metoclopramide was used in patients receiving sertraline or venlafaxine.[8]

Theoretic Infant Dose: 18.75 µg/kg/day

Relative Infant Dose: 4.3%

Adult Dose: 10-15 mg TID

Alternatives: Domperidone

T½ =	5-6 hours	M/P =	0.5-4.06
PHL =		PB =	30%
T$_{max}$ =	1-2 hours (oral)	Oral =	30-100%
MW =	300	pKa =	
Vd =			

References:
1. Kauppila A, Kivinen S, Ylikorkala O. A dose response relation between improved lactation and metoclopramide. Lancet 1981; 1(8231):1175-1177.
2. Budd SC, Erdman SH, Long DM, Trombley SK, Udall JN, Jr. Improved lactation with metoclopramide. A case report. Clin Pediatr (Phila) 1993; 32(1):53-57.

3. Kauppila A, Arvela P, Koivisto M, Kivinen S, Ylikorkala O, Pelkonen O. Metoclopramide and breast feeding: transfer into milk and the newborn. Eur J Clin Pharmacol 1983; 25(6):819-823.
4. Ehrenkranz RA, Ackerman BA. Metoclopramide effect on faltering milk production by mothers of premature infants. Pediatrics 1986; 78(4):614-620.
5. Gupta AP, Gupta PK. Metoclopramide as a lactogogue. Clin Pediatr (Phila) 1985; 24(5):269-272.
6. Ertl T, Sulyok E, Ezer E, Sarkany I, Thurzo V, Csaba IF. The influence of metoclopramide on the composition of human breastmilk. Acta Paediatr Hung 1991; 31(4):415-422.
7. Lewis PJ, Devenish C, Kahn C. Controlled trial of metoclopramide in the initiation of breast feeding. Br J Clin Pharmacol 1980; 9(2):217-219.

METOPROLOL

Trade: Toprol-XL, Lopressor
Can/Aus/UK: Apo-Metoprolol, Betaloc, Lopressor, Novo-Metoprol, Minax
Uses: Antihypertensive, beta blocker
LRC: L3
AAP: Maternal Medication Usually Compatible with Breastfeeding

At low doses, metoprolol is a very cardioselective Beta-1 blocker, and it is used for hypertension, angina, and tachyarrhythmias. In a study of 3 women 4-6 months postpartum, who received 100 mg twice daily for 4 days, the peak concentration of metoprolol ranged from 0.38 to 2.58 μmol/L, whereas the maternal plasma levels ranged from 0.1 to 0.97 μmol/L.[1] The mean milk/plasma ratio was 3.0. Assuming ingestion of 75 mL of milk at each feeding, and the maximum concentration of 2.58 μmol/L, an infant would ingest approximately 0.05 mg metoprolol at the first feeding and considerably less at subsequent feedings.

In another study of 9 women receiving 50-100 mg twice daily, the maternal plasma and milk concentrations ranged from 4-556 nmol/L and 19-1690 nmol/L respectively.[2] Using this data, the authors calculated an average milk concentration throughout the day as 280 μg/L of milk. This dose is 20-40 times less than a typical clinical dose. The milk/plasma ratio in these studies averaged 3.72.

Although the milk/plasma ratios for this drug are in general high, the maternal plasma levels are quite small so the absolute amount transferred to the infant are quite small. Although these levels are probably too low to be clinically relevant, clinicians should use metoprolol under close supervision.

Pregnancy Risk Category: B

Lactation Risk Category: L3

Adult Concerns: Hypotension, weakness, depression, bradycardia

Pediatric Concerns: None reported in several studies, but close observation for hypotension, weakness, bradycardia is advised.

Drug Interactions: Decreased effect when used with aluminum salts, barbiturates, calcium salts, cholestyramine, NSAIDs, ampicillin, rifampin, and salicylates. Beta blockers may reduce the effect of oral sulfonylureas (hypoglycemic agents). Increased toxicity/effect when used with other antihypertensives, contraceptives, MAO inhibitors, cimetidine, and numerous other products. See drug interaction reference for complete listing.

Theoretic Infant Dose: 42 µg/kg/day

Relative Infant Dose: 1.4%

Adult Dose: 100-450 mg daily

Alternatives: Propranolol

T½ =	3-7 hours	M/P =	3-3.72
PHL =		PB =	12%
T$_{max}$ =	2.5-3 hours	Oral =	40-50%
MW =	267	pKa =	9.7
Vd =	2.5-5.6		

References:
1. Liedholm H, Melander A, Bitzen PO, Helm G, Lonnerholm G, Mattiasson I, Nilsson B, Wahlin-Boll E. Accumulation of atenolol and metoprolol in human breastmilk. Eur J Clin Pharmacol 1981; 20(3):229-231.
2. Sandstrom B, Regardh CG. Metoprolol excretion into breastmilk. Br J Clin Pharmacol 1980; 9(5):518-519.
3. Kulas J, Lunell NO, Rosing U, Steen B, Rane A. Atenolol and metoprolol. A comparison of their excretion into human breastmilk. Acta Obstet Gynecol Scand Suppl 1984; 118:65-69.

METRIZAMIDE

Trade: Amipaque
Can/Aus/UK: Amipaque
Uses: Radiocontrast agent
LRC: L2
AAP: Maternal Medication Usually Compatible with Breastfeeding

Metrizamide is a radiographic contrast medium used mainly in myelography. It is water soluble and nonionic. Metrizamide contains 48% bound iodine. The iodine molecule is organically bound and is not available for uptake into breastmilk due to minimal metabolism. Following subarachnoid administration of 5.06 gm the peak plasma level of 32.9 µg/mL occurred at 6 hours. Cumulative excretion in milk increased with time but was extremely small with only 1.1 mg or 0.02% of the dose being recovered in milk within 44.3 hours.[1] The drug's high water solubility, nonionic characteristic, and its high molecular weight (789) also support minimal excretion into breastmilk. This agent is sometimes used as an oral radiocontrast agent.[2] Only minimal oral absorption occurs (< 0.4%). The authors suggest that the very small amount of metrizamide secreted in human milk is unlikely to be hazardous to the infant.

Pregnancy Risk Category: B

Lactation Risk Category: L2

Adult Concerns: Nausea, vomiting, headache, backache, neck stiffness, seizures

Pediatric Concerns: None reported in one study. Milk levels are too low, and its not orally bioavailable.

Drug Interactions: Chlorpromazine, ketamine, other phenothiazines, and any medication which lowers seizure threshold should be discontinued 5 days prior to exposure to metrizamide. Major seizures may occur. Lactic acidosis and acute renal failure may occur when used with metformin.

Theoretic Infant Dose:

Relative Infant Dose: 0.02%

Adult Dose: 5-12 mL X 1

Alternatives:

T½ =	> 24 hours	M/P =	
PHL =		PB =	
T$_{max}$ =	6 hours	Oral =	< 0.4 %
MW =	789	pKa =	
Vd =	1.3		

References:

1. Ilett KF, Hackett LP, Paterson JW, McCormick CC. Excretion of metrizamide in milk. Br J Radiol 1981; 54(642):537-538.
2. Johansen JG. Assessment of a non-ionic contrast medium (Amipaque) in the gastrointestinal tract. Invest Radiol 1978; 13(6):523-527.

METRIZOATE

Trade: Isopaque
Can/Aus/UK: Isopaque
Uses: Radiocontrast agent
LRC: L2
AAP: Maternal Medication Usually Compatible with Breastfeeding

Metrizoate is an ionic radiocontrast agent. Radiopaque agents (except barium) are iodinated compounds used to visualize various organs during X-ray, CAT scans, and other radiological procedures. These compounds are highly iodinated benzoic acid derivatives. Although under usual circumstances, iodine products are contraindicated in nursing mothers (due to ion trapping in milk), these products are unique in that they are extremely inert and are largely cleared without metabolism.

In a study of 4 women who received metrizoate 0.58 g/kg (350 mg Iodine/mL) IV, the peak level of metrizoate in milk was 14 mg/L at 3 and 6 hours post-injection.[1] The average milk concentration during the first 24 hours was only 11.4 mg/L. During the first 24 hours following injection, it is estimated that a total of 1.7 mg/kg would be transferred to the infant which is only 0.3% of the maternal dose.

As a group, radiocontrast agents are virtually unabsorbed after oral administration (< 0.1%). Metrizoate has a brief half-life of just 2 hours, and the estimated dose ingested by the infant is only 0.2% of the radiocontrast dose used clinically for various scanning procedures in infants. Although most company package inserts suggest that an infant be removed from the breast for 24 hours, no untoward effects have been reported with these products in breastfed infants. Because the amount of metrizoate transferred into milk is so small, the authors conclude that breastfeeding is acceptable after intravenously administered metrizoate.

Pregnancy Risk Category: **B**

Lactation Risk Category: **L2**

Adult Concerns: Hypersensitivity to iodine. Arrhythmias, renal failure. Volume expansion.

Pediatric Concerns: None reported via milk in one study.

Drug Interactions: Anaphylaxis.

Theoretic Infant Dose: 1.71 mg/kg/day

Relative Infant Dose: 0.3%

Adult Dose:

Alternatives:

T½ =	< 2 hours	M/P =	
PHL =		PB =	< 5%
T$_{max}$ =		Oral =	Nil
MW =	628	pKa =	
Vd =			

References:
1. Nielsen ST, Matheson I, Rasmussen JN, Skinnemoen K, Andrew E, Hafsahl G. Excretion of iohexol and metrizoate in human breastmilk. Acta Radiol 1987; 28(5):523-526.

METRONIDAZOLE

Trade: Flagyl, Metizol, Trikacide, Protostat, Noritate
Can/Aus/UK: Apo-Metronidazole, Flagyl, NeoMetric, Novo-Nidazol, Metrozine, Rozex
Uses: Antibiotic, amebicide
LRC: L2
AAP: Drugs whose effect on nursing infants is unknown but may be of concern

Metronidazole is indicated in the treatment of vaginitis due to Trichomonas Vaginalis and various anaerobic bacterial infections including Giardiasis, H. Pylori, B. Fragilis, and Gardnerella vaginalis. Metronidazole has become the treatment of choice for pediatric giardiasis (AAP).

Metronidazole absorption is time and dose dependent and also depends on the route of administration (oral vs. vaginal). Following a 2 mg oral dose, milk levels were reported to peak at 50-57 mg/L at 2 hours. Milk levels after 12 hours were approximately 19 mg/L and at 24 hours were approximately 10 mg/L.[1] The average drug concentration reported in milk at 2, 8, 12, and 12-24 hours was 45.8, 27.9, 19.1, and 12.6 mg/L respectively. If breastfeeding were to continue uninterrupted, an infant would consume 21.8 mg via breastmilk. With a 12 hour discontinuation, an infant would consume only 9.8 mg.

In a group of 12 nursing mothers receiving 400 mg three times daily, the mean milk/plasma ratio was 0.91.[2] The mean milk metronidazole concentration was 15.5 mg/L. Infant plasma metronidazole levels ranged from 1.27 to 2.41 μg/mL. No adverse effects were attributable to metronidazole therapy in these infants.

In another study in patients receiving 600 and 1200 mg daily, the average milk metronidazole concentration was 5.7 and 14.4 mg/L respectively.[3] The plasma levels of metronidazole (2 hours) at the 600 mg/d dose were 5 μg/mL (mother) and 0.8 μg/mL (infant). At the 1200 mg/d dose (2 hours), plasma levels were 12.5 μg/mL (mother) and 2.4 μg/mL (infant). The authors estimated the daily metronidazole dose received by the infant at 3.0 mg/kg with 500 mL milk intake per day, which is well below the advocated 10-20 mg/kg recommended therapeutic dose for infants.

For treating trichomoniasis, many physicians now recommend 2 gm single oral dose with an interruption of breastfeeding for 12-24 hours, then reinstitute breastfeeding. Thus far, no reports of untoward effects in breastfed infants have been published for the 2 gm STAT dose or the 250 mg three times daily for 10 day dosage regimen.

In a study of 6 women receiving 400 mg TID for 3 days, the average milk concentration was 13.5 mg/L with a milk/plasma ratio of 0.9.[4]

For intravaginal use see MetroGel. MetroGel vaginal jel produces only 2% of the mean peak serum level concentration of a 500 mg oral metronidazole tablet. The maternal plasma level following use of each dose of vaginal gel averaged only 237 μg/L, far less than orally administered tablet formulations. Milk levels following intravaginal use would probably be exceedingly low. Milk/plasma ratios although published for oral metronidazole, may be different for this route of administration.

It is true that the relative infant dose via milk is moderately high depending on the dose and timing. Infants whose mothers ingest 1.2 gm/d will receive approximately 13.5% or less of the maternal dose or approximately 2.3 mg/kg/day. Bennett has calculated the relative infant dose from 11.7% to as high as 24% of the maternal dose.[8] Heisterberg found metronidazole levels in infant plasma to be 16% and 19% of the maternal plasma levels following doses of 600 mg/d and 1200 mg/d.[3] While these levels seem significant, it is still pertinent to remember that metronidazole is a commonly used drug in premature neonates, infants, and children, and 2.3 mg/kg/d is still much less than the therapeutic dose used in infants/children (7.5-30 mg/kg/d). Thus far, virtually no adverse effects have been reported.

INTRAVENOUS STUDIES

Metronidazole is approximately 98% bioavailable orally, and it is rapidly absorbed. In one study of intravenous kinetics, the authors found peak plasma levels of 28.9 μg/mL in adults following a 500 mg TID dose.[5] In another study of oral and intravenous kinetics, the authors used 400 mg orally and 500 mg intravenously.[6] Following 400 mg orally, the C_{max} at 90 minutes was 17.4 μg/mL. Following 500 mg IV, the C_{max} at 90 minutes was 23.6 μg/mL. Reducing the IV dose to 400 mg would have given a plasma level of approximately 18.8 or an amount similar to the oral plasma level attained in the above group(17.4). From these two sets of data, it is apparent that the peak (C_{max}) following an intravenous dose is only slightly higher than that obtained following oral administration. In an elegant study of plasma kinetics of oral and IV metronidazole (both 500 mg and 2000 mg), Loft found that the AUC (500mg dose) for oral and IV treatments was virtually identical (101 vs. 100 μg/mL h respectively).[7] The C_{max} (taken from graph) for oral and IV treatments were essentially the same. In another study comparing the plasma kinetics following 800 mg doses orally and IV, Bergan[12] found that plasma levels are virtually identical at 2-3 hours after the dose. Therefore, in a breastfeeding mother receiving IV metronidazole, a brief interruption of breastfeeding for perhaps 1-2 hours would expose the infant to almost identical levels as obtained from the same dose given orally.

Data from older studies with rats and mice have shown that metronidazole is potentially mutagenic/carcinogenic. Thus far, no studies in humans have found it to be mutagenic. In fact, the opposite seems to be the finding.[9,10,11] Roe suggests that metronidazole is "essentially free of cancer risk or other serious toxic side effects".[11] Age-gender stratified analysis did not reveal any association between short-term exposure to metronidazole and cancer in humans.[10]

Pregnancy Risk Category: B

Lactation Risk Category: L2

Adult Concerns: Nausea, dry mouth, vomiting, diarrhea, abdominal discomfort. Drug may turn urine brown.

Pediatric Concerns: Numerous studies show no untoward effects. One letter to the editor suggests an infant developed diarrhea and a case of lactose intolerance. The link to metronidazole is tenuous.

Drug Interactions: Phenytoin and phenobarbital may decrease half-life of metronidazole. Alcohol may induce disulfiram-like reactions. May increase prothrombin times when used with warfarin.

Theoretic Infant Dose: 2.16 µg/kg/day

Relative Infant Dose: 12.6%

Adult Dose: 250-500 mg BID

Alternatives:

$T\frac{1}{2}$ =	8.5 hours	M/P =	1.15
PHL =	25-75 hours (full term)	PB =	10%
T_{max} =	2-4 hours	Oral =	100%
MW =	171	pKa =	
Vd =			

References:

1. Erickson SH, Oppenheim GL, Smith GH. Metronidazole in breastmilk. Obstet Gynecol 1981; 57(1):48-50.
2. Passmore CM, McElnay JC, Rainey EA, D'Arcy PF. Metronidazole excretion in human milk and its effect on the suckling neonate. Br J Clin Pharmacol 1988; 26(1):45-51.
3. Heisterberg L, Branebjerg PE. Blood and milk concentrations of metronidazole in mothers and infants. J Perinat Med 1983; 11(2):114-120.
4. Amon I, Amon K. Wirkstoffkonzentrationen von metronidazol bie schwangeren und postpartal. Fortschritte der antimikrobiellen und antineoplastischen. Chemotherapie 2004; Band 2-4:605-612.
5. Ti TY, Lee HS, Khoo YM. Disposition of intravenous metronidazole in Asian surgical patients. Antimicrob Agents Chemother 1996; 40(10):2248-2251.

6. Earl P, Sisson PR, Ingham HR. Twelve-hourly dosage schedule for oral and intravenous metronidazole. J Antimicrob Chemother 1989; 23(4):619-621.
7. Loft S, Dossing M, Poulsen HE, Sonne J, Olesen KL, Simonsen K, Andreasen PB. Influence of dose and route of administration on disposition of metronidazole and its major metabolites. Eur J Clin Pharmacol 1986; 30(4):467-473.
8. Bennett PN. Use of the monographs on drugs: In: Drugs and Human Lactation. Amsterdam, Elsevier, 1996.
9. Falagas ME, Walker AM, Jick H, Ruthazer R, Griffith J, Snydman DR. Late incidence of cancer after metronidazole use: a matched metronidazole user/nonuser study. Clin Infect Dis 1998; 26(2):384-388.
10. Fahrig R, Engelke M. Reinvestigation of in vivo genotoxicity studies in man. I. No induction of DNA strand breaks in peripheral lymphocytes after metronidazole therapy. Mutat Res 1997; 395(2-3):215-221.
11. Roe FJ. Toxicologic evaluation of metronidazole with particular reference to carcinogenic, mutagenic, and teratogenic potential. Surgery 1983; 93(1 Pt 2):158-164.
12. Bergan T, Leinebo O, Blom-Hagen T, Salvesen B. Pharmacokinetics and bioavailability of metronidazole after tablets, suppositories and intravenous administration. Scand J Gastroenterol Suppl 1984; 91:45-60.

METRONIDAZOLE TOPICAL GEL

Trade: Metrogel Topical
Can/Aus/UK: Metro-Gel, Metrogyl, Metrogel
Uses: Topical antibacterial
LRC: L3
AAP: Not reviewed

Metronidazole topical gel is primarily indicated for acne and is a gel formulation containing 0.75% metronidazole. For metronidazole kinetics and entry into human milk see metronidazole. Following topical application of 1 gm of metronidazole gel to the face (equivalent to 7.5 mg metronidazole base), the maximum serum concentration was only 66 nanograms/mL in only one of 10 patients (In three of the ten patients, levels were undetectible).[1,2] This concentration is 100 times less than the serum concentration achieved following the oral ingestion of just one 250 mg tablet. Therefore, the topical application of metronidazole gel provides only exceedingly low plasma levels in the mother and minimal to no levels in milk.

Pregnancy Risk Category: B

Lactation Risk Category: L3

Adult Concerns: Watery eyes if the gel is applied too close to eyes. Minor skin irritation, redness, milk dryness, burning.

Pediatric Concerns: None reported via milk. Milk levels would be exceedingly low to nil.

Drug Interactions: Although many known interactions with oral metronidazole are documented, due to minimal plasma levels of this preparation, they would be extremely remote.

Theoretic Infant Dose:

Relative Infant Dose:

Adult Dose: Apply topically BID

Alternatives:

$T\frac{1}{2}$ =	8.5 hours	M/P =	0.4-1.8
PHL =		PB =	10%
T_{max} =		Oral =	Complete
MW =	171	pKa =	
Vd =			

References:
1. Drug Facts and Comparisons 1996 ed. ed. St. Louis: 1996.
2. Pharmaceutical Manufacturer Prescribing Information. 1997.

METRONIDAZOLE VAGINAL GEL

Trade: Metrogel Vaginal
Can/Aus/UK: Metrogel
Uses: Antibiotic
LRC: L2
AAP: Drugs whose effect on nursing infants is unknown but may be of concern

Both topical and vaginal preparations of metronidazole contain only 0.75% metronidazole. Plasma levels following administration are exceedingly low.[1] This metronidazole vaginal product produces only 2% of the mean peak serum level concentration of a 500 mg oral metronidazole tablet. The maternal plasma level following use of each dose of vaginal gel averaged 237 µg/L compared to 12,785 µg/L following an oral 500 mg tablet. Milk levels following intravaginal use would probably be exceeding low.

Milk/plasma ratios although published for oral metronidazole, may be different for this route of administration, primarily due to the low plasma levels attained with this product. Topical and intravaginal metronidazole gels are indicated for bacterial vaginosis.

Pregnancy Risk Category: B

Lactation Risk Category: L2

Adult Concerns: Mild irritation to vaginal wall

Pediatric Concerns: None reported.

Drug Interactions: Phenytoin and phenobarbital may decrease half-life of metronidazole. Alcohol may induce disulfiram-like reactions. May increase prothrombin times when used with warfarin.

Theoretic Infant Dose:

Relative Infant Dose:

Adult Dose: 37.5 mg BID

Alternatives:

T½ =	8.5 hours	M/P =	
PHL =		PB =	10%
T$_{max}$ =	6-12 hours	Oral =	Complete
MW =	171	pKa =	
Vd =			

References:

1. Pharmaceutical Manufacturer Prescribing Information. 1996.

MEXILETINE HCL

Trade: Mexitil
Can/Aus/UK: Mexitil, Novo-Mexiletine
Uses: Antiarrhythmic
LRC: L2
AAP: Maternal Medication Usually Compatible with Breastfeeding

Mexiletine is an antiarrhythmic agent with activity similar to lidocaine. In a study on one patient who was receiving 600 mg/day in divided doses, the milk level at steady state was 0.8 mg/L, which represented at milk/plasma ratio of 1.1.[1] Mexiletine was not detected in the infant nor were untoward effects noted. In another study on day 2 to 5 postpartum, and in a patient receiving 200 mg three times daily, the mean peak concentration of mexiletine in breastmilk was 959 μg/L, and the maternal serum was 724 μg/L.[2] In this study the milk plasma ratio varied from 0.78 to 1.89 with an average of 1.45. It is unlikely this exposure would lead to untoward side effects in a breastfeeding infant.

Pregnancy Risk Category: B

Lactation Risk Category: L2

Adult Concerns: Arrhythmias, bradycardia, hypotension, tremors, dizziness

Pediatric Concerns: None reported in two studies.

Drug Interactions: Aluminum, magnesium hydroxide, atropine, and narcotics may reduce the oral absorption of mexiletine. Cimetidine may increase or decreased mexiletine plasma levels. Hydantoins such as phenytoin may increase mexiletine clearance and reduce plasma levels.

Rifampin may increase mexiletine clearance leading to lower levels. Mexiletine may reduce the clearance of caffeine by 50%. Serum theophylline levels may be increased significantly to toxic levels.

Theoretic Infant Dose: 143.85 µg/kg/day

Relative Infant Dose: 1.67 %

Adult Dose: 200 mg q 8 hours

Alternatives:

T½ =	9.2 hours	M/P =	1.45
PHL =		PB =	63%
T$_{max}$ =	2-3 hours (oral)	Oral =	90%
MW =	179	pKa =	8.4
Vd =	6-12		

References:
1. Lewis AM, Patel L, Johnston A, Turner P. Mexiletine in human blood and breastmilk. Postgrad Med J 1981; 57(671):546-547.
2. Timmis AD, Jackson G, Holt DW. Mexiletine for control of ventricular dysrhythmias in pregnancy. Lancet 1980; 2(8195 pt 1):647-648.

MICONAZOLE

Trade: Monistat IV, Monistat 3, 7
Can/Aus/UK: Micatin, Monistat, Daktarin, Daktozin, Fungo
Uses: Antifungal for candidiasis
LRC: L2
AAP: Not reviewed

Miconazole is an effective antifungal that is commonly used IV, topically, and intravaginally. After intravaginal application, approximately 1% of the dose is absorbed systemically.[1,2] After topical application, there is little or no absorption (0.1%). It is unlikely that the limited absorption of miconazole from vaginal application would produce significant milk levels. Milk concentrations following oral and IV miconazole have not been reported. Oral absorption of miconazole is poor, only 25-30%. Miconazole is commonly used in pediatric patients less than 1 year of age.

Pregnancy Risk Category: C

Lactation Risk Category: L2

Adult Concerns: Nausea, vomiting, diarrhea, anorexia, itching, rash, local irritation

Pediatric Concerns: None reported via milk.

Drug Interactions: May increase warfarin anticoagulant effect. May increase hypoglycemia of oral sulfonylureas. Phenytoin levels may be increased.

Theoretic Infant Dose:

Relative Infant Dose:

Adult Dose: 200-1200 mg TID

Alternatives:

T½ =	20-25 hours	M/P =	
PHL =		PB =	91-93%
T$_{max}$ =	Immediate (IV)	Oral =	25-30%
MW =	416	pKa =	
Vd =			

References:
1. Drug Facts and Comparisons 1995 ed. ed. St. Louis: 1995.
2. McEvoy GE. (ed):AFHS Drug Information. New York, NY: 2003.

MIDAZOLAM
Trade: Versed
Can/Aus/UK: Versed, Hypnovel
Uses: Short acting benzodiazepine sedative, hypnotic
LRC: L3
AAP: Effect on nursing infants unknown but may be of concern

Midazolam is a very short acting benzodiazepine primarily used as an induction or preanesthetic medication. The onset of action of midazolam is extremely rapid. Its potency is greater than diazepam, and its metabolic elimination is more rapid. With a plasma half-life of only 1.9 hours, it is preferred for rapid induction and maintenance of anesthesia. After oral administration of 15 mg for up to 6 days postnatally in 22 women, the mean milk/plasma ratio was 0.15 and the maximum level of midazolam in breastmilk was 9 nanogram/mL and occurred 1-2 hours after administration.[1] Midazolam and its hydroxy-metabolite were undetectable 4 hours after administration. Therefore, the amount of midazolam transferred to an infant via early milk is minimal, particularly if the baby is breastfed more than 4 hours after administration.

Pregnancy Risk Category: D

Lactation Risk Category: L3

Adult Concerns: Sedation, respiratory depression

Pediatric Concerns: None reported in several studies.

Drug Interactions: Theophylline may reduce the sedative effects of midazolam. Other CNS depressants may potentiate the depressant effects of midazolam. Cimetidine may increase plasma levels of midazolam.

Theoretic Infant Dose: 1.35 µg/kg/day

Relative Infant Dose: 0.63 %

Adult Dose: 1-2.5 mg once or twice

Alternatives: Lorazepam

T½ =	2-5 hours	M/P =	0.15
PHL =	6.5-23 hours	PB =	97%
T$_{max}$ =	20-50 minutes (oral)	Oral =	27-44%
MW =	326	pKa =	6.2
Vd =	1.0-2.5		

References:

1. Matheson I, Lunde PK, Bredesen JE. Midazolam and nitrazepam in the maternity ward: milk concentrations and clinical effects. Br J Clin Pharmacol 1990; 30(6):787-793.

MIDODRINE

Trade: Proamatine
Can/Aus/UK: Amatine, Gutron, Midon
Uses: Vasopressor / Antihypotensive agent
LRC: L3
AAP: Not reviewed

Midodrine is a vasopressor used to increase blood pressure. Midodrine is a prodrug that is metabolized to desglymidodrine. This metabolite is a long-acting alpha-1 agonist. It produces an increase in vascular tone and elevation of blood pressure. Desglymidodrine does not stimulate cardiac beta-1 receptors nor does it pass the blood-brain barrier. No data are available on its transfer to human milk, but some should be expected. This product is small in molecular weight, belongs to the phenylethylamine family, is lipophilic, and is likely to penetrate milk as do the other members of this family. Some caution is recommended.

Pregnancy Risk Category: C

Lactation Risk Category: L3

Adult Concerns: Supine hypertension, pruritus, pilomotor reactions, chills, painful urination retention, and GI symptoms have been reported. CNS reactions include headache, insomnia, stimulation, restlessness, dizziness. A vagal reflex may occur following use and produce a reflex bradycardia.

Pediatric Concerns: None reported via milk, but some caution is recommended. Observer for hypertension, insomnia, and excitement.

Drug Interactions: Additive with other adrenergic stimulants such as pseudoephedrine, ephedrine, phenylephrine, or phenylpropanolamine. Digoxin may enhance or precipitate reflex bradycardia. The concurrent use of prazosin or other alpha blockers may inhibit the effects of midodrine. Use with tricyclic antidepressants may precipitate arrhythmias and tachycardia.

Theoretic Infant Dose:

Relative Infant Dose:

Adult Dose: 10 mg 3 times daily at 4-hour intervals for orthostatic hypotension

Alternatives:

T½ =	3-4 hours (metab)	M/P =	
PHL =		PB =	
T_{max} =	1-2 hours	Oral =	93%
MW =	290	pKa =	
Vd =			

References:
1. Pharmaceutical Manufacturers Prescribing Information, 2003.

MIGLITOL
Trade: Glyset, Diastabol
Can/Aus/UK: Glyset
Uses: Anti diabetic agent
LRC: L2
AAP: Not reviewed

Miglitol is an oral alpha-glycosidase inhibitor for use in non-insulin depended diabetes mellitus. Miglitol delays the digestion of ingested carbohydrates thereby resulting in a small rise in blood glucose concentration following meals. Miglitol does not stimulate insulin release nor does it inhibit lactase nor does it induce hypoglycemia. The oral absorption of miglitol is saturable in adults in doses higher than 25 mg. A dose of 100 mg is only 50-70% absorbed orally.

The manufacturer reports that milk levels are very small. Total excretion into milk accounted for 0.02% of a 100 mg maternal dose. The estimated exposure to a nursing infant is approximately 0.4% of the maternal dose.

Pregnancy Risk Category: B

Lactation Risk Category: L2

Adult Concerns: Flatulence, soft stools, diarrhea, abdominal discomfort are the most commonly reported side effects.

Pediatric Concerns: No reports of use in breastfeeding mothers.

Drug Interactions: Glyburide may reduce plasma levels(17-25%) of miglitol.   Only small but insignificant changes were noted when coadministered with metformin.

Theoretic Infant Dose:

Relative Infant Dose: 0.4 %

Adult Dose: 50 mg three times daily

Alternatives: Metformin

T½ =	2 hours	M/P =	
PHL =		PB =	< 4%
T_{max} =	2-3 hours	Oral =	Variable
MW =	207	pKa =	5.9
Vd =	0.18		

References:
1. Pharmaceutical Manufacturers Prescribing Information, 2003.

MILK THISTLE

Trade: Holy Thistle, Lady Thistle, Marian Thistle, Silybum, Silymarin
Can/Aus/UK:
Uses: Hepatoprotectant
LRC: L3
AAP: Not reviewed

Milk Thistle has been used since 23 A.D. as a liver protectant.[1] Silymarin, a mixture of three isomeric flavonolignans, consists of Silybin, silychristin, and silidianin.[2] Silybin is the most biologically active and is believed to be a potent antioxidant and hepatoprotective agent. Silymarin is poorly soluble in water so aqueous preparations such as teas are ineffective. The oral bioavailability is likewise poor, only 23-47% is absorbed orally.   Oral forms are generally concentrated. Silymarin effects are almost exclusively on the liver and kidney and concentrates in liver cells. It is believed to inhibit oxidative damage to cells by increasing glutathione synthesis. It is believed to also stimulate the regenerative capacity of liver cells. While it has been advocated for the stimulation of milk synthesis, little evidence of efficacy exists. No data are available concerning Silymarin transfer to human milk but some probably transfers. However, it is rather devoid of reported toxicity with only brief GI intolerance and mild allergic reactions.[3,4]

Pregnancy Risk Category:

Lactation Risk Category: L3

Adult Concerns: Mild GI intolerance and allergic reactions

Pediatric Concerns: None reported via milk.

Drug Interactions:

Theoretic Infant Dose:

Relative Infant Dose:

Adult Dose: 200-400 mg daily via extracts

Alternatives:

$T\frac{1}{2}$ =		M/P =		
PHL =		PB =		
T_{max} =		Oral =	23-47%	
MW =	482	pKa =		
Vd =				

References:
1. Foster S. Milk thistle-Silybum marianum. Botanical Series No. 305. American Botanical Council, Austin, TX 1991;3-7.
2. Leung AY. Encyclopedia of Common Natural Ingredients used in Food, Drugs and Cosmetics. J Wiley and Sons, 1980.
3. Review of Natural Products Facts and Comparisons 1999.
4. Awang D. Can Pharm J Oct 1993;403-404.

MINOCYCLINE

Trade: Minocin, Dynacin, Arestin
Can/Aus/UK: Minocin, Novo-Minocycline, Akamin, Minomycin, Blemix
Uses: Tetracycline antibiotic
LRC: L2 for acute use
L4 for chronic use
AAP: Not reviewed

Minocycline is a broad spectrum tetracycline antibiotic with significant side effects in pediatric patients, including dental staining and reduced bone growth.[1,2] It is probably secreted into breastmilk in small but clinically insignificant levels. Because tetracyclines, in general, bind to milk calcium they would have reduced absorption in the infant, but minocycline may be absorbed to a greater degree than the older tetracyclines. Although most tetracyclines secreted into milk are generally bound to calcium, thus inhibiting their absorption, minocycline is poorly bound and may be better absorbed in a breastfeeding infant than the older tetracyclines. While the absolute absorption of older tetracyclines may be dramatically reduced by calcium salts, the newer doxycycline and minocycline analogs bind less and their overall absorption, while slowed, may be significantly higher than earlier versions. A dosage of tetracycline 2 gm/day for 3 days has achieved a milk/plasma ratio of 0.6 to 0.8. In another study of 5 lactating women receiving tetracycline 500 mg PO four times daily, the breastmilk concentrations ranged from 0.43 mg/L to 2.58 mg/L. Levels in infants were below the limit of detection. Because we have many other antimicrobials with similar spectrums, the use of tetracyclines in breastfeeding women is not generally recommended but not necessarily contraindicated. Short-term use (< 3 weeks) is probably safe, longer therapy should be avoided. There is little risk of permanent dental staining with only a brief exposure (several weeks).

Pregnancy Risk Category: **D**

Lactation Risk Category: **L2 for acute use**
                                      L4 for chronic use

Adult Concerns: Adverse effects include GI distress, dizziness, thyroid pigmentation, vomiting, diarrhea, nephrotoxicity, photosensitivity.

Pediatric Concerns: None via breastmilk, but pediatric side effects include decreased linear bone growth and dental staining after prolong edexposure.

Drug Interactions: Absorption may be reduced or delayed when used with dairy products, calcium, magnesium, or aluminum containing antacids, oral contraceptives, iron, zinc, sodium bicarbonate, penicillins, cimetidine. Increased toxicity may result when used with methoxyflurane anesthesia. Use with warfarin anticoagulants may increase anticoagulation.

Theoretic Infant Dose: 0.387 mg/kg/day

Relative Infant Dose: 1.35%

Adult Dose: 100 mg BID

Alternatives: Doxycycline

$T\frac{1}{2}$ =	15-20 hours	M/P =	
PHL =		PB =	76%
T_{max} =	3 hours	Oral =	90-100%
MW =	457	pKa =	
Vd =			

References:
1. Drug Facts and Comparisons 1996 ed. ed. St. Louis: 1996.
2. McEvoy GE. (ed):AFHS Drug Information. New York, NY: 2003.

MINOXIDIL

Trade: Loniten, Minodyl, Rogaine
Can/Aus/UK: Loniten, Rogaine, Apo-Gain, Minox, Regaine
Uses: Antihypertensive
LRC: L2 topically
　　　 L3 orally
AAP: Maternal Medication Usually Compatible with Breastfeeding

Minoxidil is a potent vasodilator and antihypertensive. It is also used for hair loss and baldness. When applied topically, only 1.4% of the dose is absorbed systemically. Following a dose of 7.5 mg, minoxidil was secreted into human milk in concentrations ranging from trough levels of 0.3 µg/L at 12 hours to peak levels of 41.7-55 µg/L at 1 hour following an oral dose of 7.5 mg.[1] Long-term exposure of breastfeeding infants in women ingesting oral minoxidil may not be advisable. However, in those using topical minoxidil, the limited absorption via skin would minimize systemic levels and significantly reduce risk of transfer to infant via breastmilk. It is unlikely that the amount absorbed via topical application would produce clinically relevant concentrations in breastmilk.

Pregnancy Risk Category: C

Lactation Risk Category: L2 topically
　　　　　　　　　　　　　　L3 orally

Adult Concerns: Hypotension, tachycardia, headache, weight gain, skin pigmentation, rash, renal toxicity, leukopenia

Pediatric Concerns: None reported.

Drug Interactions: Profound orthostatic hypotension when used with guanethidine. May potentiate hypotensive effect of other antihypertensives.

Theoretic Infant Dose: 8.25 µg/kg/day

Relative Infant Dose: 7.7%

Adult Dose: 10-40 mg daily
Alternatives:

T½　 =	3.5-4.2 hours	M/P =	0.75-1.0
PHL =		PB　 =	Low
T$_{max}$ =	2-8 hours	Oral =	90-95%
MW =	209	pKa =	
Vd　 =			

References:
1.　Valdivieso A, Valdes G, Spiro TE, Westerman RL. Minoxidil in breastmilk. Ann Intern Med 1985; 102(1):135.

MIRTAZAPINE
Trade: Remeron
Can/Aus/UK: Avanza, Zispin
Uses: Antidepressant
LRC: L3
AAP: Not reviewed

Mirtazapine is a unique antidepressant structurally dissimilar to the SSRIs, tricyclics, or the monoamine oxidase inhibitors. Mirtazapine has little or no serotonergic-like side effects, fewer anticholinergic side effects than amitriptyline, it produces less sexual dysfunction, and has not demonstrated cardiotoxic or seizure potential in a limited number of overdose cases.[1]

In a study of 3 women who received 45, 60, and 45 mg/day mirtazapine, the average concentration (AUC) in milk was 77, 75, and 47 µg/L, respectively.[2] The absolute infant dose was 10, 11.3, and 7.1 µg/kg/d, respectively. The relative infant dose was 1.9%, 1.1%, and 1.5% of the weight-normalized maternal dose, respectively. Mirtazapine was below the limit of quantitation in two of the infants and only 1.5 ng/mL in the second infant. The infants were meeting all developmental milestones and were without side effects.

Pregnancy Risk Category: C

Lactation Risk Category: L3

Adult Concerns: Drowsiness (54%), dizziness, dry mouth, constipation, increased appetite (17%), and weight gain (12%) have been reported.

Pediatric Concerns: None reported via milk but observe for sedation.

Drug Interactions: Enhanced impairment of cognitive function when administered with alcohol. Mirtazapine is a weak inhibitor of cytochrome P450 2D6 and others. Drugs metabolized by this enzyme system may have enhanced activity. Coadministration with benzodiazepines may reduce cognitive function.

Theoretic Infant Dose: 11.5 µg/kg/day

Relative Infant Dose: 1.9%

Adult Dose: 15-45 mg daily

Alternatives: Sertraline, venlafaxine, paroxetine

T½ =	20-40 hours	M/P =	0.76
PHL =		PB =	85%
Tmax =	2 hours	Oral =	50%
MW =	265	pKa =	
Vd =			

References:
1. Pharmaceutical Manufacturer Prescribing Information. 1999.
2. Ilett KF, Hackett LP, Kristensen JH, Rampono J. Distribution and excretion of the novel antidepressant mirtazapine in human milk. International Lactation Consultants Meeting, Sydney, July 31- August 3, 2003.

MISOPROSTOL

Trade: Cytotec
Can/Aus/UK: Cytotec
Uses: Prostaglandin hormone, gastric protectant
LRC: L3
AAP: Not reviewed

Misoprostol is a prostaglandin E1 compound that is useful in treating nonsteroidal-induced gastric ulceration. Misoprostol is absorbed orally and rapidly metabolized. Intact misoprostol is not detectable in plasma and is rapidly metabolized to misoprostol acid which is biologically active.[1] Secretion of misoprostol in milk is unlikely due to rapid maternal metabolism. However, secretion of its active metabolite is possible and could produce diarrhea in newborns although this has not been reported.

Pregnancy Risk Category: X

Lactation Risk Category: L3

Adult Concerns: Diarrhea, abdominal cramps and pain, uterine bleeding and abortion

Pediatric Concerns: None reported, but observe for diarrhea, abdominal cramps.

Drug Interactions: Levels are diminished when administered with food. Antacids reduce total bioavailability but this does not appear clinically significant.

Theoretic Infant Dose:

Relative Infant Dose:

Adult Dose: 100-200 µg QID

Alternatives:

$T\frac{1}{2}$ =	20-40 minutes	M/P =	
PHL =		PB =	80-90%
T_{max} =	14-20 minutes (oral)	Oral =	Complete
MW =	383	pKa =	
Vd =			

References:
1. Pharmaceutical Manufacturer Prescribing Information. 1995.

MITOXANTRONE

Trade: Novantrone
Can/Aus/UK: Onkotrone, Novantrone
Uses: Immunosuppressant for MS
LRC: L5
AAP: Not reviewed

Mitoxantrone is an antineoplastic agent used in the treatment of relapsing multiple sclerosis. It is a DNA-reactive agent that intercalates into DNA via hydrogen bonding, causing crosslinks. It inhibits B cell, T cell, and macrophage proliferation. Milk levels of 18 μg/L up to 28 days after the last administration have been reported by the manufacturer.[1] As this is a DNA-reactive agent, and it has a huge volume of distribution leading to prolonged plasma levels, it should not be used in breastfeeding mothers.

Pregnancy Risk Category: D

Lactation Risk Category: L5

Adult Concerns: Leukopenia and thrombocytopenia are the most common adverse effects. Cardiotoxicity, nausea, vomiting, diarrhea, mucositis, hepatotoxicity, alopecia, pruritus, phlebitis have been reported. Neuropathy and paralysis of the bowel and bladder are reported.

Pediatric Concerns: None reported but extreme caution is recommended. Probably contraindicated.

Drug Interactions: Avoid vaccinations with live or attenuated vaccines (Smallpox, Rotavirus, etc). The half-life of mitoxantrone is increased (1.8 fold) by use with valspodar.

Theoretic Infant Dose:

Relative Infant Dose:

Adult Dose: 12 mg/meter^2

Alternatives:

T½ =	23-215 hours	M/P =	
PHL =		PB =	78%
T$_{max}$ =		Oral =	Poor
MW =	517	pKa =	
Vd =	14-54		

References:
1. Pharmaceutical Manufacturer Prescribing Information.

MIVACURIUM

Trade: Mivacron
Can/Aus/UK: Mivacrom, Mevacron
Uses: Neuromuscular blocking agent
LRC: L2
AAP: Not reviewed

Mivacurium is a short-acting neuromuscular blocking agent used to relax skeletal muscles during surgery. Its duration is very short and complete recovery generally occurs in 15-30 minutes.[1,2] No data are available on its transfer to breastmilk. However, it has an exceedingly short plasma half-life and probably poor to no oral absorption. It is very unlikely that it would be absorbed by a breastfeeding infant.

Pregnancy Risk Category: C

Lactation Risk Category: L2

Adult Concerns: Flushing, hypotension, weakness

Pediatric Concerns: None reported.

Drug Interactions: Inhaled anesthetics, local anesthetics, calcium channel blockers, antiarrhythmic such as quinidine, and certain antibiotics such as amino glycosides, tetracyclines, vancomycin, and clindamycin may significantly prolong neuromuscular blockade with mivacurium.

Theoretic Infant Dose:

Relative Infant Dose:

Adult Dose: 0.1-0.15 mg/kg q 15 minutes PRN

Alternatives:

$T\frac{1}{2}$ =	< 30 minutes	M/P =	
PHL =		PB =	
T_{max} =		Oral =	Poor
MW =		pKa =	
Vd =			

References:
1. McEvoy GE. (ed):AFHS Drug Information. New York, NY: 2003.
2. Pharmaceutical Manufacturer Prescribing Information. 1995.

MMR VACCINE

Trade: MMR Vaccine, Measles - Mumps - Rubella
Can/Aus/UK:
Uses: Live attenuated triple virus vaccine
LRC: L2
AAP: Not reviewed

MMR vaccine is a mixture of live, attenuated viruses from measles, mumps, and rubella strains. It is usually administered to children at 12-15 months of age. NEVER administer to a pregnant woman. Rubella, and perhaps measles and mumps virus, are undoubtedly transferred via breastmilk and have been detected in throat swabs of 56% of breastfeeding infants.[1-4] Infants exposed to the attenuated viruses via breastmilk had only mild symptoms. If medically required, MMR vaccine can be administered early postpartum.[5] See rubella.

Pregnancy Risk Category:

Lactation Risk Category: L2

Adult Concerns: Mild symptoms, fever, flu-like symptoms

Pediatric Concerns: Mild symptoms of rubella have been reported in one newborn infant.

Drug Interactions:

Theoretic Infant Dose:

Relative Infant Dose:

Adult Dose: 0.5 mL once

Alternatives:

References:
1. Buimovici-Klein E, Hite RL, Byrne T, Cooper LZ. Isolation of rubella virus in milk after postpartum immunization. J Pediatr 1977; 91(6):939-941.
2. Losonsky GA, Fishaut JM, Strussenberg J, Ogra PL. Effect of immunization against rubella on lactation products. I. Development and characterization of specific immunologic reactivity in breastmilk. J Infect Dis 1982; 145(5):654-660.
3. Losonsky GA, Fishaut JM, Strussenberg J, Ogra PL. Effect of immunization against rubella on lactation products. II. Maternal-neonatal interactions. J Infect Dis 1982; 145(5):661-666.
4. Landes RD, Bass JW, Millunchick EW, Oetgen WJ. Neonatal rubella following postpartum maternal immunization. J Pediatr 1980; 97(3):465-467.
5. Lawrence RA. Breastfeeding: A guide for the medical profession. St. Louis: Mosby Publishers, 1994.

MOCLOBEMIDE

Trade:
Can/Aus/UK: Apo-Moclobemide, Manerix, Arima, Aurorix
Uses: MAO inhibitor, antidepressant.
LRC: L3
AAP: Not reviewed

Unlike older MAO inhibitors, moclobemide is a selective and reversible inhibitor of MAO-A isozyme and thus is not plagued with the dangerous side effects of the older MAO inhibitor families. It is an effective treatment for depression.[1] In a study by Pons in 6 lactating women, who received a single oral dose of 300 mg, the concentration of moclobemide (C_{max}) was highest at 3 hours after the dose and averaged 2.7 mg/L.[2] The average (AUC) milk concentration throughout the 12 hour period was 0.97 mg/L hour. The minimal levels of moclobemide found in milk are unlikely to produce untoward effects according to the authors.

Pregnancy Risk Category:

Lactation Risk Category: L3

Adult Concerns: Dry mouth, headache, dizziness, tremor, sweating, insomnia, and constipation

Pediatric Concerns: None reported via milk.

Drug Interactions: Serotonergic syndrome is unlikely, but possible when admixed with SSRI antidepressants, clomipramine, fluoxetine, etc. Do not coadminister with SSRIs and tricyclic antidepressants. Do not administer with meperidine (pethidine) or dextromethorphan. Sympthathomimetic hyperactivity (hypertension, headache, hyperpyrexia, arrhythmias, cerebral hemorrhage) may occur when admixed with tyramine, ephedrine, pseudoephedrine, phenylephrine, epinephrine, norepinephrine and other sympathomimetics.

Theoretic Infant Dose: 0.14 mg/kg/day

Relative Infant Dose: 3.4%

Adult Dose: 450 mg/day

Alternatives:

T½ =	1-2.2 hours	M/P =	0.72
PHL =		PB =	50%
T_{max} =	2 hours	Oral =	80%
MW =	269	pKa =	6.3
Vd =	1-2		

References:
1. Fulton B, Benfield P. Moclobemide. An update of its pharmacological properties and therapeutic use. Drugs 1996; 52(3):450-474.

2. Pons G, Schoerlin MP, Tam YK, Moran C, Pfefen JP, Francoual C, Pedarriosse AM, Chavinie J, Olive G. Moclobemide excretion in human breastmilk. Br J Clin Pharmacol 1990; 29(1):27-31.

MODAFINIL

Trade: Provigil
Can/Aus/UK: Alertec, Provigil
Uses: Wakefulness-promoting agent
LRC: L4
AAP: Not reviewed

Modafinil is a wakefulness-promoting agent used for the treatment of narcolepsy. Although its pharmacologic results are similar to amphetamines and methylphenidate (Ritalin), its method of action is unknown. No data are available on its transfer into human milk. Some caution is recommended as it is small in molecular weight and very lipid soluble, both characteristics which may ultimately lead to higher milk levels. In addition, it apparently stimulates dopamine levels. Compounds that stimulate dopamine levels in brain often reduce prolactin secretion. Milk production may suffer, but this is only supposition.

Pregnancy Risk Category: C

Lactation Risk Category: L4

Adult Concerns: May increase incidence of headache, chest pain, palpitations, dyspnea, and transient T-wave changes on ECG. CNS changes include delusions, auditory hallucinations and sleep deprivation. Diarrhea, dry mouth, nausea, and rhinitis have been reported.

Pediatric Concerns: None reported. Observe for reduced milk supply.

Drug Interactions: May increase plasma levels of diazepam, phenytoin and propranolol. Caution when used with tricyclic and SSRI antidepressants. May induce hepatic enzymes, thus reducing circulating levels of cyclosporine, theophylline, and steroidal contraceptives.

Theoretic Infant Dose:

Relative Infant Dose:

Adult Dose: 200-400 up to twice daily

Alternatives:

$T\frac{1}{2}$ =	15 hours	M/P =	
PHL =		PB =	60%
T_{max} =	2-4 hours	Oral =	Complete
MW =	273	pKa =	
Vd =	0.9		

References:
1.   Pharmaceutical Manufacturer Prescribing Information.

MOMETASONE

Trade: Elocon, Nasonex
Can/Aus/UK:
Uses: Corticosteroid
LRC: L3
AAP: Not reviewed

Mometasone is a corticosteroid primarily intended for intranasal and topical use. It is considered a medium-potency steroid, similar to betamethasone and triamcinolone. Following topical application to the skin, less than 0.7% is systemically absorbed over an 8 hour period.[1,2] It is extremely unlikely mometasone would be excreted into human milk in clinically relevant levels following topical or intranasal administration.

Pregnancy Risk Category: C

Lactation Risk Category: L3

Adult Concerns: Topically, only minimal side effects have been reported and include irritation, burning, stinging, and dermal atrophy. After nasal administration, common adverse effects include headache, pharyngitis, epistaxis, and cough.

Pediatric Concerns: None reported via milk.

Drug Interactions:

Theoretic Infant Dose:

Relative Infant Dose:

Adult Dose: Apply topically 2-3 times daily

Alternatives:

References:
1.   Pharmaceutical Manufacturer Prescribing Information. 1999.
2.   Drug Facts and Comparisons 1999 ed. ed. St. Louis: 1999.

MONTELUKAST SODIUM

Trade: Singulair
Can/Aus/UK:
Uses: Antiasthmatic agent
LRC: L3
AAP: Not reveiwed

Montelukast is a leukotriene receptor inhibitor similar to Accolate and is used as an adjunct in the treatment of asthma.   The manufacturer reports that montelukast is secreted into animal milk, but no data on human milk are available.[1] This product is cleared for use in children aged 6 and above. This product does not enter the CNS nor many other tissues. Although the milk levels in humans are unreported, they are probably quite low.

Pregnancy Risk Category: B

Lactation Risk Category: L3

Adult Concerns: Abdominal pain, fever, dyspepsia, dental pain, dizziness, headache, cough and nasal congestion, some changes in liver enzymes.

Pediatric Concerns: None reported via milk.

Drug Interactions: Phenobarbital may reduce plasma levels by 40%. Although unreported, other inhibitors of Cytochrome P450 may affect plasma levels.

Theoretic Infant Dose:

Relative Infant Dose:

Adult Dose: 10 mg daily

Alternatives: Zafirlukast

$T\frac{1}{2}$ =	2.7-5.5 hours	M/P =	
PHL =		PB =	99%
T_{max} =	2-4 hours	Oral =	64%
MW =	608	pKa =	
Vd =	0.15		

References:
1. Pharmaceutical Manufacturer Prescribing Information.

MORPHINE

Trade: Duramorph, Infumorph
Can/Aus/UK: Epimorph, Morphitec, M.O.S. MS Contin, Statex, Morphalgin, Ordine, Anamorph, Kapanol, Oramorph, Sevredol
Uses: Narcotic analgesic
LRC: L3
AAP: Maternal Medication Usually Compatible with Breastfeeding

Morphine is a potent narcotic analgesic. In a group of 5 lactating women, the highest morphine concentration in breastmilk following two epidural doses was only 82 μg/L at 30 minutes.[1] The highest breastmilk level following 15 mg IV/IM was only 0.5 mg/L although it dropped to almost 0.01 mg/L in 4 hours. In this study and following two 4 mg epidural doses, the peak milk level was 82 μg/L or a relative infant dose of 10.7%.

In another study of women receiving morphine via PCA pumps for 12-48 hours postpartum, the concentration of morphine in breastmilk ranged from 50-60 µg/L(estimated from graph).[2] None of the infants in this study were neurobehaviorally delayed at 3 days. Because of the poor oral bioavailability of morphine (26%) it is unlikely these levels would be clinically relevant in a stable breastfeeding infant.

However, data from Robieux suggests the levels transferred to the infant are higher.[3] In this study of a single patient, plasma levels in the breastfed infant were within therapeutic range (4 ng/mL) although the infant showed no untoward signs or symptoms. However, this case was somewhat unique in that the mother received daily morphine (50 mg PO every 6 hrs) during the third trimester for severe back pain. One week postpartum, the morphine was discontinued and then 5 days later reinstated due to withdrawal effects in the mother. The reported concentration in foremilk and hindmilk was 100 ng/mL and 10 ng/mL respectively and the authors suggested that the dose to the infant would be 0.8 to 12% of the maternal oral dose (0.15 to 2.41 mg/day). Although this study suggests that the amount of morphine transferred in milk can be clinically relevant, the authors calculated the infant dose from the highest milk concentration and a milk intake of 150 mL/kg/day, thus the dose of morphine to the infant would have been substantially lower (53 µg/day). This study seems flawed because the plasma levels and the doses via milk just don't correlate. That this infant showed no untoward effects, can be explained by the fact that it may have exhibited tolerance after long exposure, that the reported analgesic-therapeutic level required in neonates is actually slightly higher than in adults, or the plasma levels assayed in this infant were in error.

Infants under 1 month of age have a prolonged elimination half-life and decreased clearance of morphine relative to older infants. The clearance of morphine and its elimination begins to approach adult values by 2 months of age. In summary, morphine is probably the preferred opiate in breastfeeding mothers primarily due to its poor oral bioavailability. It is unfortunate that the clinical studies above do not necessarily suggest this. However, high doses over prolonged periods could lead to sedation and respiratory problems in newborn infants.

Pregnancy Risk Category: B

Lactation Risk Category: L3

Adult Concerns: Sedation, flushing, CNS depression, respiratory depression, bradycardia

Pediatric Concerns: None reported via milk but sedation is possible with higher doses.

Drug Interactions: Barbiturates may significantly increase respiratory and CNS depressant effects of morphine. The admixture of cimetidine has produced CNS toxicity such as confusion, disorientation, respiratory depression, apnea, and seizures when used with narcotic analgesics. Diazepam may produce cardiovascular depression when used with opiates. Phenothiazines may antagonize the analgesic effect of morphine.

Theoretic Infant Dose: 12.3 µg/kg/day

Relative Infant Dose: 10.7%

Adult Dose: 10-30 mg q 4 hours PRN

Alternatives: Codeine

T½ =	1.5-2 hours	M/P =	1.1-3.6
PHL =	13.9 hours (neonates)	PB =	35%
T$_{max}$ =	0.5-1 hours	Oral =	26%
MW =	285	pKa =	8.1
Vd =	2-5		

References:
1. Feilberg VL, Rosenborg D, Broen CC, Mogensen JV. Excretion of morphine in human breastmilk. Acta Anaesthesiol Scand 1989; 33(5):426-428.
2. Wittels B, Scott DT, Sinatra RS. Exogenous opioids in human breastmilk and acute neonatal neurobehavior: a preliminary study. Anesthesiology 1990; 73(5):864-869.
3. Robieux I, Koren G, Vandenbergh H, Schneiderman J. Morphine excretion in breastmilk and resultant exposure of a nursing infant. J Toxicol Clin Toxicol 1990; 28(3):365-370.

MOXIFLOXACIN

Trade: Avelox, Vigamox
Can/Aus/UK: Avelox
Uses: Fluoroquinolone antibiotic
LRC: L2 Ophthalmically
L3 Orally, IV
AAP: Not reviewed

Moxifloxacin is a quinolone antibiotic for use orally, intravenously, and in the eye. It is a new-generation fluoroquinolone which exhibits improved activity against S. pneumonia and other species. No data are available on its transfer into human milk so until we have data, one should opt for using ofloxacin or levofloxacin for which published data are available.

Pregnancy Risk Category: C

Lactation Risk Category: **L2 Ophthalmically**
L3 Orally, IV

Adult Concerns: Nausea and diarrhea are the most common complications following oral use in adults. It should be avoided in patients with prolonged QT intervals.

Pediatric Concerns: No reports available, but changes in gut flora, and diarrhea are possible. Complications following ophthalmic use are extremely remote as the plasma levels are very very low.

Drug Interactions: Moxifloxacin can be administered concurrently with food. Do not take with antacids containing magnesium, aluminum, sucralfate, metal cations such as iron or zinc. Wait a minimum of 4 hours after using these products.

Theoretic Infant Dose:

Relative Infant Dose:

Adult Dose: Oral = 400 mg daily

Alternatives: Ofloxacin, Levofloxacin, Ciprofloxacin

$T\frac{1}{2}$ =	9-16 hours	M/P =	
PHL =		PB =	50%
T_{max} =	1-3 hours	Oral =	90%
MW =	437	pKa =	
Vd =	1.7-3		

References:
1. Pharmaceutical Manufacturer Prescribing Information.

MUPIROCIN OINTMENT
Trade: Bactroban
Can/Aus/UK: Bactroban
Uses: Antibacterial ointment
LRC: L1
AAP: Not reviewed

Mupirocin is a topical antibiotic used for impetigo, Group A beta-hemolytic strep, and strep. Pyogenes. Mupirocin is only minimally absorbed following topical application. In one study, less than 0.3% of a topical dose was absorbed after 24 hours. Most remained adsorbed to the corneum layer of the skin. The drug is absorbed orally but it is so rapidly metabolized that systemic levels are not sustained. It is quite safe for breastfeeding mothers.

Pregnancy Risk Category: B

Lactation Risk Category: L1

Adult Concerns: Rash, irritation

Pediatric Concerns: None reported. Commonly used in pediatric patients.

Drug Interactions:

Theoretic Infant Dose:

Relative Infant Dose:

Adult Dose: Apply sparingly.

Alternatives:

T½ =	17-36 minutes	M/P =	
PHL =		PB =	
Tmax =		Oral =	Complete
MW =	501	pKa =	
Vd =			

References:

MYCOPHENOLATE

Trade: Cellcept
Can/Aus/UK: CellCept
Uses: Immunosuppressive agent
LRC: L4
AAP: Not reviewed

Mycophenolate is an immunosuppressive agent used to prevent rejection of allogenic transplants (kidney, heart, liver, intestine, limb, small bowel, etc. It is well absorbed and rapidly metabolized to MPA, the active metabolite. MPA glucuronide then subsequently enters the small intestine and is reabsorbed by enterohepatic recirculation. No data are available on its transfer into human milk. The average blood level is about 63.9 µg/mL (AUC) which is relatively high. Until we have data on human breastmilk levels this agent should be considered relatively hazardous.

Pregnancy Risk Category: C

Lactation Risk Category: L4

Adult Concerns: Increased risk for diarrhea, leukopenia, sepsis, vomiting, headache, tremor, insomnia, high risk of infections, lymphoma and other malignancies, bone marrow suppression.

Pediatric Concerns: This product is a high risk product for breastfeeding mothers. Great caution is recommended. See cyclosporin and others as alternatives.

Drug Interactions: Comcomitant use with azathioprine is not recommended. Use cautiously with drugs that affect enterohepatic recirculation, such as cholestyramine. Avoid use of live attenuated vaccines. Numerous other drug-drug reactions occur, consult other references.

Theoretic Infant Dose:

Relative Infant Dose:

Adult Dose: 1-1.5 mg orally twice daily

Alternatives: Cyclosporine

T½ =	17.9 hours	M/P =	
PHL =		PB =	97%
T$_{max}$ =	1 hour	Oral =	94% (parent)
MW =	433	pKa =	
Vd =	4		

References:
1. Pharmaceutical Manufacturers prescribing information, 2003.

NABUMETONE

Trade: Relafen
Can/Aus/UK: Relafen, Relifex
Uses: Antiinflammatory agent for arthritic pain
LRC: L3
AAP: Not reviewed

Nabumetone is a non-steroidal antiinflammatory agent for arthritic pain.[1] Immediately upon absorption, nabumetone is metabolized to the active metabolite. The parent drug is not detectable in plasma. It is not known if the nabumetone metabolite (6MNA) is secreted in human milk. It is known to be secreted into animal milk and has a very long half-life. NSAIDS are not generally recommended in nursing mothers, with the exception of ibuprofen. See ibuprofen as alternative.

Pregnancy Risk Category: C

Lactation Risk Category: L3

Adult Concerns: GI distress, nausea, vomiting, diarrhea

Pediatric Concerns: None reported via milk.   Observe for GI distress.

Drug Interactions: May prolong prothrombin time when used with warfarin. Antihypertensive effects of ACEi family may be blunted or completely abolished by NSAIDs. Some NSAIDs may block antihypertensive effect of beta blockers, diuretics. Used with cyclosporin, may dramatically increase renal toxicity. May increase digoxin, phenytoin, lithium levels. May increase toxicity of methotrexate. May increase bioavailability of penicillamine. Probenecid may increase NSAID levels.

Theoretic Infant Dose:

Relative Infant Dose:

Adult Dose: 500-1000 mg daily-BID

Alternatives: Ibuprofen

T½ =	22-30 hours	M/P =	
PHL =		PB =	99%
T$_{max}$ =	2.5 - 4 hours	Oral =	38%
MW =	228	pKa =	
Vd =			

References:
1.   Pharmaceutical Manufacturer Prescribing Information.

NADOLOL
Trade: Corgard
Can/Aus/UK: Corgard, Syn-Nadolol, Novo-Nadolol
Uses: Antihypertensive, antianginal, beta blocker
LRC: L4
AAP: Maternal Medication Usually Compatible with Breastfeeding

Nadolol is a long-acting beta adrenergic blocker used as an antihypertensive. It is secreted into breastmilk in moderately high concentrations. Following a maternal dose of 20 mg/day, breastmilk levels at 38 hours postpartum were 146 µg/L.[1]   In another study of 12 women receiving 80 mg daily the mean steady-state concentrations in milk were 357 µg/L.[2] The time to maximum concentration was 6 hours. The milk/serum ratio was reported to average 4.6. A five kg infant would receive from 2-7% of the maternal dose. The authors recommended caution with the use of this beta blocker in breastfeeding patients.   Due to its long half-life and high milk/plasma ratio, this would not be a preferred beta blocker.

Pregnancy Risk Category: C

Lactation Risk Category: L4

Adult Concerns: Hypotension, nausea, diarrhea, bradycardia, apnea, depression

Pediatric Concerns: None reported, but due to the high M/P ratio of 4.6, this product is not recommended.

Drug Interactions: Decreased effect when used with aluminum salts, barbiturates, calcium salts, cholestyramine, NSAIDs, ampicillin, rifampin, and salicylates. Beta blockers may reduce the effect of oral sulfonylureas (hypoglycemic agents). Increased toxicity/effect when used with other antihypertensives, contraceptives, MAO inhibitors, cimetidine, and numerous other products.   See   drug interaction reference for complete listing.

Theoretic Infant Dose: 53.5 µg/kg/day

Relative Infant Dose: 4.6%

Adult Dose: 40-80 mg daily

Alternatives: Propranolol, Metoprolol

T½ =	20-24 hours	M/P =	4.6
PHL =		PB =	30%
T_{max} =	2-4 hours	Oral =	20-40%
MW =	309	pKa =	9.7
Vd =	1.5-3.6		

References:

1. Fox RE, Marx C, Stark AR. Neonatal effects of maternal nadolol therapy. Am J Obstet Gynecol 1985; 152(8):1045-1046.
2. Devlin RG, Duchin KL, Fleiss PM. Nadolol in human serum and breastmilk. Br J Clin Pharmacol 1981; 12(3):393-396.

NAFCILLIN

Trade: Unipen, Nafcil
Can/Aus/UK: Unipen
Uses: Penicillin antibiotic
LRC: L1
AAP: Not reviewed

Nafcillin is a penicillin antibiotic that is poorly and erratically absorbed orally.[1] The only formulations are IV and IM. No data are available on concentration in milk but it is likely small. Oral absorption in the infant would be minimal. See other penicillins.

Pregnancy Risk Category: B

Lactation Risk Category: L1

Adult Concerns: Neutropenia, hypokalemia, pseudomembranous colitis, allergic rash

Pediatric Concerns: None reported. Observe for GI symptoms such as diarrhea. Nafcillin is frequently used in infants.

Drug Interactions: Chloramphenicol may decreased nafcillin levels. Nafcillin may inhibit efficacy of oral contraceptives. Probenecid may increase nafcillin levels. May increase anticoagulant effect of warfarin and heparin.

Theoretic Infant Dose:

Relative Infant Dose:

Adult Dose: 250-1000 mg q 4-6 hours

Alternatives:

T½ =	0.5-1.5 hours	M/P =	
PHL =	2.2-5.5 hours (neonates)	PB =	70-90%
T$_{max}$ =	30-60 minutes (IM)	Oral =	50%
MW =	436	pKa =	
Vd =			

References:
1. McEvoy GE. (ed):AFHS Drug Information. New York, NY: 2003.

NALBUPHINE

Trade: Nubain
Can/Aus/UK: Nubain
Uses: Analgesic
LRC: L2
AAP: Not reviewed

Nalbuphine is a potent narcotic analgesic similar in potency to morphine. In a group of 20 postpartum mothers who received 20 mg IM nalbuphine, the total amount of nalbuphine excreted into human milk during a 24 hour period averaged 2.3 micrograms, which is equivalent to 0.012% of the maternal dosage.[1] The mean milk/plasma ratio using the AUC was 1.2. According to the authors, an oral intake of 2.3 micrograms nalbuphine would not show any measurable plasma concentrations in the neonate. Nalbuphine is both an antagonist and agonist of opiate receptors and should not be mixed with other opiates due to interference with analgesia.

Pregnancy Risk Category: B

Lactation Risk Category: L2

Adult Concerns: Hypotension, sedation, withdrawal syndrome, respiratory depression

Pediatric Concerns: None reported via milk.

Drug Interactions: May reduce efficacy of other opioid analgesics. Barbiturates may increase CNS sedation.

Theoretic Infant Dose:

Relative Infant Dose:

Adult Dose: 10-20 mg q 3-6 hours PRN

Alternatives:

T½ =	5 hours	M/P =	1. 2
PHL =	0.86 hours	PB =	
T$_{max}$ =	2-15 minutes (IV,IM)	Oral =	16%
MW =	357	pKa =	
Vd =	2.4-7.3		

References:
1. Wischnik A, Wetzelsberger N, Lucker PW. Elimination of nalbuphine in human milk. Arzneimittelforschung 1988; 38(10):1496-1498.
2. Jaillon P, Gardin ME, Lecocq B, Richard MO, Meignan S, Blondel Y, Grippat JC, Bergnieres J, Vergnoux O. Pharmacokinetics of nalbuphine in infants, young healthy volunteers, and elderly patients. Clin Pharmacol Ther 1989; 46(2):226-233.

NALIDIXIC ACID

Trade: NegGram
Can/Aus/UK: NegGram
Uses: Urinary anti-infective
LRC: L4
AAP: Maternal Medication Usually Compatible with Breastfeeding

Nalidixic is an old urinary antiseptic and belongs to the fluoroquinolone family. In a group of 4 women receiving 1000 mg orally/day the concentration in breastmilk was approximately 5 mg/L.[1] Hemolytic anemia has been reported in one infant whose mother received 1 gm nalidixic acid 4 times daily. Use with extreme caution. A number of new and less toxic choices (ofloxacin) should preclude the use of this compound.[2]

Pregnancy Risk Category: B

Lactation Risk Category: L4

Adult Concerns: Hemolytic anemia, headache, drowsiness, blurred vision, nausea, vomiting

Pediatric Concerns: Hemolytic anemia in one infant. This is an old product that should not be used currently.

Drug Interactions: Decreased efficacy/oral bioavailability when used with antacids. Increased anticoagulation with warfarin.

Theoretic Infant Dose: 750 µg/kg/day

Relative Infant Dose: 5.2%

Adult Dose: 1 g QID

Alternatives: Norfloxacin, ofloxacin, levofloxacin

T½ =	1-2.5 hours	M/P =	0.08-0.13
PHL =		PB =	93%
T$_{max}$ =	1-2 hours	Oral =	60%
MW =	232	pKa =	
Vd =			

References:
1. Belton EM, Jones RV. Haemolytic anaemia due to nalidixic acid. Lancet 1965; 2(7414):691.
2. Drug Facts and Comparisons 1994 ed. ed. St. Louis: 1994.

NALTREXONE

Trade: Revia
Can/Aus/UK: ReVia, Nalorex
Uses: Narcotic antagonist
LRC: L1
AAP: Not reviewed

Naltrexone is a long acting narcotic antagonist similar in structure to Naloxone. Orally absorbed, it has been clinically used in addicts to prevent the action of injected heroin. It occupies and competes with all opioid medications for the opiate receptor. When used in addicts, it can induce rapid and long lasting withdrawal symptoms. Although the half-life appears brief, the duration of antagonism is long lasting (24-72 hours).[1-5] Naltrexone is quite lipid soluble, has a high pKa, and transfers into the brain easily (brain/plasma ratio = 0.81). It is readily metabolized to 6-beta-naltrexol (active) and two minor metabolites. The activity of naltrexone is believed to be mainly due to parent and 6-beta-naltrexol. In a study of one patient (60 kg) receiving 50 mg/day, the average concentration of naltrexone and 6-beta-naltrexol in milk were 1.7 and 46 µg/L.[6] The milk/plasma ratios of naltrexone and 6-beta-naltrexol were 1.9 and 3.4 respectively. The absolute infant dose was 0.26 and 6.86 µg/kg/day, respectively. The relative infant dose was 0.06 and 1.0% (range= 0.86-1.06%). The infant was reported to have achieved all expected milestones and showed no drug-related side effects. Naltrexone was undetectable in the infants' plasma and levels of 6-beta-naltrexol were only marginally detectable, at 1.1 µg/L.

Pregnancy Risk Category: C

Lactation Risk Category: L1

Adult Concerns: Rapid opiate withdrawal symptoms. Dizziness, anorexia, rash, nausea, vomiting, and hepatocellular toxicity. Liver toxicity is common at doses approximately 5 times normal or less. A Narcan challenge test should be initiated in patients prior to therapy with naltrexone.

Pediatric Concerns: None reported in one case. Plasma levels of 6-beta-naltrexol were only marginally detectable, at 1.1 µg/L.

Drug Interactions: Suppresses narcotic analgesia and sedation.

Theoretic Infant Dose: 7.1 µg/kg/day

Relative Infant Dose: 1.0%

Adult Dose: 50-150 mg daily

Alternatives:

T½ =	4-13 hours	M/P =	1.9 (3.4 metab)
PHL =		PB =	21%
T$_{max}$ =	1 hour	Oral =	96%
MW =	341	pKa =	7.9
Vd =	19		

References:
1. Bullingham RE, McQuay HJ, Moore RA. Clinical pharmacokinetics of narcotic agonist-antagonist drugs. Clin Pharmacokinet 1983; 8(4):332-343.
2. Crabtree BL. Review of naltrexone, a long-acting opiate antagonist. Clin Pharm 1984; 3(3):273-280.
3. Ludden TM, Malspeis L, Baggot JD, Sokoloski TD, Frank SG, Reuning RH. Tritiated naltrexone binding in plasma from several species and tissue distribution in mice. J Pharm Sci 1976; 65(5):712-716.
4. Verebey K, Volavka J, Mule SJ, Resnick RB. Naltrexone: disposition, metabolism, and effects after acute and chronic dosing. Clin Pharmacol Ther 1976; 20(3):315-328.
5. Wall ME, Brine DR, Perez-Reyes M. Metabolism and disposition of naltrexone in man after oral and intravenous administration. Drug Metab Dispos 1981; 9(4):369-375.
6. Chan CF, Page-Sharp M, Kristensen JH, O'Neil G, Ilett KF. Transfer of naltrexone and its metabolite 6,beta naltrexol into human milk. Journal of Human Lactation 2004; in press, accepted 28 Jan 2004.

NAPROXEN

Trade: Anaprox, Naprosyn, Aleve
Can/Aus/UK: Anaprox, Apo-Naproxen, Naprosyn, Naxen, Inza, Proxen SR, Synflex
Uses: NSAID, analgesic for arthritis
LRC: L3
  L4 for chronic use
AAP: Maternal Medication Usually Compatible with Breastfeeding

Naproxen is a popular NSAID analgesic. In a study done at steady state in one mother consuming 375 mg twice daily, milk levels ranged from 1.76-2.37 mg/L at 4 hours.[1,2] Total naproxen excretion in the infant's urine was only 0.26% of the maternal dose. Although the amount of naproxen transferred via milk is minimal, one should use with caution in nursing mothers because of its long half-life and its effect on infant cardiovascular system, kidneys, and GI tract. However, its short term use postpartum or infrequent or occasional use would not necessarily be incompatible with breastfeeding. One reported case of prolonged bleeding, hemorrhage, and acute anemia in a seven-day-old infant.[3] The relative infant dose on a weight-adjusted maternal daily dose would probably be less than 3.3%.

Pregnancy Risk Category: B

Lactation Risk Category: **L3**
L4 for chronic use

Adult Concerns: GI distress, gastric bleeding, hemorrhage

Pediatric Concerns: One reported case of prolonged bleeding, hemorrhage, and acute anemia in a seven-day-old infant.

Drug Interactions: May prolong prothrombin time when used with warfarin. Antihypertensive effects of ACEi family may be blunted or completely abolished by NSAIDs. Some NSAIDs may block antihypertensive effect of beta blockers, diuretics. Used with cyclosporin, may dramatically increase renal toxicity. May increase digoxin, phenytoin, lithium levels. May increase toxicity of methotrexate. May increase bioavailability of penicillamine. Probenecid may increase NSAID levels.

Theoretic Infant Dose: 0.35 mg/kg/day

Relative Infant Dose: 3.3%

Adult Dose: 250-500 mg BID

Alternatives: Ibuprofen

$T\frac{1}{2}$ =	12-15 hours	M/P =	0.01	
PHL =	12-15 hours	PB =	99.7%	
T_{max} =	2-4 hours	Oral =	74-99%	
MW =	230	pKa =	5.0	
Vd =	0.09			

References:
1. Jamali F, Stevens DR. Naproxen excretion in milk and its uptake by the infant. Drug Intell Clin Pharm 1983; 17(12):910-911.
2. Jamali F. et.al. Naproxen excretion in breastmilk and its uptake by sucking infant. Drug Intell Clin Pharm 1982; 16:475 (Abstr).
3. Figalgo I. et.al. Anemia aguda, rectaorragia y hematuria asociadas a la ingestion de naproxen. Anales Espanoles de Pediatrica 1989; 30:317-319.

NARATRIPTAN

Trade: Amerge
Can/Aus/UK: Naramig
Uses: Migraine headaches
LRC: L3
AAP: Not reviewed

Naratriptan is a 5-HT1D and 5-HT1B receptor stimulant and is used for treatment of acute migraine headache. No data are currently available on its transfer into human milk although the manufacturer suggests it penetrates the milk of rodents.[1] Naratriptan is a close congener of sumatriptan, only slightly better absorbed orally, and may produce few side effects in sumatriptan-sensitive patients. Some studies suggest that sumatriptan is equal to if not more effective than naratriptan.[2] Sumatriptan has been studied in breastfeeding mothers and produces minimal milk levels. See sumatriptan.

Pregnancy Risk Category: C

Lactation Risk Category: L3

Adult Concerns: Chest discomfort including pain, pressure, heaviness, tightness has been reported. Nausea, dizziness, paresthesias are infrequently reported. Cardiovascular events are rare but include hypertension, and tachyarrhythmias.

Pediatric Concerns: None reported via milk.

Drug Interactions: MAOIs can markedly increase naratriptan systemic effect and elimination including elevated plasma levels. Ergot containing drugs have caused prolonged vasospastic reactions, do not use within 24 hours after using an ergot-containing product. There have been rare reports of weakness, hyperreflexia, and incoordination with combined use with SSRIs such as fluoxetine, paroxetine, sertraline and fluvoxamine.

Theoretic Infant Dose:

Relative Infant Dose:

Adult Dose: 1-2.5 mg q 4 hours X 2-3

Alternatives: Sumatriptan

T½ =	6 hours	M/P =	
PHL =		PB =	31%
T$_{max}$ =	2-3 hours	Oral =	70%
MW =	372	pKa =	
Vd =	2.42		

References:
1. Pharmaceutical Manufacturer Prescribing Information. 1999.
2. Dahlof C, Winter P. et. al. Randomized, double-blind, placebo-controlled comparison of oral naratriptan and oral sumatriptan in the acute treatment of migraine (abstract). Neurology 1997; 48(suppl):A85-A86.

NEDOCROMIL SODIUM

Trade: Tilade
Can/Aus/UK: Tilade, Mireze
Uses: Inhaled anti-inflammatory for asthmatics
LRC: L2
AAP: Not reviewed

Nedocromil is believed to stabilize mast cells and prevent release of bronchoconstrictors in the lung following exposure to allergens. The systemic effects are minimal due to reduced plasma levels. Systemic absorption averages less than 8-17% of the total dose even after continued dosing, which is quite low.[1,2] The poor oral bioavailability of this product and the reduced side effect profile of this family of drugs suggest that it is unlikely to produce untoward effects in a nursing infant. See cromolyn as comparison.

Pregnancy Risk Category: B

Lactation Risk Category: L2

Adult Concerns: Poor taste. Dizziness, headache, nausea and vomiting, sore throat, and cough.

Pediatric Concerns: None reported via milk.

Drug Interactions:

Theoretic Infant Dose:

Relative Infant Dose:

Adult Dose: 3.5-4 mg QID

Alternatives:

$T\frac{1}{2}$ =	3.3 hours	M/P =	
PHL =		PB =	89%
T_{max} =	28 minutes	Oral =	8-17%
MW =	371	pKa =	
Vd =			

References:
1. Pharmaceutical Manufacturer Prescribing Information. 1996.
2. Drug Facts and Comparisons 1995 ed. ed. St. Louis: 1995.

NEFAZODONE HCL

Trade: Serzone
Can/Aus/UK: Serzone, Dutonin
Uses: Antidepressant
LRC: L4
AAP: Not reviewed

Nefazodone is an antidepressant similar to trazodone but structurally dissimilar from the other serotonin reuptake inhibitors. It is rapidly metabolized to three partially active metabolites that have significantly longer half-lives (1.5 to 18 hours).[1]

In a study of one patient receiving 200 mg in the morning and 100 mg at night, the infant at 9 weeks of age (2.1 kg), was admitted for drowsiness, lethargy, failure to thrive, and poor temperature control.[2] The infant was born premature at 27 weeks. The maximum milk concentration of nefazodone was 358 μg/L while the maternal plasma

C_{max} was 1270 µg/L. The concentration of the metabolites was reported to be 83 µg/L for triazoledione, 32 µg/L for HO-Nefazodone, and 18 µg/L for m-Chlorophenylpiperazine. The relative infant dose was calculated to be 0.45 % of the weight-adjusted maternal dose. The AUC milk/plasma ratio ranged from 0.02 to 0.27. Unfortunately, no infant plasma samples were taken for analysis.

Dodd et.al.[3] recently reported a M/P ratio of only 0.1 for nefazodone in a patient receiving 200 mg twice daily. This is approximately one-third of the M/P ratio(0.27) reported by Yapp. However, the Yapp study used AUC data over many points and is probably a more accurate reflection of nefazodone transfer into milk during the day.

This medication should probably not be used in breastfeeding mothers with young infants, premature infants, infants subject to apnea, or other weakened infants.

Pregnancy Risk Category: C

Lactation Risk Category: L4

Adult Concerns: Weakness, hypotension, somnolence, dizziness, dry mouth, constipation, nausea, headache

Pediatric Concerns: Drowsiness, lethargy, failure to thrive, and poor temperature control in one infant.

Drug Interactions: Sometimes fatal reactions may occur with MAOI. Plasma levels of astemizole and terfenadine may be increased. Clinically important increases in plasma concentrations of alprazolam and triazolam have been reported. Serum concentrations of digoxin have been increased by nefazodone by 29%. Haloperidol clearance decreased by 35%. Nefazodone may decrease propranolol plasma levels by as much as 30%.

Theoretic Infant Dose: 53.7 µg/kg/day

Relative Infant Dose: 1.2%

Adult Dose: 150-300 mg BID

Alternatives: Sertraline, Paroxetine, Trazodone

$T\frac{1}{2}$ =	1-4 hours	M/P =	0.1-0.27
PHL =		PB =	> 99%
T_{max} =	1 hour	Oral =	20%
MW =	507	pKa =	6.6
Vd =	0.9		

References:

1. Pharmaceutical Manufacturer Prescribing Information. 1996.
2. Yapp P, Ilett KF, Kristensen JH, Hackett LP, Paech MJ, Rampono J. Drowsiness and poor feeding in a breast-fed infant: association with nefazodone and its metabolites. Ann Pharmacother 2000; 34(11):1269-1272.

3. Dodd S, Buist A, Burrows GD, Maguire KP, Norman TR. Determination of nefazodone and its pharmacologically active metabolites in human blood plasma and breastmilk by high-performance liquid chromatography. J Chromatogr B Biomed Sci Appl 1999; 730(2):249-255.

NETILMICIN

Trade: Netromycin
Can/Aus/UK: Netromycin, Nettilin
Uses: Aminoglycoside antibiotic
LRC: L3
AAP: Not reviewed

Netilmicin is a typical aminoglycoside antibiotic (see gentamicin). Poor oral absorption limits its use to IM and IV administration although some studies suggest significant oral absorption in infancy.[1,2] Only small levels are believed to be secreted into human milk although no reports exist. See gentamicin.

Pregnancy Risk Category: D

Lactation Risk Category: L3

Adult Concerns: Kidney damage, hearing loss, changes in GI flora

Pediatric Concerns: None reported, but observe for GI symptoms such as diarrhea.

Drug Interactions: Risk of nephrotoxicity may be increased when used with cephalosporins, enflurane, methoxyflurane, and vancomycin. Auditory toxicity may increase when used with loop diuretics. The neuromuscular blocking effects of neuromuscular blocking agents may be increased when used with aminoglycosides.

Theoretic Infant Dose:

Relative Infant Dose:

Adult Dose: 1.3-2.2 mg/kg q 8 hours

Alternatives:

$T\frac{1}{2}$ =	2-2.5 hours	M/P =	
PHL =	4.5-8 hours (neonates)	PB =	< 10%
T_{max} =	30-60 minutes (IM)	Oral =	Negligible
MW =	476	pKa =	
Vd =			

References:
1. Pharmaceutical Manufacturer Prescribing Information. 1995.
2. McEvoy GE. (ed):AFHS Drug Information. New York, NY: 2003.

NEUROMUSCULAR BLOCKING AGENTS

Trade: Anectine, Mivacron, Tracrium, Nuromax, Pavulon, Arduan, RaplonZemuron, Norcuron
Can/Aus/UK:
Uses: Muscle Relaxants for surgery
LRC: L3
AAP: Not reviewed

Neuromuscular blocking agents are similar to curare and are primarily used to relax skeletal muscle during surgery.[1,2] They typically have a three phase elimination curve. The first phase elimination is rapid, averaging less than 5 minutes. The second phase half-life ranges from 7-40 minutes and a third phase half-life is 2-3 hours. It is not known if any of these agents penetrate into human milk but it is very unlikely. First they are large in molecular weight, have highly polar structures, and they are virtually excluded from most cells. Oral bioavailability is not reported, but it is likely small to nil. A brief waiting period (few hours) after surgery will eliminate most risks associated with the use of these products. See table in appendix.

Pregnancy Risk Category: C

Lactation Risk Category: L3

Adult Concerns: Adverse effects include prolonged apnea, residual muscle weakness, and allergic reactions. Other side effects include hypotension, bronchospams, cardiac arrhythmias. Histamine-related events include flushing, erythemia, pruritus, urticaria, wheezing and bronchospasm.

Pediatric Concerns: None reported via milk. They are unlikely to penetrate into milk in significant levels.

Drug Interactions: There are literally dozens of drug-drug interactions with the neuormuscular blocking agents. Consult a more thorough text.

Theoretic Infant Dose:

Relative Infant Dose:

Adult Dose: Variable depending on individual agent.

Alternatives:

$T\frac{1}{2}$ =	Variable	M/P =	
PHL =		PB =	50%
T_{max} =		Oral =	Nil
MW =	Large	pKa =	
Vd =			

References:
1. Pharmaceutical Manufacturers Package Insert, 2004.
2. Baselt RC. Disposition of toxic drugs and chemicals in man. Foster City, CA: Chemical Toxicology Institute, 2000.

NICARDIPINE

Trade: Cardene
Can/Aus/UK: Cardene
Uses: Antihypertensive, calcium channel blocker
LRC: L3
AAP: Not reviewed

Nicardipine is a typical calcium channel blocker structurally related to nifedipine. Animal studies indicate that it is secreted to some degree in breastmilk.[1] No specific data on human milk levels are available. See verapamil, nifedipine.

Pregnancy Risk Category: C

Lactation Risk Category: L3

Adult Concerns: Headache, peripheral edema, flushing, hypotension, bradycardia, gingival hyperplasia

Pediatric Concerns: None reported, but no studies available. See nifedipine as alternative.

Drug Interactions: Barbiturates may reduce bioavailability of calcium channel blockers (CCB). Calcium salts may reduce hypotensive effect. Dantrolene may increase risk of hyperkalemia and myocardial depression. H2 blockers may increase bioavailability of certain CCBs. Hydantoins may reduce plasma levels. Quinidine increases risk of hypotension, bradycardia, tachycardia. Rifampin may reduce effects of CCBs. Vitamin D may reduce efficacy of CCBs. CCBs may increase carbamazepine, cyclosporin, encainide, prazosin levels.

Theoretic Infant Dose:

Relative Infant Dose:

Adult Dose: 5-15 mg q 1 hour PRN

Alternatives: Nifedipine, Nimodipine

$T^{1/2}$ =	2-4 hours	M/P =	
PHL =		PB =	> 95%
T_{max} =	0.5-2 hours	Oral =	35%
MW =	480	pKa =	
Vd =			

References:
1. Pharmaceutical Manufacturer Prescribing Information.

NICOTINE PATCHES or GUM

Trade: Habitrol, Nicoderm, Nicotrol, ProStep
Can/Aus/UK: Habitrol, Nicoderm, Nicorette, ProStep, Nicotinell, Nicabate, Nicotinell TTS
Uses: Nicotine withdrawal systems
LRC: L2
AAP: Not reviewed

Nicotine and its metabolite cotinine are both present in milk. Fifteen lactating women (mean age, 32 years; mean weight, 72 kg) who were smokers (mean of 17 cigarettes per day) participated in a trial of the nicotine patch to assist in smoking cessation.[1] Serial milk samples were collected from the women over sequential 24-hour periods when they were smoking and when they were stabilized on the 21-mg/d, 14-mg/d, and 7-mg/d nicotine patches. Nicotine and cotinine concentrations in milk were not significantly different between smoking (mean of 17 cigarettes per day) and the 21-mg/d patch, but concentrations were significantly lower when patients were using the 14-mg/d and 7-mg/d patches than when smoking. There was also a downward trend in absolute infant dose (nicotine equivalents) from smoking or the 21-mg patch through to the 14-mg and 7-mg patches. Milk intake by the breastfed infants was similar while their mothers were smoking (585 mL/d) and subsequently when their mothers were using the 21-mg (717 mL/d), 14-mg (731 mL/d), and 7-mg (619 mL/d) patches. The authors conclude that the absolute infant dose of nicotine and its metabolite cotinine decreases by about 70% from when subjects were smoking or using the 21-mg patch to when they were using the 7-mg patch. In addition, use of the nicotine patch had no significant influence on the milk intake by the breastfed infant. Undertaking maternal smoking cessation with the nicotine patch is, therefore, a safer option than continued smoking.

With nicotine gum, maternal serum nicotine levels average 30-60% of those found in cigarette smokers. While patches (transdermal systems) produce a sustained and lower nicotine plasma level, nicotine gum may produce large variations in peak levels when the gum is chewed rapidly, fluctuations similar to smoking itself. Mothers who choose to use nicotine gum and breastfeed should be counseled to refrain from breastfeeding for 2-3 hours after using the gum product.

Nicotine has been suggested to decrease in basal prolactin production.[2,3] One study clearly suggests that cigarette smoking significantly reduces breastmilk production at two weeks postpartum from 514 mL/day in non-smokers to 406 mL/day in smoking mothers.[4] However, Ilett's well-done study above did not detect any change in milk production at all.

Therefore, the risk of using nicotine patches while breastfeeding is much less than the risk of formula feeding. Mothers should be advised to limit smoking as much as possible and to smoke only after they have fed their infant, or to switch to the use of nicotine patches.

Pregnancy Risk Category: **X if used in overdose**
                                       D if used in 3rd trimester

Lactation Risk Category: **L2**

Adult Concerns: Tachycardia, GI distress, vomiting, diarrhea, rapid heart beat, and restlessness. Smoking during pregnancy has been associated with preterm births, decreased birth weight, and an increased risk of abortion and stillbirth . The use of nicotine during the last trimester has been associated with a decrease in fetal breathing movements, possibly resulting from decreased placental perfusion induced by nicotine. However, the use of nicotine patches instead of smoking is still preferred .

Pediatric Concerns: No untoward effects were noted from nicotine patch study.

Drug Interactions: Cessation of smoking may alter response to a number of medications in ex-smokers. Including are acetaminophen, caffeine, imipramine, oxazepam, pentazocine, propranolol, and theophylline. Smoking may reduce diuretic effect of furosemide. Smoking while continuing to use patches may dramatically elevate nicotine plasma levels.

Theoretic Infant Dose:

Relative Infant Dose: 7.6-8.0%

Adult Dose: 7-21 mg daily

Alternatives:

$T\frac{1}{2}$ =	2.0 hours(non-patch)	M/P =	2.9
PHL =		PB =	4.9%
T_{max} =	2-4 hours	Oral =	30%
MW =	162	pKa =	
Vd =			

References:
1. Ilett KF, Hale TW, Page-Sharp M, Kristensen JH, Kohan R, Hackett LP. Use of nicotine patches in breast-feeding mothers: transfer of nicotine and cotinine into human milk. Clin Pharmacol Ther 2003; 74(6):516-524.
2. Benowitz NL. Nicotine replacement therapy during pregnancy. JAMA 1991; 266(22):3174-3177.
3. Matheson I, Rivrud GN. The effect of smoking on lactation and infantile colic. JAMA 1989; 261(1):42-43.
4. Hopkinson JM, Schanler RJ, Fraley JK, Garza C. Milk production by mothers of premature infants: influence of cigarette smoking. Pediatrics 1992; 90(6):934-938.

NICOTINIC ACID

Trade: Nicobid, Nicolar, Niacels, Niacin, Nicotinamide
Can/Aus/UK:
Uses: Vitamin B-3
LRC: L3
AAP: Not reviewed

Nicotinic acid, commonly called niacin, is a component of two coenzymes which function in oxidation-reduction reactions essential for tissue respiration. It is converted to nicotinamide in vivo. Although considered a vitamin, large doses(2-6 gm/day) are effective in reducing serum LDL cholesterol and triglyceride and increasing serum HDL. From numerous studies niacin content even when supplemented with moderately low amounts seems to vary from about 1.1 to 3.9 mg/L under normal circumstances.[1] Supplementation apparently does increase milk niacin levels. The concentration transferred into milk as a function of dose or following high maternal doses has not been reported, but it is presumed that elevated maternal plasma levels may significantly elevate milk levels of niacin as well. Because niacin is known to be hepatotoxic in higher doses, breastfeeding mothers should not significantly exceed the RDA.

Pregnancy Risk Category: A during 1st and 2nd trimester
C during 3rd trimester

Lactation Risk Category: L3

Adult Concerns: Flushing, peripheral dilation, itching, nausea, bloating, flatulence, vomiting. In high doses, some abnormal liver function tests.

Pediatric Concerns: None reported via milk, but do not exceed RDA.

Drug Interactions: Niacin may produce fluctuations in blood glucose levels and interfere with oral hypoglycemics. May inhibit uricosuric effects of sulfinpyrazone and probenecid. Increased toxicity (myopathy) when used with lovastatin and other cholesterol-lowering drugs.

Theoretic Infant Dose: 0.585 mg/kg/day

Relative Infant Dose:

Adult Dose: 10-20 mg daily

Alternatives:

$T\frac{1}{2}$ =	45 minutes	M/P =	
PHL =		PB =	
T_{max} =	45 minutes	Oral =	Complete
MW =	123	pKa =	4.85
Vd =			

References:
1. Pratt jp, Hamil BM, Moyer EZ, et.al. Metabolism of women during the reproductive cycle. XVIII. The effect of multivitamin supplements on the secretion of B vitamins in human milk. J Nutr 1951; 44(1):141-157.

NIFEDIPINE
Trade: Adalat, Procardia
Can/Aus/UK: Adalat, Apo-Nifed, Novo-Nifedin, Nu-Nifed, Nifecard, Nyefax, Nefensar XL
Uses: Antihypertensive calcium channel blocker
LRC: L2
AAP: Maternal Medication Usually Compatible with Breastfeeding

Nifedipine is an effective antihypertensive. It belongs to the calcium channel blocker family of drugs. Two studies indicate that nifedipine is transferred to breastmilk in varying but generally low levels. In one study in which the dose was varied from 10-30 mg three times daily, the highest concentration (53.35 µg/L) was measured at 1 hour after a 30 mg dose.[1] Other levels reported were 16.35 µg/L 60 minutes after a 20 mg dose and 12.89 µg/L 30 minutes after a 10 mg dose. The milk levels fell linearly with the milk half-lives estimated to be 1.4 hours for the 10 mg dose, 3.1 hours for the 20 dose, and 2.4 hours for the 30 mg dose. The milk concentration measured 8 hours following a 30 mg dose was 4.93 µg/L. In this study, using the highest concentration found and a daily intake of 150 mL/kg of human milk, the amount of nifedipine intake would only be 8 µg/kg/day (less than 1.8% of the therapeutic pediatric dose). The authors conclude that the amount ingested via breastmilk poses little risk to an infant.

In another study, concentrations of nifedipine in human milk 1 to 8 hours after 10 mg doses varied from < 1 to 10.3 µg/L (median 3.5 µg/L) in six of eleven patients.[2] In this study, milk levels three days after discontinuing medication ranged from < 1 to 9.4 µg/L. The authors concluded the exposure to nifedipine through breastmilk is not significant. In a study by Penny and Lewis, following a maternal dose of 20 mg nifedipine daily for 10 days, peak breastmilk levels at 1 hour were 46 µg/L.[3] The corresponding maternal serum level was 43 µg/L. From this data the authors suggest a daily intake for an infant would be approximately 6.45 µg/kg/day.

Nifedipine has been found clinically useful for nipple vasospasm. Because of the similarity to Raynaud's Phenomenon, sustained release formulations providing 30-60 mg per day are suggested.

Pregnancy Risk Category: C
Lactation Risk Category: L2

Adult Concerns: Headache, peripheral edema, gingival hyperplasia, hypotension. Distortion of smell and taste.

Pediatric Concerns: None reported via milk.

Drug Interactions: Barbiturates may reduce bioavailability of calcium channel blockers (CCB). Calcium salts may reduce hypotensive effect. Dantrolene may increase risk of hyperkalemia and myocardial depression. H2 blockers may increase bioavailability of certain CCBs. Hydantoins may reduce plasma levels. Quinidine increases risk of hypotension, bradycardia, tachycardia. Rifampin may reduce effects of CCBs. Vitamin D may reduce efficacy of CCBs. CCBs may increase carbamazepine, cyclosporin, encainide, prazosin levels.

Theoretic Infant Dose: 8 µg/kg/day
Relative Infant Dose: 1.8%

Adult Dose: 10-20 mg TID

Alternatives: Nimodipine

T½ =	1.8-7 hours	M/P =	1.0
PHL =	26.5(neonatal)	PB =	92-98%
T$_{max}$ =	45 minutes - 4 hours	Oral =	50%
MW =	346	pKa =	
Vd =			

References:
1. Ehrenkranz RA, Ackerman BA, Hulse JD. Nifedipine transfer into human milk. J Pediatr 1989; 114(3):478-480.
2. Manninen AK, Juhakoski A. Nifedipine concentrations in maternal and umbilical serum, amniotic fluid, breastmilk and urine of mothers and offspring. Int J Clin Pharmacol Res 1991; 11(5):231-236.
3. Penny WJ, Lewis MJ. Nifedipine is excreted in human milk. Eur J Clin Pharmacol 1989; 36(4):427-428.

NIMODIPINE

Trade: Nimotop
Can/Aus/UK: Nimotop
Uses: Antihypertensive, calcium channel
LRC: L2
AAP: Not reviewed

Nimodipine is a calcium channel blocker although it is primarily used in preventing cerebral artery spasm and improving cerebral blood flow. Nimodipine is effective in reducing neurologic deficits following subarachnoid hemorrhage, acute stroke, and severe head trauma. It is also useful in prophylaxis of migraine.

In one study of a patient 3 days postpartum who received 60 mg every 4 hours for one week, breastmilk levels paralleled maternal serum levels with a milk/plasma ratio of approximately 0.33.[1] The highest milk concentration reported was approximately 3.5 µg/L while the maternal plasma was approximately 16 µg/L.

In another study [2], a 36 year old mother received a total dose of 46 mg IV over 24 hours. Nimodipine concentration in milk was much lower than in maternal serum, with a milk/serum ratio of 0.06 to 0.15. During IV infusion, nimodipine concentrations in milk raised initially to 2.2 µg/L and stabilized at concentrations between 0.87 and 1.6 µg/L of milk. Assuming a daily milk intake of 150 mg/kg, an infant would ingest approximately 0.063 to 0.705 µg/kg/day or 0.008 to 0.092% of the weight-adjusted dose administered to the mother.

Pregnancy Risk Category: C

Lactation Risk Category: L2

Adult Concerns: Hypotension, diarrhea, nausea, cramps

Pediatric Concerns: None reported via milk in two studies.

Drug Interactions: When used with adenosine, prolonged bradycardia may result. Use with amiodarone may lead to sinus arrest and AV block. H2 blockers may increase bioavailability of nimodipine. Beta blockers may increase cardiac depression.   May increase carbamazepine levels with admixed.   May increase cyclosporine, digoxin, quinidine plasma levels.   May increase theophylline effects. Used with fentanyl, it may increase hypotension.

Theoretic Infant Dose: 0.24 µg/kg/day

Relative Infant Dose: 0.03%

Adult Dose: 60 mg q 4 hours

Alternatives: Verapamil, Nifedipine

$T\frac{1}{2}$ =	9 hours	M/P =	0.06 to 0.33
PHL =		PB =	95%
T_{max} =	1 hour	Oral =	13%
MW =	418	pKa =	
Vd =	0.94		

References:
1.   Tonks AM. Nimodipine levels in breastmilk. Aust N Z J Surg 1995; 65(9):693-694.
2.   Carcas AJ, Abad-Santos F, de Rosendo JM, Frias J. Nimodipine transfer into human breastmilk and cerebrospinal fluid. Ann Pharmacother 1996; 30(2):148-150.

NISOLDIPINE

Trade: Sular
Can/Aus/UK: Syscor
Uses: Antihypertensive
LRC: L3
AAP: Not reviewed

Nisoldipine is a typical calcium channel blocker antihypertensive.[1] No data are available on its transfer into human milk. For alternatives see nifedipine and verapamil. Due to its poor oral bioavailability, presence of lipids which reduce its absorption and high protein binding, it is unlikely to penetrate milk and be absorbed by the infant (undocumented).

Pregnancy Risk Category: C

Lactation Risk Category: L3

Adult Concerns: Hypotension, bradycardia, peripheral edema

Pediatric Concerns: None reported via milk. Observe for hypotension, sedation although unlikely.

Drug Interactions: Barbiturates may reduce bioavailability of calcium channel blockers (CCB). Calcium salts may reduce hypotensive effect. Dantrolene may increase risk of hyperkalemia and myocardial depression. H2 blockers may increase bioavailability of certain CCBs. Hydantoins may reduce plasma levels. Quinidine increases risk of hypotension, bradycardia, tachycardia. Rifampin may reduce effects of CCBs. Vitamin D may reduce efficacy of CCBs. CCBs may increase carbamazepine, cyclosporin, encainide, prazosin levels.

Theoretic Infant Dose:

Relative Infant Dose:

Adult Dose: 20-40 mg daily
Alternatives: Nifedipine, Verapamil, Nimodipine

$T\frac{1}{2}$ =	7-12 hours	M/P =	
PHL =		PB =	99%
T_{max} =	6-12 hours	Oral =	5%
MW =	388	pKa =	
Vd =	4		

References:
1. Pharmaceutical Manufacturer Prescribing Information.

NITRAZEPAM

Trade: Mogadon
Can/Aus/UK: Mogadon, Nitrazadon, Alodorm, Atempol, Nitrodos
Uses: Sedative, hypnotic
LRC: L2 (short term)
AAP: Not reviewed

Nitrazepam is a typical benzodiazepine (Valium family) used as a sedative. In a study of 9 women who received 5 mg nitrazepam at night, the concentration in milk increased over a period of 5 days from 30 nmol/L to 48 nmol/L over 5 days.[1] The mean milk/plasma ratio after 7 hours was 0.27 in 32 paired samples and did not vary from day 1 to day 5. The mean concentration of nitrazepam in milk was 13 µg/L and the C_{max} was 0.20 µg/L. Nitrazepam levels in a 6 day old infant were below the limits of detection. No adverse effects were noted in the infants breastfed for 5 days.

Pregnancy Risk Category:

Lactation Risk Category: L2 (short term)

Adult Concerns: Sedation, disorientation

Pediatric Concerns: None reported, but observe for sedation.

Drug Interactions:

Theoretic Infant Dose: 1.95 µg/kg/day

Relative Infant Dose: 2.7%

Adult Dose: 5-10 mg daily
Alternatives: Alprazolam, Lorazepam

$T\frac{1}{2}$ =	30 hours	M/P =	0.27
PHL =		PB =	90%
T_{max} =	0.5 - 5 hours	Oral =	53-94%
MW =	281	pKa =	3.2, 10.8
Vd =	2-5		

References:
1. Matheson I, Lunde PK, Bredesen JE. Midazolam and nitrazepam in the maternity ward: milk concentrations and clinical effects. Br J Clin Pharmacol 1990; 30(6):787-793.

NITRENDIPINE

Trade: Baypress
Can/Aus/UK:
Uses: Calcium channel blocker, antihypertensive
LRC: L2
AAP: Not reviewed

Nitrendipine is a typical calcium channel antihypertensive. In a group of 3 breastfeeding mothers who received 20 mg/d for 5 days, nitrendipine was excreted in breastmilk at peak concentrations ranging from 4.3 to 6.5 μg/L 1-2 h after acute dosing while its inactive pyridine metabolite ranged from 6.9 to 11.9 μg/L.[1] After 5 days of dosing, the C_{max} remained in the same range and the breastmilk/plasma ratio for nitrendipine was 0.2 to 0.5. On the fourth day of continuous dosing, average concentrations of nitrendipine from 24 hour collections of the milk were 1.1 to 3.8 μg/L. Thus, nitrendipine and its metabolite are excreted in very low concentrations in human breastmilk. Based on a maternal dose of 20 mg daily, a newborn infant would ingest an average of 1.7 μg/d of nitrendipine or a relative dose of 0.095%.

Pregnancy Risk Category:

Lactation Risk Category: L2

Adult Concerns: Headache, hypotension, peripheral edema, cardiac arrhythmias, fatigue

Pediatric Concerns: None reported via milk.

Drug Interactions: Barbiturates may reduce bioavailability of calcium channel blockers (CCB). Calcium salts may reduce hypotensive effect. Dantrolene may increase risk of hyperkalemia and myocardial depression. H2 blockers may increase bioavailability of certain CCBs. Hydantoins may reduce plasma levels. Quinidine increases risk of hypotension, bradycardia, tachycardia. Rifampin may reduce effects of CCBs. Vitamin D may reduce efficacy of CCBs. CCBs may increase carbamazepine, cyclosporin, encainide, prazosin levels.

Theoretic Infant Dose: 0.27 μg/kg/day

Relative Infant Dose: 0.09%

Adult Dose: 10-80 mg/day

Alternatives: Nifedipine, Nimodipine

T½ =	8-11 hours	**M/P =**	0.2-0.5
PHL =		**PB =**	98%
T$_{max}$ =	1-2 hours	**Oral =**	16-20%
MW =	360	**pKa =**	
Vd =			

References:
1.   White WB, Yeh SC, Krol GJ. Nitrendipine in human plasma and breastmilk. Eur J Clin Pharmacol 1989; 36(5):531-534.

NITROFURANTOIN

Trade: Furadantin, Macrodantin, Furan, Macrobid
Can/Aus/UK: Apo-Nitrofurantoin, Macrodantin, Nephronex, Furadantin
Uses: Urinary antibiotic
LRC: L2 ·
AAP: Maternal Medication Usually Compatible with Breastfeeding

Nitrofurantoin is an old urinary tract antimicrobial. It is secreted in breastmilk but in very small amounts. In one study of 20 women receiving 100 mg four times daily, none was detected in milk.[1] In another group of nine nursing women who received 100-200 mg every 6 hours, nitrofurantoin was undetectable in the milk of those treated with 100 mg and only trace amounts were found in those treated with 200 mg (0.3-0.5 mg/L milk).[2] In these two patients the milk/plasma ratio ranged from 0.27 to 0.31.

In a well-done study of 4 breastfeeding mothers who ingested 100 mg nitrofurantoin with a meal, the milk/serum ratio averaged 6.21 suggesting an active transfer into milk.[3] Regardless of an active transfer, the average milk concentration throughout the day (AUC) was only 1.3 mg/L. According to the authors, the estimated dose an infant would ingest was 0.2 mg/kg/day or 6.8% of the weight-adjusted maternal dose if they consumed 200 mg/d nitrofurantoin. The therapeutic dose administered to infants is 5-7 mg/kg/day.

Use with caution in infants with G6PD or in infants less than 1 month of age with hyperbilirubinemia, due to displacement of bilirubin from albumin binding sites.

Pregnancy Risk Category: B

Lactation Risk Category: L2

Adult Concerns: Nausea, vomiting, brown urine, hemolytic anemia, hepatotoxicity

Pediatric Concerns: None reported via milk, however, do not use in infants with G6PD or in infants less than 1 month of age.

Drug Interactions: Anticholinergics increase nitrofurantoin bioavailability by delaying gastric emptying and increasing absorption. Magnesium salts may delay or decrease absorption. Uricosurics may increase nitrofurantoin levels by decreasing renal clearance.

Theoretic Infant Dose: 0.195 mg/kg/day

Relative Infant Dose: 6.8%

Adult Dose: 50-100 mg QID

Alternatives:

T½ =	20-58 minutes	M/P =	0.27-6.2
PHL =		PB =	20-60%
T$_{max}$ =	4.9 hours	Oral =	94%
MW =	238	pKa =	7.2
Vd =			

References:
1. Hosbach RH, Foster RB. Absence of nitrofurantoin from human milk. JAMA 1967; 202(11):1057.
2. Varsano I, Fischl J, Shochet SB. The excretion of orally ingested nitrofurantoin in human milk. J Pediatr 1973; 82(5):886-887.
3. Gerk PM, Kuhn RJ, Desai NS, McNamara PJ. Active transport of nitrofurantoin into human milk. Pharmacotherapy 2001; 21(6):669-675.

NITROGLYCERIN, NITRATES, NITRITES

Trade: Nitrostat, Nitrolingual, Nitrogard, Amyl Nitrite, Nitrong, Nitro-Bid, NitroglynMinitran, Nitro-Dur
Can/Aus/UK: Nitrong SR, Nitrol, Transderm-Nitro, Nitro-Dur, Anginine, Nitrolingual Spray, Nitradisc, Deponit
Uses: Vasodilator
LRC: L4
AAP: Not reviewed

Nitroglycerin is a rapid and short acting vasodilator used in angina and other cardiovascular problems including congestive heart failure. Nitroglycerin, as well as numerous other formulations (amyl nitrate, isorbide dinitrate, etc) all work by release of the nitrite and nitrate molecule. Nitrates come in numerous formulations, some for acute use (sublingual), others are more sustained (Nitro-Dur). Nitrates and Nitrites are derived from multiple sources, including medications in the form of nitroglycerin, or isorbide dinitrate, or from food and water sources. Elevated nitrate levels in drinking water in the USA are common in rural areas. Numerous cases of nitrate-induced methemoglobinemia have been reported in infants exposed to well water with high levels of nitrates when they were fed foods/formulas prepared with contaminated water. Only one case of a breastfed infant has been reported and it is questionable.[1] Thus far, it is less certain that the oral ingestion of nitrates can penetrate into human milk in clinically relevant amounts.

Two studies suggest that while nitrates/nitrites are well absorbed orally in the mother (approx. 50%), little seems to be transported to human milk. In a study by Dusdieker,[2] following a mean total nitrate intake from diet and water of 46.6, 168.1, and 272 mg/day, milk levels only averaged 4.4, 5.1, and 5.2 mg/L respectively. Thus higher maternal intake did not necessarily correlate with higher milk levels. The authors conclude that mothers who ingest nitrate of 100 mg/day or less do not produce milk with elevated nitrate levels.

In a study by Green[3], milk levels were not different from maternal plasma levels. Thus it is apparent that even at relatively high rates of ingestion, nitrate levels do not concentrate in milk and may not be high enough to harm an infant. However, these studies were done using nitrates in water and may not correlate with the ingestion of high and prolonged concentrations of nitrates from medications administered orally, buccally, or transcutaneously. No studies have been found comparing milk nitrates with oral nitroglycerine or isorbide dinitrate.

While it is apparent that milk levels are not high following the ingestion of oral nitrates, infants younger than 6 months are most at risk from nitrate intoxication because of their susceptibility to methemoglobinemia.[4]

In another study of 59 women living in regions with high nitrate levels, breastmilk levels of nitrates and nitrites were 2.83 mg/L and 0.46 mg/L respectively, while those living in low nitrate regions were 2.75 mg/L and 0.32 mg/L respectively.[5] They were not significantly different. Breastfeed with caution at higher doses and with prolonged exposure. Observe the infant for methemoglobinemia.

Pregnancy Risk Category: C

Lactation Risk Category: L4

Adult Concerns: Postural hypotension, flushing, headache, weakness, drug rash, exfoliative dermatitis, bradycardia, nausea, vomiting, methemoglobinemia (overdose), sweating

Pediatric Concerns: None are reported via milk.   Observe for methemoglobinemia.

Drug Interactions: IV nitroglycerin may counteract the effects of heparin.   Increased toxicity when used with alcohol, beta-blockers. Calcium channel blockers may increase hypotensive effect of nitrates.

Theoretic Infant Dose:

Relative Infant Dose:

Adult Dose: 1.3-6.5 mg BID

Alternatives:

T½ =	1-4 minutes	M/P =	
PHL =		PB =	60%
T$_{max}$ =	2-20 minutes	Oral =	Complete
MW =	227	pKa =	
Vd =			

References:
1. Donahoe WE. Cyanosis in infants with nitrates in drinking water as a cause. Pediatrics 1949; 3:308.
2. Dusdieker LB, Stumbo PJ, Kross BC, Dungy CI. Does increased nitrate ingestion elevate nitrate levels in human milk? Arch Pediatr Adolesc Med 1996; 150(3):311-314.
3. Green LC, Tannenbaum SR, Fox JG. Nitrate in human and canine milk. N Engl J Med 1982; 306(22):1367-1368.
4. Johnson CJ, Kross BC. Continuing importance of nitrate contamination of groundwater and wells in rural areas. Am J Ind Med 1990; 18(4):449-456.
5. Paszkowski T, Sikorski R, Kozak A, Kowalski B, Jakubik J. [Contamination of human milk with nitrates and nitrites]. Pol Tyg Lek 1989; 44(46-48):961-963.

NITROPRUSSIDE

Trade: Nitropress
Can/Aus/UK: Nipride
Uses: Hypotensive agent
LRC: L4
AAP: Not reviewed

Nitroprusside is a rapid acting hypotensive agent of short duration (1-10 minutes). Besides rapid hypotension, nitroprusside is converted metabolically to cyanogen (cyanide radical) which is potentially toxic. Although rare, significant thiocyanate toxicity can occur at higher doses (> 2 µg/kg/minutes) and longer durations of exposure (> 1-2 days).[1] When administered orally, nitroprusside is reported to not be active although one report suggests a modest hypotensive effect. No data are available on transfer of nitroprusside nor thiocyanate into human milk. The half-life of the thiocyanate metabolite is approximately 3 days. Because the thiocyanate metabolite is orally bioavailable, some caution is advised if the mother has received nitroprusside for more than 24 hours.[2]

Pregnancy Risk Category: C

Lactation Risk Category: L4

Adult Concerns: Hypotension, methemoglobinemia, headache, drowsiness, cyanide toxicity, hypothyroidism, nausea, vomiting

Pediatric Concerns: None reported but caution is urged due to thiocyanate metabolite.

Drug Interactions: Clonidine may potentiate the hypotensive effect of nitroprusside.   May reduce Iodine-131 uptake and induce hypothyroidism.

Theoretic Infant Dose:

Relative Infant Dose:

Adult Dose: 0.3-10 µg/kg/minute X 10 minutes

Alternatives:

T½ =	3-4 minutes	M/P =	
PHL =		PB =	
T$_{max}$ =	1-2 minutes	Oral =	Poor
MW =		pKa =	
Vd =			

References:
1.   Page IH, Corcoran AC, Dustan HP, Koppanyi T. Cardiovascular actions of sodium nitroprusside in animals and hypertensive patients. Circulation 1955; 11(2):188-198.
2.   Benitz WE, Malachowski N, Cohen RS, Stevenson DK, Ariagno RL, Sunshine P. Use of sodium nitroprusside in neonates: efficacy and safety. J Pediatr 1985; 106(1):102-110.

NITROUS OXIDE
Trade:
Can/Aus/UK: Entonox
Uses: Anesthetic gas
LRC: L3
AAP: Not reviewed

Nitrous oxide is a weak anesthetic gas.   It provides good analgesia and a weak anesthesia.   It is rapidly eliminated from the body due to rapid exchange with nitrogen via the pulmonary alveoli (within minutes).[1]   A rapid recovery generally occurs in 3-5 minutes.   Due to poor lipid solubility,   uptake by adipose tissue is relatively poor, and only insignificant traces of nitrous oxide circulate in blood after discontinuing inhalation of the gas.   No data exists on the entry of nitrous oxide into human milk.   Ingestion of nitrous oxide orally via milk is unlikely.   Chronic exposure may lead to elevated risks of fetal malformations, abortions, and bone marrow toxicity (particular in dental care workers).[2]

Pregnancy Risk Category:

Lactation Risk Category: L3

Adult Concerns: Chronic exposure can produce bone marrow suppression, headaches, hypotension and bradycardia

Pediatric Concerns: None reported via milk.

Drug Interactions:

Theoretic Infant Dose:

Relative Infant Dose:

Adult Dose: Inhalation 30% with 70% oxygen

Alternatives:

T½ =	< 3 minutes	M/P =	
PHL =		PB =	
T$_{max}$ =	15 minutes	Oral =	Poor
MW =	44	pKa =	
Vd =			

References:
1. General Anesthetics. In: Drug Evaluations Annual 1995 American Medical Association, 1995.
2. Adriani J. General Anesthetics. In: Clinical Management of Poisoning and Drug Overdose. W.B. Saunders & Co., 1983.

NIZATIDINE

Trade: Axid
Can/Aus/UK: Axid, Apo-Nizatidine, Tazac
Uses: Reduces gastric acid secretion
LRC: L2
AAP: Not reviewed

Nizatidine is an antisecretory, histamine-2 antagonist that reduces stomach acid secretion. In one study of 5 lactating women using a dose of 150 mg, milk levels of nizatidine were directly proportional to circulating maternal serum levels, yet were very low.[1] Over a 12 hour period 96 µg (less than 0.1% of dose) was secreted into the milk. No effects on infant have been reported.

Pregnancy Risk Category: C

Lactation Risk Category: L2

Adult Concerns: Headache, GI distress

Pediatric Concerns: None reported.

Drug Interactions: Elevated salicylate levels may occur when nizatidine is used with high doses of salicylates.

Theoretic Infant Dose:

Relative Infant Dose:

Adult Dose: 150-300 mg daily

Alternatives: Famotidine

T½ =	1.5 hours	M/P =	
PHL =		PB =	35%
T$_{max}$ =	0.5-3 hours	Oral =	94%
MW =	331	pKa =	
Vd =			

References:
1. Obermeyer BD, Bergstrom RF, Callaghan JT, Knadler MP, Golichowski A, Rubin A. Secretion of nizatidine into human breastmilk after single and multiple doses. Clin Pharmacol Ther 1990; 47(6):724-730.

NORELGESTROMIN + ETHINYL ESTRADIOL
Trade: Ortho Evra
Can/Aus/UK:
Uses: Patch combination contraceptive
LRC: L3
AAP: Not reviewed

Ortho Evra is a new combination progestin and estrogen-containing patch.[1] It delivers approximately 150 μg/day norelgestromin and 20 μg/d ethinyl estradiol to the plasma compartment of the female. Small amounts of estrogens and progestins are known to pass into milk, but long-term follow-up of children whose mothers used combination hormal contraceptives while breastfeeding has shown no deleterious effects on infants. Estrogen-containing contraceptives may interfere with milk production by decreasing the quantity and quality of milk production.

Pregnancy Risk Category:

Lactation Risk Category: L3

Adult Concerns: Side effects include: breast tenderness and enlargement, headache, nausea , menstrual changes, abdominal cramps and bloating, vaginal discharge and irritation at the site of application.

Pediatric Concerns: Potential reduction of daily milk production due to estrogen content.

Drug Interactions: Same as with all combination oral contraceptives. Effectiveness may be reduced if co-administered with certain antibiotics, antifungals, anticonvulsants, protease inhibitors, or other drugs that affect hepatic metabolism.   Other drugs include: St. John's Wort, barbiturates, griseofulvin, rifampin, phenytoin, and carbamazepine.

Theoretic Infant Dose:

Relative Infant Dose:

Adult Dose: Applied for 7 days times 3 per month.

Alternatives: Norethindrone

References:
1.   Pharmaceutical Manufacturer Prescribing Information.

NORETHINDRONE

Trade: Aygestin, Norlutate, Micronor, Nor-Q.D.
Can/Aus/UK: Micronor, Norlutate, Norethisterone, Brevinor
Uses: Progestin for oral contraceptives.
LRC: L1
AAP: Not reviewed

Norethindrone is a typical synthetic progestational agent that is used for oral contraception and other endocrine functions. It is believed to be secreted into breastmilk in small amounts. It produces a dose-dependent suppression of lactation at higher doses, although somewhat minimal at lower doses. It may reduce lactose content and reduce overall milk volume and nitrogen/protein content, resulting in lower infant weight gain although these effects are unlikely if doses are kept low.[1-5] Progestin-only mini pills are preferred oral contraceptives in breastfeeding mothers.

Pregnancy Risk Category: X

Lactation Risk Category: L1

Adult Concerns: Changes in menstruation, breakthrough bleeding, nausea, abdominal pain, edema, breast tenderness

Pediatric Concerns: None reported via milk.

Drug Interactions: Rifampin may reduce the plasma level of norethindrone possibly decreasing its effect.

Theoretic Infant Dose:

Relative Infant Dose:

Adult Dose: 0.35-5 mg daily
Alternatives:

T½ =	4-13 hours	M/P =	
PHL =		PB =	97%
T$_{max}$ =	1-2 hours	Oral =	60%
MW =	298	pKa =	
Vd =			

References:
1.   Kora SJ. Effect of oral contraceptives on lactation. Fertil Steril 1969; 20(3):419-423.
2.   Miller GH, Hughes LR. Lactation and genital involution effects of a new low-dose oral contraceptive on breast-feeding mothers and their infants. Obstet Gynecol 1970; 35(1):44-50.

3. Karim M, Ammar R, el Mahgoub S, el Ganzoury B, Fikri F, Abdou I. Injected progestogen and lactation. Br Med J 1971; 1(742):200-203.
4. Lonnerdal B, Forsum E, Hambraeus L. Effect of oral contraceptives on composition and volume of breastmilk. Am J Clin Nutr 1980; 33(4):816-824.
5. Laukaran VH. The effects of contraceptive use on the initiation and duration of lactation. Int J Gynaecol Obstet 1987; 25 Suppl:129-142.

NORETHYNODREL

Trade: Enovid
Can/Aus/UK:
Uses: Progestational agent
LRC: L2
AAP: Maternal Medication Usually Compatible with Breastfeeding

Norethynodrel is a synthetic progestational agent used in oral contraceptives. Limited or no effects on infant. May decrease volume of breastmilk to some degree in some mothers if therapy is initiated too soon after birth and if dose is too high.[1-3] See norethindrone, medroxyprogesterone.

Pregnancy Risk Category: X

Lactation Risk Category: L2

Adult Concerns: Changes in menstruation, breakthrough bleeding, nausea, abdominal pain, edema, breast tenderness

Pediatric Concerns: None reported. May suppress lactation.

Drug Interactions:

Theoretic Infant Dose:

Relative Infant Dose:

Adult Dose:

Alternatives:

$T\frac{1}{2}$ =		M/P =	
PHL =		PB =	
T_{max} =		Oral =	
MW =	298	pKa =	
Vd =			

References:
1. Booker DE, Pahl IR. Control of postpartum breast engorgement with oral contraceptives. Am J Obstet Gynecol 1967; 98(8):1099-1101.
2. Laukaran VH. The effects of contraceptive use on the initiation and duration of lactation. Int J Gynaecol Obstet 1987; 25 Suppl:129-142.
3. Kora SJ. Effect of oral contraceptives on lactation. Fertil Steril 1969; 20(3):419-423.

NORFLOXACIN

Trade: Noroxin
Can/Aus/UK: Noroxin
Uses: Fluoroquinolone antibiotic
LRC: L3
AAP: Not reviewed

Although other members in the fluoroquinolone family are secreted into breastmilk (see ciprofloxacin, ofloxacin), only limited data are available on this drug.[1] Wise has suggested that norfloxacin is not present in breastmilk. [2] The manufacturer's product information states that doses of 200 mg do not produce detectable concentrations in milk although this was a single dose.[3] Of the fluoroquinolone family, norfloxacin, levofloxacin, or perhaps ofloxacin may be preferred over others for use in a breastfeeding mother.

Pregnancy Risk Category: **C**

Lactation Risk Category: **L3**

Adult Concerns: Nausea, vomiting, GI dyspepsia, depression, dizziness, pseudomembranous colitis in pediatric patients.

Pediatric Concerns: None reported via milk. Observe for diarrhea.

Drug Interactions: Decreased absorption with antacids. Quinolones cause increased levels of caffeine, warfarin, cyclosporine, theophylline. Cimetidine, probenecid, azlocillin increase norfloxacin levels. Increased risk of seizures when used with foscarnet.

Theoretic Infant Dose:

Relative Infant Dose:

Adult Dose: 400 mg BID

Alternatives: Ofloxacin, levofloxacin

T½ =	3.3 hours	M/P =	
PHL =		PB =	20%
T$_{max}$ =	1-2 hours	Oral =	30-40%
MW =	319	pKa =	
Vd =			

References:
1. Harmon T, Burkhart G, Applebaum H. Perforated pseudomembranous colitis in the breast-fed infant. J Pediatr Surg 1992; 27(6):744-746.
2. Wise R. Norfloxacin--a review of pharmacology and tissue penetration. J Antimicrob Chemother 1984; 13 Suppl B:59-64.
3. Pharmaceutical Manufacturer Prescribing Information. 1999.

NORTRIPTYLINE

Trade: Aventyl, Pamelor
Can/Aus/UK: Aventyl, Norventyl, Apo-Nortriptyline, Allegron
Uses: Tricyclic antidepressant
LRC: L2
AAP: Drugs whose effect on nursing infants is unknown but may be of concern

Nortriptyline (NT) is a tricyclic antidepressant and is the active metabolite of amitriptyline (Elavil). In one patient receiving 125 mg or nortriptyline at bedtime, milk concentrations of NT averaged 180 µg/L after 6-7 days of administration.[1] Based on these concentrations, the authors estimate the average daily infant exposure would be 27 µg/kg/d. The relative dose in milk would be 1.5% of the maternal dose. Several other authors have been unable to detect NT in maternal milk nor the serum of infants after prolonged exposure.[2,3] So far no untoward effects have been noted.

Pregnancy Risk Category: D

Lactation Risk Category: L2

Adult Concerns: Sedation, dry mouth, constipation, urinary retention, blurred vision

Pediatric Concerns: None reported in several studies.

Drug Interactions: Phenobarbital may reduce effect of nortriptyline. Nortriptyline blocks the hypotensive effect of guanethidine. May increase toxicity of nortriptyline when used with clonidine. Dangerous when used with MAO inhibitors, other CNS depressants. May increase anticoagulant effect of coumadin, warfarin. SSRIs (Prozac, Zoloft,etc) should not be used with or soon after nortriptyline or other TCAs due to serotonergic crisis.

Theoretic Infant Dose: 27 µg/kg/day

Relative Infant Dose: 1.5%

Adult Dose: 25 mg TID-QID

Alternatives: Imipramine

$T\frac{1}{2}$ =	16-90 hours	M/P =	0.87-3.71
PHL =		PB =	92%
T_{max} =	7-8.5 hours	Oral =	51%
MW =	263	pKa =	9.7
Vd =	20-57		

References:

1. Matheson I, Skjaeraasen J. Milk concentrations of flupenthixol, nortriptyline and zuclopenthixol and between-breast differences in two patients. Eur J Clin Pharmacol 1988; 35(2):217-220.

2. Wisner KL, Perel JM. Serum nortriptyline levels in nursing mothers and their infants. Am J Psychiatry 1991; 148(9):1234-1236.
3. Brixen-Rasmussen L, Halgrener J, Jorgensen A. Amitriptyline and nortriptyline excretion in human breastmilk. Psychopharmacology (Berl) 1982; 76(1):94-95.

NYSTATIN

Trade: Mycostatin, Nilstat
Can/Aus/UK: Mycostatin, Nadostine, Nilstat, Candistatin, Nystan
Uses: Antifungal
LRC: L1
AAP: Not reviewed

Nystatin is an antifungal primarily used for candidiasis topically and orally. The oral absorption of nystatin is extremely poor, and plasma levels are undetectable after oral administration.[1] The likelihood of secretion into milk is remote due to poor maternal absorption. It is frequently administered directly to neonates in neonatal units for candidiasis. In addition, absorption into infant circulation equally unlikely. Dose: neonates= 100,000 units; children=200,000 units, 400,000-600,000 units in older children, administered four times daily. Current studies suggest that resistance to nystatin is growing.

Pregnancy Risk Category: B

Lactation Risk Category: L1

Adult Concerns: Bad taste, diarrhea, nausea, vomiting

Pediatric Concerns: None reported. Nystatin is commonly used in infants.

Drug Interactions:

Theoretic Infant Dose:

Relative Infant Dose:

Adult Dose: 500,000-1 million units TID

Alternatives: Fluconazole

T½ =		M/P =	
PHL =		PB =	
T$_{max}$ =		Oral =	Poor
MW =		pKa =	
Vd =			

References:

1. Rothermel P, Faber M. Drugs in breastmilk: a consumer's guide. Birth and Family J 1975; 2:76-78.

OCTREOTIDE ACETATE AND 111-INDIUM OCTREOTIDE

Trade: Sandostatin Lar, Octreoscan, 111-Indium Octreotide, Octreotide Acetate
Can/Aus/UK:
Uses: Somatostatin analog
LRC: L3
       L4 for radioactive product
AAP: Radioactive compound that requires temporary cessation of breastfeeding

Octreotide (Sandostatin LAR) is a long acting form consisting of microspheres containing octreotide. Octreotide is a close analog of and provides activity similar to the natural hormone somatostatin. Like somatostatin, it also suppresses LH response to GnRH, decreases splanchnic blood flow, and inhibits release of serotonin, gastrin, vasoactive intestinal peptide, secretin, motilin, and pancreatic polypeptide. It is used to treat acromegaly and carcinoid tumors. This product, if present in milk, would not likely be absorbed to any degree.

Radioactive 111-Indium Octreotide (OctreoScan):
OctreoScan® is an imaging agent that can help find primary and metastatic neuroendocrine tumors. The concentration of radioactive octreotide in breastmilk in a 10 weeks postpartum woman was measured at daily intervals for three days after injection of 5.3 mCi (196 MBq) of 111-Indium-octreotide (OctreoScan).[1] The disappearance of radiolabeled octreotide from the breastmilk exhibited a bi-exponential pattern with a maximum concentration of 14.2 nCi (0.54 kBq) per 125 mL feeding at 4 hours. The maximum reading was 8.3 mrem x h(-1) (0.83 mSv x h(-1)) immediately after administration. This decreased rapidly (85%) due to rapid urinary clearance by 24 hours.

Breastmilk content of radio-active octreotide and external surveys at the breast surface were determined at 3 hour intervals for up to 10 days. Assuming an infant is breastfed for the first 10 days following therapy, the internal and external dose equivalents would be 22.97 mrem (0.23 mSv) and 27.86 mrem (0.28 mSv) respectively, for a total of 50.83 mrem (0.5 mSv). In this paper, the patient resumed breastfeeding on day 10 when the newborn received a total dose equivalent of 1.55 mrem (0.016 mSv). The 10 day waiting period used in this study was based on very conservative assumptions and assumed 100% of the ingested 111-In is orally bioavailable. However, oral indium has been shown to be poorly absorbed from the gastrointestinal tract (approximately 0.15%), which suggests the infant's dose could be considerably less. The authors suggest that a briefer interruption deserves attention.

Pregnancy Risk Category: B

Lactation Risk Category: L3
                          L4 for radioactive product

Adult Concerns: May inhibit gallbladder contractility and decrease bile secretion. Hypoglycemia or hyperglycemia, hypothyroidism may result. Bradycardia, arrhythmias in acromegalic patients. Numerous other adverse effects, consult package insert.

Pediatric Concerns: None reported via milk.

Drug Interactions: May reduce absorption of cyclosporin and other drugs by altering oral absorption. Patients receiving insulin, oral hypoglycemic agents, beta blockers, and other drugs may require dosage adjustment of these therapeutic agents.

Theoretic Infant Dose:

Relative Infant Dose:

Adult Dose: 50 mg TID (non-depo form)

Alternatives:

$T\frac{1}{2}$ =	1.7 hours	M/P =	
PHL =		PB =	65%
T_{max} =	0.4 hours	Oral =	0.15
MW =	1019	pKa =	
Vd =	13.6		

References:

1.   Castronovo FP, Jr., Stone H, Ulanski J. Radioactivity in breastmilk following 111In-octreotide. Nucl Med Commun 2000; 21(7):695-699.

OFLOXACIN

Trade: Floxin
Can/Aus/UK: Floxin, Ocuflox, Tarivid
Uses: Fluoroquinolone antibiotic
LRC: L2
AAP: Maternal Medication Usually Compatible with Breastfeeding

Ofloxacin is a typical fluoroquinolone antimicrobial. Breastmilk concentrations are reported equal to maternal plasma levels. In one study in lactating women who received 400 mg oral doses twice daily, drug concentrations in breastmilk averaged 0.05-2.41 mg/L in milk (24 hrs and 2 hrs post-dose respectively).[1] The drug was still detectable in milk 24 hours after a dose. The fluoroquinolones are becoming more popular in pediatrics due to recent studies and reviews showing their safe use.[2] It is very unlikely that arthropathy would ensue following the dose received via milk. The only probable risk is a change in gut flora, diarrhea, and a remote risk of overgrowth of C. Difficile. Ofloxacin levels in breastmilk are consistently lower (37%) than ciprofloxacin. If a fluoroquinolone is required, ofloxacin, levofloxacin, or norfloxacin are probably the better choices for breastfeeding mothers.

Pregnancy Risk Category: C

Lactation Risk Category: L2

Adult Concerns: Nausea, vomiting, diarrhea, abdominal cramps, GI bleeding

Pediatric Concerns: None reported, but caution recommended. Observe for diarrhea.

Drug Interactions: Decreased absorption with antacids. Quinolones cause increased levels of caffeine, warfarin, cyclosporine, theophylline. Cimetidine, probenecid, azlocillin may increase ofloxacin levels. Increased risk of seizures when used with foscarnet.

Theoretic Infant Dose: 0.3615 mg/kg/day

Relative Infant Dose: < 3.1%

Adult Dose: 200-400 mg BID

Alternatives: Norfloxacin, Trovafloxacin

$T\frac{1}{2}$ =	5-7 hours	M/P =	0.98-1.66
PHL =		PB =	32%
T_{max} =	0.5-2 hours	Oral =	98 %
MW =	361	pKa =	
Vd =	1.4		

References:

1. Giamarellou H, Kolokythas E, Petrikkos G, Gazis J, Aravantinos D, Sfikakis P. Pharmacokinetics of three newer quinolones in pregnant and lactating women. Am J Med 1989; 87(5A):49S-51S.
2. Ghaffar F, McCracken GH. Quinolones in Pediatrics. In: Hooper DC, Rubinstein E, editors. Quinolone Antimicrobial Agents. Washington, D.C.: ASM Press, 2003: 343-354.

OLANZAPINE
Trade: Zyprexa, Symbyax
Can/Aus/UK: Zyprexa
Uses: Antipsychotic
LRC: L2
AAP: Not reviewed

Olanzapine is a typical antipsychotic agent structurally similar to clozapine and may be used for treating schizophrenia.[1] It is rather unusual in that it blocks serotonin receptors rather than dopamine receptors.

In a recent and excellent study of seven mother-infant nursing pairs receiving a median dose of olanzine of 7.5 mg/day (range = 5-20 mg/day), the median infant dose ingested via milk was approximately 1.02% of the maternal dose.[2] The median milk/plasma AUC ratio was 0.38. Olanzapine was not detected in the plasma of six infants tested. All infants were healthy and experienced no observable side effects. The maximum relative infant dose was approximately 1.2%.

Another case of its use in lactating women has been briefly mentioned. No levels were reported but it did not produce complications in the infant.[3]

The new product Symbyax contains both fluoxetine and olanzapine for treatment of Bipolar Depression.

Pregnancy Risk Category: C

Lactation Risk Category: L2

Adult Concerns: Agitation, dizziness, somnolence, constipation, weight gain, elevated liver enzymes

Pediatric Concerns: None reported in one excellent study. Probably safe.

Drug Interactions: Ethanol may potentiate the effects of olanzapine. Fluvoxamine may inhibit olanzapine metabolism. Carbamazepine may increase clearance of olanzapine by 50%.   Levodopa may antagonize the effect of olanzapine.

Theoretic Infant Dose: 1.1 µg/kg/day

Relative Infant Dose: 1.2%

Adult Dose: 5-10 mg daily
Alternatives: Risperidone, Haloperidol

$T\frac{1}{2}$ =	21-54 hours	M/P =	0.38
PHL =		PB =	93%
T_{max} =	5-8 hours	Oral =	> 57%
MW =	312	pKa =	5.0, 7.4
Vd =	14.3		

References:
1. Pharmaceutical Manufacturer Prescribing Information. 1997.
2. Croke S, Buist A, Hackett LP, Ilett KF, Norman TR, Burrows GD. Olanzapine excretion in human breastmilk: estimation of infant exposure. Int J Neuropsychopharmacol 2002; 5(3):243-247.
3. Goldstein DJ, Corbin LA, Fung MC. Olanzapine-exposed pregnancies and lactation: early experience. J Clin Psychopharmacol 2000; 20(4):399-403.

OLMISARTAN MEDOXOMIL

Trade: Benicar, Benicar HCT
Can/Aus/UK:
Uses: Antihypertensive
LRC: L3 in older infants
AAP: Not reviewed

Olmisartan(Benicar) and Olmesartan plus Hydrochlorthiazide(Benicar HCT) are antihypertensives.[1] Olmesartan is an angiotensin II receptor antagonist and hydrochlorothiazide is a diuretic. Olmesartan medoxomil is a prodrug and is rapidly metabolized in the GI tract to the active Olmesartan antihypertensive. It effectively blocks the angiotensin II receptor site. While it is different from the ACE inhibitors, it effectively produces the same end result, hypotension. Use in pregnancy is contraindicated. No data are available on its transfer to human milk but its use in newborn infants could be risky.

Pregnancy Risk Category: **C in first trimester**
                                       D in 2nd and 3rd trimester

Lactation Risk Category: **L3 in older infants**

Adult Concerns: Adverse effects include dizziness and low blood pressure

Pediatric Concerns: None via milk. No data are available.

Drug Interactions: No major drug-drug interaction are noted with exception of its use with adrenergics.

Theoretic Infant Dose:

Relative Infant Dose:

Adult Dose: 20-40 mg daily

Alternatives: Captopril, enalapril

$T\frac{1}{2}$ =	13 hours	M/P =	
PHL =		PB =	
T_{max} =	1-2 hours	Oral =	26%
MW =	558	pKa =	
Vd =	0.24		

References:
1. Pharmaceutical Manufacturers prescribing information, 2003.

OLOPATADINE OPHTHALMIC

Trade: Patanol
Can/Aus/UK: Patanol, Opatanol
Uses: Ophthalmic antihistamine
LRC: L2
AAP: Not reviewed

Olopatadine is a selective H1-receptor antagonist and inhibitor of histamine release from mast cells. It is used topically in the eye. Kinetic studies by the manufacturer suggest that absorption is low in adults and that plasma levels are undetectable in most cases(< 0.5 ng/mL).[1] Samples in which olopatadine was found in the plasma compartment were at 2 hours and were < 1.3 ng/mL. Because adult plasma levels are so low, it is extremely unlikely any would be detectable in human milk. No data are available reporting levels in human milk but the risk is probably quite low.

Pregnancy Risk Category: C

Lactation Risk Category: L2

Adult Concerns: Headaches have been reported in 7% of patients.Asthenia, blurred vision, burning, dry eye, redness, lid edema, pruritis and rhinitis have been reported.

Pediatric Concerns: None reported via milk.

Drug Interactions:

Theoretic Infant Dose:

Relative Infant Dose:

Adult Dose: One drop in affected eye twice daily.

Alternatives:

$T\frac{1}{2}$ =	3 hours	M/P =	
PHL =		PB =	
T_{max} =	2 hours	Oral =	
MW =	373	pKa =	
Vd =			

References:
1. Pharmaceutical Manufacturers Prescribing Information, 2003.

OLSALAZINE

Trade: Dipentum
Can/Aus/UK: Dipentum
Uses: Anti-inflammatory
LRC: L3
AAP: Not reviewed

Olsalazine is converted to 5-aminosalicylic acid (mesalamine:5-ASA) in the gut which has anti-inflammatory activity in ulcerative colitis.[1] After oral administration, only 2.4% is systemically absorbed while the majority is metabolized in the GI tract to 5-ASA. 5-ASA is slowly and poorly absorbed. Plasma levels are exceedingly small (1.6-6.2 mmol/L), the half-life very short, and protein binding is very high. In rodents fed up to 20 times the normal dose, olsalazine produced growth retardation in pups. In one study of a mother who received a single 500 mg dose of olsalazine, acetylated-5-ASA achieved concentrations of 0.6, 0.86, and 1.24 µmol/L in breastmilk at 10, 14, and 24 hours respectively.[2] Olsalazine, olsalazine-S, and 5-ASA were undetectable in breastmilk. While clinically significant levels in milk are remote, infants should be closely monitored for gastric changes such as diarrhea.

Pregnancy Risk Category: C

Lactation Risk Category: L3

Adult Concerns: Watery diarrhea, dyspepsia, diarrhea, nausea, pain/cramping, headache

Pediatric Concerns: None specifically reported with this product, but observe for diarrhea and cramping if used for longer periods.

Drug Interactions:

Theoretic Infant Dose: 62.25 µg/kg/day

Relative Infant Dose: 0.87%

Adult Dose: 500 mg BID

Alternatives:

T½ =	0.9 hours	M/P =	
PHL =		PB =	> 99%
Tmax =	1-2 hours	Oral =	2.4% (olsalazine)
MW =	346	pKa =	
Vd =			

References:

1. Drug Facts and Comparisons 1995 ed. ed. St. Louis: 1995.
2. Miller LG, Hopkinson JM, Motil KJ, Corboy JE, Andersson S. Disposition of olsalazine and metabolites in breastmilk. J Clin Pharmacol 1993; 33(8):703-706.

OMEPRAZOLE

Trade: Prilosec
Can/Aus/UK: Prilosec, Losec
Uses: Reduces gastric acid secretion
LRC: L2
AAP: Not reviewed

Omeprazole is a potent inhibitor of gastric acid secretion. In a study of one patient receiving 20 mg omeprazole daily, the maternal serum concentration was negligible until 90 minutes after ingestion and then reached 950 nM at 240 minutes.[1] The breastmilk concentration of omeprazole began to rise minimally at 90 minutes after ingestion but peaked after 180 minutes at only 58 nM, or less than 7% of the highest serum level. Omeprazole milk levels were essentially flat over 4 hours of observation.

Omeprazole is extremely acid labile with a half-life of 10 minutes at pH values below 4.[2] Virtually all omeprazole ingested via milk would probably be destroyed in the stomach of the infant prior to absorption.

Pregnancy Risk Category: C

Lactation Risk Category: L2

Adult Concerns: Headache, diarrhea, elevated liver enzymes

Pediatric Concerns: None reported via milk in one case.

Drug Interactions: Administration of Omeprazole and clarithromycin may result in increased plasma levels of omeprazole. Omeprazole produced a 130% increase in the half-life of diazepam, reduced the plasma clearance of phenytoin by 15%, and increased phenytoin half-life by 27%. May prolong the elimination of warfarin.

Theoretic Infant Dose:

Relative Infant Dose:

Adult Dose: 20 mg BID

Alternatives: Famotidine, Nizatidine

$T^{1/2}$ =	1 hour	M/P =	
PHL =		PB =	95%
T_{max} =	0.5-3.5 hours	Oral =	30-40%
MW =	345	pKa =	
Vd =			

References:

1. Marshall JK, Thompson AB, Armstrong D. Omeprazole for refractory gastroesophageal reflux disease during pregnancy and lactation. Can J Gastroenterol 1998; 12(3):225-227.
2. Pilbrant A, Cederberg C. Development of an oral formulation of omeprazole. Scand J Gastroenterol Suppl 1985; 108:113-120.

ONDANSETRON

Trade: Zofran
Can/Aus/UK: Zofran
Uses: Antiemetic
LRC: L2
AAP: Not reviewed

Ondansetron is used clinically for reducing the nausea and vomiting associated with chemotherapy. It has occasionally been used during pregnancy without effect on the fetus.[1,2] It is available for oral and IV administration. Ondansetron is secreted in animal milk but no data on humans are available. Four studies of ondansetron use in pediatric patients 4-18 years of age are available.

Pregnancy Risk Category: B

Lactation Risk Category: L2

Adult Concerns: Headache, drowsiness, malaise, clonic-tonic seizures, and constipation

Pediatric Concerns: None reported via milk.

Drug Interactions: The clearance and half-life of ondansetron may be changed when used with barbiturates, carbamazepine, rifampin, phenytoin.

Theoretic Infant Dose:

Relative Infant Dose:

Adult Dose: 8 mg BID

Alternatives:

$T\frac{1}{2}$ =	3.6 hours	M/P =		
PHL =	2.7 hours	PB =	70-76%	
T_{max} =	1.7, 3.1 (IV,PO)	Oral =	56-66%	
MW =	293	pKa =		
Vd =				

References:

1. Pharmaceutical Manufacturer Prescribing Information. 1996.
2. Spratto GR. In: Nurse's Drug Reference. Albany, NY: Delmar Publishers Inc., 1995.

ORAL CONTRACEPTIVES

Trade: Norinyl, Norlestin, Ovral, Ortho-Novum
Can/Aus/UK: Nornyl, Cilest, Brevinor
Uses: Contraceptive
LRC: L3
AAP: Maternal Medication Usually Compatible with Breastfeeding

Oral contraceptives, particularly those containing estrogens, tend to reduce lactose production, hence reducing volume of milk produced.[1] Quality (fat content) may similarly be reduced; although, one recent study of the fat, energy, protein, and lactose concentration in milk of mothers using oral contraceptives showed no effect of contraceptives.[4] The earlier oral contraceptives are started, the greater the negative effect on lactation.[2,3] Suppression of breastmilk production with estrogen-progestin contraceptives is well-known, is more prevalent early postpartum, and is common. Although it was previously believed that waiting for 6 weeks would preclude breastfeeding problems, this is apparently not accurate. Numerous examples of supply problems have occurred months postpartum in some patients.

Suggest that the mother establish a good flow (60-90 days) prior to beginning oral contraceptives. If necessary, use only LOW DOSE combination oral contraceptives with 35-50 μg of estrogen, or better, progestin-only mini pills. Suggest alternates such as progestin-only oral contraceptives (rather than Depo-Provera) so that if a supply problem occurs, the patient can easily withdraw from the medication. Use Depo-Provera in those patients who have used it previously and have not experienced breastmilk supply problems or in those who have used progestin-only mini pills without problems. Attempt to wait for 6 weeks postpartum prior to using Depo-Provera.

The progestins and estrogens present in breastmilk are quite low and numerous studies confirm that they have minimal or no effect on sexual development in infants.

Pregnancy Risk Category: X

Lactation Risk Category: L3

Adult Concerns: Reduced milk production, particularly with estrogen containing preparations, but also rarely with progestin only products.

Pediatric Concerns: None reported via milk. May suppress lactation, reducing weight gain of infant.

Drug Interactions: Barbiturates, hydantoins, and rifampin, may increase the clearance of oral contraceptives resulting in decreased effectiveness of the OC. Co-administration of griseofulvin, penicillin, or tetracyclines with OC s may decrease the efficacy of oral contraceptives possibly due to altered gut metabolism. May increase or decrease anticoagulant efficacy. Co-administration with cyclosporine, or carbamazepine may result in decreased OC efficacy.

Theoretic Infant Dose:

Relative Infant Dose:

Adult Dose:

Alternatives: Norethindrone

References:
1.   Booker DE, Pahl IR. Control of postpartum breast engorgement with oral contraceptives. Am J Obstet Gynecol 1967; 98(8):1099-1101.
2.   Laukaran VH. The effects of contraceptive use on the initiation and duration of lactation. Int J Gynaecol Obstet 1987; 25 Suppl:129-142.
3.   Kora SJ. Effect of oral contraceptives on lactation. Fertil Steril 1969; 20(3):419-423.
4.   Costa TH, Dorea JG. Concentration of fat, protein, lactose and energy in milk of mothers using hormonal contraceptives. Ann Trop Paediatr 1992; 12(2):203-209.

ORPHENADRINE CITRATE

Trade: Norflex, Banflex, Norgesic, Myotrol
Can/Aus/UK: Disipal, Norflex, Orfenace, Norgesic
Uses: Muscle relaxant
LRC: L3
AAP: Not reviewed

Orphenadrine is an analog of Benadryl.[1]   It is primarily used as a muscle relaxant although its primary effects are anticholinergic. No data are available on its secretion into breastmilk.

Pregnancy Risk Category: C

Lactation Risk Category: L3

Adult Concerns: Agitation, aplastic anemia, dizziness, tremor, dry mouth, nausea, constipation

Pediatric Concerns: None reported due to limited studies.

Drug Interactions: Increased anticholinergic side effects may be noted when used with amantadine.   Orphenadrine may reduce therapeutic efficacy of phenothiazine family.

Theoretic Infant Dose:

Relative Infant Dose:

Adult Dose: 100 mg BID

Alternatives:

T½ =	14 hours	M/P =	
PHL =		PB =	
T_max =	2-4 hours	Oral =	95%
MW =	269	pKa =	
Vd =			

References:
1. McEvoy GE. (ed):AFHS Drug Information. New York, NY: 2003.

OSELTAMIVIR PHOSPHATE
Trade: Tamiflu
Can/Aus/UK: Tamiflu
Uses: Anti-viral for influenza A and B
LRC: L3
AAP: Not reviewed

Tamiflu is indicated for the treatment of uncomplicated acute illness due to influenza A and B infection in adults who have been symptomatic for no more than 2 days. Tamiflu is an oral viral neuraminidase inhibitor, which blocks or prevents viral seeding or release from infected cells and prevents viral aggregation. It is only moderately effective and is believed to reduce symptoms by only 1.3 days and only if treatment is instituted within 2 days of infection. It is approximately 75% bioavailable following oral administration. The peak maternal plasma concentration is only 551 nanograms/mL following a 75 mg oral dose. It is not known if it transfers into human milk, but the levels would likely be incredibly low due to the low maternal plasma levels. However, due to its limited efficacy (reduces length of illness by 1.3 days), its use in breastfeeding mothers is probably not warranted, unless in high-risk patients with other severe medical conditions.

Pregnancy Risk Category: C

Lactation Risk Category: L3

Adult Concerns: Nausea and vomiting are most common. Diarrhea, bronchitis, abdominal pain are less common.

Pediatric Concerns: None reported via milk.

Drug Interactions: None yet reported.

Theoretic Infant Dose:

Relative Infant Dose:

Adult Dose: 75 mg twice daily for 5 days.

Alternatives:

T½ =	6-10 hours	M/P =	
PHL =		PB =	42%
Tmax =		Oral =	75%
MW =	312	pKa =	
Vd =	0.37		

References:
1. Manufacturers Product Information. 1999. Roche Laboratories.

OSMOTIC LAXATIVES

Trade: Milk Of Magnesia, Fleet Phospho-Soda, Citrate Of Magnesia, Epsom Salt
Can/Aus/UK: Acilac, Citromag, Fleet Phosph-Soda, Sorbilax, Duphalac
Uses: Laxatives
LRC: L1
AAP: Not reviewed

Osmotic or Saline laxatives comprise a large number of magnesium and phosphate compounds, but all work similarly in that they osmotically pull and retain water in the GI tract, thus functioning as laxatives. Because they are poorly absorbed, they largely stay in the GI tract and are eliminated without significant systemic absorption.[1,2] The small amount of magnesium and phosphate salts absorbed are rapidly cleared by the kidneys. Products considered osmotic laxatives include: Milk of Magnesia, Epsom Salts, Citrate of Magnesia, Fleets Phospho-soda, and other sodium phosphate compounds.

Because milk electrolytes and ion concentrations are tightly controlled by the maternal alveolar cell, the secretion of higher than normal levels into milk is rare and unlikely. It is not known for certainty if these products enter milk in higher levels than are normally present but it is very unlikely.

Pregnancy Risk Category: C

Lactation Risk Category: L1

Adult Concerns: Diarrhea, nausea, vomiting, hypocalcemia, hypermagnesemia

Pediatric Concerns: None reported via milk.

Drug Interactions: May reduce absorption of anticoagulants such as coumarin, and dicoumarol.

Theoretic Infant Dose:

Relative Infant Dose:

Adult Dose:

Alternatives:

T½ =		M/P =
PHL =		PB =
T$_{max}$ =		Oral = Poor
MW =		pKa =
Vd =		

References:
1. Drug Facts and Comparisons 1997 ed. ed. St. Louis: 1997.
2. Pharmaceutical Manufacturer Prescribing Information. 1997.

OXAPROZIN

Trade: Daypro
Can/Aus/UK: Daypro
Uses: Nonsteroidal analgesic
LRC: L3
AAP: Not reviewed

Oxaprozin belongs to the NSAID family of analgesics and is reputed to have lesser GI side effects than certain others.[1] Although its long half-life could prove troublesome in breastfed infants, it is probably poorly transferred to human milk. No data on transfer into human milk are available although it is known to transfer into animal milk.

Pregnancy Risk Category: C

Lactation Risk Category: L3

Adult Concerns: Headache, nausea, abdominal pain, gastric bleeding, diarrhea, vomiting, bleeding, constipation

Pediatric Concerns: None reported, but ibuprofen preferred in absence of data.

Drug Interactions: May prolong prothrombin time when used with warfarin. Antihypertensive effects of ACEi family may be blunted or completely abolished by NSAIDs. Some NSAIDs may block antihypertensive effect of beta blockers, diuretics. Used with cyclosporin, may dramatically increase renal toxicity. May increase digoxin, phenytoin, lithium levels. May increase toxicity of methotrexate. May increase bioavailability of penicillamine. Probenecid may increase NSAID levels.

Theoretic Infant Dose:

Relative Infant Dose:

Adult Dose: 600-1200 mg daily

Alternatives: Ibuprofen, celecoxib

T½ =	42-50 hours	M/P =	
PHL =		PB =	99%
T_{max} =	3-5 hours	Oral =	95%
MW =	293	pKa =	
Vd =			

References:
1. Pharmaceutical Manufacturer Prescribing Information.

OXAZEPAM
Trade: Serax
Can/Aus/UK: Apo-Oxazepam, Novoxapam, Serax, Zapex, Alepam, Murelax, Serepax, Oxanid
Uses: Benzodiazepine antianxiety drug
LRC: L3
AAP: Not reviewed

Oxazepam is a typical benzodiazepine (See Valium) and is used in anxiety disorders. Of the benzodiazepines, oxazepam is the least lipid soluble, which accounts for its low levels in milk. In one study of a patient receiving 10 mg three times daily for 3 days, the concentration of oxazepam in breastmilk was relatively constant between 24 and 30 µg/L from the evening of the first day.[1] The milk/plasma ratio ranged from 0.1 to 0.33.

Pregnancy Risk Category: D

Lactation Risk Category: L3

Adult Concerns: Sedation

Pediatric Concerns: None reported in one study.

Drug Interactions: May increase sedation when used with CNS depressants such as alcohol, barbiturates, opioids. Cimetidine may decrease metabolism and clearance of oxazepam. Cisapride can dramatically increase plasma levels of diazepam. SSRIs (fluoxetine, sertraline, paroxetine) can dramatically increase benzodiazepine levels by altering clearance, thus leading to sedation . Digoxin plasma levels may be increased.

Theoretic Infant Dose: 4.5 µg/kg/day

Relative Infant Dose: 1.04%

Adult Dose: 10-30 mg TID-QID

Alternatives:

T½ =	12 hours	M/P =	0.1-0.33
PHL =	22 hours	PB =	97%
T$_{max}$ =	1-2 hours	Oral =	97%
MW =	287	pKa =	1.7,11.6
Vd =	0.7-1.6		

References:
1. Wretlind M. Excretion of oxazepam in breastmilk. Eur J Clin Pharmacol 1987; 33(2):209-210.

OXCARBAZEPINE
Trade: Trileptal
Can/Aus/UK: Trileptal
Uses: Anticonvulsant
LRC: L3
AAP: Not reviewed

Oxcarbazepine is a derivative of carbamazepine and is used in the treatment of partial seizures in adults and as adjunctive therapy in the treatment of partial seizures in children. It is rapidly metabolized to a longer half-life active metabolite 10-hydroxy-carbazepine (MHD). In a brief and somewhat incomplete study of a pregnant patient who received 300 mg three times daily while pregnant, plasma levels were studied in her infant for the first 5 days postpartum while the infant was breastfeeding.[1] While no breastmilk levels were reported, plasma levels of MHD were essentially the same as the mothers immediately after delivery, suggesting complete transfer transplacentally of the drug. However, while breastfeeding for the next 5 days, plasma levels of MHD in the infant declined significantly from approximately 7 µg/mL to 0.2 µg/mL on the fifth day. The decay of MHD concentrations in neonatal plasma during the first 4 days postpartum indicated first order elimination. The plasma MHD levels on day 5 amounted to 7% of those on day 1 postpartum (93% drop in 5 days). The authors estimated the milk/plasma ratio to be 0.5. No neonatal side effects were reported by the authors.

Pregnancy Risk Category: C

Lactation Risk Category: L3

Adult Concerns: Cognitive symptoms include psychomotor slowing, difficulty with concentration, speech or language problems, somnolence or fatigue, ataxia and gait disturbances. Hyponatremia

Pediatric Concerns: None reported in one study.

Drug Interactions: Slight increases in other anticonvulsant plasma levels have been reported and include phenobarbital, phenytoin. A reduction in plasma levels of oxcarbazepine have been reported with admixed with phenobarbital, carbamazepine, phenytoin, etc. Major reductions in plasma levels of estrogens and other hormonal contraceptives has been reported and may render oral contraceptives less effective.

Theoretic Infant Dose:

Relative Infant Dose:

Adult Dose: 300-600 mg BID

Alternatives: Carbamazepine

T½ =	9 hours MHD	M/P =	0.5
PHL =		PB =	40%
Tmax =	4.5 hours	Oral =	Complete
MW =	252	pKa =	
Vd =	0.7		

References:
1.   Bulau P, Paar WD, von Unruh GE. Pharmacokinetics of oxcarbazepine and 10-hydroxy-carbazepine in the newborn child of an oxcarbazepine-treated mother. Eur J Clin Pharmacol 1988; 34(3):311-313.

OXYBUTYNIN

Trade: Ditropan
Can/Aus/UK: Ditropan, Apo-Oxybutynin, Oxybutyn
Uses: Anticholinergic, antispasmodic
LRC: L3
AAP: Not reviewed

Oxybutynin is an anticholinergic agent used to provide antispasmodic effects for conditions characterized by involuntary bladder spasms and reduces urinary urgency and frequency. It has been used in children down to 5 years of age at doses of 15 mg daily.[1]

No data on transfer of this product into human milk are available. But oxybutynin is a tertiary amine which is poorly absorbed orally (only 6%). Further, the maximum plasma levels (C_{max}) generally attained are less than 31.7 nanogram/mL.[2] If one were to assume a theoretical M/P ratio of 1.0 (which is probably unreasonably high) and a daily ingestion of 1 Liter of milk, then the theoretical dose to the infant would be < 2 micrograms/day, a dose that would be clinically irrelevant to even a neonate.

Pregnancy Risk Category: B
Lactation Risk Category: L3

Adult Concerns: Nausea, dry mouth, constipation, esophagitis, urinary hesitancy, flushing and urticaria. Palpitations, somnolence, hallucinations infrequently occur.

Pediatric Concerns: Suppression of lactation has been reported by the manufacturer.

Drug Interactions: May potentiate the anticholinergic effect of biperiden and other anticholinergics such as the tricyclic antidepressants. May counteract the effects of cisapride and metoclopramide.

Theoretic Infant Dose:

Relative Infant Dose:

Adult Dose: 5 mg BID-QID

Alternatives:

$T\frac{1}{2}$ =	1-2 hours	M/P =	
PHL =		PB =	
T_{max} =	3-6 hours	Oral =	6%
MW =	393	pKa =	6.96
Vd =			

References:
1. Pharmaceutical Manufacturer Prescribing Information. 1997.
2. Douchamps J, Derenne F, Stockis A, Gangji D, Juvent M, Herchuelz A. The pharmacokinetics of oxybutynin in man. Eur J Clin Pharmacol 1988; 35(5):515-520.

OXYCODONE

Trade: Tylox, Percodan, Oxycontin, Roxicet, Endocet, Roxiprin, Percocet
Can/Aus/UK: Supeudol, Endone, Proladone
Uses: Narcotic analgesic
LRC: L3
AAP: Not reviewed

Oxycodone is similar to hydrocodone and is a mild analgesic somewhat stronger than codeine. Small amounts are secreted in breastmilk. Following a dose of 5-10 mg every 4-7 hours, maternal levels peaked at 1-2 hours, and analgesia persisted for up to 4 hours.[1] Reported milk levels range from < 5 to 226 µg/L. Maternal plasma levels were 14-35 µg/L. The authors suggest a milk/plasma ratio of approximately 3.4. No reports of untoward effects in infants have been found although sedation is a possibility in some infants. Endocet, Percocet, Roxicet and Roxiprin are all just formulations of oxycodone and acetaminophen.

Pregnancy Risk Category: B

Lactation Risk Category: L3

Adult Concerns: Drowsiness, sedation, nausea, vomiting, constipation

Pediatric Concerns: None reported via milk but observe for sedation.

Drug Interactions: Cigarette smoking increases effect of codeines. Increased toxicity/sedation when used with CNS depressants, phenothiazines, tricyclic antidepressants, other opiates, guanabenz, MAO inhibitors, neuromuscular blockers.

Theoretic Infant Dose: 33.9 μg/kg/day

Relative Infant Dose: 3.9%

Adult Dose: 5 mg q 6 hours

Alternatives: Codeine

T½ =	3-6 hours	M/P =	3.4
PHL =		PB =	
T$_{max}$ =	1-2 hours	Oral =	50%
MW =	315	pKa =	8.5
Vd =	1.8-3.7		

References:
1. Marx CM, Pucin F, Carlson JD. et.al. Oxycodone excretion in human milk in the puerperium. Drug Intel Clin 1986; 20:474.

OXYTOCIN

Trade: Pitocin
Can/Aus/UK: Toesen, Syntocinon, Syntometrine
Uses: Labor induction
LRC: L2
AAP: Not reviewed

Oxytocin is an endogenous nonapeptide hormone produced by the posterior pituitary and has uterine and myoepithelial muscle cell stimulant properties, as well as vasopressive and antidiuretic effects. Prepared synthetically, it is bioavailable via IV and intranasal applications. It is destroyed orally by chymotrypsin in the stomach of adults and systemically by the liver. It is known to be secreted in small amounts into human milk. Takeda reported that mean oxytocin concentrations in human milk at postpartum day 1 to 5 were 4.5, 4.7, 4.0, 3.2, and 3.3 microunits/mL respectively.[1] The oral absorption in neonates is unknown but probably minimal.

Intranasal sprays (Syntocinon) contained 40 IU/mL with a recommended typical dose being one spray (3 drops) in each nostril to induce letdown. This is roughly equivalent to 2 IU per drop or a total dose of approximately 12 IU per letdown dose. Although oxytocin is secreted in small amounts in breastmilk, no untoward effects have been noted. However, chronic use of intranasal oxytocin may lead to dependence and should be limited to the first week postpartum. See index for intranasal formulation.

Pregnancy Risk Category:

Lactation Risk Category: L2

Adult Concerns: Hypotension, hypertension, water intoxication and excessive uterine contractions, uterine hypertonicity, spasm, etc. May induce bradycardia, arrhythmias, intracranial hemorrhage, neonatal jaundice.

Pediatric Concerns: None via breastmilk.

Drug Interactions: When used within 3-4 hours of cyclopropane

Theoretic Infant Dose:

Relative Infant Dose:

Adult Dose: 40-80 units daily

Alternatives:

T½ =	3-5 minutes	M/P =	
PHL =		PB =	
T$_{max}$ =		Oral =	Minimal
MW =	>1000	pKa =	
Vd =			

References:
1. Takeda S, Kuwabara Y, Mizuno M. Concentrations and origin of oxytocin in breastmilk. Endocrinol Jpn 1986; 33(6):821-826.

PACLITAXEL
Trade: Taxol
Can/Aus/UK: Paxene, Taxol, Anzatax
Uses: Antineoplastic agent
LRC: L5
AAP: Not reviewed

Paclitaxel is a diterpene plant product with antineoplastic activity that is derived from the bark of the western yew tree. It is an antimicrotubule agent that promotes assembly of dimeric tubulin, which is stable to depolymerization.[1] It is a large molecular weight, highly lipophilic agent with only minimal kinetic data available. It is not known if paclitaxel enters milk but due to the extraordinary toxicity and lipophilicity of this compound, it would be inadvisable to breastfeed while under therapy with this drug.

Pregnancy Risk Category: D

Lactation Risk Category: L5

Adult Concerns: Anaphylaxis and severe hypersensitivity reactions including fatal dyspnea and hypotension, and angioedema have been reported. Neutropenia, leukopenia, abnormal ECG, myalgia, arthralgia, nausea, vomiting, and diarrhea.

Pediatric Concerns: None reported via milk, but extreme caution is recommended.

Drug Interactions: Increased myelosuppression when admixed with cisplatin. Increased levels of doxorubicin when admixed with paclitaxel.

Theoretic Infant Dose:

Relative Infant Dose:

Adult Dose: 135-175 mg/m² q 3 weeks

Alternatives:

T½ =	13-52 hours	M/P =	
PHL =		PB =	89-98%
T_max =		Oral =	
MW =	853	pKa =	
Vd =	688 L/sq meter		

References:
1. Pharmaceutical Manufacturer Prescribing Information. 1999.

PAMIDRONATE
Trade: Aredia
Can/Aus/UK:
Uses: Bisphosphonate bone-resorption inhibitor.
LRC: L2
AAP: Not reviewed

Pamidronate is an inhibitor of bone-resorption.   Although its mechanism of action is obscure, it possibly absorbs to the calcium phosphate crystal in bone and blocks dissolution (reabsorption) of this mineral component in bone, thus reducing turnover of bone calcium. A 39 year-old patient presented in the first month of pregnancy with reflex sympathetic dystrophy.   Because she wished to continue breastfeeding, she was treated with monthly IV doses of pamidronate (30 mg).   Following the first dose, breastmilk was assayed for pamidronate content.   After infusion, breastmilk was pumped and collected into two portions: 0-24 hours and 25-48 hours.   None was detected (limit of detection, 0.4 micromol/L).   The authors suggested that pamidronate could be considered safe for use in lactating women. Pamidronate is poorly absorbed (0.3% to 3% of a dose) after oral administration and thus any present in milk would not likely be absorbed by the infant.

Pregnancy Risk Category: C

Lactation Risk Category: L2

Adult Concerns: Adverse effects include fever and malaise, anemia (6%), leukopenia, thrombocytopenia, hypertension, hypocalcemia, abdominal pain, anorexia, constipation, nausea and vomiting. Numerous other side effects, consult package insert.

Pediatric Concerns: None reported via milk.

Drug Interactions: None reported.

Theoretic Infant Dose:

Relative Infant Dose:

Adult Dose: 60 to 90 milligrams as a single intravenous infusion.

Alternatives:

$T\frac{1}{2}$ =	28 hours	M/P =	
PHL =		PB =	
T_{max} =		Oral =	0.3% to 3%
MW =	369	pKa =	
Vd =			

References:

1. Siminoski K, Fitzgerald AA, Flesch G, Gross MS. Intravenous pamidronate for treatment of reflex sympathetic dystrophy during breast feeding. J Bone Miner Res 2000; 15(10):2052-2055.

PANTOPRAZOLE

Trade: Protonix
Can/Aus/UK: Pantoloc
Uses: Suppresses gastric acid production
LRC: L2
AAP: Not reviewed

Pantoprazole is a proton-pump inhibitor similar to omeprazole (Prilosec). It is used primarily to suppress acid production in the stomach for treatment of gastroesophageal reflux or peptic ulcer disease. The pharmaceutical manufacturer reports 0.02% of an administered dose is excreted into milk.[1] As with all the proton-pump inhibitors, pantoprazole is virtually unstable in an acid milieu and when presented in milk, it would be highly unstable in the infant's stomach. If any were present in milk, it would be largely degraded prior to absorption. See omeprazole for an alternative.

Pregnancy Risk Category: B

Lactation Risk Category: L2

Adult Concerns: Headache, diarrhea, flatulence, and rash

Pediatric Concerns: None reported via milk.

Drug Interactions: None reported.

Theoretic Infant Dose:

Relative Infant Dose:

Adult Dose: 40-80 mg daily

Alternatives: Omeprazole

T½ =	1 hour	M/P =		
PHL =		PB =	98%	
T_{max} =	2.4 hours	Oral =	77%	Enteric coated
MW =	432	pKa =		
Vd =	0.32			

References:
1.   Pharmaceutical Manufacturer Prescribing Information. 2003.

PAREGORIC
Trade:
Can/Aus/UK:
Uses: Opiate analgesic used for diarrhea.
LRC: L3
AAP: Not reviewed

Paregoric is camphorated tincture of opium, and contains approximately 2 mg morphine per 5cc (teaspoonful) in 45% alcohol.[1] It is frequently used for diarrhea and in the past for withdrawal symptoms in neonates (Tincture of Opium is now preferred). Because the active ingredient is morphine, see morphine for breastfeeding indications. Due to its camphor content, the pediatric use of paregoric is discouraged.

Pregnancy Risk Category: B

Lactation Risk Category: L3

Adult Concerns: Sedation, constipation, apnea, nausea, vomiting

Pediatric Concerns: None reported. See morphine.

Drug Interactions: See morphine.

Theoretic Infant Dose:

Relative Infant Dose:

Adult Dose: 5-10 mL (2-4 mg morphine) BID-QID

Alternatives:

T½ =	1.5-2 hours	M/P =	1.1-3.6
PHL =	13.9 hours(neonatal)	PB =	35%
T$_{max}$ =	0.5-1 hours	Oral =	26%
MW =		pKa =	
Vd =			

References:
1. Drug Facts and Comparisons 1995 ed. ed. St. Louis: 1995.

PAROXETINE

Trade: Paxil
Can/Aus/UK: Paxil, Aropax 20, Seroxat
Uses: Antidepressant, serotonin reuptake inhibitor
LRC: L2
AAP: Drugs whose effect on nursing infants is unknown but may be of concern

Paroxetine is a typical serotonin reuptake inhibitor. Although it undergoes hepatic metabolism, the metabolites are not active. Paroxetine is exceedingly lipophilic and distributes throughout the body with only 1% remaining in plasma. In one case report of a mother receiving 20 mg/day paroxetine at steady state[1], the breastmilk level at peak (4 hrs) was 7.6 µg/L. While the maternal paroxetine dose was 333 µg/kg, the maximum daily dose to the infant was estimated at 1.14 µg/kg or 0.34% of the maternal dose.

In two studies of 6 and 4 nursing mothers respectively,[2] the mean dose of paroxetine received by the infants in the first study was 1.13% (range 0.5-1.7) of the weight adjusted maternal dose. The mean M/P (AUC) was 0.39 (range 0.32-0.51) while the predicted M/P was 0.22.

In the second study, the mean dose of paroxetine received by the infants was 1.25% (range 0.38-2.24%) of the weight adjusted maternal dose with a mean M/P of 0.96 (range 0.31-3.33). The drug was not detected in the plasma of 7 of the 8 infants studied and was detected (< 4 mg/L) in only one infant. No adverse effects were observed in any of the infants.

In a recent study of 16 mothers by Stowe, paroxetine levels in milk were low and varied according to maternal dose.[3] Milk/plasma ratios varied from 0.056 to 1.3. Milk levels ranged from approximately 17 µg/L, 45 µg/L, 70 µg/L, 92 µg/L, and 101 µg/L in mothers receiving a dose of 10, 20, 30, 40, and 50 mg/day respectively. Levels of paroxetine were below the limit of detection (< 2 ng/mL) in all 16 infants.

In a study of 6 women receiving 20-40 mg/day, the milk/plasma ratio ranged from 0.39 to 1.11 but averaged 0.69.[4] The average estimated dose to the infants ranged from 0.7 to 2.9% of the weight-adjusted maternal dose. In a seventh patient, and based on area-under-the-curve data, the milk/plasma ratio was 0.69 at a dose of 20 mg and 0.72 at a dose of 40 mg/day. The estimated dose to the infant was 1.0% and 2.0% of the weight-adjusted maternal dose at 20 and 40 mg respectively. Paroxetine levels in milk averaged 44.3 and 78.5 µg/L over 6 hours following 20 and 40 mg doses respectively. No adverse reactions or unusual behaviors were noted in any of the infants.

In another study of 24 breastfeeding mothers who received an average dose of 17.6 mg/d (range 10-40 mg/d) the average level of paroxetine in maternal serum and milk was 45.2 ng/mL and 19.2 µg/L respectively.[5] The average milk/plasma ratio was 0.53. The authors estimated the average infant dose to be 2.88 µg/kg/d or 2.88% of the weight-adjusted maternal dose. All infant serum levels were below the limit of detection.

These studies generally conclude that paroxetine can be considered relatively 'safe' for breastfeeding infants as the absolute dose transferred is quite low. Plasma levels in the infant were generally undetectable. Recent data suggests that a neonatal withdrawal syndrome may occur in newborns exposed in utero to paroxetine[6] although there is significant difficulty in differentiating between withdrawal and toxicity.[7] Symptoms include jitteriness, vomiting, irritability, hypoglycemia, and necrotizing enterocolitis.

Pregnancy Risk Category: **B**

Lactation Risk Category: **L2**

Adult Concerns: Sedation, headache, dry mouth, dizziness, nausea, insomnia, constipation, seizures. Use in children and adolescents suggests increased risk of suicide.

Pediatric Concerns: Numerous studies suggest minimal to no effect on breastfed infants. A neonatal withdrawal effect (early postnatally) may following in utero exposure. Most studies show minimal to no plasma levels in breastfed infants.

Drug Interactions: Decreased effect with phenobarbital and phenytoin. Increased toxicity with alcohol, cimetidine, MAO inhibitors (serotonergic syndrome). Increased effect with fluoxetine, tricyclic antidepressants, sertraline, phenothiazines, warfarin.

Theoretic Infant Dose: 15.1 µg/kg/day

Relative Infant Dose: 2.1%

Adult Dose: 20-50 mg daily

Alternatives: Sertraline

T½ =	21 hours	M/P =	0.056-1.3
PHL =		PB =	95%
Tmax =	5-8 hours	Oral =	Complete
MW =	329	pKa =	
Vd =	3-28		

References:
1. Spigset O, Carleborg L, Norstrom A, Sandlund M. Paroxetine level in breastmilk. J Clin Psychiatry 1996; 57(1):39.
2. Begg EJ, Duffull SB, Saunders DA, Buttimore RC, Ilett KF, Hackett LP, Yapp P, Wilson DA. Paroxetine in human milk. Br J Clin Pharmacol 1999; 48(2):142-147.
3. Stowe ZN, Cohen LS, Hostetter A, Ritchie JC, Owens MJ, Nemeroff CB. Paroxetine in human breastmilk and nursing infants. Am J Psychiatry 2000; 157(2):185-189.
4. Ohman R, Hagg S, Carleborg L, Spigset O. Excretion of paroxetine into breastmilk. J Clin Psychiatry 1999; 60(8):519-523.
5. Misri S, Kim J, Riggs KW, Kostaras X. Paroxetine levels in postpartum depressed women, breastmilk, and infant serum. J Clin Psychiatry 2000; 61(11):828-832.
6. Stiskal JA, Kulin N, Koren G, Ho T, Ito S. Neonatal paroxetine withdrawal syndrome. Arch Dis Child Fetal Neonatal Ed 2001; 84(2):F134-F135.
7. Isbister GK, Dawson A, Whyte IM, Prior FH, Clancy C, Smith AJ. Neonatal paroxetine withdrawal syndrome or actually serotonin syndrome? Arch Dis Child Fetal Neonatal Ed 2001; 85(2):F147-F148.

PEMOLINE

Trade: Cylert
Can/Aus/UK: Cylert, Kethamed, Ronyl
Uses: CNS stimulant for attention deficit disorder.
LRC: L4
AAP: Not reviewed

Pemoline is a specialized CNS stimulate qualitatively similar to amphetamine and Ritalin.[1] At present there are no data available on its transfer into human milk, but it is likely due to its low molecular weight. Maternal peak level occurs 2-4 hours after dose. Serum half-life in children (5-12 yrs) is less than that of adults.

Pregnancy Risk Category: C

Lactation Risk Category: L4

Adult Concerns: Agitation, excitement, elevated liver enzymes, weight loss, insomnia, tachycardia

Pediatric Concerns: None reported, but observe for agitation, excitement, insomnia.

Drug Interactions: May reduce effect of insulin. Increased toxicity when used with other CNS depressants, CNs stimulants.

Theoretic Infant Dose:

Relative Infant Dose:

Adult Dose: 50-200 mg daily

Alternatives:

$T\frac{1}{2}$ =	12 hours	M/P =		
PHL =	7-8.6 hours	PB =	50%	
T_{max} =	2-4 hours	Oral =	Complete	
MW =	176	pKa =	10.5	
Vd =	0.22-0.59			

References:
1. Drug Facts and Comparisons 1995 ed. ed. St. Louis: 1995.

PENCICLOVIR

Trade: Denavir
Can/Aus/UK: Vectavir
Uses: Antiviral agent.
LRC: L3
AAP: Not reviewed

Penciclovir is an antiviral agent for the treatment of cold sores (herpes simplex labialis) of the lips and face and occasionally for herpes zoster (Shingles).[1] Following topical administration, plasma levels are undetectable.[2] Because oral bioavailability is nil and maternal plasma levels are undetectable following topical therapy, it is extremely unlikely that detectable amounts would transfer into human milk or be absorbable by an infant.

Pregnancy Risk Category: B

Lactation Risk Category: L3

Adult Concerns: Following topical application only mild erythema was occasionally observed.

Pediatric Concerns: None reported.

Drug Interactions: None reported.

Theoretic Infant Dose:

Relative Infant Dose:

Adult Dose: Topical application q 2 hours

Alternatives:

T½ =	2.3 hours	M/P =	
PHL =		PB =	< 20%
T$_{max}$ =		Oral =	1.5%
MW =		pKa =	
Vd =			

References:
1. Hodge RA, Perkins RM. Mode of action of 9-(4-hydroxy-3-hydroxymethylbut-1-yl)guanine (BRL 39123) against herpes simplex virus in MRC-5 cells. Antimicrob Agents Chemother 1989; 33(2):223-229.
2. Pharmaceutical Manufacturer Prescribing Information.

PENICILLAMINE

Trade: Cuprimine, Depen
Can/Aus/UK: Cuprimine, Depen, D-Penamine, Distamine, Pendramine
Uses: Used in arthritis, autoimmune syndromes
LRC: L4
AAP: Not reviewed

Penicillamine is a potent chelating agent used to chelate copper, iron, mercury, lead, and other metals. It is also used to suppress the immune response in rheumatoid arthritis and other immunologic syndromes. It is extremely dangerous during pregnancy. Safety has not been established during lactation. Penicillamine is a potent drug that requires constant observation and care by attending physicians. Recommend discontinuing lactation if this drug is mandatory.[1]

Pregnancy Risk Category: D

Lactation Risk Category: L4

Adult Concerns: Anorexia, nausea, vomiting, diarrhea, alteration of taste, elevated liver enzymes, kidney damage

Pediatric Concerns: None reported, but caution is recommended.

Drug Interactions: An increased risk of serious hematologic and renal reactions may occur if used with gold therapy, antimalarial, or other cytotoxic drugs. The absorption of penicillamine is decreased by 35% when used with iron salts. The absorption of penicillamine is decreased by 66% when used with antacids. Digoxin plasma levels may be reduced.

Theoretic Infant Dose:

Relative Infant Dose:

Adult Dose: 250-500 mg QID

Alternatives:

T½ =	1.7-3.2 hours	M/P =	
PHL =		PB =	
Tmax =	1 hour	Oral =	Complete
MW =	149	pKa =	
Vd =			

References:
1. Ostensen M, Husby G. Antirheumatic drug treatment during pregnancy and lactation. Scand J Rheumatol 1985; 14(1):1-7.

PENICILLIN G

Trade: Pfizerpen
Can/Aus/UK: Crystapen, Megacillin, Bicillin L-A, Ayercillin
Uses: Antibiotic
LRC: L1
AAP: Maternal Medication Usually Compatible with Breastfeeding

Penicillins generally penetrate into breastmilk in small concentrations which is largely determined by class. Following IM doses of 100,000 units, the milk/plasma ratios varied between 0.03 - 0.13.[1,2] Milk levels varied from 7 units to 60 units/L. Possible side effects in infants would include alterations in GI flora or allergic responses in a hypersensitive infant. Compatible with breastfeeding in non-hypersensitive infants.

Pregnancy Risk Category: B

Lactation Risk Category: L1

Adult Concerns: Changes in GI flora, allergic rashes

Pediatric Concerns: None reported via milk, but observe for changes in GI flora, diarrhea.

Drug Interactions: Probenecid may increase penicillin levels. Tetracyclines may decrease penicillin effectiveness.

Theoretic Infant Dose:

Relative Infant Dose:

Adult Dose: 1.2-2.4 million units daily
Alternatives:

T½ =	< 1.5 hours	M/P =	0.03-0.13
PHL =		PB =	60-80%
Tmax =	1-2 hours	Oral =	15-30%
MW =	372	pKa =	
Vd =			

References:
1. Matsuda S. Transfer of antibiotics into maternal milk. Biol Res Pregnancy Perinatol 1984; 5(2):57-60.

2. Greene H, Burkhart B, Hobby G. Excretion of penicillin human milk following partiturition. Am J Obstet Gynecol 1946; 51:732.

PENTAZOCINE

Trade: Talwin, Talacen
Can/Aus/UK: Talwin, Fortral, Fortral
Uses: Analgesic
LRC: L3
AAP: Not reviewed

Pentazocine is a synthetic opiate and is also an opiate antagonist. Once absorbed it undergoes extensive hepatic metabolism and only small amounts achieve plasma levels.[1] It is primarily used as a mild analgesic. No data are available on transfer into breastmilk.

Pregnancy Risk Category: B

Lactation Risk Category: L3

Adult Concerns: Sedation, respiratory depression, nausea, vomiting, dry mouth, taste alteration

Pediatric Concerns: None reported due to limited studies.

Drug Interactions: May reduce the analgesic effect of other opiate agonists such as morphine. Increased toxicity when used with tripelennamine can be lethal. Increased toxicity when used with CNS depressants such as phenothiazines, sedatives, hypnotics, or alcohol.

Theoretic Infant Dose:

Relative Infant Dose:

Adult Dose: 50-100 mg q 3-4 hours PRN

Alternatives:

T½ =	2-3 hours	M/P =	
PHL =		PB =	60%
T$_{max}$ =	1-3 hours	Oral =	18%
MW =	285	pKa =	9.0
Vd =	4.4-7.8		

References:
1. McEvoy GE. (ed):AFHS Drug Information. New York, NY: 2003.

PENTOBARBITAL

Trade: Nembutal
Can/Aus/UK: Nembutal, Nova-Rectal, Novo-Pentobarb, Barbopen, Carbrital, Lethobarb
Uses: Sedative, hypnotic.
LRC: L3
AAP: Not reviewed

Pentobarbital is a short acting barbiturate primarily used at a sedative. Following a dose of 100 mg for 3 days, the concentration of pentobarbital 19 hours after the last dose was 0.17 mg/L.[1] The effect of short acting barbiturates on the breastfed infant is unknown, but significant tolerance and addiction can occur.[2-4] Use caution if used in large amounts. No reported harmful effects breastfeeding infants.

Pregnancy Risk Category: D

Lactation Risk Category: L3

Adult Concerns: Sedation, respiratory arrest, tachycardia, physical dependence

Pediatric Concerns: None reported, but observe for sedation, dependence.

Drug Interactions: Barbiturates may decrease the antimicrobial activity of metronidazole. Phenobarbital may significantly reduce the serum levels and half-life of quinidine. Barbiturates decrease theophylline levels. The clearance of verapamil may be increased and its bioavailability decreased.

Theoretic Infant Dose: 25.5 µg/kg/day

Relative Infant Dose: 1.7%

Adult Dose: 20-40 mg BID-QID

Alternatives:

T½ =	15-50 hours	M/P =	
PHL =		PB =	35-45%
T$_{max}$ =	30-60 minutes(oral)	Oral =	95%
MW =	248	pKa =	7.9
Vd =	0.5-1.0		

References:
1. Wilson JT, Brown RD, Cherek DR, Dailey JW, Hilman B, Jobe PC, Manno BR, Manno JE, Redetzki HM, Stewart JJ. Drug excretion in human breastmilk: principles, pharmacokinetics and projected consequences. Clin Pharmacokinet 1980; 5(1):1-66.
2. Tyson RM, Shrader EA, Perlman HH. Drugs transmitted through breastmilk. II Barbiturates. J Pediatr 1938; 14:86-90.
3. Kaneko S, Sato T, Suzuki K. The levels of anticonvulsants in breastmilk. Br J Clin Pharmacol 1979; 7(6):624-627.

4. Horning MG. Identification and quantification of drugs and drug metabolites in human milk using GC-MS-COM methods. Mod Probl Pediatr 1975; 15:73-79.

PENTOSAN POLYSULFATE

Trade: Elmiron
Can/Aus/UK: Elmiron
Uses: Urinary tract analgesic
LRC: L2
AAP: Not reviewed

Pentosan polysulfate is a negatively-charged synthetic sulfated polysaccharide with Heparin-like properties although it is used as a urinary tract analgesic. It is structurally related to dextran sulfate with a molecular weight of 4000-6000 daltons. Pentosan adheres to the bladder wall mucosa and may act as a buffer to control cell permeability preventing irritating solutes in the urine from reaching the cell membrane.[1,2] Although no data are available on its transfer into human milk, its large molecular weight and its poor oral bioavailability would largely preclude the transfer and absorption of clinically relevant amounts in breastfed infants.

Pregnancy Risk Category: B

Lactation Risk Category: L2

Adult Concerns: Alopecia areata. Weak anticoagulant (1/15 th activity of heparin). Mildly hepatoxic. Headache, depression, insomnia, pruritus, urticaria, diarrhea, nausea, vomiting, etc. have been reported.

Pediatric Concerns: None reported via milk. Unlikely to enter milk.

Drug Interactions: May increase bleeding time when used with cisapride.

Theoretic Infant Dose:

Relative Infant Dose:

Adult Dose: 100 mg TID

Alternatives:

$T^{1/2}$ =	< 5 hours	M/P =	
PHL =		PB =	
T_{max} =	3 hours	Oral =	3%
MW =	6000	pKa =	
Vd =			

References:
1. Wagner WH. Hoe/Bay 946--a new compound with activity against the AIDS virus. Arzneimittelforschung 1989; 39(1):112-113.

2. Asmal AC, Leary WP, Carboni J, Lockett CJ. The effects of sodium pentosan polysulphate on peripheral metabolism. S Afr Med J 1975; 49(27):1091-1094.

PENTOXIFYLLINE

Trade: Trental
Can/Aus/UK: Trental, Apo-Pentoxifylline
Uses: Reduces blood viscosity
LRC: L2
AAP: Not reviewed

Pentoxifylline and its metabolites improve the flow properties of blood by decreasing its viscosity. It is a methylxanthine derivative similar in structure to caffeine and is extensively metabolized although the metabolites do not have long half-lives. In a group of 5 breastfeeding women who received a single 400 mg dose, the mean milk/plasma ratio was 0.87 for the parent compound.[1] The milk/plasma ratios for the metabolites were lower: 0.54, 0.76, and 1.13. Average milk concentration at 2 hours following the dose was 73.9 µg/L.

Pregnancy Risk Category: C

Lactation Risk Category: L2

Adult Concerns: Bleeding. Dyspepsia, bloating, diarrhea, nausea, vomiting, bad taste, dyspnea

Pediatric Concerns: None reported.

Drug Interactions: Bleeding, and prolonged prothrombin times when used with coumarins. Use with other theophylline containing products leads to increased theophylline plasma levels.

Theoretic Infant Dose: 11.08 µg/kg/day

Relative Infant Dose: 0.19%

Adult Dose: 400 mg TID

Alternatives:

T½ =	0.4-1.6 hours	M/P =	
PHL =		PB =	
T$_{max}$ =	1 hour	Oral =	Complete
MW =	278	pKa =	
Vd =			

References:
1. Witter FR, Smith RV. The excretion of pentoxifylline and its metabolites into human breastmilk. Am J Obstet Gynecol 1985; 151(8):1094-1097.

PERMETHRIN

Trade: Nix, Elimite, A-200, Pyrinex, Pyrinyl, Acticin
Can/Aus/UK: Nix, Lyclear, Pyrifoam, Quellada
Uses: Insecticide, scabicide
LRC: L2
AAP: Not reviewed

Permethrin is a synthetic pyrethroid structure of the natural ester pyrethrum, a natural insecticide, and is used to treat lice, mites, and fleas. Permethrin absorption through the skin following application of a 5% cream is reported to be less than 2%.[1] Permethrin is rapidly metabolized by serum enzymes to inactive metabolites and rapidly excreted in the urine. Overt toxicity is very low. It is not known if permethrin is secreted in human milk although it has been found in animal milk after injection of significant quantities IV. In spite of its rapid metabolism, some residuals are sequestered in fat tissue.

To use, recommend that the hair be washed with detergent, then saturated with permethrin liquid for 10 minutes before rinsing with water. One treatment is all that is required. At 14 days, a second treatment may be required if viable lice are seen. Elimite cream is generally recommended for scabies infestations and should be applied head to toe for 8-12 hours. Reapplication may be needed in 7 days if live mites appear.

Pregnancy Risk Category: B

Lactation Risk Category: L2

Adult Concerns: Itching, rash, skin irritation. Dyspnea has been reported in one patient.

Pediatric Concerns: None via milk.

Drug Interactions:

Theoretic Infant Dose:

Relative Infant Dose:

Adult Dose:

Alternatives:

T½ =		M/P =
PHL =		PB =
T$_{max}$ =		Oral =
MW =	391	pKa =
Vd =		

References:
1. Pharmaceutical Manufacturer Prescribing Information.

PERPHENAZINE AND AMITRIPTYLINE

Trade: Triavil, Etrafon
Can/Aus/UK:
Uses: Phenothiazine antipsychotic and antidepressant
LRC: L3
AAP: Drugs whose effect on nursing infants is unknown but may be of concern

Commonly combined in the USA with amitriptyline it is called Etrafon or Triavil. For information on amitriptyline see individual monograph.

Perphenazine is a phenothiazine derivative used as an antipsychotic or sedative. In a study of one patient receiving either 16 or 24 mg/day of perphenazine divided in two doses at 12 hr intervals, milk levels were 2.1 μg/L and 3.2 μg/L respectively.[1] The authors estimated the dose to the infant at 1.06 μg (0.3 μg/kg) or 1.59 μg (0.45 μg/kg) respective of dose. Serum perphenazine levels in the mother drawn 12 hours after doses of 16 or 24 mg/d were 2.0 and 4.9 ng/mL respectively. Hence milk/plasma ratios were approximately 1.1 and 0.7 respective of the dose. The authors estimate the dose to be approximately 0.1% of the weight-adjusted maternal dose. The authors report that during a 3 month exposure, the infant thrived and had no adverse response to the medication.

Pregnancy Risk Category: C

Lactation Risk Category: L3

Adult Concerns: Sedation, extrapyramidal symptoms, tardive dyskinesia, anticholinergic symptoms, postural hypotension, obstructive jaundice

Pediatric Concerns: None reported via milk. Observe for sedation. Rate of SIDS may be increased in infants exposed to phenothiazines.

Drug Interactions: Anticholinergics used to control extrapyramidal side effects may reduce oral absorption of perphenazine and antagonize the behavioral and antipsychotic effects of the drug. They may also enhance the anticholinergic side effects. Enhanced cardiotoxicity with cisapride. Check drug reference for numerous others.

Theoretic Infant Dose: 0.48 μg/kg/day (perphenazine)

Relative Infant Dose: 0.14 % (perphenazine)

Adult Dose: 12-64 mg daily

Alternatives:

T½ =	8-12 hours	M/P =	1.1
PHL =		PB =	
Tmax =	3 hours	Oral =	Complete
MW =	403	pKa =	7.8
Vd =	10-35		

References:
1. Olesen OV, Bartels U, Poulsen JH. Perphenazine in breastmilk and serum. Am J Psychiatry 1990; 147(10):1378-1379.

PHENAZOPYRIDINE HCL
Trade: Pyridium, Eridium, Azo-Standard
Can/Aus/UK: Phenazo, Pyridium, Pyronium, Uromide
Uses: Urinary tract analgesic
LRC: L3
AAP: Not reviewed

Phenazopyridine is an azo dye that is rapidly excreted in the urine, where it exerts a topical analgesic effect on urinary tract mucosa.[1] Pyridium is only moderately effective and produces a reddish-orange discoloration of the urine. It may also ruin contact lenses. It is not known if pyridium transfers into breastmilk, but it probably does to a limited degree. This product, due to limited efficacy, should probably not be used in lactating women although it is doubtful that it would be harmful to an infant. This product is highly colored and can stain clothing. Stains can be removed by soaking in a solution of 0.25% sodium dithionite.

Pregnancy Risk Category: B

Lactation Risk Category: L3

Adult Concerns: Anemia, nausea, vomiting, diarrhea, colored urine, methemoglobinemia, hepatitis, GI distress

Pediatric Concerns: None reported via lactation.

Drug Interactions:

Theoretic Infant Dose:

Relative Infant Dose:

Adult Dose: 100-200 mg TID

Alternatives:

T½ =		M/P =	
PHL =		PB =	
Tmax =		Oral =	Complete
MW =	250	pKa =	
Vd =			

References:
1. Drug Facts and Comparisons 1994 ed. ed. St. Louis: 1994.

PHENCYCLIDINE

Trade: Pcp, Angel Dust
Can/Aus/UK:
Uses: Hallucinogen
LRC: L5
AAP: Contraindicated by the American Academy of Pediatrics in Breastfeeding Mothers

Phencyclidine, also called Angel Dust, is a potent and extremely dangerous hallucinogen. High concentrations are secreted into breastmilk (> 10 times plasma level) of mice.[1] Continued secretion into milk occurs over long periods of time (perhaps months). One patient who consumed PCP 41 days prior to lactating had a milk level of 3.90 μg/L.[2] EXTREMELY DANGEROUS TO NURSING INFANT. PCP is stored for long periods in adipose tissue. Urine samples are positive for 14-30 days in adults and probably longer in infants. The infant could test positive for PCP long after maternal exposure, particularly if breastfeeding. Definitely contraindicated.

Pregnancy Risk Category: X

Lactation Risk Category: L5

Adult Concerns: Hallucinations, psychosis

Pediatric Concerns: Significant concentrations would likely transfer to infant. Extremely dangerous.

Drug Interactions:

Theoretic Infant Dose:

Relative Infant Dose:

Adult Dose:

Alternatives:

$T\frac{1}{2}$ =	24-51 hours	M/P =		> 10
PHL =		PB =		65%
T_{max} =	Immediate	Oral =		Complete
MW =	243	pKa =		8.5
Vd =	5.3-7.5			

References:
1. Nicholas JM, Lipshitz J, Schreiber EC. Phencyclidine: its transfer across the placenta as well as into breastmilk. Am J Obstet Gynecol 1982; 143(2):143-146.
2. Kaufman KR, Petrucha RA, Pitts FN, Jr., Weekes ME. PCP in amniotic fluid and breastmilk: case report. J Clin Psychiatry 1983; 44(7):269-270.

PHENOBARBITAL

Trade: Luminal
Can/Aus/UK: Barbilixir, Phenobarbitone, Gardenal
Uses: Long acting barbiturate sedative, anticonvulsant
LRC: L3
AAP: Drugs associated with significant side effects and should be given with caution

Phenobarbital is a long half-life barbiturate frequently used as an anticonvulsant in adults and during the neonatal period. Its long half-life in infants may lead to significant accumulation and blood levels higher than mother although this is infrequent. During the first 3-4 weeks of life, phenobarbital is poorly absorbed by the neonatal GI tract. However, protein binding by neonatal albumin is poor, 36-43%, as compared to the adult, 51%. Thus, the volume of distribution is higher in neonates and the tissue concentrations of phenobarbital may be significantly higher. The half-life in premature infants can be extremely long (100-500 hours) and plasma levels must be closely monitored. Although varied, milk/plasma ratios vary from 0.46 to 0.6.[1-3] In one study, following a dose of 30 mg four times daily, the milk concentration of phenobarbital averaged 2.74 mg/L 16 hours after the last dose.[3] The dose an infant would receive was estimated at 2-4 mg/day.[4] Phenobarbital should be administered with caution and close observation of infant is required, including plasma drug levels. One should generally expect the infant's plasma level to be approximately 30-40% of the maternal level.

Pregnancy Risk Category: D

Lactation Risk Category: L3

Adult Concerns: Drowsiness, sedation, ataxia, respiratory depression, withdrawal symptoms

Pediatric Concerns: Phenobarbital sedation has been reported but is infrequent. Expect infant plasma levels to approximate one-third (or lower) of maternal plasma level. Withdrawal symptoms have been reported.

Drug Interactions: Barbiturates may decrease the antimicrobial activity of metronidazole. Phenobarbital may significantly reduce the serum levels and half-life of quinidine. Barbiturates decrease theophylline levels. The clearance of verapamil may be increased and its bioavailability decreased.

Theoretic Infant Dose: 0.411 mg/kg/day

Relative Infant Dose: 23.9%

Adult Dose: 100-200 mg daily

Alternatives:

T½ =	53-140 hours	M/P =	0.4-0.6
PHL =	36-144 hours	PB =	51%
T$_{max}$ =	8-12 hours	Oral =	80% (Adult)
MW =	232	pKa =	7.2
Vd =	0.5-0.6		

References:
1. Tyson RM, Shrader EA, Perlman HH. Drugs transmitted through breastmilk. II Barbiturates. J Pediatr 1938; 14:86-90.
2. Kaneko S, Sato T, Suzuki K. The levels of anticonvulsants in breastmilk. Br J Clin Pharmacol 1979; 7(6):624-627.
3. Nau H, Kuhnz W, Egger HJ, Rating D, Helge H. Anticonvulsants during pregnancy and lactation. Transplacental, maternal and neonatal pharmacokinetics. Clin Pharmacokinet 1982; 7(6):508-543.
4. Horning MG. Identification and quantification of drugs and drug metabolites in human milk using GC-MS-COM methods. Mod Probl Pediatr 1975; 15:73-79.

PHENTERMINE
Trade: Fastin, Zantryl, Ionamin, Adipex-P
Can/Aus/UK: Ionamin, Duromine, Ponderax caps
Uses: Appetite suppressant
LRC: L4
AAP: Not reviewed

Phentermine is an appetite suppressant structurally similar to the amphetamine family. As such, it frequently produces CNS stimulation.[1] No data are available on transfer to human milk. This product has a very small molecular weight (149) and would probably transfer into human milk in significant quantities and could produce stimulation, anorexia, tremors, and other CNS side effects in the newborn. The use of this product in breastfeeding mothers would be difficult to justify and is not advised.

Pregnancy Risk Category: C

Lactation Risk Category: L4

Adult Concerns: Hypertension, tachycardia, palpitations, nervousness, tremulousness, insomnia, dizziness, depression, headache, cerebral infarct, paranoid psychosis, heat stroke, nausea, vomiting, physical dependence as evidenced by withdrawal syndrome.

Pediatric Concerns: Growth impairment has been reported from direct use of phentermine in children age 3-15 years.

Drug Interactions: Decreased effect of guanethidine, CNS depressants. Increased toxicity of MAO inhibitors, other stimulants.

Theoretic Infant Dose:

Relative Infant Dose:

Adult Dose: 8 mg TID

Alternatives:

T½ =	7-20 hours	M/P =	
PHL =		PB =	
Tmax =	8 hours	Oral =	Complete
MW =	149	pKa =	
Vd =			

References:
1. Silverstone T. Appetite suppressants. A review. Drugs 1992; 43(6):820-836.

PHENYLEPHRINE

Trade: Neo-Synephrine, Ak-Dilate, Vicks Sinex Nasal
Can/Aus/UK: Mydfrin, Dionephrine, Albalone, Fenox
Uses: Decongestant
LRC: L3
AAP: Not reviewed

Phenylephrine is a sympathomimetic most commonly used as a nasal decongestant due to its vasoconstrictive properties but also for treatment of ocular uveitis, inflammation, and glaucoma as a mydriatic agent to dilate the pupil during examinations and for cardiogenic shock.[1]   Phenylephrine is a potent adrenergic stimulant, and systemic effects (tachycardia, hypertension, arrhythmias), although rare, have occurred following ocular administration in some sensitive individuals. Phenylephrine is most commonly added to cold mixtures and nasal sprays for use in respiratory colds, flu, and congestion. Numerous pediatric formulations are in use, and it is generally considered safe in pediatric patients.

No data are available on its secretion into human milk. It is likely that small amounts will probably be transferred, but due to the poor oral bioavailability (< 38%), it is not likely that it would produce clinical effects in a breastfed infant unless the maternal doses were quite high.

Pregnancy Risk Category: C

Lactation Risk Category: L3

Adult Concerns: Local ocular irritation, transient tachycardia, hypertension, and sympathetic stimulation

Pediatric Concerns: None reported via milk.

Drug Interactions: Concomitant use with other sympathomimetics may exacerbate cardiovascular effects of phenylephrine. This includes albuterol, amitriptyline, other tricyclic antidepressants, MAO inhibitors, furazolidone, guanethidine, and others. Increased effect when used with oxytocic drugs.

Theoretic Infant Dose:

Relative Infant Dose:

Adult Dose: 1-10 mg IM

Alternatives: Pseudoephedrine

$T\frac{1}{2}$ =	2-3 hours	M/P =	
PHL =		PB =	
T_{max} =	10-60 minutes	Oral =	38%
MW =	203	pKa =	
Vd =	0.57		

References:
1. Pharmaceutical Manufacturer Prescribing Information.

PHENYLPROPANOLAMINE
Trade: Dexatrim, Acutrim
Can/Aus/UK: Caldomine-DH, Dimetapp, Eskornade
Uses: Adrenergic, nasal decongestant, anorexiant.
LRC: L2
AAP: Not reviewed

Phenylpropanolamine is an adrenergic compound frequently used in nasal decongestants and also diet pills, although no longer in the USA. It produces significant constriction of nasal mucosa and is a common ingredient in cold preparations. No data are available on its secretion into human milk, but due to its low molecular weight and its rapid entry past the blood-brain-barrier, it should be expected. It has recently been withdrawn from the US market.

Pregnancy Risk Category: C

Lactation Risk Category: L2

Adult Concerns: Hypertension, bradycardia, AV block, arrhythmias, paranoia, seizures, psychosis, tremor, excitement, insomnia, seizures, anorexia, and physical dependence

Pediatric Concerns: None reported via milk but observe for excitement, loss of appetite, insomnia.

Drug Interactions: Hypertensive crisis when admixed with MAO inhibitors. Increased toxicity (pressor effects) with beta blockers. Decreased effect of antihypertensives.

Theoretic Infant Dose:

Relative Infant Dose:

Adult Dose: 12.5-25 mg q 4-6 hours

Alternatives:

T½ =	5.6 hours	M/P =		
PHL =		PB =	Low	
T$_{max}$ =	1 hour	Oral =	100%	
MW =	188	pKa =	9.1	
Vd =	4.5			

References:

PHENYTOIN

Trade: Dilantin
Can/Aus/UK: Dilantin, Novo-Phenytoin, Epanutin
Uses: Anticonvulsant
LRC: L2
AAP: Maternal Medication Usually Compatible with Breastfeeding

Phenytoin is an old and efficient anticonvulsant. It is secreted in small amounts into breastmilk. The effect on infant is generally considered minimal if the levels in the maternal circulation are kept in low-normal range (10 µg/mL). Phenytoin levels peak in milk at 3.5 hours.

In one study of 6 women receiving 200-400 mg/day, plasma concentrations varied from 12.8 to 78.5 µmol/L, while their milk levels ranged from 1.61 to 2.95 mg/L.[1] The milk/plasma ratios were low, ranging from 0.06 to 0.18. In only two of these infants were plasma concentrations of phenytoin detectible (0.46 and 0.72 µmol/L). No untoward effects were noted in any of these infants.

Others have reported milk levels of 6 µg/mL[2] or 0.8 µg/mL[3]. Although the actual concentration in milk varies significantly between studies, the milk/plasma ratio appears relatively similar at 0.13 to 0.45. Breastmilk concentrations varied from 0.26 to 1.5 mg/L depending on the maternal dose.

In a mother receiving 250 mg twice daily, milk levels were 0.26 and the milk/plasma ratio was 0.45.[4] The maternal plasma level of phenytoin was 0.58. In another study of two patients receiving 300-600 mg/d, the average milk level was 1.9 mg/L.[5] The maximum observed milk level was 2.6 mg/L.

The neonatal half-life of phenytoin is highly variable for the first week of life. Monitoring of the infant's plasma may be useful; although, it is not definitely required. All of the current studies indicate rather low levels of phenytoin in breastmilk and minimal plasma levels in breastfeeding infants.

Pregnancy Risk Category: D

Lactation Risk Category: L2

Adult Concerns: Sedation, hypertrophied gums, ataxia, liver toxicity

Pediatric Concerns: Only one case of methemoglobinemia, drowsiness, and poor sucking has been reported. Most other studies suggest no problems.

Drug Interactions: Increased effects of phenytoin may occur when used with: amiodarone, benzodiazepines, chloramphenicol, cimetidine, disulfiram, ethanol, fluconazole (azoles), isoniazid, metronidazole, omeprazole, sulfonamides, valproic acid, TCAs, ibuprofen. Decreased effects of phenytoin may occur when used with: barbiturates, carbamazepine, rifampin, antacids, charcoal, sucralfate, folic acid, laxapine, nitrofurantoin, pyridoxine. May others have been reported, please consult more complete reference.

Theoretic Infant Dose: 0.44 mg/kg/day

Relative Infant Dose: 7.7%

Adult Dose: 300 mg daily

Alternatives:

T½ =	6-24 hours	M/P =	0.18-0.45
PHL =	20-160 hours(premature)	PB =	89%
T_{max} =	4-12 hours	Oral =	70-100%
MW =	252	pKa =	8.3
Vd =	0.5-0.8		

References:

1. Steen B, Rane A, Lonnerholm G, Falk O, Elwin CE, Sjoqvist F. Phenytoin excretion in human breastmilk and plasma levels in nursed infants. Ther Drug Monit 1982; 4(4):331-334.
2. Svensmark O, Schiller PJ, Buchthal F. 5, 5-Diphenylhydantoin (dilantin) blood levels after oral or intravenous dosage in man. Acta Pharmacol Toxicol (Copenh) 1960; 16:331-346.
3. Kaneko S, Sato T, Suzuki K. The levels of anticonvulsants in breastmilk. Br J Clin Pharmacol 1979; 7(6):624-627.
4. Rane A, Garle M, Borga O, Sjoqvist F. Plasma disappearance of transplacentally transferred diphenylhydantoin in the newborn studied by mass fragmentography. Clin Pharmacol Ther 1974; 15(1):39-45.
5. Mirkin BL. Diphenylhydantoin: placental transport, fetal localization, neonatal metabolism, and possible teratogenic effects. J Pediatr 1971; 78(2):329-337.

PHYTONADIONE

Trade: Phytonadione, Aquamephyton, Konakion, Mephyton, Vitamin K1
Can/Aus/UK: Konakion
Uses: Vitamin K1
LRC: L1
AAP: Maternal Medication Usually Compatible with Breastfeeding

Vitamin K1 is often used to reverse the effects of oral anticoagulants and to prevent hemorrhagic disease of the newborn (HDN).[1-3] The use of vitamin K has long been accepted primarily because it reduces the decline of the vitamin K dependent coagulation factors II, VII, IX, and X. A single IM injection of 0.5 to 1 mg or an oral dose of 1-2 mg during the neonatal period is recommended by the AAP. Although controversial, it is generally recognized that exclusive breastfeeding may not provide sufficient vitamin K1 to provide normal clotting factors, particularly in the premature infant or those with malabsorptive disorders. Vitamin K concentration in breastmilk is normally low (< 5-20 ng/mL), and most infants are born with low coagulation factors (30-60% of normal). Although vitamin K is transferred to human milk, the amount may not be sufficient to prevent hemorrhagic disease of the newborn. Vitamin K requires the presence of bile and other factors for absorption, and neonatal absorption may be slow or delayed due to the lack of requisite gut factors.

Pregnancy Risk Category: C

Lactation Risk Category: L1

Adult Concerns: Adverse effects include hemolytic anemia, thrombocytopenia, thrombosis, hypotension, prothrombin abnormalities, pruritus, and cutaneous reactions. Anaphylaxis.

Pediatric Concerns: Vitamin K transfer to milk is low.

Drug Interactions: Decreased effect when used with coumarin/warfarin anticoagulants.

Theoretic Infant Dose: 3 ng/kg/day

Relative Infant Dose:

Adult Dose: 65 µg daily

Alternatives:

T½ =		M/P =	
PHL =	26-193 hours	PB =	
T$_{max}$ =	12 hours	Oral =	Complete
MW =	450	pKa =	
Vd =			

References:
1. Olson JA. Recommended dietary intakes (RDI) of vitamin K in humans. Am J Clin Nutr 1987; 45(4):687-692.
2. Lane PA, Hathaway WE. Vitamin K in infancy. J Pediatr 1985; 106(3):351-359.
3. Vitamin and mineral supplement needs in normal children in the United States Pediatrics 1980; 66(6):1015-1021.

PILOCARPINE

Trade: Isopto Carpine, Pilocar, Akarpine, Ocusert Pilo
Can/Aus/UK: Minims Pilocarpine, Ocusert-Pilo
Uses: Intraocular hypotensive
LRC: L3
AAP: Not reviewed

Pilocarpine is a direct acting cholinergic agent used primarily in the eyes for treatment of open-angle glaucoma. The ophthalmic dose is approximately 1 mg or less per day, while the oral adult dose is approximately 15-30 mg daily.[1,2] It is not known if pilocarpine enters milk, but it probably does in low levels due to its minimal plasma level. It is not likely that an infant would receive a clinical dose via milk, but this is presently unknown. Side effects would largely include diarrhea, gastric upset, excessive salivation, and other typical cholinergic symptoms.

Pregnancy Risk Category: C

Lactation Risk Category: L3

Adult Concerns: Common side effects from ophthalmic use include burning or itching, blurred vision, poor night vision, headaches. Following oral use, excessive sweating may occur.

Pediatric Concerns: None reported via milk but observe for vomiting, epigastric distress, abdominal cramping and diarrhea.

Drug Interactions: A decreased response when added with anticholinergic agents. Diprivan and pilocarpine may increase myopia and increase blurred vision. Sulfacetamide ophthalmic solutions may precipitate pilocarpine prior to absorption and should not be used together.

Theoretic Infant Dose:

Relative Infant Dose:

Adult Dose: 5-10 mg TID

Alternatives:

T½ =	0.76-1.55 hours	M/P =	
PHL =		PB =	0%
Tmax =	1.25 hours	Oral =	Good
MW =	208	pKa =	7.15
Vd =			

References:
1. Drug Facts and Comparisons 1999 ed. ed. St. Louis: 1999.
2. Pharmaceutical Manufacturer Prescribing Information. 1999.

PIMECROLIMUS
Trade: Elidel
Can/Aus/UK: Elidel
Uses: Cytokine inhibitor used for atopic dermatitis.
LRC: L2
       L4 on nipple.
AAP: Not reviewed

Pimecrolimus is a topical agent used as a cytokine inhibitor for atopic dermatitis. While its mechanism of action is unknown, it inhibits the release of various inflammatory cytokines for T cells and many others. Systemic absorption following topical application is minimal with reported blood concentrations consistently below 0.5 ng/milliliter following twice-daily application of the 1% cream.[1] Oral absorption is unreported, but probably low to moderate as plasma levels of 54 ng/mL have been reported following twice daily oral doses of 30 mg.[2] Pimecrolimus is cleared for use in pediatric patients 2 years and older.

No data are available on its transfer to human milk, but because the maternal plasma levels are so low, it is extremely remote that this agent would penetrate milk in clinically relevant amounts. However, its use on or around the nipples should be avoided as the clinical dose absorbed orally in the infant could be significant.

Pregnancy Risk Category: C

Lactation Risk Category: L2
                             L4 on nipple

Adult Concerns: Adverse reactions include excessive skin warmth and burning. Elevated risk of skin infection (varicella zolster virus infection, herpes simplex virus infection, or eczema herpeticum) and skin cancer is possible. Hives or itching, swelling of the face, tightness in the chest, and fever have been reported.

Pediatric Concerns: None reported via milk. It is commonly used in children 2 years old and greater. It is unlikely to penetrate milk in clinically relevant amounts. Should not be used directly on the nipple, or areola.

Drug Interactions:

Theoretic Infant Dose:

Relative Infant Dose:

Adult Dose: Apply twice daily to skin.

Alternatives:

T½ =		M/P =	
PHL =		PB =	87%
Tmax =		Oral =	Moderate
MW =	810	pKa =	
Vd =			

References:
1. Pharmaceutical Manufacturers prescribing information, 2003.
2. Harper J, Green A, Scott G, Gruendl E, Dorobek B, Cardno M, Burtin P. First experience of topical SDZ ASM 981 in children with atopic dermatitis. Br J Dermatol 2001; 144(4):781-787.

PIMOZIDE

Trade: Orap
Can/Aus/UK: Orap
Uses: Potent tranquilizer
LRC: L4
AAP: Not reviewed

Pimozide is a potent neuroleptic agent primarily used for Tourette's syndrome and chronic schizophrenia which induces a low degree of sedation.[1,2]   No data are available on the secretion of pimozide into breastmilk.   Must weigh benefit to mother with possible dangers to child. Suggest extreme caution.

Pregnancy Risk Category: C

Lactation Risk Category: L4

Adult Concerns: Extrapyramidal symptoms, anorexia, weight loss, GI distress, seizures

Pediatric Concerns: None reported but caution is urged.   No pediatric studies are found.

Drug Interactions: Increases toxicity of alfentanil, CNS depressants, guanabenz, and MAO inhibitors. Do not use with macrolide antibiotics such as clarithromycin, erythromycin, azithromycin and dirithromycin, due to two reported deaths.

Theoretic Infant Dose:

Relative Infant Dose:

Adult Dose: 7-16 mg daily
Alternatives:

T½ =	55 hours		M/P =	
PHL =	66 hours		PB =	
T$_{max}$ =	6-8 hours		Oral =	> 50%
MW =	462		pKa =	
Vd =				

References:
1. Pharmaceutical Manufacturer Prescribing Information. 1996.
2. Drug Facts and Comparisons 1996 ed. ed. St. Louis: 1996.

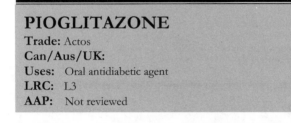

PIOGLITAZONE
Trade: Actos
Can/Aus/UK:
Uses: Oral antidiabetic agent
LRC: L3
AAP: Not reviewed

Pioglitazone is a thiazolidinediones family oral antidiabetic agent similar to troglitazone and rosiglitazone.[1]   It acts primarily by increasing insulin sensitivity.   In essence, the insulin receptor is activated reducing insulin resistance.   This family also decreases hepatic gluconeogenesis and increases insulin-dependent muscle glucose uptake.   They do not increase the release or secretion of insulin.   No data are available on its entry into human milk.

Pregnancy Risk Category: C

Lactation Risk Category: L3

Adult Concerns: Hypoglycemia, upper respiratory tract infection, headache, sinusitis, myalgia, elevated liver enzymes.   Elevated CPK. Edema, anemia, and pharyngitis have been reported but are rare.

Pediatric Concerns: None reported via milk, but no data are available.

Drug Interactions: May reduce plasma levels of oral contraceptives, estrogens, and progestins by 30% which could lead to loss of contraception.

Theoretic Infant Dose:

Relative Infant Dose:

Adult Dose: 15-30 mg once daily

Alternatives:

T½ =	16-24 hours	M/P =	
PHL =		PB =	> 99%
T$_{max}$ =	2 hours	Oral =	
MW =	392	pKa =	
Vd =	0.63		

References:
1. Pharmaceutical Manufacturer Prescribing Information.

PIPERACILLIN

Trade: Zosyn, Pipracil
Can/Aus/UK: Pipracil, Pipril, Tazocin
Uses: Penicillin antibiotic.
LRC: L2
AAP: Not reviewed

Piperacillin is an extended-spectrum penicillin. It is not absorbed orally and must be given IM or IV. Piperacillin, when combined with tazobactam sodium, is called Zosyn.[1] Tazobactam is a penicillin-like inhibitor of the enzyme beta lactamase and has few clinical effects. Concentrations of piperacillin secreted into milk are believed to be extremely low.[2] Its poor oral absorption would limit its absorption.

Pregnancy Risk Category: B

Lactation Risk Category: L2

Adult Concerns: Allergic skin rash, blood dyscrasias, diarrhea, nausea, vomiting, kidney toxicity, changes in GI flora

Pediatric Concerns: None reported via milk.

Drug Interactions: Tetracyclines may reduce penicillin effectiveness. Probenecid may increase penicillin levels.

Theoretic Infant Dose:

Relative Infant Dose:

Adult Dose: 4-5 g BID-TID

Alternatives:

T½ =	0.6-1.3 hours	M/P =	
PHL =	3.6 hours(neonate)	PB =	30 %
T$_{max}$ =	30 - 50 minutes	Oral =	Poor
MW =	518	pKa =	
Vd =			

References:
1. Pharmaceutical Manufacturer Prescribing Information. 1996.
2. Chaplin S, Sanders GL, Smith JM. Drug excretion in human breastmilk. Adv Drug React Ac Pois Rev 1982; 1:255-287.

PIRBUTEROL ACETATE
Trade: Maxair
Can/Aus/UK: Maxair, Evirel
Uses: Bronchodilator for asthmatics
LRC: L2
AAP: Not reviewed

Pirbuterol is a classic beta-2 drug (similar to albuterol) for dilating pulmonary bronchi in asthmatic patients. It is administered by inhalation and, occasionally, orally.[1] Plasma levels are all but undetectable with normal inhaled doses. No data exists on levels in milk, but they would probably be minimal if administered via inhalation. Oral preparations would provide much higher plasma levels and would be associated with a higher risk for breastfeeding infants.

Pregnancy Risk Category: C

Lactation Risk Category: L2

Adult Concerns: Irritability, tremors, dry mouth, excitement, palpitations, and tachycardia

Pediatric Concerns: None reported via milk, but observe for irritability, tremors.

Drug Interactions: Decreased effect when used with beta blockers. Increased toxicity with other beta agonists, MAOi, and TCAs.

Theoretic Infant Dose:

Relative Infant Dose:

Adult Dose: 0.2-0.4 mg q 4-6 hours

Alternatives:

$T\frac{1}{2}$ =	2-3 hours	M/P =	
PHL =		PB =	
T_{max} =	5 minutes(Aerosol)	Oral =	Complete
MW =	240	pKa =	
Vd =			

References:
1. Pharmaceutical Manufacturer Prescribing Information. 1993, 1994.

PIROXICAM

Trade: Feldene
Can/Aus/UK: Apo-Piroxicam, Feldene, Novo-Pirocam, Candyl, Mobilis, Pirox
Uses: Non-steroidal analgesic for arthritis
LRC: L2
AAP: Maternal Medication Usually Compatible with Breastfeeding

Piroxicam is a typical nonsteroidal antiinflammatory commonly used in arthritics. In one patient taking 40 mg/day, breastmilk levels were 0.22 mg/L at 2.5 hours after dose.[1] In another study of long-term therapy in four lactating women receiving 20 mg/day, the mean piroxicam concentration in breastmilk was 78 µg/L which is approximately 1-3% of the maternal plasma concentration.[2] The daily dose ingested by the infant was calculated to average 3.5% of the weight-adjusted maternal dose of piroxicam. Even though piroxicam has a very long half-life, this report suggests its use to be safe in breastfeeding mothers.

Pregnancy Risk Category: B

Lactation Risk Category: L2

Adult Concerns: Gastric distress, GI bleeding, constipation, vomiting, edema, dizziness, liver toxicity

Pediatric Concerns: None reported via milk in several studies.

Drug Interactions: May prolong prothrombin time when used with warfarin. Antihypertensive effects of ACEi family may be blunted or completely abolished by NSAIDs. Some NSAIDs may block antihypertensive effect of beta blockers, diuretics. Used with cyclosporin, may dramatically increase renal toxicity. May increase digoxin, phenytoin, lithium levels. May increase toxicity of methotrexate. May increase bioavailability of penicillamine. Probenecid may increase NSAID levels.

Theoretic Infant Dose: 11.7 µg/kg/day

Relative Infant Dose: 4.1%

Adult Dose: 20 mg daily

Alternatives: Ibuprofen

$T\frac{1}{2}$ =	30-86 hours	M/P =	0.008-.013
PHL =		PB =	99.3%
T_{max} =	3-5 hours	Oral =	Complete
MW =	331	pKa =	5.1
Vd =	0.31		

References:
1. Ostensen M. Piroxicam in human breastmilk. Eur J Clin Pharmacol 1983; 25(6):829-830.
2. Ostensen M, Matheson I, Laufen H. Piroxicam in breastmilk after long-term treatment. Eur J Clin Pharmacol 1988; 35(5):567-569.

POLIO VACCINE, ORAL

Trade: Vaccine - Live Oral Trivalent Polio
Can/Aus/UK:
Uses: Vaccine
LRC: L2
AAP: Not reviewed

Oral polio vaccine is a mixture of three, live, attenuated oral polio viruses.[1] Human milk contains oral polio antibodies consistent with that of the maternal circulation.[2] Early exposure of the infant may reduce production of antibodies in the infant later on. Immunization of infant prior to 6 weeks of age is not recommended due to reduced antibody production. At this age, the effect of breastmilk antibodies on the infant's development of antibodies is believed minimal. Wait until infant is 6 weeks of age before immunizing mother.

Pregnancy Risk Category: C

Lactation Risk Category: L2

Adult Concerns: Rash, fever

Pediatric Concerns: None reported via milk.

Drug Interactions: May have inadequate response when used with immunosuppressants. Cholera vaccine may reduce seroconversion rate when coadministered, wait at least 30 days.

Theoretic Infant Dose:

Relative Infant Dose:

Adult Dose:

Alternatives:

References:
1. Pharmaceutical Manufacturer Prescribing Information. 1996.
2. Adcock E, Greene H. Poliovirus antibodies in breast-fed infants. Lancet 1971; 2(7725):662-663.

POLYETHYLENE GLYCOL-ELECTROLYTE SOLUTIONS

Trade: Golytely, Col-Lav, Colovage, Colyte, Ocl
Can/Aus/UK: PegLyte
Uses: Bowel evacuant
LRC: L3
AAP: Not reviewed

PEG-ES is a polyethylene glycol-3350 saline laxative.[1]   It is a non-absorbable solution used as an osmotic agent to cleanse the bowel. It is completely non-absorbed from the adult GI tract and would not likely penetrate human milk.   This product is often used in children and infants prior to GI surgery. Although no data are available on transfer into human milk, it is very unlikely that enough maternal absorption would occur to produce milk levels.

Pregnancy Risk Category: C

Lactation Risk Category: L3

Adult Concerns: Diarrhea, bad taste, intestinal fullness. Do not use in GI obstruction, gastric retention, bowel preformation, toxic colitis, megacolon, or ileus.

Pediatric Concerns: None reported via milk.

Drug Interactions: Due to intense diarrhea produced, it would dramatically reduce oral absorption of any other orally administered medicine.

Theoretic Infant Dose:

Relative Infant Dose:

Adult Dose: 240 mL q 10 minutes up to 4 L

Alternatives:

T½ =		M/P =	
PHL =		PB =	
T$_{max}$ =		Oral =	None
MW =		pKa =	
Vd =			

References:
1.   Pharmaceutical Manufacturer Prescribing Information. 1996.

POLYMYXIN B SULFATE

Trade: Polysporin, Bacitracin, Ak-Spore, Akorn, Aerosporin, Neosporin, Cortisporin
Can/Aus/UK: Aerosporin, Aerocortin
Uses: Antibacterial
LRC: L2
AAP: Not reviewed

Polymyxin B is a commonly used topical, ophthalmic, and rarely injectable antibiotic. Most commonly used with other antibiotics including neomycin and corticosteroids (hydrocortisone), it is commonly used to treat conjunctivitis, blepharitis, keratitis, and other topical infections. It primarily covers most gram negative bacteria and some gram positive. It has been used in infants via injection (40,000 units/kg/d) but this is extremely rare. When applied ophthalmically, it is almost completely unabsorbed into surrounding tissues.

No data are available on its transfer to human milk. However, when used topically it is very unlikely enough would be absorbed transcutaneously to produce plasma or milk levels. Orally, it would be largely destroyed by the gastric acid in the infant as it is very unstable in acidic milieu. When applied topically to nipples in small amounts it is unlikely to produce problems in a breastfed infant.

Pregnancy Risk Category: B

Lactation Risk Category: L2

Adult Concerns: Plasma concentrations exceeding 5 μg/mL in adults may produce paresthesias, dizziness, weakness, drowsiness, ataxia, etc. But these are only seen following IM, IV, or intrathecal injections, not via topical application.

Pediatric Concerns: The adult observations are rarely seen in children.

Drug Interactions: Additive effects when polymyxin is added to neuromuscular blockers. Incompatible with acids, alkali solutions, amphotericin B solutions.

Theoretic Infant Dose:

Relative Infant Dose:

Adult Dose: Topical: 10,000-25,000 units/mL

Alternatives:

T½ =	6 hours	M/P =	
PHL =		PB =	Low
T$_{max}$ =	2 hours	Oral =	Minimal
MW =	Large	pKa =	
Vd =			

References:

POTASSIUM IODIDE
Trade: SSKI
Can/Aus/UK:
Uses: Antithyroid agent, Expectorant
LRC: L4
AAP: Not reviewed

Potassium iodide is frequently used to suppress thyroxine secretion in hyperthyroid patients. Iodide salts are known to be secreted into milk in high concentrations.[1,2] Milk/plasma ratios as high at 23 have been reported. Iodides are sequestered in the thyroid gland at high levels and can potentially cause severe thyroid depression in a breastfed infant.[1] Use with extreme caution if at all. Combined with the fact that it is a poor expectorant and that it is concentrated in breastmilk, it is not recommended in breastfeeding mothers.

Pregnancy Risk Category: D

Lactation Risk Category: L4

Adult Concerns: Thyroid depression, goiter, GI distress, rash, GI bleeding, fever, weakness

Pediatric Concerns: Thyroid suppression may occur. Do not use doses higher than RDA.

Drug Interactions:

Theoretic Infant Dose:

Relative Infant Dose:

Adult Dose: 5-10 mg daily

Alternatives:

$T\frac{1}{2}$ =		M/P =	23
PHL =		PB =	
T_{max} =		Oral =	Complete
MW =	166	pKa =	
Vd =			

References:
1. Delange F, Chanoine JP, Abrassart C, Bourdoux P. Topical iodine, breastfeeding, and neonatal hypothyroidism. Arch Dis Child 1988; 63(1):106-107.
2. Postellon DC, Aronow R. Iodine in mother's milk. JAMA 1982; 247(4):463.

POVIDONE IODIDE

Trade: Betadine, Iodex, Operand, Pharmadine
Can/Aus/UK: Betadine, Proviodine, Isodine, Viodine, Minidine
Uses: Special chelated iodine antiseptic
LRC: L4
AAP: Maternal Medication Usually Compatible with Breastfeeding

Povidone iodide is a chelated form of iodine. It is primarily used as an antiseptic and antimicrobial. When placed on the adult skin, very little is absorbed. When used intravaginally, significant and increased plasma levels of iodine have been documented. In a study of 62 pregnant women who used povidone-iodine douches, significant increases in plasma iodine were noted, and a seven fold increase in fetal thyroid iodine content was reported.[1] Topical application to infants has resulted in significant absorption through the skin. Once plasma levels are attained in the mother, iodide rapidly sequester in human milk at high milk/plasma ratios.[2,3] See potassium iodide. High oral iodine intake in mothers is documented to produce thyroid suppression in breastfed infants.[2] Use with extreme caution or not at all. Repeated use of povidone iodide is not recommended in nursing mothers or their infants.

Pregnancy Risk Category: D

Lactation Risk Category: L4

Adult Concerns: Iodine toxicity, hypothyroidism, goiter, neutropenia

Pediatric Concerns: Transfer of absorbed iodine could occur leading to neonatal thyroid suppression. Avoid if possible.

Drug Interactions:

Theoretic Infant Dose:

Relative Infant Dose:

Adult Dose:

Alternatives:

$T\frac{1}{2}$ =		M/P =	> 23
PHL =		PB =	
T_{max} =		Oral =	Complete
MW =		pKa =	
Vd =			

References:

1. Mahillon I, Peers W, Bourdoux P, Ermans AM, Delange F. Effect of vaginal douching with povidone-iodine during early pregnancy on the iodine supply to mother and fetus. Biol Neonate 1989; 56(4):210-217.
2. Delange F, Chanoine JP, Abrassart C, Bourdoux P. Topical iodine, breastfeeding, and neonatal hypothyroidism. Arch Dis Child 1988; 63(1):106-107.
3. Postellon DC, Aronow R. Iodine in mother's milk. JAMA 1982; 247(4):463.

PRAMIPEXOLE

Trade: Mirapex
Can/Aus/UK: Mirepexin
Uses: Dopamine agonist for Parkinson's disease
LRC: L4
AAP: Not reviewed

Pramipexole is a nonergot dopamine agonist for use in treating the symptoms of Parkinson's disease.[1] While rodent studies showed rather high levels in milk, rat studies simply don't correlate with humans. No human studies are available concerning levels in milk. Regardless, pramipexole is known to reduce the secretion of prolactin, and it is possible that it could significantly reduce milk synthesis. This product should probably not be used in breastfeeding mothers.

Pregnancy Risk Category: C

Lactation Risk Category: L4

Adult Concerns: Adverse events include falling asleep during the day. Such events may occur without warning. Other adverse effects include dizziness, insomnia, extrapyramidal symptoms, headache, nausea, vomiting, constipation, dry mouth, postural hypotension, and confusion.

Pediatric Concerns: None reported via milk, but inhibition of prolactin secretion could severely reduce milk production.

Drug Interactions: Cimetidine produced a 50% increase in pramipexole levels. Dopamine antagonists such as metoclopramide, domperidone, and others may significantly interfere with the activity of pramipexole.

Theoretic Infant Dose:

Relative Infant Dose:

Adult Dose: 1.5-4.5 mg/day

Alternatives:

T½ =	8 hours	M/P =	
PHL =		PB =	15%
Tmax =	2 hours	Oral =	> 90%
MW =	302	pKa =	
Vd =	7.14		

References:
1. Pharmaceutical Manufacturers prescribing information, 2003.

PRAVASTATIN

Trade: Pravachol
Can/Aus/UK: Pravachol, Lipostat
Uses: Lowers blood cholesterol
LRC: L3
AAP: Not reviewed

Pravastatin belongs to the HMG-CoA reductase family of cholesterol lowering drugs.[1] Small amounts are believed to be secreted into human milk but the levels were unreported. The effect on an infant is unknown, but it could reduce cholesterol synthesis. Atherosclerosis is a chronic process, and discontinuation of lipid-lowering drugs during pregnancy and lactation should have little to no impact on the outcome of long-term therapy of primary hypercholesterolemia. Cholesterol and other products of cholesterol biosynthesis are essential components for fetal and neonatal development, and the use of cholesterol-lowering drugs would not be advisable under any circumstances.

Pregnancy Risk Category: X

Lactation Risk Category: L3

Adult Concerns: Leukopenia, elevated liver enzymes, depression, neuropathy, etc.

Pediatric Concerns: None reported via milk but studies are limited.

Drug Interactions: The anticoagulant effect of warfarin may be increased. Use with bile acid sequestrants may reduce pravastatin bioavailability by 50%. May increased toxicities of cyclosporine. Concurrent use of niacin may increase risk of severe myopathy.

Theoretic Infant Dose:

Relative Infant Dose:

Adult Dose: 10-20 mg daily

Alternatives:

T½ =	77 hours	M/P =	
PHL =		PB =	50%
Tmax =	1-1.5 hours	Oral =	17%
MW =	446	pKa =	
Vd =			

References:
1. Pharmaceutical Manufacturer Prescribing Information.

PRAZEPAM

Trade: Centrax
Can/Aus/UK: Centrax
Uses: Antianxiety agent
LRC: L3
AAP: Drugs whose effect on nursing infants is unknown but may be of concern

Prazepam is a typical benzodiazepine that belongs to the Valium family. It has a long half-life in adults. Peak plasma level occurs 6 hrs post-dose.[1] An active metabolite with a longer half-life is produced. No data are available on transfer into human milk. Most benzodiazepines have high milk/plasma ratios and transfer into milk readily. Observe infant closely for sedation. See diazepam.

Pregnancy Risk Category: D

Lactation Risk Category: L3

Adult Concerns: Sedation, hypotension, depression

Pediatric Concerns: None reported via milk, but benzodiazepines may induce sedation in breastfed infants.

Drug Interactions: May decrease effect of levodopa. May produce increased toxicity when used with other CNS depressants, disulfiram, cimetidine, anticoagulants, and digoxin.

Theoretic Infant Dose:

Relative Infant Dose:

Adult Dose: 10 mg TID

Alternatives: Lorazepam, Alprazolam

$T^{1/2}$ =	30-100 hours	M/P =	
PHL =		PB =	> 70%
T_{max} =	6 hours	Oral =	Complete
MW =	325	pKa =	2.7
Vd =	12-14		

References:
1. Drug Facts and Comparisons 1995 ed. ed. St. Louis: 1995.

PRAZIQUANTEL

Trade: Biltricide
Can/Aus/UK: Biltricide
Uses: Anthelmintic
LRC: L2
AAP: Not reviewed

Praziquantel is a trematodicide used for treatment of schistosome infections and infestations of liver flukes. In a study of 10 women who received 1.) a single dose of 50 mg/kg or 2.) 20 mg/kg three times daily, milk and plasma levels were determined at multiple time intervals over the next 32 hours.[1] In group one, the average milk concentration was 0.190 mg/L.   In group 2, the average milk concentration was 0.198 mg/L. Throughout the duration of this study, the infants in group 1 ingested 27.4 µg and those in group 2 ingested 25.6 µg of praziquantel. On average, the plasma concentrations were four times higher than milk concentrations.   Using these data, the relative infant dose would be approximately 0.05% of the maternal dose in both groups. These values are probably too low to harm an infant.

Pregnancy Risk Category: B

Lactation Risk Category: **L2**

Adult Concerns: Fever, dizziness, headache, abdominal pain, drowsiness, and malaise

Pediatric Concerns: None reported via milk.

Drug Interactions: May increase levels of albendazole when admixed. Carbamazine, dexamethasone, and phenytoin may decrease praziquantel AUC significantly.   Cimetidine may increase plasma levels by 300%.

Theoretic Infant Dose: 29.7 µg/kg/day

Relative Infant Dose: 0.05%

Adult Dose: 10-25 mg/kg BID-TID X 1 day

Alternatives:

T½ =	0.8-3 hours	M/P =	0.25%
PHL =		PB =	80%
Tmax =	1-3 hours	Oral =	80%
MW =	312	pKa =	
Vd =			

References:

1.   Leopold G, Ungethum W, Groll E, Diekmann HW, Nowak H, Wegner DH. Clinical pharmacology in normal volunteers of praziquantel, a new drug against schistosomes and cestodes. An example of a complex study covering both tolerance and pharmacokinetics. Eur J Clin Pharmacol 1978; 14(4):281-291.

PRAZOSIN

Trade: Minipress
Can/Aus/UK: Minipress, Apo-Prazo, Novo-Prazin, Pressin, Hypovasl
Uses: Strong antihypertensive
LRC: L4
AAP: Not reviewed

Prazosin is a selective alpha-1-adrenergic antagonist used to control hypertension. It is structurally similar to doxazosin and terazosin.[1,2] Antihypertensives may reduce breastmilk production, and prazosin may do likewise. Others in this family (doxazosin) are known to concentrate in milk. Exercise extreme caution when administering to nursing mothers.

Pregnancy Risk Category: C

Lactation Risk Category: L4

Adult Concerns: Leukopenia, tachycardia, hypotension, dizziness, fainting, headache, edema, diarrhea, urinary frequency

Pediatric Concerns: None reported via milk, but some in this family are concentrated in milk. Observe extreme caution.

Drug Interactions: Beta blockers may enhance acute postural hypotensive reaction. The antihypertensive action of prazosin may be decreased by NSAIDs. Verapamil appears to increase serum prazosin levels. The antihypertensive effect of clonidine may be decreased when used with Prazosin.

Theoretic Infant Dose:

Relative Infant Dose:

Adult Dose: 3-7.5 mg BID

Alternatives:

$T\frac{1}{2}$ =	2-3 hours	M/P =	
PHL =		PB =	97%
T_{max} =	2-3 hours	Oral =	
MW =	383	pKa =	6.5
Vd =	0.6		

References:
1. Drug Facts and Comparisons 1994 ed. ed. St. Louis: 1994.
2. Pharmaceutical Manufacturer Prescribing Information. 1993, 1994.

PREDNICARBATE

Trade: Dermatop
Can/Aus/UK:
Uses: High potency steroid ointment
LRC: L3
AAP: Not reviewed

Prednicarbate is a high potency steroid ointment. Its absorption via skin surfaces is exceedingly low, even in infants. Its oral absorption is not reported but would probably be equivalent to prednisolone, or higher. If recommended for topical application on the nipple, other less potent steroids should be suggested including hydrocortisone or triamcinolone. If applied to the nipple, only extremely small amounts should be applied.

Pregnancy Risk Category: C

Lactation Risk Category: L3

Adult Concerns: Symptoms of adrenal steroid suppression, fluid retention, gastric erosions

Pediatric Concerns: None reported via milk.

Drug Interactions:

Theoretic Infant Dose:

Relative Infant Dose:

Adult Dose:

Alternatives:

T½ =		M/P =
PHL =		PB =
T$_{max}$ =		Oral =
MW =	488	pKa =
Vd =		

References:

PREDNISONE - PREDNISOLONE
Trade: Prednisone, Prednisolone
Can/Aus/UK:
Uses: Steroid, corticosteroid
LRC: L2
AAP: Not reviewed

Small amounts of most corticosteroids are secreted into breastmilk. Following a 10 mg oral dose of prednisone, peak milk levels of prednisolone and prednisone were 1.6 μg/L and 2.67 μg/L respectively.[1] In a group of 10 women who received 10-80 mg/d prednisolone, the milk levels were only 5-25% of the maternal serum levels.[2]

In one patient who received 80 mg/day prednisolone, the C_{max} at 1 hour was 317 μg/L. The AUC average milk concentration in this mother was 156 μg/L over 6 hours.[2] This is significantly less than 2% of the weight-normalized maternal dose. Because this last estimate was only determined over 6 hours and this dose was administered once each 24 hours, the total daily estimate would be much less than the 2% estimate.

In another study of a single patient who received 120 mg prednisone/day, the total combined steroid levels (prednisone + prednisolone) peaked at 2 hours.[3] The peak level of combined steroid was 627 μg/L. Assuming the infant received 120 mL of milk every 4 hours, the total possible ingestion would only be 47 μg/day.

In a group of 7 women who received radioactive labeled prednisolone 5 mg, the total recovery per liter of milk during the 48 hours after the dose was 0.14%.[4]

In small doses, most steroids are certainly not contraindicated in nursing mothers. Whenever possible use low-dose alternatives such as aerosols or inhalers. Following administration, wait at least 4 hrs if possible prior to feeding infant to reduce exposure. With high doses, particularly for longer periods, steroids could potentially produce problems in infants. Brief applications of high dose steroids are probably not contraindicated as the overall exposure is low.

Pregnancy Risk Category: C

Lactation Risk Category: L2

Adult Concerns: Gastric distress, gastric ulceration, glaucoma, thinning skin

Pediatric Concerns: None reported via milk. Limit degree and duration of exposure if possible. Use inhaled or intranasal steroids to reduce exposure. Short-term use is safe.

Drug Interactions: Decreased effect when used with barbiturates, phenytoin, rifampin.

Theoretic Infant Dose: 23.4 µg/kg/day

Relative Infant Dose: 2.0%

Adult Dose: 5-120 mg/day

Alternatives:

T½ =	24+ hours	M/P =	0.25
PHL =		PB =	75%
T$_{max}$ =	1 hour (milk)	Oral =	Complete
MW =	346	pKa =	
Vd =			

References:
1. Katz FH, Duncan BR. Letter: Entry of prednisone into human milk. N Engl J Med 1975; 293(22):1154.
2. Ost L, Wettrell G, Bjorkhem I, Rane A. Prednisolone excretion in human milk. J Pediatr 1985; 106(6):1008-1011.
3. Berlin CM, Kaiser DG, Demmers L. Excretion of prednisone and prednisolone in human milk. Pharmacologist 1979; 21:264.
4. McKenzie SA, Selley JA, Agnew JE. Secretion of prednisolone into breastmilk. Arch Dis Child 1975; 50(11):894-896.

PRIMAQUINE PHOSPHATE
Trade:
Can/Aus/UK: Primacin, Primaquine phosphate
Uses: Antimalarial
LRC: L3
AAP: Not reviewed

Primaquine is a typical antimalarial medication that is primarily used as chemoprophylaxis after the patient has returned from the region of exposure with the intention of preventing relapses of plasmodium vivax and/or ovale. It is used in pediatric patients at a dose of 0.3 mg/kg/day for 14 days.[1-3] No data are available on its transfer into human milk. Maternal plasma levels are rather low, only 53-107 nanogram/mL, suggesting that milk levels might be rather low as well.

Pregnancy Risk Category: C

Lactation Risk Category: L3

Adult Concerns: Blood dyscrasias including granulocytopenia, anemia, leukocytosis, methemoglobinemia. Arrhythmia, hypertension, abdominal pain, cramps, visual (ocular) disturbances.

Pediatric Concerns: None reported from milk.

Drug Interactions: Elevated risk of blood dyscrasias with aurothioglucose. May reduce plasma levels of oral contraceptives.

Theoretic Infant Dose:

Relative Infant Dose:

Adult Dose: 15 mg daily

Alternatives:

T½ =	4-7 hours	M/P =	
PHL =		PB =	
T$_{max}$ =	1-2 hours	Oral =	96%
MW =	259	pKa =	
Vd =			

References:

1. Mihaly GW, Ward SA, Edwards G, Orme ML, Breckenridge AM. Pharmacokinetics of primaquine in man: identification of the carboxylic acid derivative as a major plasma metabolite. Br J Clin Pharmacol 1984; 17(4):441-446.
2. Mihaly GW, Ward SA, Edwards G, Nicholl DD, Orme ML, Breckenridge AM. Pharmacokinetics of primaquine in man. I. Studies of the absolute bioavailability and effects of dose size. Br J Clin Pharmacol 1985; 19(6):745-750.
3. Bhatia SC, Saraph YS, Revankar SN, Doshi KJ, Bharucha ED, Desai ND, Vaidya AB, Subrahmanyam D, Gupta KC, Satoskar RS. Pharmacokinetics of primaquine in patients with P. vivax malaria. Eur J Clin Pharmacol 1986; 31(2):205-210.

PRIMIDONE

Trade: Mysoline
Can/Aus/UK: Apo-Primidone, Mysoline, Sertan, Misolyne
Uses: Anticonvulsant
LRC: L3
AAP: Drugs associated with significant side effects and should be given with caution

Primidone is metabolized in adults to several derivatives including phenobarbital. After chronic therapy, levels of phenobarbital rise to a therapeutic range. Hence, problems for the infant would not only include primidone but, subsequently, phenobarbital. In one study of 2 women receiving primidone, the steady-state concentrations of primidone in neonatal serum via ingestion of breastmilk were 0.7 and

2.5 µg/mL.[1] The steady-state "phenobarbital" levels in neonatal serum were between 2.0 to 13.0 µg/mL. The calculated dose of phenobarbital per day received by each infant ranged from 1.8 to 8.9 mg/day. Some sedation has been reported particularly during the neonatal period. See phenobarbital.

Pregnancy Risk Category: D

Lactation Risk Category: L3

Adult Concerns: Sedation, apnea, reduced suckling

Pediatric Concerns: Some sedation, during neonatal period.

Drug Interactions: Acetazolamide may decrease primidone plasma levels. Co-administration of carbamazepine may lower primidone and phenobarb concentrations and elevate carbamazepine concentrations. Use of phenytoin may reduce primidone concentrations. Primidone concentrations may be increased when used with isoniazid. The clearance of primidone may be decreased with nicotinamide.

Theoretic Infant Dose: 0.375 mg/kg/day

Relative Infant Dose:

Adult Dose: 250 mg TID

Alternatives:

T½ =	10-21 hours (primidone)	M/P =	0.72
PHL =		PB =	< 20%
T$_{max}$ =	0.5-5 hours	Oral =	90%
MW =	218	pKa =	
Vd =	0.5-1.0		

References:
1. Kuhnz W, Koch S, Helge H, Nau H. Primidone and phenobarbital during lactation period in epileptic women: total and free drug serum levels in the nursed infants and their effects on neonatal behavior. Dev Pharmacol Ther 1988; 11(3):147-154.

PROCAINAMIDE

Trade: Pronestyl, Procan
Can/Aus/UK: Pronestyl, Procan SR, Apo-Procainamide
Uses: Antiarrhythmic
LRC: L3
AAP: Maternal Medication Usually Compatible with Breastfeeding

Procainamide is an antiarrhythmic agent. Procainamide and its active metabolite are secreted into breastmilk in moderate concentrations. In one patient receiving 500 mg four times daily, the breastmilk levels of procainamide at 0, 3, 6, 9, and 12 hours were 5.3, 3.9, 10.2, 4.8, and 2.6

mg/L respectively.[1] The milk/serum ratio varied from 1.0 at 12 hours to 7.3 at 6 hours post-dose (mean = 4.3). The milk levels averaged 5.4 mg/L for parent drug and 3.5 mg/L for metabolite. Although levels in milk are still too small to provide significant blood levels in an infant, one should use with caution.

Pregnancy Risk Category: C

Lactation Risk Category: L3

Adult Concerns: Nausea, vomiting, liver toxicity, blood dyscrasias, hypotension

Pediatric Concerns: None reported via milk. Observe for liver toxicity, hypotension, but very unlikely.

Drug Interactions: Propranolol may increase procainamide serum levels. Cimetidine and ranitidine appear to increase bioavailability of procainamide. Use with lidocaine may increase cardio depressant action of procainamide.

Theoretic Infant Dose: 1.53 mg/kg/day

Relative Infant Dose: 5.4%

Adult Dose: 500-1000 mg q 4-6 hours

Alternatives:

T½ =	3.0 hours	M/P =	1-7.3
PHL =	13.5 hours (neonate)	PB =	16%
Tmax =	0.75-2.5 hours	Oral =	75-90%
MW =	271	pKa =	9.2
Vd =	3.3-4.8		

References:
1. Pittard WB, III, Glazier H. Procainamide excretion in human milk. J Pediatr 1983; 102(4):631-633.

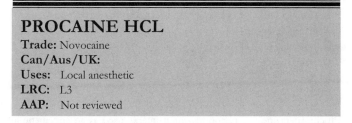

PROCAINE HCL
Trade: Novocaine
Can/Aus/UK:
Uses: Local anesthetic
LRC: L3
AAP: Not reviewed

Procaine is an ester-type local anesthetic with low potential for systemic toxicity and short duration of action.[1] Procaine is generally used for infiltration or local anesthesia, peripheral nerve block, or rarely, spinal anesthesia. Procaine is rapidly metabolized by plasma pseudocholinesterase to p-aminobenzoic acid.[2] No data are available on its transfer to human milk, but it is unlikely. Most other local anesthetics (see bupivacaine, lidocaine) penetrate milk only poorly, and it is likely that procaine, due to its brief plasma half-life, would produce even lower milk levels. Due to its ester bond, it would be poorly bioavailable.

Pregnancy Risk Category: C

Lactation Risk Category: L3

Adult Concerns: High plasma concentrations of PROCAINE due to excessive dosage, or inadvertent intravascular injection may result in systemic adverse effects involving the cardiovascular and central nervous systems including nervousness, drowsiness, or blurred vision. Allergic reactions due to the p-aminobenzoic acid metabolite have been reported and may produce urticaria and edema.

Pediatric Concerns: None reported via milk.

Drug Interactions:

Theoretic Infant Dose:

Relative Infant Dose:

Adult Dose: 350-600 mg X 1

Alternatives:

T½ =	7.7 minutes	M/P =	
PHL =		PB =	5.8%
T_{max} =		Oral =	Poor
MW =	236	pKa =	9.1
Vd =			

References:
1. Drug Facts and Comparisons 1999 ed. ed. St. Louis: 1999.
2. McEvoy GE. (ed): AFHS Drug Information. New York, NY: 1999.

PROCHLORPERAZINE

Trade: Compazine
Can/Aus/UK: Prorazin, Stemetil, Nu-Prochlor, Buccastem
Uses: Antiemetic, tranquilizer-sedative
LRC: L3
AAP: Not reviewed

Prochlorperazine is a phenothiazine primarily used as an antiemetic in adults and pediatric patients.[1] There are no data yet concerning breastmilk levels, but other phenothiazine derivatives enter milk in small amounts. Because infants are extremely hypersensitive to these compounds, suggest caution in younger infants. This product may also increase prolactin levels.[2] See promethazine as a safer alternative.

Pregnancy Risk Category: C

Lactation Risk Category: **L3**

Adult Concerns: Sedation, extrapyramidal effects, seizures, weight gain, liver toxicity

Pediatric Concerns: None reported via milk, but caution is recommended.

Drug Interactions: May have increased toxicity when used with other CNS depressants, anticonvulsants. Epinephrine may cause hypotension.

Theoretic Infant Dose:

Relative Infant Dose:

Adult Dose: 5-10 mg TID-QID

Alternatives: Promethazine

T½ =	10-20 hours	M/P =	
PHL =		PB =	90%
T$_{max}$ =	3.4-9.9 (oral)	Oral =	Complete
MW =	374	pKa =	
Vd =			

References:
1. Drug Facts and Comparisons 1995 ed. ed. St. Louis: 1995.
2. McEvoy GE. (ed):AFHS Drug Information. New York, NY: 2003.

PROGESTERONE

Trade: Crinone, Prometrium
Can/Aus/UK: Crinone, Gesterol, Cyclogest, Gestone
Uses: Progestational agent
LRC: L3
AAP: Maternal Medication Usually Compatible with Breastfeeding

Progesterone is a naturally occurring steroid (progestin) that is secreted by the ovary, placenta, and adrenal gland. Oral administration is hampered by rapid and extensive intestinal and liver metabolism leading to poorly sustained serum concentrations and poor bioavailability.[1] As progesterone is virtually unabsorbed orally, the vaginal route has become the most established way to deliver natural progesterone because it is easily administered, avoids liver first-pass metabolism, and has no systemic side-effects. Absorption through the vagina produces higher uterine levels and is called the 'uterine first-pass effect'. A study by Levine[2] suggests the area under the curve is about 38 times less with oral administration as with progesterone vaginal gel (Crinone). Thus fewer systemic effects are noted.

With the use of progesterone in breastfeeding mothers, two principles are of paramount interest. What effect does it have on milk production and the components of milk? Does it transfer into milk in high enough levels to affect the infant directly? In general, there is significant confusion in the literature as to the effect of progestins on milk composition, but the compositional changes do not appear major, volume is normal or higher, and some authors report minor changes in lipid and protein content.[3-5] However, the majority of the studies are with other progestins (e.g. medroxyprogesterone). Shaaban studied the effect of an intravaginal progesterone ring(10 mg/d) in 120 women and found no changes in growth and development of the infant or breastfeeding performance of the study participants.[6] The author suggests the ring adds a measure of safety because the amount of steroid present in milk would be effectively absorbed from the infant's gut.

The effect of progesterones on milk production is poorly studied. Early postpartum, while progestin receptors are still present in the breast, administering progestins may actually suppress milk production just as it does in the pregnant women. This has been seen occasionally in patients early postpartum. Several days to a week later, most progestin receptors disappear from the lactocyte, and breast tissues become relatively immune to the effects of progestins. Thus it is advisable to wait as long as possible postpartum prior to instituting therapy with progesterone to avoid reducing the milk supply.

The effect of progesterone therapy on the nursing infant is generally unknown, but it is believed minimal to none as natural progesterone is poorly bioavailable to the infant via milk. Several cases of gynecomastia in infants have been reported but are extremely rare.

Pregnancy Risk Category:

Lactation Risk Category: **L3**

Adult Concerns: Bloating, cramps, pain, dizziness, headache, nausea, breast pain, constipation, diarrhea, nausea, somnolence, breast enlargement

Pediatric Concerns: None reported. Not bioavailable.

Drug Interactions: May increase estrogen levels when co-administered with estrogen-containing tablets. Increased doxorubicin-induced neutropenia when co-administered. Ketoconazole may increase levels of progesterone.

Theoretic Infant Dose:

Relative Infant Dose:

Adult Dose: 90 mg daily

Alternatives:

T½ =	13-18 hours	M/P =	
PHL =		PB =	99%
T_{max} =	6 hours	Oral =	Low
MW =	314	pKa =	
Vd =			

References:
1. Levy T, Gurevitch S, Bar-Hava I, Ashkenazi J, Magazanik A, Homburg R, Orvieto R, Ben Rafael Z. Pharmacokinetics of natural progesterone administered in the form of a vaginal tablet. Hum Reprod 1999; 14(3):606-610.
2. Naqvi HM, Baseer A. Milk composition changes--a simple and non-invasive method of detecting ovulation in lactating women. J Pak Med Assoc 2001; 51(3):112-115.
3. Rodriguez-Palmero M, Koletzko B, Kunz C, Jensen R. Nutritional and biochemical properties of human milk: II. Lipids, micronutrients, and bioactive factors. Clin Perinatol 1999; 26(2):335-359.
4. Costa TH, Dorea JG. Concentration of fat, protein, lactose and energy in milk of mothers using hormonal contraceptives. Ann Trop Paediatr 1992; 12(2):203-209.
5. Sas M, Gellen JJ, Dusitsin N, Tunkeyoon M, Chalapati S, Crawford MA, Drury PJ, Lenihan T, Ayeni O, Pinol A. An investigation on the influence of steroidal contraceptives on milk lipid and fatty acids in Hungary and Thailand. WHO Special Programme of Research, Development and Research Training in Human Reproduction. Task Force on oral contraceptives. Contraception 1986; 33(2):159-178.
6. Shaaban MM. Contraception with progestogens and progesterone during lactation. J Steroid Biochem Mol Biol 1991; 40(4-6):705-710.

PROMETHAZINE
Trade: Phenergan, Promethegan
Can/Aus/UK: Histanil, Phenergan, PMS Promethazine, Avomine
Uses: Phenothiazine used as antihistamine
LRC: L2
AAP: Not reviewed

Promethazine is a phenothiazine that is primarily used for nausea, vomiting, and motion sickness. It has been used safely for many years in adult and pediatric patients for vomiting, particularly associated with pregnancy. No data are available on the transfer of promethazine into milk, but small amounts probably do transfer. However, this product has been safely used in many pediatric conditions, and it is unlikely to produce untoward effects in older infants. Observe for sedation, particularly in younger infants. Long term followup (6 years) has found no untoward effects on development.[1]

Pregnancy Risk Category: C

Lactation Risk Category: L2

Adult Concerns: Sedation, apnea, extrapyramidal symptoms

Pediatric Concerns: None reported via breastmilk, but promethazine has been implicated in SIDs. Some caution is recommended.

Drug Interactions: Epinephrine may cause significant decrease in blood pressure.

Theoretic Infant Dose:

Relative Infant Dose:

Adult Dose: 12.5-25 mg q 4-6 hours

Alternatives:

T½ =	12.7 hours	M/P =	
PHL =		PB =	76-80%
Tmax =	2.7	Oral =	25%
MW =	284	pKa =	9.1
Vd =	9-19		

References:
1. Kris EB. Children born to mothers maintained on pharmacotherapy during pregnancy and postpartum. Recent Adv Biol Psychiatry 1961; 4:180-187.

PROPAFENONE
Trade: Rythmol
Can/Aus/UK: Arythmol
Uses: Antiarrhythmic agent
LRC: L2
AAP: Not reviewed

Propafenone is a class 1C antiarrhythmic agent with structural similarities to propranolol. In a mother receiving 300 mg three times daily and at 3 days postpartum, maternal serum levels of propafenone and 5-OH-propafenone(active metabolite) were 219 µg/L and 86 µg/L respectively. The breastmilk level of propafenone and 5-OH-propafenone was 32 µg/L and 47 µg/L respectively. The milk/plasma ratios for drug and metabolite were 0.15 and 0.54 respectively. The authors estimate that the daily intake of drug and active metabolite in their infant (3.3 kg) would have been 16 µg and 24 µg per day respectively.

Pregnancy Risk Category: C

Lactation Risk Category: L2

Adult Concerns: Adverse effects include dizziness, unusual taste, first degree AV block, intraventricular conduction delay, nausea and/or vomiting, and constipation. In addition, dyspnea, CHF, and proarrhythmia has been reported. Less frequently , hepatotoxicity, agranulocytosis, leukopenia, and positive ANA have been reported. Other side effects include sexual dysfunction.

Pediatric Concerns: None reported via milk. Levels are quite low.

Drug Interactions: Increased levels with cimetidine, beta blockers, quinidine, warfarin, cyclosporin, and other drugs metabolized by this enzyme. Rifampin may reduce levels of propafenone.

Theoretic Infant Dose: 11.8 µg/kg/day

Relative Infant Dose: 0.09%

Adult Dose: 150-225 mg TID

Alternatives:

T½ =	2-10 hours	M/P =	0.15
PHL =		PB =	85-97%
T$_{max}$ =	2-3 hours	Oral =	12%
MW =		pKa =	
Vd =	4		

References:

1. Libardoni M, Piovan D, Busato E, Padrini R. Transfer of propafenone and 5-OH-propafenone to foetal plasma and maternal milk. Br J Clin Pharmacol 1991; 32(4):527-528.

PROPOFOL

Trade: Diprivan
Can/Aus/UK: Diprivan
Uses: Preanesthetic sedative
LRC: L2
AAP: Not reviewed

Propofol is an IV sedative hypnotic agent for induction and maintenance of anesthesia. It is particularly popular in various pediatric procedures. Although the terminal half-life is long, it is rapidly distributed out of the plasma compartment to other peripheral compartments (adipose) so that anesthesia is short (3-10 minutes). Propofol is incredibly lipid soluble. However, only very low concentrations of propofol have been found in breastmilk. In one study of 3 women who received propofol 2.5 mg/kg IV followed by a continuous infusion, the breastmilk levels ranged from 0.04 to 0.74 mg/L.[1] The second breastmilk level, obtained 24 hours after delivery, contained only 6% of the 4-hour sample. Similar levels (0.12-0.97 mg/L) were noted by Schmitt in colostrum samples obtained 4-8 hours after induction with propofol.[2] From these data it is apparent that only minimal levels of propofol is transferred to human milk. No data are available on the oral absorption of propofol. Propofol is rapidly cleared from the neonatal circulation.[1]

Pregnancy Risk Category: B

Lactation Risk Category: L2

Adult Concerns: Sedation, apnea

Pediatric Concerns: None reported in several studies.

Drug Interactions: Anaphylactoid reactions when used with atracurium. May potentiate the neuromuscular blockade of vecuronium. May be additive with other CNS depressants. Theophylline may antagonize the effect of propofol.

Theoretic Infant Dose: 0.11 mg/kg/day

Relative Infant Dose: 4.4%

Adult Dose: 6-12 mg/kg/hour

Alternatives: Midazolam

T½ =	1-3 days	M/P =	
PHL =		PB =	99%
T$_{max}$ =	Instant (IV)	Oral =	
MW =	178	pKa =	11.0
Vd =	60		

References:
1. Dailland P, Cockshott ID, Lirzin JD, Jacquinot P, Jorrot JC, Devery J, Harmey JL, Conseiller C. Intravenous propofol during cesarean section: placental transfer, concentrations in breastmilk, and neonatal effects. A preliminary study. Anesthesiology 1989; 71(6):827-834.
2. Schmitt JP, Schwoerer D, Diemunsch P, Gauthier-Lafaye J. [Passage of propofol in the colostrum. Preliminary data]. Ann Fr Anesth Reanim 1987; 6(4):267-268.

PROPOXYPHENE

Trade: Darvocet N, Propacet, Darvon

Can/Aus/UK: Darvon-N, Novo-Propoxyn, Dextropropoxyphene, Capadex, Paradex, Di-Gesic, Doloxene, Progesic

Uses: Mild narcotic analgesic

LRC: L2

AAP: Maternal Medication Usually Compatible with Breastfeeding

Propoxyphene is a mild narcotic analgesic similar in efficacy to aspirin. The amount secreted into milk is extremely low and is generally too low to produce effects in infant (< 1 mg/day).[1] Maternal plasma levels peak at 2 hours. Propoxyphene is metabolized to norpropoxyphene (which has weaker CNS effects). Adult half-life= 6-12 hrs (propoxyphene),

30-36 hrs (norpropoxyphene). Thus far, no reports of untoward effects in infants have been reported.

Pregnancy Risk Category: **C**

Lactation Risk Category: **L2**

Adult Concerns: Nausea, respiratory depression, sedation, agitation, seizures, anemia, liver toxicity, withdrawal symptoms

Pediatric Concerns: None reported but observe for sedation.

Drug Interactions: Additive sedation may occur when used with CNS depressants such as barbiturates. Carbamazepine levels may be increased. Use with cimetidine may produce CNS toxicity such as confusion, disorientation, apnea, seizures.

Theoretic Infant Dose:

Relative Infant Dose:

Adult Dose: 65 mg q 4 hours PRN

Alternatives: Ibuprofen, Acetaminophen

T½ =	6-12 hours (propoxyphene)	M/P =	
PHL =		PB =	78%
T$_{max}$ =	2 hours	Oral =	Complete
MW =	339	pKa =	6.3
Vd =	12-26		

References:
1. Catz CS, Giacoia GP. Drugs and breastmilk. Pediatr Clin North Am 1972; 19(1):151-166.

PROPRANOLOL
Trade: Inderal
Can/Aus/UK: Detensol, Inderal, Novo-Pranol, Deralin, Cardinol
Uses: Beta-blocker, antihypertensive
LRC: L2
AAP: Maternal Medication Usually Compatible with Breastfeeding

Propranolol is a popular beta blocker used in treating hypertension, cardiac arrhythmia, migraine headache, and numerous other syndromes. In general, the maternal plasma levels are exceedingly low, hence the milk levels are low as well. Milk/plasma ratios are generally less than one. In one study of 3 patients, the average milk concentration was only 35.4 µg/L after multiple dosing intervals. The milk/plasma ratio varied from 0.33 to 1.65.[1] Using these data, the authors suggest that an infant would receive only 70 µg/Liter of milk per day, which is < 0.1% of the maternal dose.

In another study of a patient receiving 20 mg twice daily, milk levels varied from 4 to 20 µg/L with an estimated average dose to infant of 3 µg/day.[2] In another patient receiving 40 mg four times daily, the peak concentration occurred at 3 hours after dosing.[3] Milk levels varied from zero to 9 µg/L.

After a 30 day regimen of 240 mg/day propranolol, the pre-dose and post dose concentration in breastmilk was 26 and 64 µg/L respectively.[3] No symptoms or signs of beta blockade were noted in this infant. The above amounts in milk would likely be clinically insignificant. Long term exposure has not been studied, and caution is urged. Of the beta blocker family, propranolol is probably preferred in lactating women.

Pregnancy Risk Category: C

Lactation Risk Category: L2

Adult Concerns: Bradycardia, asthmatic symptoms, hypotension, sedation, weakness, hypoglycemia

Pediatric Concerns: None reported via breastmilk in numerous studies.

Drug Interactions: Decreased effect when used with aluminum salts, barbiturates, calcium salts, cholestyramine, NSAIDs, ampicillin, rifampin, and salicylates. Beta blockers may reduce the effect of oral sulfonylureas (hypoglycemic agents). Increased toxicity/effect when used with other antihypertensives, contraceptives, MAO inhibitors, cimetidine, and numerous other products. See   drug interaction reference for complete listing.

Theoretic Infant Dose: 9.6 µg/kg/day

Relative Infant Dose: 0.28%

Adult Dose: 160-240 mg daily
Alternatives: Metoprolol

$T\frac{1}{2}$ =	3-5 hours	M/P =	0.5
PHL =		PB =	90%
T_{max} =	60-90 minutes	Oral =	30%
MW =	259	pKa =	9.5
Vd =	3-5		

References:

1.   Smith MT, Livingstone I, Hooper WD, Eadie MJ, Triggs EJ. Propranolol, propranolol glucuronide, and naphthoxylactic acid in breastmilk and plasma. Ther Drug Monit 1983; 5(1):87-93.
2.   Taylor EA, Turner P. Anti-hypertensive therapy with propranolol during pregnancy and lactation. Postgrad Med J 1981; 57(669):427-430.
3.   Bauer JH, Pape B, Zajicek J, Groshong T. Propranolol in human plasma and breastmilk. Am J Cardiol 1979; 43(4):860-862.

PROPYLTHIOURACIL

Trade: PTU
Can/Aus/UK: Propyl-Thyracil
Uses: Antithyroid
LRC: L2
AAP: Maternal Medication Usually Compatible with Breastfeeding

Propylthiouracil reduces the production and secretion of thyroxine by the thyroid gland. Only small amounts are secreted into breastmilk. Reports thus far suggest that levels absorbed by infant are too low to produce side effects.[1] In one study of nine patients given 400 mg doses, mean serum and milk levels were 7.7 mg/L and 0.7 mg/L respectively.[2] No changes in infant thyroid have been reported. PTU is the best of antithyroid medications for use in lactating mothers. Monitor infant thyroid function (T4, TSH) carefully during therapy.

Pregnancy Risk Category: D

Lactation Risk Category: L2

Adult Concerns: Hypothyroidism, liver toxicity, aplastic anemia, anemia

Pediatric Concerns: None reported, but observe closely for thyroid function.

Drug Interactions: Activity of oral anticoagulants may be potentiated by PTU associated anti-vitamin K activity.

Theoretic Infant Dose: 0.105 mg/kg/day

Relative Infant Dose: 1.84%

Adult Dose: 100 mg TID

Alternatives:

$T\frac{1}{2}$ =	1-2 hours	M/P =	0.1
PHL =		PB =	80%
T_{max} =	1-1.5 hours	Oral =	50-95%
MW =	170	pKa =	
Vd =			

References:
1.   Cooper DS. Antithyroid drugs: to breast-feed or not to breast-feed. Am J Obstet Gynecol 1987; 157(2):234-235.
2.   Kampmann JP, Johansen K, Hansen JM, Helweg J. Propylthiouracil in human milk. Revision of a dogma. Lancet 1980; 1(8171):736-737.

693

PSEUDOEPHEDRINE

Trade: Sudafed, Halofed, Novafed
Can/Aus/UK: Eltor, Pseudofrin, Sudafed, Balminil, Contac
Uses: Decongestant
LRC: L3 for acute use
L4 for chronic use
AAP: Maternal Medication Usually Compatible with Breastfeeding

Pseudoephedrine is an adrenergic compound primarily used as a nasal decongestant. It is secreted into breastmilk but in low levels. In a study of 3 lactating mothers who received 60 mg of pseudoephedrine, the milk/plasma ratio was as high as 2.6-3.9.[1] The average pseudoephedrine milk level over 24 hours was 264 µg/L. The calculated dose that would be absorbed by the infant was still very low (0.4 to 0.6% of the maternal dose).

In a study of eight lactating women who received a single 60 mg dose of pseudoephedrine, the 24 hour milk production was reduced by 24% from 784 mL/d in the placebo period to 623 mL/d in the pseudoephedrine period. While this study was done with a single 60 mg dose, if the normal dosing rate of 60 mg four times daily was used, the estimated infant dose of pseudoephedrine would have been 4.3% of the weight-adjusted maternal dose. While these results are preliminary, it is apparent that mothers in late-stage lactation may be more sensitive to pseudoephedrine and have greater loss in milk production. Therefore breastfeeding mothers with poor or marginal milk production should be exceedingly cautious in using pseudoephedrine.

Pregnancy Risk Category: C

Lactation Risk Category: **L3 for acute use**
L4 for chronic use

Adult Concerns: Irritability, agitation, anorexia, stimulation, insomnia, hypertension, tachycardia

Pediatric Concerns: One case of irritability via milk. Reduced milk production has been reported. Mothers with marginal production should avoid this medication.

Drug Interactions: May have increased toxicity when used with MAOI.

Theoretic Infant Dose: 39.6 µg/kg/day

Relative Infant Dose: 4.3%

Adult Dose: 60 mg q 4-6 hours

Alternatives:

T½ =	< 4 hours	M/P =	2.6-3.3
PHL =		PB =	
T$_{max}$ =	0.5-1 hours	Oral =	90%
MW =	165	pKa =	9.7
Vd =			

References:
1. Findlay JW, Butz RF, Sailstad JM, Warren JT, Welch RM. Pseudoephedrine and triprolidine in plasma and breastmilk of nursing mothers. Br J Clin Pharmacol 1984; 18(6):901-906.
2. Aljazaf K, Hale TW, Ilett KF, Hartmann PE, Mitoulas LR, Kristensen JH, Hackett LP. Pseudoephedrine: effects on milk production in women and estimation of infant exposure via breastmilk. Br J Clin Pharmacol 2003; 56(1):18-24.

PYRANTEL

Trade: Pin-Rid, Reese's Pinworm, Antiminth, Pin-X
Can/Aus/UK: Combantrin, Early Bird
Uses: Anthelmintic
LRC: L3
AAP: Not reviewed

Pyrantel is an anthelmintic used to treat pinworm, hookworm, and round worm infestations. It is only minimally absorbed orally, with the majority being eliminated in feces. Peak plasma levels are generally less than 0.05 to 0.13 μg/mL and occur prior to 3 hours. Reported side effects are few and minimal. No data on transfer of pyrantel in human milk are available, but due to minimal oral absorption and low plasma levels, it is unlikely that breastmilk levels would be clinically relevant. Generally it is administered as a single dose.

Pregnancy Risk Category: C

Lactation Risk Category: L3

Adult Concerns: Side effects are generally minimal and include headache, dizziness, somnolence, insomnia, nausea, vomiting, abdominal cramps, diarrhea, and pain. Only moderate changes in liver enzymes have been noted without serious hepatotoxicity.

Pediatric Concerns: None reported via milk.

Drug Interactions: Pyrantel and piperazine should not be mixed because they are antagonistic. Pyrantel increases theophylline plasma levels.

Theoretic Infant Dose:

Relative Infant Dose:

Adult Dose: 11 mg/kg X 2 over two weeks

Alternatives:

T½ =		M/P =	
PHL =		PB =	
T$_{max}$ =	< 3 hours	Oral =	< 50%
MW =	206	pKa =	
Vd =			

References:

PYRAZINAMIDE

Trade: Pyrazinamide, D-50, Mk-56
Can/Aus/UK: PMS-pyrazinamide, Tebrazid, Zinamide
Uses: Antitubercular antibiotic
LRC: L3
AAP: Not reviewed

Pyrazinamide is a typical antituberculosis antibiotic used as first-line therapy in tuberculosis infections. In one patient, three hours following an oral dose of 1000 mg, peak milk levels were 1.5 mg/Liter of milk.[1] Peak maternal plasma levels at 2 hours were 42 µg/mL.

Pregnancy Risk Category: C

Lactation Risk Category: L3

Adult Concerns: The most common side effect is hepatotoxicity, nausea and vomiting. Transient increases in liver enzymes, including fever, anorexia, malaise, jaundice, and liver tenderness have been reported.   Hyperuricemia including gout has been reported. Maculopapular rashes, arthralgia, acne, and numerous other side effects have been noted.

Pediatric Concerns: None reported via milk.

Drug Interactions:

Theoretic Infant Dose: 0.225 mg/kg/day

Relative Infant Dose: 1.58%

Adult Dose: 15-30 mg/kg daily

Alternatives:

T½ =	9-10 hours	M/P =	
PHL =		PB =	17%
T$_{max}$ =	2 hours	Oral =	Complete
MW =	123	pKa =	
Vd =			

References:
1.   Holdiness MR. Antituberculosis drugs and breast-feeding. Arch Intern Med 1984; 144(9):1888.

PYRIDOSTIGMINE

Trade: Mestinon, Regonol
Can/Aus/UK: Mestinon, Regonol
Uses: Anticholinesterase muscle stimulant
LRC: L2
AAP: Maternal Medication Usually Compatible with Breastfeeding

Pyridostigmine is a potent cholinesterase inhibitor used in myasthenia gravis to stimulate muscle strength. In a group of 2 mothers receiving from 120-300 mg/day, breastmilk concentrations varied from 5 to 25 µg/Liter.[1] The calculated milk/plasma ratios varied from 0.36 to 1.13. No cholinergic side effects were noted and no pyridostigmine was found in the infants plasma.

Because the oral bioavailability is so poor (10-20%), the actual dose received by the breastfed infant would be significantly less than the above concentrations. Please note the dosage is highly variable and may be as high as 600 mg/day in divided doses. The authors estimated total daily intake at 0.1% or less of the maternal dose.

Pregnancy Risk Category: C

Lactation Risk Category: L2

Adult Concerns: Nausea, vomiting, salivation, sweating, weakness, asthmatic symptoms, muscle cramps, fasciculations, constricted pupils

Pediatric Concerns: None reported in one study of two infants.

Drug Interactions: Increased effect of neuromuscular blockers such as succinylcholine. Increased toxicity with edrophonium.

Theoretic Infant Dose: 3.75 µg/kg/day

Relative Infant Dose: 0.08%

Adult Dose: 60-180 mg BID-QID

Alternatives:

$T\frac{1}{2}$ =	3.3 hours	M/P =	0.36-1.13
PHL =		PB =	0%
T_{max} =	1-2 hours	Oral =	10-20%
MW =	261	pKa =	
Vd =			

References:

1. Hardell LI, Lindstrom B, Lonnerholm G, Osterman PO. Pyridostigmine in human breastmilk. Br J Clin Pharmacol 1982; 14(4):565-567.

PYRIDOXINE

Trade: Vitamin B-6, Hexa-Betalin
Can/Aus/UK: Hexa-Betalin, Pyroxin, Comploment continus
Uses: Vitamin B-6
LRC: L2
      L4 in high doses
AAP: Maternal Medication Usually Compatible with Breastfeeding

Pyridoxine is vitamin B-6. The recommended daily allowance for non-pregnant women is 1.6 mg/day. Pyridoxine is secreted in milk in direct proportion to the maternal intake, and concentrations in milk vary from 123 to 314 ng/mL depending on the study. Pyridoxine is required in slight excess during pregnancy and lactation, and most prenatal vitamin supplements contain from 12-25 mg/day. Very high doses (600 mg/day) suppress prolactin secretion and therefore production of breastmilk.[1,2] Although, these data have been refuted in two studies where high doses of pyridoxine failed to suppress prolactin levels or lactation.[3,4]

However, it is not advisable to use in excess of 25 mg/day. One study clearly indicates that pyridoxine readily transfers into breastmilk and that B-6 levels in milk correlate closely with maternal intake.[5] Breastfeeding mothers who are deficient in pyridoxine should be supplemented with modest amounts (< 25 mg/day).

Pregnancy Risk Category: A

Lactation Risk Category: L2
      L4 in high doses

Adult Concerns: Reduced milk production, sensory neuropathy, GI distress, sedation

Pediatric Concerns: Excessive oral doses have been reported to produce sedation, hypotonia and respiratory distress in infants, although none have been reported via breastmilk.

Drug Interactions: Decreased serum levels with levodopa, phenobarbital, and phenytoin.

Theoretic Infant Dose: 47.1 µg/kg/day

Relative Infant Dose:

Adult Dose: 1.6 mg daily

Alternatives:

		M/P =	
T½ =	15-20 days	M/P =	
PHL =		PB =	
T_{max} =	1-2 hours	Oral =	Complete
MW =	205	pKa =	
Vd =			

References:
1. Marcus RG. Suppression of lactation with high doses of pyridoxine. S Afr Med J 1975; 49(52):2155-2156.
2. Foukas MD. An antilactogenic effect of pyridoxine. J Obstet Gynaecol Br Commonw 1973; 80(8):718-720.
3. de Waal JM, Steyn AF, Harms JH, Slabber CF, Pannall PR. Failure of pyridoxine to suppress raised serum prolactin levels. S Afr Med J 1978; 53(8):293-294.
4. Canales ES, Soria J, Zarate A, Mason M, Molina M. The influence of pyridoxine on prolactin secretion and milk production in women. Br J Obstet Gynaecol 1976; 83(5):387-388.
5. Kang-Yoon SA, Kirksey A, Giacoia G, West K. Vitamin B-6 status of breast-fed neonates: influence of pyridoxine supplementation on mothers and neonates. Am J Clin Nutr 1992; 56(3):548-558.

PYRIMETHAMINE

Trade: Daraprim
Can/Aus/UK: Daraprim, Fansidar, Maloprim
Uses: Antimalarial, folic acid antagonist
LRC: L4
AAP: Maternal Medication Usually Compatible with Breastfeeding

Pyrimethamine is a folic acid antagonist that has been used for prophylaxis of malaria. Maternal peak plasma levels occur 2-6 hours post-dose.[1] Pyrimethamine is secreted into human milk. In a group of mothers receiving 25, 50, and 75 mg/day of pyrimethamine for 10 days, the peak concentration was 3.3 mg/L.[2] An infant would receive an estimated dose of 3-4 mg in a 48 hr period (following 75 mg maternal dose). A number of reports of carcinogenesis in adults are available and indicate that infants should not be exposed to this medication.

Pregnancy Risk Category: C

Lactation Risk Category: L4

Adult Concerns: Anemia, blood dyscrasias, folate deficiency states, carcinogenesis, insomnia, headache, anorexia, vomiting, megaloblastic anemia, leukopenia

Pediatric Concerns: None reported, but possible carcinogenesis may preclude its use in breastfed infants.

Drug Interactions: Use of pyrimethamine with other antifolate drugs (methotrexate, sulfonamides, TMP-SMZ) may increase the risk of bone marrow suppression and folate deficiency states.

Theoretic Infant Dose: 0.495 mg/kg/day

Relative Infant Dose: 46.2%

Adult Dose: 25 mg q week

Alternatives:

T½ =	96 hours	M/P =	0.2-0.43
PHL =		PB =	87%
T$_{max}$ =	2-6 hours	Oral =	Complete
MW =	249	pKa =	
Vd =			

References:
1. Pharmaceutical Manufacturer Prescribing Information. 1996.
2. CLYDE DF, PRESS J, SHUTE GT. Transfer of pyrimethamine in human milk. J Trop Med Hyg 1956; 59(12):277-284.

QUAZEPAM
Trade: Doral, Dormalin
Can/Aus/UK:
Uses: Sedative, hypnotic
LRC: L2
AAP: Drugs whose effect on nursing infants is unknown but may be of concern

Quazepam is a long half-life benzodiazepine (Valium-like) medication used as a sedative and hypnotic. It is selectively metabolized to several metabolites that have even longer half-lives. In a study of four breastfeeding mothers who received a single 15 mg dose of quazepam, the average milk/plasma ratio (AUC) was 4.18.[1] The C_{max} of quazepam in milk occurred at 3 hours and was 95.8 µg/L, and over the 48 hours only 11.59 µg quazepam was recovered. The average concentration (AUC) of quazepam equivalents over 48 hours was 19.6 µg/L. However, including metabolites, the authors suggest that 17.1 µg of quazepam equivalents or 0.11% of the administered dose was recovered in milk. The authors estimated that 28.7 µg quazepam equivalents, or 0.19% of the quazepam dose would be excreted in breastmilk every 24 hours.

Pregnancy Risk Category: X

Lactation Risk Category: L2

Adult Concerns: Drowsiness, sedation

Pediatric Concerns: None reported via breastmilk. Observe for sedation.

Drug Interactions: May increase sedation when used with CNS depressants such as alcohol, barbiturates, and opioids. Cimetidine may decrease metabolism and clearance of benzodiazepines. Valproic may displace BZs from binding sites thus increasing sedative effects. SSRIs (fluoxetine, sertraline, paroxetine) can dramatically increase BZs levels by altering clearance, thus leading to sedation .

Theoretic Infant Dose: 2.94 µg/kg/day

Relative Infant Dose: 0.19%

Adult Dose: 15 mg daily

Alternatives: Lorazepam, Alprazolam

T½ =	39 hours	M/P =	4.18
PHL =		PB =	> 95%
T$_{max}$ =	2 hours	Oral =	Complete
MW =	387	pKa =	
Vd =			

References:
1. Hilbert JM, Gural RP, Symchowicz S, Zampaglione N. Excretion of quazepam into human breastmilk. J Clin Pharmacol 1984; 24(10):457-462.

QUETIAPINE FUMARATE
Trade: Seroquel
Can/Aus/UK:
Uses: Antipsychotic drug
LRC: L4
AAP: Not reviewed

Quetiapine (Seroquel) is indicated for the treatment of psychotic disorders.[1] It works similarly to other antipsychotic agents by inhibiting dopamine and serotonin receptors. It has some affinity for histamine receptors, which may account for its sedative properties. It has been shown to increase the incidence of seizures, prolactin levels, and to lower thyroid levels in adults. At present, there are no data on the transmission of quetiapine into human milk, but it has been found in rodent milk. Until we know more, this product should be considered risky for breastfeeding women.

Pregnancy Risk Category: C

Lactation Risk Category: L4

Adult Concerns: The side effects of quetiapine are similar to other anti-psychotic drugs and include sedation, tardive dyskinesia, seizures, priapism, hypothermia, dysphagia, hyperprolactinemia, orthostatic hypotension, cataracts, and hypothyroidism.

Pediatric Concerns: None reported via milk, but caution is recommended.

Drug Interactions: Phenytoin increases clearance of quetiapine significantly (5X). Other drugs which increase clearance include: cimetidine, thioridazine, and other P450 3a inhibitors. Lorazepam levels may be reduced by 20% when used with quetiapine.

Theoretic Infant Dose:

Relative Infant Dose:

Adult Dose: 300-400 mg daily

Alternatives:

T½ =	6 hours	M/P =		
PHL =		PB =	83%	
T$_{max}$ =	1.5 hours	Oral =	100%	
MW =	883	pKa =		
Vd =	10			

References:
1. Pharmaceutical Manufacturer Prescribing Information. 1999.

QUINACRINE
Trade: Atabrine
Can/Aus/UK:
Uses: Antimalarial, giardiasis
LRC: L4
AAP: Not reviewed

Quinacrine was once used for malaria but has been replaced by other preparations. It is primarily used for giardiasis.[1,2]   Small to trace amounts are secreted into milk. No known harmful effects except in infants with G6PD deficiencies. However, quinacrine is eliminated from the body very slowly, requiring up to 2 months for complete elimination. Quinacrine levels in liver are extremely high. Accumulation in infant is likely due to slow rate of excretion. Caution is urged.

Pregnancy Risk Category: C

Lactation Risk Category: L4

Adult Concerns: GI distress, liver toxicity, seizures, aplastic anemia, retinopathy

Pediatric Concerns: None reported via milk, but accumulation may occur after prolonged exposure. Use with caution.

Drug Interactions: Primaquine toxicity is increased by quinacrine. Concomitant use is contraindicated.

Theoretic Infant Dose:

Relative Infant Dose:

Adult Dose: 100 mg TID

Alternatives:

T½ =	>5 days	M/P =	
PHL =		PB =	High
T$_{max}$ =	1-3 hours	Oral =	Complete
MW =	400	pKa =	
Vd =			

References:
1. Drug Facts and Comparisons 1994 ed. ed. St. Louis: 1994.
2. McEvoy GE. (ed): AFHS Drug Information. 1992.

QUINAPRIL
Trade: Accupril, Accuretic
Can/Aus/UK: Accupril, Asig, Accupro
Uses: ACE inhibitor, antihypertensive
LRC: L2
　　　 L4 if used early postpartum
AAP: Not reviewed

Quinapril is an angiotensin converting enzyme inhibitor (ACE) used as an antihypertensive. Accuretic products also contain the diuretic hydrochlorothiazide. Once in the plasma compartment, quinapril is rapidly converted to quinaprilat, the active metabolite. In a study of 6 women who received 20 mg/d the milk/plasma ratio for quinapril was 0.12.[1] Quinapril was not detected in milk after 4 hours. No quinaprilat (metabolite) was detected in any of the milk samples. The estimated 'dose' of quinapril that would be received by the infant was 1.6% of the maternal dose, adjusted for respective weights. The authors suggest that quinapril appears to be 'safe' during breastfeeding although, as always, the risk:benefit ratio should be considered when it is to be given to a nursing mother. ACE inhibitors are generally contraindicated during pregnancy due to increased fetal morbidity.

Pregnancy Risk Category: D

Lactation Risk Category: L2
　　　　　　　　　　　　L4 if used early postpartum

Adult Concerns: Cough, hypotension, nausea, vomiting

Pediatric Concerns: None reported in one study. Levels are so low this agent is probably quite safe in most instances.

Drug Interactions: Probenecid increases plasma levels of ACEi. ACEi and diuretics have additive hypotensive effects. Antacids reduce bioavailability of ACE inhibitors. NSAIDS reduce hypotension of ACE inhibitors. Phenothiazines increase effects of ACEi. ACEi increase digoxin and lithium plasma levels. May elevate potassium levels when potassium supplementation is added.

Theoretic Infant Dose:

Relative Infant Dose: 1.6%

Adult Dose: 20-80 mg daily

Alternatives: Captopril, Enalapril

T½ =	2 hours	M/P =	0.12
PHL =		PB =	97%
T$_{max}$ =	2 hours	Oral =	Complete
MW =	474	pKa =	
Vd =			

References:
1. Begg EJ, Robson RA, Gardiner SJ, Hudson LJ, Reece PA, Olson SC, Posvar EL, Sedman AJ. Quinapril and its metabolite quinaprilat in human milk. Br J Clin Pharmacol 2001; 51(5):478-481.

QUINIDINE

Trade: Quinaglute, Quinidex
Can/Aus/UK: Apo-Quinidine, Cardioquin, Novo-Quinidin, Kinidin Durules, Kiditard
Uses: Antiarrhythmic agent
LRC: L2
AAP: Maternal Medication Usually Compatible with Breastfeeding

Quinidine is used to treat cardiac arrhythmias. Three hours following a dose of 600 mg, the level of quinidine in the maternal serum was 9.0 mg/L, and the concentration in her breastmilk was 6.4 mg/L.[1] Subsequently, a level of 8.2 mg/L was noted in breastmilk. Quinidine is selectively stored in the liver. Long-term use could expose an infant to liver toxicity. Monitor liver enzymes.

Pregnancy Risk Category: C

Lactation Risk Category: L2

Adult Concerns: Blood dyscrasias, hypotension, thrombocytopenia, depression, fever

Pediatric Concerns: None reported, but observe for changes in liver function.

Drug Interactions: Quinidine levels may be elevated with amiodarone, certain antacids, cimetidine, or verapamil. Digoxin plasma levels may be increased with quinidine. Quinidine may increase anticoagulant levels with used with warfarin. Quinidine levels or effect may be reduced when used with barbiturates, nifedipine, rifampin, sucralfate, or phenytoin. Effects of procainamide may be dangerously increased when used with quinidine. Clearance of TCAs may be decreased by quinidine.

Theoretic Infant Dose: 1.23 mg/kg/day

Relative Infant Dose: 14.35%

Adult Dose: 200-400 mg TID-QID

Alternatives:

T½ =	6-8 hours	M/P =	0.71
PHL =		PB =	87%
T$_{max}$ =	1-2 hours	Oral =	80%
MW =	324	pKa =	4.2,8.3
Vd =	1.8-3.0		

References:
1. Hill LM, Malkasian GD, Jr. The use of quinidine sulfate throughout pregnancy. Obstet Gynecol 1979; 54(3):366-368.

QUININE

Trade: Quinamm
Can/Aus/UK: Novo-Quinine, Biquinate, Myoquin, Quinbisul, Quinate
Uses: Antimalarial
LRC: L2
AAP: Maternal Medication Usually Compatible with Breastfeeding

Quinine is a cinchona alkaloid primarily used in malaria prophylaxis and treatment. Small to trace amounts are secreted into milk. No reported harmful effects have been reported except in infants with G6PD deficiencies. In a study of 6 women receiving 600-1300 mg/day, the concentration of quinine in breastmilk ranged from 0.4 to 1.6 mg/L at 1.5 to 6 hours postdose.[1] The authors suggest these levels are clinically insignificant. In another study, with maternal plasma concentrations of 0.5 to 8 mg/L, the milk/plasma ratio ranged from 0.11 to 0.53.[2] The total daily consumption by a breastfed infant was estimated to be 1-3 mg/day.

Pregnancy Risk Category: D

Lactation Risk Category: L2

Adult Concerns: Blood dyscrasias, thrombocytopenia, retinal toxicity, tongue discoloration, kidney damage

Pediatric Concerns: None reported via breastmilk in several studies.

Drug Interactions: Aluminum containing antacid may delay or decrease absorption. Quinine may depress vitamin K dependent clotting factors. Therefore increasing warfarin effects. Cimetidine may reduce quinine clearance. Digoxin serum levels may be increased. Do not use with mefloquine.

Theoretic Infant Dose: 0.24 mg/kg/day

Relative Infant Dose: 1.29%

Adult Dose: 650 mg q 8 hours

Alternatives:

T½ =	11 hours	M/P =	0.11-0.53
PHL =		PB =	93%
T$_{max}$ =	1-3 hours	Oral =	76%
MW =	324	pKa =	4.3,8.4
Vd =	1.8-3.0		

References:
1. Terwillinger WG, Hatcher RA. The elimination of morphine and quinine in human milk. Surg Gynecol Obstet 1934; 58:823.
2. Phillips RE, Looareesuwan S, White NJ, Silamut K, Kietinun S, Warrell DA. Quinine pharmacokinetics and toxicity in pregnant and lactating women with falciparum malaria. Br J Clin Pharmacol 1986; 21(6):677-683.

QUINUPRISTIN AND DALFOPRISTIN

Trade: Synercid
Can/Aus/UK:
Uses: Antimicrobial
LRC: L3
AAP: Not reviewed

Synercid is a streptogramin antibacterial agent for intravenous use only. It is indicated for the treatment of vancomycin-resistant enterococcus faecium as well as for treatment of susceptible staph aureus. It has some use against methicillin-resistant organisms. No data are available on its transfer to human milk. However, due to its acidity and large molecular weight, milk levels will probably be low.

Pregnancy Risk Category: B

Lactation Risk Category: L3

Adult Concerns: This product is well-tolerated. Infusion site problems such as pain and erythema have been reported. Headache, GI disturbances, and elevated liver enzymes reported. Arthralgia, myalgia have been reported.

Pediatric Concerns: None reported via milk.

Drug Interactions: Synercid inhibits cytochrome P450 3A4. Thus numerous interactions with other drugs metabolized by this enzyme. A partial list includes: cyclosporin, midazolam, nifedipine, and terfenadine. Check numerous other drug interactions with alternate drug source.

Theoretic Infant Dose:

Relative Infant Dose:

Adult Dose: 7.5 mg/kg q 8 h

Alternatives:

T½ =	1-3 hours	M/P =	
PHL =		PB =	32%q + 56%d
T$_{max}$ =	1 hour	Oral =	Nil
MW =	1022	pKa =	
Vd =	0.45q and 0.24d		

References:

1.   Pharmaceutical Manufacturer Prescribing Information.

RABEPRAZOLE

Trade: Aciphex
Can/Aus/UK:
Uses: Antisecretory, antacid
LRC: L3
AAP: Not reviewed

Rabeprazole is an antisecretory proton pump inhibitor similar to omeprazole (Prilosec). Rodent studies suggest a high milk/plasma ratio, but as we know, these do not correlate well with humans. No data are available in humans. Further, rabeprazole is only 52% bioavailable in adults when enteric coated due to its instability in gastric acids. As presented in milk, it would be virtually destroyed in the infants stomach prior to absorption.

Pregnancy Risk Category: B

Lactation Risk Category: L3

Adult Concerns: Asthenia, fever, allergies, malaise, chest pain, photosensitivity. Myalgia, arthritis, leg cramps, and bone pain have been reported.

Pediatric Concerns: None reported via milk.

Drug Interactions: None are reported.

Theoretic Infant Dose:

Relative Infant Dose:

Adult Dose: 20 mg daily

Alternatives: Omeprazole

T½ =	1-2 hours	M/P =	
PHL =		PB =	96.3
T$_{max}$ =	2-5 hours	Oral =	52% (enteric)
MW =	381	pKa =	
Vd =			

References:
1. Pharmaceutical Manufacturer Prescribing Information.

RABIES INFECTION
Trade: Rabies Infection
Can/Aus/UK:
Uses: Viral infection
LRC:
AAP: Not reviewed

Rabies is an acute rapidly progressing illness caused by an RNA-containing virus that is usually fatal. Infection is via other warm-blooded mammals. Incubation is prolonged and can be up to 4-6 weeks.[1] The virus multiplies locally, passes into local neurons and progressively ascends to the central nervous system. The virus is seldom found in the plasma compartment. The issue of breastfeeding following exposure to an animal bite is contentious and somewhat obscure. Person to person transmission has not been documented nor has there been documentation of transmission of the rabies virus into human milk.[2,3] If a breastfeeding woman is exposed to the rabies virus, she should receive the human rabies immune globulin and begin the vaccination series.[4] Most sources agree that once immunization has begun, the mother can continue breastfeeding. For a thorough review, see reference 4.

References:
1. American Academy of Pediatrics. In: Pickering LK, ed. 2000 Red Book: Report of the Committee on Infectious Diseases. 25th ed. ed. Elk Grove Village, IL: 2000.
2. Lawrence RA. Breastfeeding: A guide for the medical profession. St. Louis: Mosby Publishers, 1994.
3. Hall TG. Diseases Transmitted from Animal to Man. Springfield, IL: Thomas, 1963.
4. Meerwood A, Philipp B. Breastfeeding: Conditions and Diseases. 1st ed. Amarillo, TX: Pharmasoft Publishing L.P., 2001.

RABIES VACCINE
Trade: Imovax Rabies Vaccine
Can/Aus/UK:
Uses: Vaccination for rabies.
LRC: L3
AAP: Not reviewed

Rabies vaccine is prepared from inactivated rabies virus. No data are available on transmission to breastmilk. Even if transferred to breastmilk, it is unlikely to produce untoward effects.[1]

Pregnancy Risk Category:

Lactation Risk Category: L3

Adult Concerns: Rash, anaphylactoid reactions, nausea, vomiting, diarrhea, etc.

Pediatric Concerns: No untoward effect reported.

Drug Interactions:

Theoretic Infant Dose:

Relative Infant Dose:

Adult Dose: 1 mL X 3 over 21-28 days

Alternatives:

References:
1.   Pharmaceutical Manufacturer Prescribing Information. 1995.

RADIOPAQUE AGENTS

Trade: Omnipaque, Conray, Cholebrine, Telepaque, Oragrafin, Bilivist, HypaqueOptiray, Radiocontrast Agents

Can/Aus/UK:

Uses: Radiocontrast agents

LRC: L2

AAP: Some approved by the American Academy of Pediatrics for use in breastfeeding mothers

Radiocontrast or radiopaque agents are opaque to X-rays and are used to visualize blood vessels in various tissues. Barium sulfate was one of the original agents used, while organic iodinated compounds are used primarily in CAT scans and for various X-ray procedures. While iodinated products in general are contraindicated in breastfeeding mothers due to the high milk transfer of iodine, in these products the iodine is covalently bound to the organic molecule and is metabolically stable and essentially not bioavailable. For the most part, these organic radiocontrast agents are rapidly excreted without significant metabolism, and the amount of elemental iodine released is minimal.[1] Virtually all of these agents have very short plasma half-lives (< 1 h), and for those studied, milk concentrations are extremely low (see table below).[2,3,4,5,6] Of the minimal amount in milk, virtually none is bioavailable to the infant as these agents are largely unabsorbed orally. According to several manufacturers, less than 0.005% of the iodine is free. These contrast agents are in essence pharmacologically inert, not metabolized, unabsorbed, and are rapidly excreted by the kidney (80-90% with 24 hrs). See appendix for tables.

Pregnancy Risk Category:

Lactation Risk Category: L2

Adult Concerns: GI distress, rash, anaphylaxis

Pediatric Concerns: None reported via milk. Commonly used in pediatric patients for diagnostic purposes.

Drug Interactions:

Theoretic Infant Dose:

Relative Infant Dose:

Adult Dose:

Alternatives:

$T\frac{1}{2}$ =	20-90 minutes	M/P =	
PHL =		PB =	0-10%
T_{max} =	< 1 hour	Oral =	Minimal
MW =		pKa =	
Vd =			

References:

1. Pharmaceutical Manufacturer Prescribing Information. 1993.
2. Nielsen ST, Matheson I, Rasmussen JN, Skinnemoen K, Andrew E, Hafsahl G. Excretion of iohexol and metrizoate in human breastmilk. Acta Radiol 1987; 28(5):523-526.
3. HOLMDAHL KH. Cholecystography during lactation. Acta Radiol 1956; 45(4):305-307.
4. Ilett KF, Hackett LP, Paterson JW, McCormick CC. Excretion of metrizamide in milk. Br J Radiol 1981; 54(642):537-538.
5. Rofsky NM, Weinreb JC, Litt AW. Quantitative analysis of gadopentetate dimeglumine excreted in breastmilk. J Magn Reson Imaging 1993; 3(1):131-132.
6. FitzJohn TP, Williams DG, Laker MF, Owen JP. Intravenous urography during lactation. Br J Radiol 1982; 55(656):603-605.

RAMIPRIL

Trade: Altace
Can/Aus/UK: Altace, Ramace, Tritace
Uses: ACE inhibitor, antihypertensive
LRC: L3
AAP: Not reviewed

Ramipril is rapidly metabolized to ramiprilat which is a potent ACE inhibitor with a long half-life. It is used in hypertension. ACE inhibitors can cause increased fetal and neonatal morbidity and should not be used in pregnant women. Ingestion of a single 10 mg oral dose produced an undetectable level in breastmilk.[1,2] However, animal studies have indicated that ramiprilat is transferred into milk in concentrations about one-third of those found in serum, but animal studies (lactation) are always high and do not at all correlate with humans. Only 0.25% of the total dose is estimated to penetrate into milk.

Pregnancy Risk Category: D

Lactation Risk Category: L3

Adult Concerns: Hypotension, cough, nausea, vomiting, dizziness

Pediatric Concerns: None reported via milk. Observe for hypotension.

Drug Interactions: Probenecid increases plasma levels of ACEi. ACEi and diuretics have additive hypotensive effects. Antacids reduce bioavailability of ACE inhibitors. NSAIDS reduce hypotension of ACE inhibitors. Phenothiazines increase effects of ACEi. ACEi increase digoxin and lithium plasma levels. May elevate potassium levels when potassium supplementation is added.

Theoretic Infant Dose:

Relative Infant Dose: 0.25%

Adult Dose: 2.5-20 mg daily
Alternatives: Captopril, Enalapril

T½ =	13-17 hours	M/P =	
PHL =		PB =	56%
T$_{max}$ =	2-4 hours	Oral =	60%
MW =	417	pKa =	
Vd =			

References:
1. Pharmaceutical Manufacturer Prescribing Information. 1996.
2. Ball SG, Robertson JI. Clinical pharmacology of ramipril. Am J Cardiol 1987; 59(10):23D-27D.

RANITIDINE

Trade: Zantac
Can/Aus/UK: Apo-Ranitidine, Novo-Ranidine, Zantac, Nu-Ranit
Uses: Reduces gastric acid secretion
LRC: L2
AAP: Not reviewed

Ranitidine is a prototypical histamine-2 blocker used to reduce acid secretion in the stomach. It has been widely used in pediatrics without significant side effects primarily for gastroesophageal reflux (GER). Following a dose of 150 mg for four doses, concentrations in breastmilk were 0.72, 2.6, and 1.5 mg/L at 1.5, 5.5, and 12 hours respectively.[1] The milk/serum ratios varied from 6.81, 8.44 to 23.77 at 1.5, 5.5, and 12 hours respectively. Although the milk/plasma ratios are quite high, using these data, an infant would ingest at most 0.4 mg/kg/d. This amount is quite small considering the pediatric dose currently recommended is 2-4 mg/kg/24 hours. See nizatidine or famotidine for alternatives.

Pregnancy Risk Category: B

Lactation Risk Category: L2

Adult Concerns: Side effects are generally minimal and include headache, GI distress, and dizziness.

Pediatric Concerns: None reported via milk. Although ranitidine is concentrated in milk, the overall dose is less than therapeutic.

Drug Interactions: Ranitidine may decrease the renal clearance of procainamide. May decrease oral absorption of diazepam. Ranitidine may increase the hypoglycemic effect of glipizide or glyburide. Ranitidine may reduce warfarin clearance, thus increasing anticoagulation.

Theoretic Infant Dose: 0.39 mg/kg/day

Relative Infant Dose: 4.55%

Adult Dose: 150 mg BID

Alternatives: Famotidine, Nizatidine

$T\frac{1}{2}$ =	2-3 hours	M/P =	1.9-6.7
PHL =		PB =	15%
T_{max} =	1-3 hours	Oral =	50%
MW =	314	pKa =	2.3,8.2
Vd =	1.6-2.4		

References:
1. Kearns GL, McConnell RF, Jr., Trang JM, Kluza RB. Appearance of ranitidine in breastmilk following multiple dosing. Clin Pharm 1985; 4(3):322-324.

REMIFENTANIL

Trade: Ultiva
Can/Aus/UK: Ultiva
Uses: Opioid analgesic
LRC: L3
AAP: Not reviewed

Remifentanil is a new opioid analgesic similar in potency and use as fentanyl. It is primarily metabolized by plasma and tissue esterases (in adults and neonates) and has an incredibly short elimination half-life of only 10-20 minutes, with an effective biological half-life of only 3 to 10 minutes.[1] Unlike other fentanyl analogs, the half-life of remifentanil does not increase with prolonged administration. Although remifentanil has been found in rodent milk, no data are available on its transfer into human milk. It is cleared for use in children > 2 years of age. As an analog of fentanyl, breastmilk levels should be similar and probably exceedingly low. In addition, remifentanil metabolism is not dependent on liver function and should be exceedingly short even in neonates. Due to its kinetics and brief half-life and its poor oral bioavailability, it is unlikely this product will produce clinically relevant levels in human breastmilk.

Pregnancy Risk Category: C

Lactation Risk Category: L3

Adult Concerns: Nausea, hypotension, sedation, vomiting, bradycardia

Pediatric Concerns: None reported via milk. Not orally bioavailable.

Drug Interactions: May potentiate the effects of other opioids.

Theoretic Infant Dose:

Relative Infant Dose:

Adult Dose: 0.25-0.4 µg/kg/minute

Alternatives:

T½ =	10-20 minutes	M/P =		
PHL =		PB =	70%	
T$_{max}$ =		Oral =	Poor	
MW =	412	pKa =	7.07	
Vd =	0.1			

References:
1.   Pharmaceutical Manufacturer Prescribing Information. 1997.

REPAGLINIDE

Trade: Prandin
Can/Aus/UK: Gluconorm, Novonorm
Uses: Antidiabetic agent
LRC: L4
AAP: Not reviewed

Repaglinide is a non-sulfonyluric hypoglycemic agent that lowers blood glucose levels in Type 2 non-insulin dependent diabetics by stimulating the release of insulin from functional beta cells. No data are available on its transfer to human milk, but rodent studies suggest that it may transfer into milk and induce hypoglycemic and skeletal changes in young animals via milk. Unfortunately, no dosing regimens were mentioned in these studies, so it is not known if normal therapeutic doses would produce such changes in humans. Dosing of repaglinide is rather unique, with doses taken prior to each meal due to its short half-life and according to the need of each patient. At this point, we do not know if it is safe for use in breastfeeding patients. But if it is used, the infant should be closely monitored for hypoglycemia and should not be fed until at least several hours after the dose to reduce exposure.

Pregnancy Risk Category: C

Lactation Risk Category: L4

Adult Concerns: In adults, hypoglycemia and headache were the most common side effects.

Pediatric Concerns: Hypoglycemia in animal studies via milk, but doses were not mentioned.

Drug Interactions: Metabolism and increased effect may occur when used with azole antifungals such as ketoconazole, itraconazole, and other drugs which inhibit liver enzymes such as erythromycin. Decreased effect may result following use of rifampin, troglitazone, barbiturates, and carbamazepine. Reduced protein binding and increased effect may result when repaglinide is used with NSAIDs, salicylates, sulfonamides, etc. Numerous other drugs may interfere with the hypoglycemic effect. Check a drug interaction reference for a complete listing. Use with gemfibrozil (Lopid) may cause a significant reduction in blood glucose levels.

Theoretic Infant Dose:

Relative Infant Dose:

Adult Dose: 0.5-4 mg BID-QID

Alternatives:

$T\frac{1}{2}$ =	1 hour	M/P =		
PHL =		PB =	98%	
T_{max} =	1 hour	Oral =	56%	
MW =		pKa =		
Vd =	31			

References:
1. Pharmaceutical Manufacturer Prescribing Information. 1999.
2. Drug Facts and Comparisons 1999 ed. ed. St. Louis: 1999.

RESERPINE

Trade: Raudixin, Serpasil
Can/Aus/UK: Serpasil, Adelphane, Abicol
Uses: Antihypertensive
LRC: L4
AAP: Not reviewed

Reserpine is an old and seldom used antihypertensive. Reserpine is known to be secreted into human milk although the levels are unreported.[1-3] Increased respiratory tract secretions, severe nasal congestion, cyanosis, and loss of appetite can occur. Some reports suggest no observable effect but should use with extreme caution if at all. Because safer, more effective products are available, reserpine should be avoided in lactating patients.

Pregnancy Risk Category: C

Lactation Risk Category: L4

Adult Concerns: Hypotonia, sedation, hypotension, nasal congestion, diarrhea, nausea, vomiting

Pediatric Concerns: None reported via milk, but observe for nasal stuffiness, sedation, hypotonia. Use with caution.

Drug Interactions: Reserpine may decrease the effect of other sympathomimetics.   May increase effect of MAOI and tricyclic antidepressants.

Theoretic Infant Dose:

Relative Infant Dose:

Adult Dose: 125-250 µg daily-BID

Alternatives:

T½ =	50-100 hours	M/P =	
PHL =		PB =	96%
T$_{max}$ =	2 hours	Oral =	40%
MW =	609	pKa =	
Vd =			

References:
1. O'Brien TE. Excretion of drugs in human milk. Am J Hosp Pharm 1974; 31(9):844-854.
2. Vorherr H. Drug excretion in breastmilk. Postgrad Med 1974; 56(4):97-104.
3. Anderson PO. Drugs and breast feeding. Semin Perinatol 1979; 3(3):271-278.

RHO (D) IMMUNE GLOBULIN

Trade: Rhogam, Gamulin Rh, Hyprho-D, Mini-Gamulin Rh
Can/Aus/UK:
Uses: Immune globulin
LRC: L2
AAP: Not reviewed

RHO(D) immune globulin is an immune globulin prepared from human plasma containing high concentrations of Rh antibodies. Only trace amounts of anti-Rh are present in colostrum and none in mature milk in women receiving large doses of Rh immune globulin.   No untoward effects have been reported.   Most immunoglobulins are destroyed in the gastric acidity of the newborn infant.   Rh immune globulins are not contraindicated in breastfeeding mothers.[1]

Pregnancy Risk Category:

Lactation Risk Category: L2

Adult Concerns: Infrequent allergies, discomfort at injection site.

Pediatric Concerns: None reported via milk.

Drug Interactions:

Theoretic Infant Dose:

Relative Infant Dose:

Adult Dose: 300 µg X 1-2

Alternatives:

T½ =	24 days	M/P =	
PHL =		PB =	
T$_{max}$ =		Oral =	None
MW =		pKa =	
Vd =			

References:
1. Lawrence RA. Breastfeeding: A guide for the medical profession. St. Louis: Mosby Publishers, 1994.

RIBAVIRIN

Trade: Virazole, Rebetol
Can/Aus/UK: Virazole, Virazide
Uses: Antiviral agent.
LRC: L4
AAP: Not reviewed

Ribavirin is a synthetic nucleoside used as an antiviral agent and is effective in a wide variety of viral infections.[1]   It has heretofore been used acutely in respiratory syncytial virus infections in infants without major complications. However, its current use in breastfeeding patients for treatment of Hepatitis C infections, when combined with interferon alfa (Rebetron) for periods up to one year, may be more problematic as high concentrations of ribavirin could accumulate in the breastfed infant. No data are available on its transfer to human milk, but it is probably low and its oral bioavailability is low as well. However, ribavirin concentrates in peripheral tissues and in the red blood cells in high concentrations over time (Vd= 802)[2]. Its elimination half-life at steady state averages 298 hours, which reflects slow elimination from nonplasma compartments. Red cell concentrations on average are 60 fold higher than plasma levels and may account for the occasional hemolytic anemia. It is likely the acute exposure of a breastfed infant would produce minimal side effects. However, chronic exposure over 6-12 months may be more risky, so caution is recommended.

Pregnancy Risk Category: X

Lactation Risk Category: L4

Adult Concerns: Rash, conjunctivitis, hemolytic anemia, congestive heart failure, seizures, asthenia, hypotension, bradycardia, reticulocytosis, bronchospasm, pulmonary edema, etc. Ribavirin may be a potent teratogen. Nursing personnel exposed to inhaled ribavirin should avoid environmental exposure.

Pediatric Concerns: None yet reported via breastmilk.

Drug Interactions:

Theoretic Infant Dose:

Relative Infant Dose:

Adult Dose: 12.5 L mist/minute (190 µg/L) 12-18 hours daily

Alternatives:

$T\frac{1}{2}$ =	298 hours (SS)	M/P =	
PHL =		PB =	0%
T_{max} =	1.5 hours	Oral =	44%
MW =	244	pKa =	
Vd =	40.4		

References:
1. Pharmaceutical Manufacturer Prescribing Information. 1999.
2. Lertora JJ, Rege AB, Lacour JT, Ferencz N, George WJ, VanDyke RB, Agrawal KC, Hyslop NE, Jr. Pharmacokinetics and long-term tolerance to ribavirin in asymptomatic patients infected with human immunodeficiency virus. Clin Pharmacol Ther 1991; 50(4):442-449.

RIBAVIRIN + INTERFERON ALFA-2B

Trade: Rebetron
Can/Aus/UK:
Uses: Antivirals for Hepatitis C treatment
LRC: L4
AAP: Not reviewed

Rebetron is a combination product containing the antiviral Ribavirin and the immunomodulator drug called interferon alfa-2b. This new combination product is indicated for the long-term treatment of hepatitis C. The typical dose for an individual < 75 kg consists of 1000 mg ribavirin daily in divided doses and 3 million units of interferon three times weekly.

Ribavirin is a synthetic nucleoside used as an antiviral agent and is effective in a wide variety of viral infections. It has heretofore been used acutely in respiratory syncytial virus infections in infants without major complications. However, its current use in breastfeeding patients for treatment of Hepatitis C infections, when combined with interferon alfa (Rebetron) for periods up to one year, may be more problematic as high concentrations of ribavirin could accumulate in the breast fed infant over time. No data are available on its transfer to human milk, but it is probably low and its oral bioavailability is low as well. However, ribavirin concentrates in peripheral tissues and in the red blood cells in high concentrations over time (Vd= 802).[1] Its elimination half-life at steady state averages 298 hours, which reflects slow elimination from nonplasma compartments. Red cell concentrations on average are 60 fold higher than plasma levels and may account for the occasional hemolytic anemia. It is likely that acute exposure of a breastfed infant would produce minimal side effects. However, chronic exposure over 12 months may be more risky, so caution is recommended.

Very little is known about the secretion of interferons in human milk although some interferons are known to be secreted normally and may contribute to the antiviral properties of human milk. However, interferons are large in molecular weight (16-28,000 daltons) which would limit their transfer into human milk. Following treatment with a massive dose of 30 million units IV of interferon alpha in a breastfeeding patient, the amount of interferon alpha transferred into human milk was 894, 1004, 1551, 1507, 788, 721 IU at 0 (baseline), 2, 4, 8, 12, and 24 hours respectively.[2] Hence, even following a massive dose, no change in breastmilk levels were noted. One thousand international units is roughly equivalent to 500 nanograms of interferon. So it is unlikely that the interferon in Rebetron would transfer to milk or the infant in amounts clinically relevant.

Rebetron is extremely dangerous to a fetus and is extremely teratogenic at doses even 1/20th of the above therapeutic doses. Pregnancy must be strictly avoided if this product is used in either the male or female partner. Due to the long half-life of this product, pregnancy should be avoided for at least 6 months following use.

Pregnancy Risk Category: X

Lactation Risk Category: L4

Adult Concerns: Anemia, insomnia, depression, and irritability are common.   Headache, fatigue, rigors, fever, flu-like symptoms, dizziness, nausea, myalgia, insomnia, and numerous other symptoms are typical.

Pediatric Concerns: None reported via breastmilk, but caution is recommended.

Drug Interactions:

Theoretic Infant Dose:

Relative Infant Dose:

Adult Dose:

Alternatives:

T½ = PHL = T~max~ = MW = Vd =	298 hours	M/P = PB = Oral = pKa =

References:

1. Lertora JJ, Rege AB, Lacour JT, Ferencz N, George WJ, VanDyke RB, Agrawal KC, Hyslop NE, Jr. Pharmacokinetics and long-term tolerance to ribavirin in asymptomatic patients infected with human immunodeficiency virus. Clin Pharmacol Ther 1991; 50(4):442-449.
2. Kumar AR, Hale TW, Mock RE. Transfer of interferon alfa into human breastmilk. J Hum Lact 2000; 16(3):226-228.

RIBOFLAVIN

Trade: Vitamin B-2
Can/Aus/UK: Abdec, Accomin
Uses: Vitamin B2
LRC: L1
AAP: Maternal Medication Usually Compatible with Breastfeeding

Riboflavin is a B complex vitamin, also called Vitamin B-2. Riboflavin is absorbed by the small intestine by a well established transport mechanism. It is easily saturable, so excessive levels are not absorbed. Riboflavin is transported into human milk in concentrations proportional to dietary intake but generally averaged 400 ng/mL.[1] Maternal supplementation is permitted if dose is small (2 mg/day). No untoward effects have been reported.

Pregnancy Risk Category: A

Lactation Risk Category: L1

Adult Concerns: Yellow colored urine

Pediatric Concerns: None reported via milk.

Drug Interactions:

Theoretic Infant Dose: 60 ng/kg/day

Relative Infant Dose:

Adult Dose: 1-4 mg daily

Alternatives:

T½ =	14 hours	M/P =	
PHL =		PB =	
T_max =	Rapid	Oral =	Complete
MW =	376	pKa =	
Vd =			

References:
1. Deodhar AD, Hajalakshmi R, Ramakrishnan CV. Studies on human lactation. III. Effect of dietary vitamin supplementation on vitamin contents of breastfmilk. Acta Paediatr 1964; 53:42-48.

RIFAMPIN

Trade: Rifadin, Rimactane
Can/Aus/UK: Rifadin, Rimactane, Rofact, Rifampicin, Rimycin,
Uses: Antitubercular drug
LRC: L2
AAP: Maternal Medication Usually Compatible with Breastfeeding

Rifampin is a broad spectrum antibiotic with particular activity against tuberculosis. It is secreted into breastmilk in very small levels. One report indicates that following a single 450 mg oral dose, maternal plasma levels averaged 21.3 mg/L, and milk levels averaged 3.4 - 4.9 mg/L.[1] Vorherr reported that after a 600 mg dose of rifampin, peak plasma levels were 50 mg/L while milk levels were 10-30 mg/L.[2]

Pregnancy Risk Category: C

Lactation Risk Category: L2

Adult Concerns: Hepatitis, anemia, headache, diarrhea, pseudomembranous colitis

Pediatric Concerns: None reported via milk.

Drug Interactions: Rifampin is known to reduce the plasma level of a large number of drugs including: acetaminophen, anticoagulants, barbiturates, benzodiazepines, beta blockers, contraceptives, corticosteroids, cyclosporine, digitoxin, phenytoin, methadone, quinidine, sulfonylureas, theophylline, verapamil, and a large number of others.

Theoretic Infant Dose: 0.735 mg/kg/day

Relative Infant Dose: 11.43%

Adult Dose: 600 mg daily

Alternatives:

720

T½ =	3.5 hours	M/P =	0.16-0.23
PHL =	2.9 hours	PB =	80%
T$_{max}$ =	2-4 hours	Oral =	90-95%
MW =	823	pKa =	
Vd =			

References:
1. Lenzi E, Santuari S. Preliminary observations on the use of a new semi-synthetic rifamycin derivative in gynecology and obstetrics. Atti Accad Lancisiana Roma 1969; 13(suppl 1):87-94.
2. Vorherr H. Drug excretion in breastmilk. Postgrad Med 1974; 56(4):97-104.

RIMANTADINE HCL
Trade: Flumadine
Can/Aus/UK:
Uses: Antiviral, anti-influenza A
LRC: L3
AAP: Not reviewed

Rimantadine is an antiviral agent primarily used for influenza A infections. It is concentrated in rodent milk.[1] Levels in animal milk 2-3 hours after administration were approximately twice those of the maternal serum, suggesting a milk/plasma ratio of about 2. Manufacturer alludes to toxic side effects but fails to state them. No side effects yet reported in breastfeeding infants. Rimantadine is, however, indicated for prophylaxis of influenza A in pediatric patients > 1 year of age.

Pregnancy Risk Category: C

Lactation Risk Category: L3

Adult Concerns: Gastrointestinal distress, nervousness, fatigue, and sleep disturbances

Pediatric Concerns: None reported via milk.

Drug Interactions: The use of acetaminophen significantly reduces rimantadine plasma levels by 11%. Peak plasma levels of rimantadine were reduce 10% by aspirin. Rimantadine clearance was reduced by 16% when used with cimetidine.

Theoretic Infant Dose:

Relative Infant Dose:

Adult Dose: 100 mg BID

Alternatives:

T½ =	25.4 hours	M/P =	2
PHL =		PB =	40%
Tmax =	6 hours	Oral =	92%
MW =	179	pKa =	
Vd =			

References:
1. Pharmaceutical Manufacturer Prescribing Information. 1996.

RISEDRONATE
Trade: Actonel
Can/Aus/UK: Actonel
Uses: Prevents bone resorption
LRC: L3
AAP: Not reviewed

Risedronate is a bisphosphonate that slows the dissolution of hydroxyapatite crystals in the bone, thus reducing bone calcium loss in certain syndromes such as Paget's syndrome. Its penetration into milk is possible due to its small molecular weight, but it has not yet been reported except in rats. However, due to the presence of fat and calcium in milk, its oral bioavailability in infants would be exceedingly low. However, the presence of this product in an infant's growing bones is concerning, and due caution is recommended.

Pregnancy Risk Category: C

Lactation Risk Category: L3

Adult Concerns: Nausea, diarrhea, flatulence, gastritis, arthralgia have been reported.

Pediatric Concerns: None via milk.

Drug Interactions: Oral products containing calcium or magnesium will significantly reduce oral bioavailability. Take on empty stomach.

Theoretic Infant Dose:

Relative Infant Dose:

Adult Dose: 30 mg/d for 2 months

Alternatives:

T½ =	480 hours	M/P =	
PHL =		PB =	24%
Tmax =	1 hour	Oral =	0.63%
MW =	305	pKa =	
Vd =	6.3		

References:
1. Pharmaceutical Manufacturer Prescribing Information.

RISPERIDONE
Trade: Risperdal
Can/Aus/UK: Risperdal
Uses: Antipsychotic
LRC: L3
AAP: Not reviewed

Risperidone is a potent antipsychotic agent belonging to a new chemical class and is a dopamine and serotonin antagonist. Risperidone is metabolized to an active metabolite, 9-hyrdoxyrisperidone. In a study of one patient receiving 6 mg/day of risperidone at steady state, the peak plasma level of approximately 130 μg/L occurred 4 hours after an oral dose.[1] Peak milk levels of risperidone and 9-hydroxyrisperidone were approximately 12 μg/L and 40 μg/L respectively. The estimated daily dose of risperidone and metabolite (risperidone equivalents) was 4.3% of the weight-adjusted maternal dose. The milk/plasma ratios calculated from areas under the curve over 24 hours were 0.42 and 0.24 respectively for risperidone and 6-hydroxyrisperidone.

In another study, the transfer of risperidone and 9-hydroxyrisperidone into milk was studied in 2 breastfeeding women and one woman with risperidone-induced galactorrhea.[2] In case 2 (risperidone= 42.1 μg/kg/d), the average concentration of risperidone and 9-hydroxyrisperidone in milk (Cav) was 2.1 and 6 μg/L respectively. The relative infant dose was 2.8% of the maternal dose. In case 3 (risperidone= 23.1μg/kg/d), the average concentration of risperidone and 9-hydroxyrisperidone in milk (Cavg) was 0.39 and 7.06 μg/L respectively. The milk/plasma ratio determined in 2 women was <0.5 for both risperidone compounds. The relative infant "doses" were 2.3%, 2.8%, and 4.7% (as risperidone equivalents) of the maternal weight-adjusted doses in these three cases. Risperidone and 9-hydroxyrisperidone were not detected in the plasma of the 2 breastfed infants studied, and no adverse effects were noted.

Pregnancy Risk Category: C

Lactation Risk Category: L3

Adult Concerns: Risks include neuroleptic malignant syndrome, tardive dyskinesia, myocardial arrhythmias, orthostatic hypotension, seizures, hyperprolactinemia, somnolence. Galactorrhea has been reported.

Pediatric Concerns: None reported via milk.

Drug Interactions: Do not use with alcohol. May enhance the hypotensive response of other antihypertensives. May antagonize the effect of levodopa. Carbamazepine or clozapine may increase clearance of risperidone.

Theoretic Infant Dose: 1.2 μg/kg/day

Relative Infant Dose: 2.8%

Adult Dose: 3 mg BID

Alternatives:

T½ =	3-20 hours	M/P =	0.42
PHL =		PB =	90%
Tmax =	3-17 hours	Oral =	70-94%
MW =	410	pKa =	
Vd =			

References:

1. Hill RC, McIvor RJ, Wojnar-Horton RE, Hackett LP, Ilett KF. Risperidone distribution and excretion into human milk: case report and estimated infant exposure during breast-feeding. J Clin Psychopharmacol 2000; 20(2):285-286.
2. Ilett KF, Hackett LP, Kristensen JH, Vaddadi KS, Gardiner SJ, Begg EJ. Transfer of risperidone and 9-hydroxyrisperidone into human milk. Ann Pharmacother 2004; 38(2):273-276.

RITODRINE

Trade: Pre-Par, Yutopar
Can/Aus/UK: Yutopar
Uses: Adrenergic agent
LRC: L3
AAP: Not reviewed

Ritodrine is primarily used to reduce uterine contractions in premature labor due to its beta-2 adrenergic effect on uterine receptors.[1] No data are available on its transfer to human milk.

Pregnancy Risk Category: B

Lactation Risk Category: L3

Adult Concerns: Fetal and maternal tachycardia, hypertension, lethargy, sleepiness, ketoacidosis, pulmonary edema

Pediatric Concerns: None reported via milk.

Drug Interactions: Use cautiously with steroids due to pulmonary edema. Acebutolol and other beta blockers would block efficacy of ritodrine. Use with atropine may lead to systemic exaggerated hypertension. Use with bupivacaine has lead to extreme hypotension. Numerous other interactions are listed, please review.

Theoretic Infant Dose:

Relative Infant Dose:

Adult Dose: 10-20 mg q 4-6 hours

Alternatives:

T½ =	15 hours	M/P =	
PHL =		PB =	32%
T$_{max}$ =	40-60 minutes	Oral =	30%
MW =	287	pKa =	9
Vd =	0.7		

References:
1. Gandar R, de Zoeten LW, van der Schoot JB. Serum level of ritodrine in man. Eur J Clin Pharmacol 1980; 17(2):117-122.

RIZATRIPTAN

Trade: Maxalt
Can/Aus/UK: Maxalt
Uses: Antimigraine
LRC: L3
AAP: Not reviewed

Rizatriptan is a selective serotonin receptor agonist, similar in effect to sumatriptan.[1] It is primarily indicated for acute migraine headache treatment. No data are available on its transfer into human milk, but it is concentrated in rodent milk (M/P=5). Until we have clear breastmilk data, the kinetics of this drug may predispose to higher milk levels, and sumatriptan may be preferred.

Pregnancy Risk Category: C

Lactation Risk Category: L3

Adult Concerns: Do not use in patients with ischemic heart disease, coronary artery vasospasm, or significant underlying cardiac disease. Rizatriptan should not be used within 24 hours of an ergot alkaloid, dihydroergotamine, or methysergide. Side effects include chest pain, paresthesia, dry mouth, nausea, dizziness, and somnolence.

Pediatric Concerns: None reported via milk, but caution is recommended.

Drug Interactions: Plasma levels may be increased when used with a MAO inhibitor or shortly thereafter.   Concurrent use of propranolol produced a 70% increase in plasma level of rizatriptan. No interactions were noted with nadolol or metoprolol.

Theoretic Infant Dose:

Relative Infant Dose:

Adult Dose: 5-10 mg orally, repeat only after 2 hours

Alternatives: Sumatriptan

T½ =	2-3 hours	M/P =		
PHL =		PB =	14%	
T$_{max}$ =	1-1.5 hours	Oral =	45%	
MW =	269	pKa =		
Vd =	2			

References:
1. Pharmaceutical Manufacturer Prescribing Information. 1999.

ROFECOXIB
Trade: Vioxx
Can/Aus/UK: Vioxx
Uses: NSAID analgesic
LRC: L3
AAP: Not reviewed

Rofecoxib is a new NSAID useful for pain relief in arthritic patients. It is one of the newer Cyclooxigenase-2 (COX-2) inhibitors. The COX-2 inhibitors claim to reduce GI symptoms in users as they do not inhibit the COX-1 enzyme in the gastrointestinal tract. The manufacturer reports that in rodents, the milk/plasma ratio was approximately 1, but this was using doses as high as 6-18 times that used in humans. It is not known if this drug is secreted into human milk. A suitable alternative is celecoxib.

Pregnancy Risk Category: C

Lactation Risk Category: L3

Adult Concerns: Abdominal pain, fatigue, dizziness, diarrhea, headache

Pediatric Concerns: None reported via milk but observe for GI cramping, distress, diarrhea.

Drug Interactions: May reduce efficacy of ACE inhibitors with elevation of blood pressure. Increased plasma concentrations of rofecoxib result when coadministered with cimetidine. May increase lithium levels and reduce the efficacy of diuretics. May increase plasma concentrations of methotrexate by 23%. Rifampin may increase rofecoxib plasma levels by 50%. When added to warfarin therapy, may increase INR by 8%.

Theoretic Infant Dose:

Relative Infant Dose:

Adult Dose: 12.5 to 25 mg once daily

Alternatives: Ibuprofen, celecoxib

T½ =	17 hours	M/P =	
PHL =		PB =	87%
T$_{max}$ =	2-3 hours	Oral =	93%
MW =	314	pKa =	
Vd =	1.3 L/kg		

References:
1. Pharmaceutical Manufacturer Prescribing Information. 1999.

ROPINIROLE

Trade: Requip
Can/Aus/UK: Requip
Uses: Dopamine agonist used in Parkinson's disease
LRC: L4
AAP: Not reviewed

Ropinirole is a nonergot dopamine agonist for use in treating the symptoms of Parkinson's disease. Ropinirole inhibits prolactin production in humans and could potentially inhibit lactation. No human studies are available concerning levels in milk. Regardless, ropinirole is known to reduce the secretion of prolactin, and it is possible that it could significantly reduce milk synthesis. This product should probably not be used in breastfeeding mothers.

Pregnancy Risk Category: C

Lactation Risk Category: L4

Adult Concerns: Adverse events include significant and inexplicable sonmolence(40% incidence). Other side effects include sweating, asthenia, chest pain, fatigue, pain, leg edema, syncope, orthostatic hypotension, dizziness, dyspepsia, nausea, and vomiting.

Pediatric Concerns: None reported via milk as we have no studies, but ropinirole is known to inhibit prolactin secretion and could potentially reduce milk synthesis. Great caution is recommended.

Drug Interactions: Inhibitors of CYP1A2 may potently alter the clearance of ropinirole. Caution is recommended Dopamine antagonists such as metoclopramide, domperidone, phenothiazines, butyrophenones, and others may significantly interfere with the activity of pramipexole. Ciprofloxacin increased ropinole AUC by 84%. Estrogens reduced the oral clearance of ropinirole by 36%

Theoretic Infant Dose:

Relative Infant Dose:

Adult Dose: 0.25 mg TID

Alternatives:

T½ =	6 hours	M/P =	
PHL =		PB =	40%
T$_{max}$ =	1-2 hours	Oral =	55%
MW =		pKa =	
Vd =	7.5		

References:
1. Pharmaceutical Manufacturers prescribing information, 2003.

ROPIVACAINE

Trade: Naropin
Can/Aus/UK: Naropin
Uses: Local anesthetic
LRC: L2
AAP: Not reviewed

Ropivacaine is a newer local anesthetic commonly used as a regional anesthetic and for epidural infusions. It is believed to produce less hypotension when compared to bupivacaine. No data are available on its transfer into human milk, but the manufacture suggests it is probably much lower than the infant receives in utero. This agent is commonly used in obstetrics and probably poses few if any problems to a breastfeeding infant.

Pregnancy Risk Category: B

Lactation Risk Category: L2

Adult Concerns: Adverse effects following epidural administration include hypotension, tachycardia, shivering, urinary retention, vomiting, nausea, headache, and back pain

Pediatric Concerns: None reported in breastmilk. This agent is commonly used in obstetrics and is unlikely to affect and infant via milk.

Drug Interactions: Fluvoxamine and other CYP1A2 inhibitors may reduce plasma clearance of ropivacaine metabolites by 70%. CYP2A4 inhibitors such as ketoconazole may reduce clearance of ropivacaine as well.

Theoretic Infant Dose:

Relative Infant Dose:

Adult Dose: Epidural = 75-150 mg

Alternatives: Bupivacaine

T½ =	4.2 hours (epidural)	M/P =	
PHL =		PB =	94%
T$_{max}$ =	43 minutes (epidural)	Oral =	
MW =	328	pKa =	8.07
Vd =	0.58		

References:
1. Pharmaceutical Manufacturers prescribing information, 2003.

ROSIGLITAZONE

Trade: Avandia
Can/Aus/UK:
Uses: Oral antidiabetic agent
LRC: L3
AAP: Not reviewed

Rosiglitazone is an oral antidiabetic agent which acts primarily by increasing insulin sensitivity. In essence, the insulin receptor is activated reducing insulin resistance. It also decreases hepatic gluconeogenesis and increases insulin-dependent muscle glucose uptake. It does not increase the release of or secretion of insulin. No data are available on its entry into human milk. The maximum plasma concentration following a 2 mg dose is only 156 nanograms/mL.[1] Assuming a dose of 2 mg every 12 hours and a theoretical milk/plasma ratio of 1.0 (which is probably high), an infant would likely ingest about 23.4 µg/kg/day via milk. In a 5 kg infant, this would be approximately 2.8% of the maternal dose. But these data are only theoretical.

Pregnancy Risk Category: C

Lactation Risk Category: L3

Adult Concerns: Elevated liver enzymes in small percentage of patients. Hypoglycemia, increased body weight gain, edema, anemia.

Pediatric Concerns: None via milk, but it has not been studied.

Drug Interactions: Metformin may enhance hypoglycemic effect. Rosiglitazone may reduce effectiveness of oral contraceptives containing estrogen and progestins by reducing plasma levels of these hormones. These changes could result in loss of contraception. Consider a higher dose contraceptive. Rosiglitazone may reduce cyclosporine levels.

Theoretic Infant Dose:

Relative Infant Dose:

Adult Dose: 2-8 mg daily

Alternatives:

T½ =	3-4 hours	M/P =	
PHL =		PB =	99.8%
Tmax =	1 hour	Oral =	99%
MW =	357	pKa =	6.8
Vd =	0.25		

References:
1. Pharmaceutical Manufacturer Prescribing Information.

RUBELLA VIRUS VACCINE, LIVE
Trade: Meruvax, Rubella Vaccine, Measles Vaccine
Can/Aus/UK:
Uses: Live attenuated (measles) vaccine
LRC: L2
AAP: Not reviewed

Rubella virus vaccine contains a live attenuated virus. The American College of Obstetricians and Gynecologists and the CDC currently recommend the early postpartum immunization of women who show no or low antibody titers to rubella. At least four studies have found rubella virus to be transferred via milk although presence of clinical symptoms was not evident.[1-3] Rubella virus has been cultured from the throat of one infant while another infant was clinically ill with minor symptoms and serologic evidence of rubella infection.[4] In general, the use of rubella virus vaccine in mothers of full-term, normal infants has not been associated with untoward effects and is generally recommended.[5]

Pregnancy Risk Category: X

Lactation Risk Category: L2

Adult Concerns: Burning, stinging, lymphadenopathy, rash, malaise, sore throat, etc.

Pediatric Concerns: One case report of rash, vomiting, and mild rubella infection.

Drug Interactions: Immunosuppressants and immune globulins may reduce immunogenicity. Concurrent use of interferon may reduce antibody response.

Theoretic Infant Dose:

Relative Infant Dose:

Adult Dose: 0.5 mL X 1

Alternatives:

References:
1. Buimovici-Klein E, Hite RL, Byrne T, Cooper LZ. Isolation of rubella virus in milk after postpartum immunization. J Pediatr 1977; 91(6):939-941.

2. Losonsky GA, Fishaut JM, Strussenberg J, Ogra PL. Effect of immunization against rubella on lactation products. I. Development and characterization of specific immunologic reactivity in breastmilk. J Infect Dis 1982; 145(5):654-660.
3. Losonsky GA, Fishaut JM, Strussenberg J, Ogra PL. Effect of immunization against rubella on lactation products. II. Maternal-neonatal interactions. J Infect Dis 1982; 145(5):661-666.
4. Landes RD, Bass JW, Millunchick EW, Oetgen WJ. Neonatal rubella following postpartum maternal immunization. J Pediatr 1980; 97(3):465-467.
5. Lawrence RA. Breastfeeding: A guide for the medical profession. St. Louis: Mosby Publishers, 1994.

SACCHARIN

Trade: Saccharin
Can/Aus/UK:
Uses: Sweetener
LRC: L3
AAP: Not reviewed

In one group of 6 women who received 126 mg (per 12 oz drink) every 6 hours for 9 doses, milk levels varied greatly from < 200 µg/L after 1 dose to 1.765 mg/L after 9 doses.[1]   Under these dosing conditions, saccharin levels appear to accumulate over time. Half-life in serum and milk were 4.84 hrs and 17.9 hrs respectively after 3 days. Even after such doses, these milk levels are considered minimal. Moderate intake should be compatible with nursing.

Pregnancy Risk Category: C

Lactation Risk Category: L3

Adult Concerns:

Pediatric Concerns: None reported via milk.

Drug Interactions:

Theoretic Infant Dose: 0.26475

Relative Infant Dose: 3.68%

Adult Dose:

Alternatives:

T½ =	4.84 hours	M/P =	
PHL =		PB =	
T$_{max}$ =		Oral =	Complete
MW =	183	pKa =	
Vd =			

References:
1. Egan PC, Marx CM. et.al. Saccharin excretion in mature human milk. Drug Intell Clin Pharm 1984; 18:511.

SAGE

Trade: Sage, Dalmatian, Spanish Sage
Can/Aus/UK:
Uses: Herbal product
LRC: L4
AAP: Not reviewed

Salvia officinalis L. (Dalmatian sage) and Salvia lavandulaefolia Vahl (Spanish sage) are the most common of the species. Extracts and teas have been used to treat digestive disorders (antispasmodic), as an antiseptic and astringent, for treating diarrhea, gastritis, sore throat, and other maladies.[1] The dried and smoked leaves have been used for treating asthma symptoms. These uses are largely unsubstantiated in the literature.

Sage extracts have been found to be strong antioxidants and with some antimicrobial properties (staph. aureus) due to the phenolic acid salvin content. Sage oil has antispasmodic effects in animals and this may account for its moderating effects on the GI tract. For the most part, sage is relatively nontoxic and nonirritating. Ingestion of significant quantities may lead to cheilitis, stomatitis, dry mouth, or local irritation.[2]

Due to drying properties and pediatric hypersensitivity to anticholinergics, sage should be used with some caution in breastfeeding mothers.

Pregnancy Risk Category:

Lactation Risk Category: L4

Adult Concerns: Observe for typical anticholinergic effects such as cheilitis, stomatitis, dry mouth, or local irritation.

Pediatric Concerns: None reported but observe for dry mouth, stomatitis, cheilitis.

Drug Interactions:

Theoretic Infant Dose:

Relative Infant Dose:

Adult Dose:

Alternatives:

References:
1. Leung AY. Encyclopedia of Common Natural Ingredients used in Food, Drugs and Cosmetics. J Wiley and Sons, 1980.
2. Bissett NG. In: Herbal Drugs and Phytopharmaceuticals. Medpharm Scientific Publishers, CRC Press, Boca Raton, 1994.

SALINE LAXATIVES
Trade: Phillips Milk Of Magnesia, Fleet, Visicol, Tridate, X-Prep
Can/Aus/UK:
Uses: Laxative
LRC: L2
AAP: Maternal Medication Usually Compatible with Breastfeeding

Saline laxatives work by retaining water content in the GI tract. Saline laxatives come in two forms, magnesium salts and phosphate-containing salt forms. Neither are substantially absorbed in normal individuals, but instead most is retained in the gut. Magnesium and phosphate salts absorbed systemically would be rapidly eliminated by the kidneys in normal individuals. Caution is recommended in individuals with cardiovascular or renal anomalies.

Magnesium Forms(Milk of Magnesia, Citrate of Magnesia, Phillips Milk of Magnesia, etc.): Magnesium citrate, magnesium hydroxide, and magnesium sulfate compose the usual forms of magnesium laxatives. Only 15-30% of magnesium salts may be absorbed from the GI tract. The remaining is retained in the intestinal lumen and keeps water in the intestinal lumen thus producing a laxative effect.

Phosphate Forms (Fleet, Visicol): Sodium phosphate solutions containing both dibasic sodium phosphate and monobasic sodium phosphate are used to empty the bowel prior to colonoscopy and other procedures. Approximately 1-20% of the sodium and phosphate in such preparations is absorbed.

It is very unlikely that the use of these saline laxatives would increase maternal plasma levels high enough to induce changes in electrolyte content of human milk. While we do not have specific data on the use of higher doses of "oral" magnesium salts or of the phosphates, the lactocyte controls the microelectrolyte concentrations of milk closely. Minute changes in maternal levels, which could potentially occur following the use of these laxatives, would not likely alter milk content of these electrolytes.

Pregnancy Risk Category:

Lactation Risk Category: L2

Adult Concerns: Diarrhea, gut cramping, hyperphosphatemia, and serious electrolyte disturbances have been reported in some patients at increased risk for electrolyte disturbances. With magnesium salts, especially in renally impaired patients, hypotension, cardiac arrhythmias or arrest, loss of deep tendon reflexes, and confusion may occur.

Pediatric Concerns: None reported via milk.

Drug Interactions: May reduce oral bioavailability of many drugs.

Theoretic Infant Dose:

Relative Infant Dose:

Adult Dose: Highly variable.

Alternatives:

T½ =		M/P =	
PHL =		PB =	
T$_{max}$ =		Oral =	33%
MW =		pKa =	
Vd =			

References:
1. AHFS Drug Information. Bethesda, Md; American Society of Health System Pharmacists, 2003.

SALMETEROL XINAFOATE

Trade: Serevent
Can/Aus/UK: Serevent
Uses: Long acting beta adrenergic bronchodilator
LRC: L2
AAP: Not reviewed

Salmeterol is a long acting beta-2 adrenergic stimulant used as a bronchodilator in asthmatics. Maternal plasma levels of salmeterol after inhaled administration are very low (85-200 pg/mL) or undetectable.[1] Studies in animals have shown that plasma and breastmilk levels are very similar. Oral absorption of both salmeterol and the xinafoate moiety are good. The terminal half-life of salmeterol is 5.5 hrs, xinafoate is 11 days. No reports of use in lactating women are available.

Pregnancy Risk Category: C

Lactation Risk Category: L2

Adult Concerns: Tremor, dizziness, hypertension

Pediatric Concerns: None reported via milk, but studies are limited.

Drug Interactions: Use with MAOI may result in severe hypertension, severe headache, and hypertensive crisis. Tricyclic antidepressants may potentiate the pressure response. The pressure response of salmeterol may be reduced by lithium.

Theoretic Infant Dose: 0.3 µg/kg/day

Relative Infant Dose:

Adult Dose: 50 µg BID

Alternatives:

T½ =	5.5 hours	M/P =	1.0
PHL =		PB =	98%
T$_{max}$ =	10 - 45 minutes	Oral =	Complete
MW =		pKa =	
Vd =			

References:
1. Pharmaceutical Manufacturer Prescribing Information. 1996.

SCOPOLAMINE

Trade: Transderm Scope
Can/Aus/UK: Transderm-V, Buscopan, Benacine, Scopoderm TTS
Uses: Anticholinergic
LRC: L3
AAP: Maternal Medication Usually Compatible with Breastfeeding

Scopolamine is a typical anticholinergic used primarily for motion sickness and preoperatively to produce amnesia and decrease salivation.[1-3] Scopolamine is structurally similar to atropine but is known for its prominent CNS effects including reducing motion sickness. There are no reports on its transfer into human milk, but due to its poor oral bioavailability it is generally believed to be minimal.

Pregnancy Risk Category: C

Lactation Risk Category: L3

Adult Concerns: Blurred vision, dry mouth, drowsiness, constipation, confusion, drowsiness, bradycardia, hypotension, dermatitis

Pediatric Concerns: None via milk. Observe for anticholinergic symptoms such as drowsiness, dry mouth.

Drug Interactions: Decreased effect of acetaminophen, levodopa, ketoconazole, digoxin. GI absorption of the following drugs may be altered: ketoconazole, digoxin, potassium supplements, acetaminophen, levodopa.

Theoretic Infant Dose:

Relative Infant Dose:

Adult Dose: 0.3-0.6 mg once

Alternatives:

T½ =	2.9 hours	M/P =	
PHL =		PB =	
T$_{max}$ =	1 hour	Oral =	27%
MW =	303	pKa =	7.55
Vd =	1.4		

References:
1. Lacy C. Drug information handbook. Lexi-Comp Inc. Cleveland, OH, 1996.
2. Drug Facts and Comparisons 1996 ed. ed. St. Louis: 1996.
3. Pharmaceutical Manufacturer Prescribing Information. 1997.

SECOBARBITAL

Trade: Seconal
Can/Aus/UK: Novo-Secobarb, Seconal
Uses: Short acting barbiturate sedative
LRC: L3
AAP: Maternal Medication Usually Compatible with Breastfeeding

Secobarbital is a sedative, hypnotic barbiturate. It is probably secreted into breastmilk although levels are unknown and may be detectable in milk for 24 hours or longer.[1-3] Recommend mothers delay breastfeeding for 3-4 hours to reduce possible transfer to infant if exposure to this barbiturate is required.

Pregnancy Risk Category: D

Lactation Risk Category: L3

Adult Concerns: Respiratory depression, sedation, addiction

Pediatric Concerns: None reported via milk, but observer for sedation.

Drug Interactions:

Theoretic Infant Dose:

Relative Infant Dose:

Adult Dose: 100 mg daily
Alternatives:

T½ =	15-40 hours	M/P =	
PHL =		PB =	30-45%
Tmax =	2-4 hours	Oral =	90%
MW =	260	pKa =	7.9
Vd =	1.6-1.9		

References:
1. Tyson RM, Shrader EA, Perlman HH. Drugs transmitted through breastmilk. II Barbiturates. J Pediatr 1938; 14:86-90.
2. Kaneko S, Sato T, Suzuki K. The levels of anticonvulsants in breastmilk. Br J Clin Pharmacol 1979; 7(6):624-627.
3. Wilson JT, Brown RD, Cherek DR, Dailey JW, Hilman B, Jobe PC, Manno BR, Manno JE, Redetzki HM, Stewart JJ. Drug excretion in human breastmilk: principles, pharmacokinetics and projected consequences. Clin Pharmacokinet 1980; 5(1):1-66.

SELENIUM SULFIDE

Trade: Selsun, Exsel, Head And Shoulders, Selsun Blue
Can/Aus/UK:
Uses: Topical antimicrobial
LRC: L3
AAP: Not reviewed

Selenium sulfide is an anti-infective compound with mild antibacterial and antifungal activity. It is commonly used for Tinea Versicolor and seborrheic dermatitis such as dandruff. Selenium is not apparently absorbed significantly through intact skin but is absorbed by damaged skin or open lesions.[1] There are no data on its transfer into human milk. If used properly on undamaged skin, it is very unlikely that enough would be absorbed systemically to produce untoward effects in a breastfed infant. Do not apply directly to nipple as enhanced absorption by the infant could occur.

Pregnancy Risk Category:

Lactation Risk Category: L3

Adult Concerns: Changes in hair color and loss of hair have been reported. Extensive washing of hair reduces the incidence of these problems. Extensive systemic absorption can occur with application to broken skin. Nausea, vomiting, diarrhea.

Pediatric Concerns: None reported via milk. Do not apply directly to nipple.

Drug Interactions:

Theoretic Infant Dose:

Relative Infant Dose:

Adult Dose: Apply topic twice weekly

Alternatives: Topical Clotrimazole, itraconazole

References:
1. McEvoy GE. (ed): AFHS Drug Information. New York, NY: 1999.

SENNA LAXATIVES

Trade: Senokot, Senexon, Ex Lax, Senna-Gen, Black-Draught, Fletcher's Castoria, Agoral
Can/Aus/UK:
Uses: Laxative
LRC: L3
AAP: Maternal Medication Usually Compatible with Breastfeeding

Senna is a potent, proven laxative. Anthraquinones, its key ingredient, are believed to increase bowel activity due to secretion of anthraquinones into the colon. Side effects such as abdominal cramping and colic are unpredictable with homemade varieties of this plant. Most sources recommend taking a standardized formulation commonly available. This product is only recommended for short use, such as 10 days. Do not use for intestinal obstruction, or appendicitis, or abdominal pain of unknown origin. Senna laxatives are occasionally used in postpartum women to alleviate constipation. In one study of 23 women who received Senokot (100mg containing 8.602 mg of Sennosides A and B), no sennoside A or B was detectable in their milk. [1] Of 15 mothers reporting loose stools, two infants had loose stools.

Pregnancy Risk Category:

Lactation Risk Category: L3

Adult Concerns: Diarrhea, abdominal cramps, dark colored urine, chronic diarrhea, fluid loss

Pediatric Concerns: Several infants had loose stools although no drug was detected in milk.

Drug Interactions:

Theoretic Infant Dose:

Relative Infant Dose:

Adult Dose: 100 mg daily

Alternatives:

References:
1. Werthmann MW, Jr., Krees SV. Quantitative excretion of Senokot in human breastmilk. Med Ann Dist Columbia 1973; 42(1):4-5.

SERTRALINE

Trade: Zoloft
Can/Aus/UK: Zoloft, Lustral
Uses: Antidepressant
LRC: L2
AAP: Drugs whose effect on nursing infants is unknown but may be of concern

Sertraline is a typical serotonin reuptake inhibitor similar to Prozac and Paxil, but unlike Prozac, the longer half-life metabolite of sertraline is only marginally active. In one study of a single patient taking 100 mg of sertraline daily for 3 weeks postpartum, the concentration of sertraline in milk was 24, 43, 40, and 19 μg/Liter of milk at 1, 5, 9, and 23 hours respectively following the dose.[1]   The maternal plasma levels of sertraline after 12 hours was 48 ng/mL. Sertraline plasma levels in the infant at three weeks were below the limit of detection (< 0.5 ng/mL) at 12 hours post-dose.   Routine pediatric evaluation after 3 months revealed a neonate of normal weight who had achieved the appropriate developmental milestones.

In another study of 3 breastfeeding patients who received 50-100 mg sertraline daily, the maternal plasma levels ranged from 18.4 to 95.8 ng/mL, whereas the plasma levels of sertraline and its metabolite, desmethylsertraline, in the three breastfed infants was below the limit of detection (< 2 ng/mL).[2]   Milk levels were not measured. Desmethylsertraline is poorly active, less than 10% of the parent sertraline.

Another recent publication reviewed the changes in platelet serotonin levels in breastfeeding mothers and their infants who received up to 100 mg of sertraline daily.[3] Mothers treated with sertraline had significant decreases in their platelet serotonin levels, which is expected. However, there was no change in platelet serotonin levels in breastfed infants of mothers consuming sertraline, suggesting that only minimal amounts of sertraline are actually transferred to the infant. This confirms other studies.

Studies by Stowe of eleven mother/infant pairs (maternal dose = 25-150 mg/day) further suggest minimal transfer of sertraline into human milk.[4] From this superb study, the concentration of sertraline peaked in the milk at 7-8 hours and the metabolite (desmethylsertraline) at 5-11 hours.   The   reported   concentrations   of   sertraline   and desmethylsertraline in breastmilk were 17-173 μg/L and 22-294 μg/L respectively. The reported dose of sertraline to the infant via milk varied from undetectable (5 of 11) to 0.124 mg/day in one infant. The infant's serum concentration of sertraline varied from undetectable to 3.0 ng/mL but was undetectable in 7 of 11 patients. No developmental abnormalities were noted in any of the infants studied.

In a study of eight women taking sertraline (1.05 mg/kg/d) the mean milk/plasma ratio was 1.93 and 1.64 for sertraline and N-desmethylsertraline.[5] Infant exposure estimated from actual milk produced was 0.2% and 0.3% of the weight-adjusted maternal dose for sertraline and N-desmethylsertraline (sertraline equivalents) respectively. Assuming a 150 mL/kg/d intake, infant exposure was significantly greater at 0.90% and 1.32% for sertraline and N-desmethylsertraline respectively. Neither sertraline nor its N-desmethyl metabolite could be detected in plasma samples from the four infants tested. No adverse effects were observed in any of the eight infants and all had achieved normal developmental milestones.

Sertraline is a potent inhibitor of 5-HT transporter function both in the CNS and platelets. One recent study assessed the effect of sertraline on platelet 5-HT transporter function in 14 breastfeeding mothers (dose = 25-200 mg/d) and their infants to determine if even low levels of sertraline exposure could perhaps lead to changes in the infant's blood platelet 5-HT levels and, therefore, CNS serotonin levels.[6] While a significant reduction in platelet levels of 5-HT were noted in the mothers, no changes in 5-HT levels were noted in the 14 infants. Thus, it appears that at typical clinical doses, maternal sertraline has a minimal effect on platelet 5-HT transport in breastfeeding infants.

These studies generally confirm that the transfer of sertraline and its metabolite to the infant is minimal, and that attaining clinically relevant plasma levels in infants is remote at maternal doses less than 150 mg/day. A thorough review of antidepressant use in breastfeeding mothers is available.[7]

Pregnancy Risk Category: B

Lactation Risk Category: L2

Adult Concerns: Diarrhea, nausea, tremor, and increased sweating

Pediatric Concerns: Of the cases reported in the literature, only one infant developed benign neonatal sleep at age 4 months which spontaneously resolved at 6 months. Its relationship, if any, to sertraline is unknown.

Drug Interactions: All SSRIs inhibit Cytochrome P450 enzymes and may inhibit metabolism of desipramine, dextromethorphan, encainide, haloperidol, metoprolol, etc. May induce serotonergic hyperstimulation when added too soon after MAO inhibitors, tricyclic antidepressants, and lithium. May displace warfarin from binding sites increasing anticoagulation. Two recent cases of serotonin-like reactions (agitation, dysarthria, diapyhoresis and extrapyramidal movement disorder) have been reported when metoclopramide was used in patients receiving sertraline or venlafaxine.[7]

Theoretic Infant Dose: 21.45 µg/kg/day

Relative Infant Dose: 2.2%

Adult Dose: 50-200 mg daily

Alternatives: Paroxetine

T½ =	26-65 hours	M/P =	0.89
PHL =		PB =	98%
T$_{max}$ =	7-8 hours	Oral =	Complete
MW =	306	pKa =	
Vd =	20		

References:

1. Altshuler LL, Burt VK, McMullen M, Hendrick V. Breastfeeding and sertraline: a 24-hour analysis. J Clin Psychiatry 1995; 56(6):243-245.
2. Mammen OK, Perel JM, Rudolph G, Foglia JP, Wheeler SB. Sertraline and norsertraline levels in three breastfed infants. J Clin Psychiatry 1997; 58(3):100-103.
3. Epperson CN. et.al. Sertraine and Breastfeeding. NEJM 1997; 336(16):1189-1190.
4. Stowe ZN, Owens MJ, Landry JC, Kilts CD, Ely T, Llewellyn A, Nemeroff CB. Sertraline and desmethylsertraline in human breastmilk and nursing infants. Am J Psychiatry 1997; 154(9):1255-1260.
5. Kristensen JH, Ilett KF, Dusci LJ, Hackett LP, Yapp P, Wojnar-Horton RE, Roberts MJ, Paech M. Distribution and excretion of sertraline and N-desmethylsertraline in human milk. Br J Clin Pharmacol 1998; 45(5):453-457.
6. Epperson N, Czarkowski KA, Ward-O'Brien D, Weiss E, Gueorguieva R, Jatlow P, Anderson GM. Maternal sertraline treatment and serotonin transport in breast-feeding mother-infant pairs. Am J Psychiatry 2001; 158(10):1631-1637.
7. Wisner KL, Perel JM, Findling RL. Antidepressant treatment during breast-feeding. Am J Psychiatry 1996; 153(9):1132-1137.

SEVOFLURANE

Trade: Ultane
Can/Aus/UK:
Uses: Anesthetic gas
LRC: L3
AAP: Not reviewed

Sevoflurane is a gaseous halogenated general anesthetic drug that is particularly popular because of its rapid wash-out. Average patient "time to emergence" is approximately 8.2 minutes. It is commonly used in adult and pediatric patients and is used in cesarean sections. The manufacturer states that, while the concentration of sevoflurane have not been measured in breastmilk, they are probably of no clinical importance 24 hours after anesthesia. Because of its rapid wash-out, sevoflurane concentrations in milk are predicted to be below those found with many other volatile anesthatics.[1] Sevoflurane follows a three term exponential decay with half-lives of 11min (18% of the dose in plasma compartment), 1.8 hours (15% from muscle compartment), and 20 hours (6% from fat compartment).[2] Small (3%) amounts of sevoflurane are metabolized and result in plasma levels that average 36 uM/liter. Levels reported are temporary and completely dissipate by 6 days. The fluoride ion released is not high enough to be contraindicated to breastfeeding. Further, the oral absorption of fluoride in infants is believed poor as it is chelated with calcium ions orally in milk.

While no data on levels of sevoflurane in breastmilk are available, this product, due to its rapid clearance from the body (100 fold drop in 120 minutes), should not pose a problem for continued breastfeeding soon after exposure.

Pregnancy Risk Category: **B**

Lactation Risk Category: **L3**

Adult Concerns: Malignant hyperthermia, bradycardia, agitation, laryngospasm, shivering, hypotension, etc. Check anesthesia text for more.

Pediatric Concerns: None reported via milk. Milk levels are likely insignificant, and oral bioavailability is unlikely.

Drug Interactions: Sevoflurane increases intensity and duration of neuromuscular blockade by nondepolarizing muscle relaxants.

Theoretic Infant Dose:

Relative Infant Dose:

Adult Dose: Variable

Alternatives:

$T\frac{1}{2}$ =	1.8-3.8 hours	M/P =	
PHL =		PB =	0%
T_{max} =		Oral =	
MW =	200	pKa =	
Vd =	0.5		

References:
1. Pharmaceutical Manufacturer Prescribing Information.
2. Holaday DA, Smith FR. Clinical characteristics and biotransformation of sevoflurane in healthy volunteers. Anesthesiology 1981; 54:100-106.

SIBUTRAMINE

Trade: Meridia
Can/Aus/UK: Meridia
Uses: Appetite suppressant
LRC: L4
AAP: Not reviewed

Sibutramine is a nonamphetamine appetite suppressant. Due to its effect on serotonin and norepinephrine reuptake, it is considered an antidepressant as well. Sibutramine is rather small in molecular weight, active in the CNS, extremely lipid soluble, and has two 'active' metabolites with long half-lives (14-16 hours).[1-3] Although no data are available on its transfer into human milk, the pharmacokinetics of this drug theoretically suggest that it might have a rather high milk/plasma ratio and could enter milk in significant levels. Until we know more, a risk assessment may not support the use of this product in breastfeeding mothers.

Pregnancy Risk Category: C

Lactation Risk Category: L4

Adult Concerns: Adult side effects include headache, insomnia, back pain, flu-like syndrome, abdominal pain, seizures (rarely), and elevated liver enzymes. Cardiovascular events include tachycardia, hypertension.

Pediatric Concerns: None reported via milk. Caution is recommended.

Drug Interactions: Use of Sibutramine with drugs that may increase blood pressure (decongestants, cough and cold remedies) could be hazardous. Do not use with MAO inhibitors. Do not admix with drugs that inhibit cytochrome P450 enzymes in the liver (ketoconazole, cimetidine, erythromycin (minor effect).

Theoretic Infant Dose:

Relative Infant Dose:

Adult Dose: 5-15 mg daily

Alternatives:

T½ =	12.5-21.8 hours	M/P =	
PHL =		PB =	94%
Tmax =	3-4 hours	Oral =	77%
MW =	334	pKa =	
Vd =			

References:
1. Lean ME. Sibutramine--a review of clinical efficacy. Int J Obes Relat Metab Disord 1997; 21 Suppl 1:S30-S36.

2. Stock MJ. Sibutramine: a review of the pharmacology of a novel anti-obesity agent. Int J Obes Relat Metab Disord 1997; 21 Suppl 1:S25-S29.
3. Pharmaceutical Manufacturer Prescribing Information.

SILDENAFIL
Trade: Viagra
Can/Aus/UK: Viagra
Uses: For erectile dysfunction
LRC: L3
AAP: Not reviewed

Sildenafil is an inhibitor of nitrous oxide metabolism, thus increasing levels of nitrous oxide, smooth muscle relaxation, and an increased flow of blood in the corpus cavernosum of the penis.[1]   While not currently indicated for women, illicit use is increasing. No data are available on the transfer of sildenafil into human milk, but it is unlikely that significant transfer will occur due to its larger molecular weight and short half-life.   However, caution is recommended in breastfeeding mothers. While not reported, persistent abnormal erections (priapism) could potentially occur in male infants.

Pregnancy Risk Category: B

Lactation Risk Category: L3

Adult Concerns: Changes in visual color perception is common. Other side effects include headache, flushing, dyspepsia, nasal congestion, and hypotension.

Pediatric Concerns: None reported via milk.   If used, observe for priapism in male infants.

Drug Interactions: Do not admix with any form of nitrate, including nitroglycerine.   Because it is metabolized by cytochrome P450 CYP3A4 and 2C9, increased plasma levels may result when admixed with azole antifungals, erythromycins, cimetidine and other such enzyme inhibitors. Serious prolonged erections have been reported with the co-administration of dihydrocodeine.

Theoretic Infant Dose:

Relative Infant Dose:

Adult Dose: 50 mg daily

Alternatives:

T½ =	4 hours	M/P =	
PHL =		PB =	96%
T$_{max}$ =	60 minutes	Oral =	40%
MW =	666	pKa =	
Vd =	1.5		

References:
1.   Pharmaceutical Manufacturer Prescribing Information. 1999.

SILICONE BREAST IMPLANTS
Trade:
Can/Aus/UK:
Uses: Silicone mammoplasty
LRC:
AAP: Not reviewed

Augmentation mammoplasty with silicone implants is no longer available in the USA. In general, placement of the implant behind the breast seldom produces interruption of vital ducts, nerve supply, or blood supply. Most women have been able to breastfeed. Breast reduction surgery, on the other hand, has been found to produce significant interruption of the nervous supply (particularly the ductile tissue), leading to a reduced ability to lactate.

Silicone transfer to breastmilk has been studied in one group of 15 lactating mothers with bilateral silicone breast implants.[1] Silicon levels were measured in breastmilk, whole blood, cow's milk, and 26 brands of infant formula. Comparing implanted women to controls, mean silicon levels were not significantly different in breastmilk (55.45 +/- 35 and 51.05 +/- 31 ng/mL respectively) or in blood (79.29 +/- 87 and 103.76 +/- 112 ng/mL respectively. Mean silicon level measured in store-bought cow's milk was 708.94 ng/mL and that for 26 brands of commercially available infant formula was 4402.5 ng/mL (ng/mL = parts per billion). The authors concluded that lactating women with silicone implants are similar to control women with respect to levels of silicon in their breastmilk and blood. From these studies, silicon levels are 10 times higher in cow's milk and even higher in infant formulas.

It is not known for certain if ingestion of leaking silicone by a nursing infant is dangerous. Although one article has been published showing esophageal strictures, it has subsequently been recalled by the author. Silicone by nature is extremely inert and is unlikely to be absorbed in the GI tract by a nursing infant although good studies are lacking. Silicone is a ubiquitous substance, found in all foods, liquids, etc.

Pregnancy Risk Category:

Lactation Risk Category:

Adult Concerns:

Pediatric Concerns: None reported via milk.

Drug Interactions:

Theoretic Infant Dose:

Relative Infant Dose:

Adult Dose: N/A

Alternatives:

References:
1. Semple JL, Lugowski SJ, Baines CJ, Smith DC, McHugh A. Breastmilk contamination and silicone implants: preliminary results using silicon as a proxy measurement for silicone. Plast Reconstr Surg 1998; 102(2):528-533.

SILVER SULFADIAZINE

Trade: Silvadene, SSD Cream, Thermazene
Can/Aus/UK: Flamazine, Dermazin, SSD, Silvazine
Uses: Topical antimicrobial cream
LRC: L3
AAP: Not reviewed

Silver sulfadiazine is a topical antimicrobial cream primarily used for reducing sepsis in burn patients. The silver component is not absorbed from the skin.[1] Sulfadiazine is partially absorbed. After prolonged therapy of large areas, sulfadiazine levels in plasma may approach therapeutic levels. Although sulfonamides are known to be secreted into human milk, they are not particularly problematic except in the newborn period when they may produce kernicterus.

Pregnancy Risk Category: B

Lactation Risk Category: L3

Adult Concerns: Allergic rash, renal failure, crystalluria

Pediatric Concerns: None reported, but studies are limited. Observe caution during the neonatal period.

Drug Interactions:

Theoretic Infant Dose:

Relative Infant Dose:

Adult Dose:

Alternatives:

$T\frac{1}{2}$ =	10 hours (sulfa)	M/P =	
PHL =		PB =	
T_{max} =		Oral =	Complete
MW =		pKa =	
Vd =			

References:
1. McEvoy GE. (ed):AFHS Drug Information. New York, NY: 2003.

SIMVASTATIN

Trade: Zocor
Can/Aus/UK: Zocor, Lipex
Uses: Reduces cholesterol
LRC: L3
AAP: Not reviewed

Simvastatin is an HMG-CoA reductase inhibitor that reduces the production of cholesterol in the liver. Like lovastatin, simvastatin reduces blood cholesterol levels. Others in this family are known to be secreted into human and rodent milk, but no data are available on simvastatin.[1] It is likely that milk levels will be low because less than 5% of simvastatin reaches the plasma, most being removed first-pass by the liver.

Atherosclerosis is a chronic process and discontinuation of lipid-lowering drugs during pregnancy and lactation should have little to no impact on the outcome of long-term therapy of primary hypercholesterolemia. Cholesterol and other products of cholesterol biosynthesis are essential components for fetal and neonatal development, and the use of cholesterol-lowering drugs would not be advisable under any circumstances.

Pregnancy Risk Category: X

Lactation Risk Category: L3

Adult Concerns: GI distress, headache, hypotension, elevated liver enzymes

Pediatric Concerns: None reported.

Drug Interactions: Increased toxicity when added to gemfibrozil (myopathy, myalgia, etc), clofibrate, niacin (myopathy), erythromycin, cyclosporine, oral anticoagulants (elevated bleeding time).

Theoretic Infant Dose:

Relative Infant Dose:

Adult Dose: 5-10 mg daily

Alternatives:

$T\frac{1}{2}$ =	Long	M/P =	
PHL =		PB =	95%
T_{max} =	1.3-2.4 hours	Oral =	Poor
MW =	419	pKa =	
Vd =			

References:
1. Drug Facts and Comparisons 1995 ed. ed. St. Louis: 1995.

SINCALIDE
Trade: Kinevac
Can/Aus/UK:
Uses: Diagnostic agent for cholecystography
LRC: L3
AAP: Not reviewed

Kinevac is a chol cystopancreatic-gastrointestinal hormone peptide which when injected produces a substantial contracture of the gall bladder. Sincalide is therefore used to assess biliary and gall bladder function. No data are available on the transfer of this peptide into human milk, but due to its molecular weight it is extremely unlikely significant quantities would ever reach the milk compartment. It has a brief but unreported half-life.

Pregnancy Risk Category: B

Lactation Risk Category: L3

Adult Concerns: Adverse effects include GI and abdominal pain, nausea, the urge to deficate, flushing, dizziness, and cramping.

Pediatric Concerns: None reported via milk. While it is unlikely to enter milk, a brief interruption of breastfeeding (1-2 hours) would preclude any possible side effects.

Drug Interactions:

Theoretic Infant Dose:

Relative Infant Dose:

Adult Dose: 0.02 μg/kg over 30 seconds.

Alternatives:

$T\frac{1}{2}$ =	Brief	M/P =	
PHL =		PB =	
T_{max} =		Oral =	Nil
MW =	1143	pKa =	
Vd =			

References:
1. Pharmaceutical Manufacturers Package Insert, 2003.

SIROLIMUS
Trade: Rapamune, Rapamycin, Nsc-226080
Can/Aus/UK: Rapamune
Uses: Immunosuppressant
LRC: L4
AAP: Not reviewed

Sirolimus is an immunosuppressant sometimes used in combination with cyclosporin in renal transplants. No data are available on its transfer to human milk. Average plasma levels are quite low (264 ng x hr/mL) and the drug is strongly attached to cellular components and plasma levels are low. It is not likely it will penetrate milk in levels that are significant. However, it is a potent inhibitor of the enzyme 70 K S6 kinase, which is stimulated in breast tissue by prolactin. This agent, in rodent mammary tissue, strongly inhibits milk component production.[1] It could potentially suppress milk production in lactating mothers and caution is recommended.

Pregnancy Risk Category: C

Lactation Risk Category: L4

Adult Concerns: Anemia, thrombocytopenia, leukopenia, hypertension, headache, hyperlipidemia, hypophosphatemia, urinary tract infection, interstitial pneumonitis

Pediatric Concerns: None via milk, but reduced milk production could occur.

Drug Interactions: Drugs which inhibit cytochrome P450 3A4 may significantly increase levels of sirolimus. These include: bromocriptine, carbamazepine, cimetidine, cisapride, clarithromycin, clotrimazole, danazol, diltiazem, erythromycin, fluconazole, fosphenytoin, metoclopramide, etc. Co-administration with cyclosporine may increase levels of sirolimus. Numerous other drug-drug contraindications may exist, consult drug interaction reference.

Theoretic Infant Dose:

Relative Infant Dose:

Adult Dose: 2 mg/d

Alternatives:

T½ =	57-63 hours	M/P =	
PHL =		PB =	
T$_{max}$ =	1-3 hours	Oral =	15%
MW =	914	pKa =	
Vd =	12		

References:
1. Hang J, Rillema JA. Effect of rapamycin on prolactin-stimulated S6 kinase activity and milk product formation in mouse mammary explants. Biochim Biophys Acta 1997; 1358(2):209-214.

SMALLPOX VACCINE
Trade: Smallpox Vaccine, Dryvax
Can/Aus/UK:
Uses: Vaccine for vaccinia virus.
LRC: L4
AAP: Not reviewed

Smallpox is a viral syndrome caused by infection with the vaccinia virus. The smallpox vaccine contains a live but attenuated (weakened) preparation of vaccinia virus. The reconstituted vaccine contains approximately 100 million infectious vaccinia viruses per mL. Introduction of potent smallpox vaccine into the superficial layers of the skin results in viral multiplication, immunity, and cellular hypersensitivity. With the primary vaccination, a papule appears at the site of vaccination on the 2nd to 5th day. It then becomes a pustule surrounded by erythema and induration. The erythema and swelling then subside after about 10 days and the crust forms. Secretions from the lesions are capable of inoculating other individuals and care should be exercised around pregnant women, infants, and particularly premature infants. No data are available suggesting the degree of transmission into human milk, but it is likely to enter milk to some degree. Infants are at increased risk from vaccinia infections and the use of smallpox vaccine in infants is contraindicated unless it is an emergency situation. Although the use of the smallpox vaccine in children is not recommended in non-emergent situations, it was safely used in the past. The product information suggests that pregnant and breastfeeding mothers should not receive the vaccination under non-emergent conditions. However, there are no absolute contraindications regarding vaccination of a person with a "high-risk exposure" to smallpox. In breastfeeding mothers who are not at high risk, the use of smallpox vaccinations is not justified(Center of Disease Control).

Pregnancy Risk Category: C

Lactation Risk Category: L4

Adult Concerns: Adverse effects include fever, lymphadema, urticaria, secondary pyogenic infections, vesicular rash.

Pediatric Concerns: No data are available on its use in breastfeeding mothers or its transfer into human milk. However, vaccinia virus is likely transmitted via milk and is probably infectious. Its use in breastfeeding mothers is not recommended in non-emergent situations.

Drug Interactions:

Theoretic Infant Dose:

Relative Infant Dose:

Adult Dose:

Alternatives:

References:
1. Pharmaceutical Manufacturers prescribing information, 2003.

SOMATREM, SOMATROPIN
Trade: Human Growth Hormone, Nutropin, Humatrope, Growth Hormone, Saizen
Can/Aus/UK: Protropin, Humatrope, Norditropin, Somatropin, Genotropin
Uses: Human growth hormone
LRC: L3
AAP: Not reviewed

Somatrem and somatropin are purified polypeptide hormones of recombinant DNA origin. It is a large protein. They are structurally similar or identical to human growth hormone (hGH). One study in 16 women indicates that hGH treatment for 7 days stimulated breastmilk production by 18.5% (verses 11.6% in controls) in a group of normal lactating women.[1] No adverse effects were noted. Leukemia has occurred in a small number of children receiving hGH, but the relationship is uncertain. Because it is a peptide of 191 amino acids and its molecular weight is so large, its transfer into milk is very unlikely. Further, its oral absorption would be minimal to nil.

Pregnancy Risk Category: C

Lactation Risk Category: L3

Adult Concerns: Some fatalities have been reported in pediatric patients with Prader-Willi syndrome. Hypothyroidism and hypoglycemia have been reported.

Pediatric Concerns: None reported via milk. Absorption is very unlikely.

Drug Interactions:

Theoretic Infant Dose:

Relative Infant Dose:

Adult Dose: 0.1-0.3 mg/kg q week

Alternatives:

T½ =		M/P =	
PHL =		PB =	
T$_{max}$ =	7.5 hours	Oral =	Poor
MW =	22,124	pKa =	
Vd =			

References:
1. Milsom SR, Breier BH, Gallaher BW, Cox VA, Gunn AJ, Gluckman PD. Growth hormone stimulates galactopoiesis in healthy lactating women. Acta Endocrinol (Copenh) 1992; 127(4):337-343.

SOTALOL

Trade: Betapace
Can/Aus/UK: Sotacor, Apo-Sotalol, Rylosol, Cardol
Uses: Antihypertensive, beta-blocker
LRC: L3
AAP: Maternal Medication Usually Compatible with Breastfeeding

Sotalol is a typical beta blocker antihypertensive with low lipid solubility. It is secreted into milk in high levels. Sotalol concentrations in milk ranged from 4.8 to 20.2 mg/L (mean= 10.5 mg/L) in 5 mothers.[1] The mean maternal dose was 433 mg/day. Although these milk levels appear high, no evidence of toxicity was noted in 12 infants.

Pregnancy Risk Category: B

Lactation Risk Category: L3

Adult Concerns: Bradycardia, hypotension, sedation, poor sucking

Pediatric Concerns: None reported via milk, but observe for sedation, bradycardia, hypotension, weakness.

Drug Interactions: Decreased effect when used with aluminum salts, barbiturates, calcium salts, cholestyramine, NSAIDs, ampicillin, rifampin, and salicylates. Beta blockers may reduce the effect of oral sulfonylureas (hypoglycemic agents). Increased toxicity/effect when used with other antihypertensives, contraceptives, MAO inhibitors, cimetidine, and numerous other products. See drug interaction reference for complete listing.

Theoretic Infant Dose: 1.57 mg/kg/day

Relative Infant Dose: 25.4%

Adult Dose: 80-160 mg BID

Alternatives: Propranolol, Metoprolol

T½ =	12 hours	M/P =	5.4
PHL =		PB =	0%
T$_{max}$ =	2.5 - 4 hours	Oral =	90-100%
MW =	272	pKa =	8.3,9.8
Vd =	1.6-2.4		

References:
1. O'Hare MF, Murnaghan GA, Russell CJ, Leahey WJ, Varma MP, McDevitt DG. Sotalol as a hypotensive agent in pregnancy. Br J Obstet Gynaecol 1980; 87(9):814-820.

SPIRONOLACTONE
Trade: Aldactone
Can/Aus/UK: Aldactone, Novospiroton, Spiractin
Uses: Potassium sparing diuretic
LRC: L2
AAP: Maternal Medication Usually Compatible with Breastfeeding

Spironolactone is metabolized to canrenone, which is known to be secreted into breastmilk. In one mother receiving 25 mg of spironolactone at 2 hours postdose the maternal serum and milk concentrations of canrenone were 144 and 104 μg/L respectively.[1] At 14.5 hours, the corresponding values for serum and milk were 92 and 47 μg/L respectively. Milk/plasma ratios varied from 0.51 at 14.5 hrs, to 0.72 at 2 hours.

Pregnancy Risk Category: D

Lactation Risk Category: L2

Adult Concerns: Nausea, vomiting, elevated serum potassium, hepatitis

Pediatric Concerns: None reported via milk, but suppression of milk supply is possible but unlikely.

Drug Interactions: Use with anticoagulants may reduce the anticoagulant effect. Use with potassium preparations may increase potassium levels in plasma. Use with ACE inhibitors may elevate serum potassium levels. The diuretic effect of spironolactone may be decreased by use with salicylates.

Theoretic Infant Dose: 15.6 μg/kg/day

Relative Infant Dose: <4.3%

Adult Dose: 50-100 mg daily
Alternatives:

T½ =	10-35 hours	M/P =	0.51-0.72
PHL =		PB =	> 90%
T$_{max}$ =	1-2 hours	Oral =	70%
MW =	417	pKa =	
Vd =			

References:
1. Phelps DL, Karim Z. Spironolactone: relationship between concentrations of dethioacetylated metabolite in human serum and milk. J Pharm Sci 1977; 66(8):1203.

ST. JOHN'S WORT
Trade: St. John's Wort
Can/Aus/UK:
Uses: Antidepressant
LRC: L2
AAP: Not reviewed

St. John's Wort (hypericum perforatum L.) consists of the whole fresh or dried plant or its components containing not less than 0.04% naphthodianthrones of the hypericin group. Hypericum contains many biologically active compounds and most researchers consider its effect due to a combination of constituents rather than any single component.[1] However, the naphthodianthrones hypericin and pseudohypericin and numerous flavonoids have stimulated the most interest as antidepressants and antivirals. Following doses of (3 x 300 mg/day), peak steady state concentrations of hypericin and pseudohypericin were 8.5 ng/mL and 5.8 ng/mL respectively.[2] Concentrations in the brain appear to be the least of all compartments. Hypericum has become increasingly popular for the treatment of depression following results from numerous studies showing efficacy.

In vitro studies have indicated that hypericin inhibits monoamine oxidase (MAO) and catechol-o-methyltransferase (COMT), the enzymes responsible for the breakdown of neurotransmitters.[3] MAO inhibitors have in the past been subject to severe restrictions due to their dangers. Thus far, the amount of hypericin present in human tissues does not appear to inhibit MAO in adults although no data are available on MAO inhibition in infants. Hypericin is presently in Phase I clinical trials as an antiviral agent as well, with potential use in herpes, HIV, and other viral infections. Although there is great interest in this phytomedicine, a number of deficiencies in the clinical trails have been pointed out.[4,5] They include poorly characterized depressed patient populations, heterogeneity of diagnoses, etc, but a number of current studies underway should clarify these deficiencies.

Several new studies show that St. John's Wort may significantly stimulate Cytochrome P450 3A4, which is a major drug metabolizing enzyme in the liver.[6-10] Following such induction, major reductions (50% or more) in plasma levels of a number of important drugs have been reported and include: cyclosporin, midazolam, indinavir, and possibly numerous other drugs. Patients taking anticonvulsants and other critically important drugs should be advised about the possible interaction with these medications leading to major reductions in plasma levels. Patients should always advise their physicians of their use of St. John's Wort.

In a recent prospective, observational, cohort study of the safety of SJW in 33 breastfeeding mothers, along with matched controls, no significant differences were found in maternal or infant demographics or maternal adverse effects following treatment with SJW.[11] In another study of a single patient receiving 3 daily doses of Jarsin 300, hypericin levels in milk were undetectable (< 0.2 ng/mL).[12] Hyperforin levels in milk ranged from 0.58 to 18.2 ng/mL. Maternal plasma levels of hypericin and hyperforin were 10.71 and 154 ng/mL respectively. Both components were undetectable in the plasma of the infant. No side effects of any kind were noted in the infant and the Denver Developmental Screen was normal.

Pregnancy Risk Category:

Lactation Risk Category: L2

Adult Concerns: Caution, because of uterotonic effects, hypericum should not be used in pregnant patients. Dry mouth, dizziness, constipation, and confusion have been infrequently reported. Overt toxicity is generally considered quite low. Photosensitization in fair-skinned people has been noted. No teratogenic effects has been documented.

Pediatric Concerns: None reported in two studies. Probably safe.

Drug Interactions: May prolong narcotic-induced sedation and sleeping times. May reduce barbiturate-induced sleeping times. A recent report in Lancet suggests St. John's wort may induce the cytochrome P-450 enzyme system. The data indicates an interaction between St. John's wort and the HIV-1 protease inhibitor, Indinavir, where indinavir AUC was reduced by a mean of 57%. In addition, trough concentrations of indinavir at 8 hours were reduced by 81%. Another report indicates acute rejection episodes in two heart transplant patients who had initiated St. John's wort for depression. Although each patient recovered after the St. John's wort was discontinued, this again implicates P-450 induction activity of St. John's wort. SJW may decrease digoxin plasma levels (AUC) by 25%, and theophylline levels significantly.

Theoretic Infant Dose:

Relative Infant Dose:

Adult Dose: 300mg TID dry-powdered (0.3% hypericin)

Alternatives: Sertraline, Paroxetine

T½ =	26.5 hours	M/P =
PHL =		PB =
T$_{max}$ =	5.9 hours	Oral =
MW =	504	pKa =
Vd =		

References:
1. Upton R. St. John's Wort. American Herbal Pharmacopoeia and Therapeutic Compendium 1997.
2. Stock S, Holzl J. Pharmacokinetic tests of (14C)-labeled hypericin and pseudohypericin from Hypericum perforatum and serum kinetics of hyperich in man. Planta Medica 1991; 57(suppl 2):A61.
3. Bladt S, Wagner H. Inhibition of MAO by fractions and constituents of hypericum extract. J Geriatr Psychiatry Neurol 1994; 7 Suppl 1:S57-S59.
4. Ernst E. St. John's Wort, an anti-depressant? A systematic, criteria-based review. Phytomedicine 1995; 2:47-71.
5. Linde K, Ramirez G, Mulrow CD, Pauls A, Weidenhammer W, Melchart D. St John's wort for depression--an overview and meta-analysis of randomised clinical trials. BMJ 1996; 313(7052):253-258.
6. Durr D, Stieger B, Kullak-Ublick GA, Rentsch KM, Steinert HC, Meier PJ, Fattinger K. St John's Wort induces intestinal P-glycoprotein/MDR1 and intestinal and hepatic CYP3A4. Clin Pharmacol Ther 2000; 68(6):598-604.
7. Barone GW, Gurley BJ, Ketel BL, Lightfoot ML, Abul-Ezz SR. Drug interaction between St. John's wort and cyclosporine. Ann Pharmacother 2000; 34(9):1013-1016.
8. Obach RS. Inhibition of human cytochrome P450 enzymes by constituents of St. John's Wort, an herbal preparation used in the treatment of depression. J Pharmacol Exp Ther 2000; 294(1):88-95.
9. Roby CA, Anderson GD, Kantor E, Dryer DA, Burstein AH. St John's Wort: effect on CYP3A4 activity. Clin Pharmacol Ther 2000; 67(5):451-457.
10. De Smet PA, Touw DJ. Safety of St John's wort (Hypericum perforatum). Lancet 2000; 355(9203):575-576.
11. Lee A, Minhas R, Matsuda N et al. The safety of St. John's wort (Hypericum perforatum) during breastfeeding. J Clin Psychiatry. 2003;64:966-968.
12. Klier CM, Schafer MR, Schmid-Siegel B et al. St. John's wort (Hypericum perforatum)--is it safe during breastfeeding? Pharmacopsychiatry. 2002;35:29-30.

STREPTOMYCIN
Trade:
Can/Aus/UK: Streptobretin, Streptotriad
Uses: Antibiotic
LRC: L3
AAP: Maternal Medication Usually Compatible with Breastfeeding

Streptomycin is an aminoglycoside antibiotic from the same family as gentamycin. It is primarily administered IM or IV although it is seldom used today with exception of the treatment of tuberculosis. One report suggests that following a 1 g dose (IM), levels in breastmilk were 0.3 to 0.6 mg/L (2-3% of plasma level).[1] Another report suggests that only 0.5% of a 1 gm IM dose is excreted in breastmilk within 24 hours.[2] Because the oral absorption of streptomycin is very poor, absorption by infant is probably minimal (unless premature or early neonate).

Pregnancy Risk Category: D

Lactation Risk Category: L3

Adult Concerns: Deafness, anemia, kidney toxicity

Pediatric Concerns: None reported via milk, but observe for changes in GI flora.

Drug Interactions: Increased toxicity when used with certain penicillins, cephalosporins, amphotericin B, loop diuretics, and neuromuscular blocking agents.

Theoretic Infant Dose: 0.09 mg/kg/day

Relative Infant Dose: 0.6%

Adult Dose: 1-2 g daily

Alternatives:

T½ =	2.6 hours	M/P =	0.12-1.0
PHL =	4-10 hours (neonates)	PB =	34%
Tmax =	1-2 hours (IM)	Oral =	Poor
MW =	582	pKa =	
Vd =			

References:
1. Wilson J. Drugs in Breastmilk. New York: ADIS Press 1981.
2. Snider DE, Jr., Powell KE. Should women taking antituberculosis drugs breast-feed? Arch Intern Med 1984; 144(3):589-590.

STRONTIUM-89 CHLORIDE
Trade: Metastron
Can/Aus/UK:
Uses: Radioactive product for bone pain
LRC: L5
AAP: Not reviewed

Metastron behaves similarly to calcium. It is rapidly cleared from plasma and sequestered into bone where its radioactive emissions relieve metastatic bone pain.[1] Radioactive half-life is 50.5 days. Transfer into milk is unreported but likely. This radioactive product is too dangerous to use in lactating mothers.

Pregnancy Risk Category: D

Lactation Risk Category: L5

Adult Concerns: Severe bone marrow suppression, septicemia

Pediatric Concerns: None reported via milk. But this product is probably too dangerous to use with breastfed infants.

Drug Interactions:

Theoretic Infant Dose:

Relative Infant Dose:

Adult Dose: 4 mCi q 90 days

Alternatives:

$T\frac{1}{2}$ =	50.5 days	M/P =	
PHL =		PB =	
T_{max} =	Immediate (IV)	Oral =	
MW =	159	pKa =	
Vd =			

References:
1.   Drug Facts and Comparisons 1995 ed. ed. St. Louis: 1995.

SUCCIMER

Trade: Chemet
Can/Aus/UK:
Uses: Lead Chelator for lead poisoning
LRC: L3
AAP: Not reviewed

Succimer is a chelating agent containing dimercaptosuccinic acid. It is commonly used to chelate and increase the urinary excretion of lead.[1] While removing lead is important, some chelators (EDTA) are noted for increasing the plasma levels of lead and promoting its migration to neural and other tissues. In the instance of a breastfeeding woman, this could theoretically increase milk lead levels. However, succimer as studied in rodents has been found to increase the urinary elimination of lead without redistribution of lead to other compartments (this would theoretically include milk).[2] While we do not have studies of succimer transfer into human milk, due to its low pKa of succimer, it is unlikely that lead, chelated to succimer, would transfer into human milk. But this is not known for sure. Clinical studies in succimer-treated patients indicate that lead levels reach their lowest point after 4-5 days of therapy with succimer.[3] If breastfeeding patients were to pump and discard milk for 5 days while under therapy with succimer, it would significantly remove the risk of lead transfer into milk(if this occurs?). However, more data is required before breastfeeding can be recommended following the use of succimer.

Pregnancy Risk Category: C

Lactation Risk Category: L3

Adult Concerns: Nausea, vomiting, diarrhea, appetite loss, thrombocytosis, intermittent eosinophilia,   arrhythmias, neutropenia, drowsiness, dizziness, neuropathies, headache, rash, and paresthesias

Pediatric Concerns: None reported.

Drug Interactions:

Theoretic Infant Dose:

Relative Infant Dose:

Adult Dose: 30 milligrams/kilogram/day for 5 days

Alternatives:

$T\frac{1}{2}$ =	2-48 hours	M/P =	
PHL =		PB =	
T_{max} =	1-2 hours	Oral =	Complete
MW =	182	pKa =	3.0
Vd =			

References:
1. Pharmaceutical Manufacturer Prescribing Information.
2. Graziano JH, Lolacono NJ, Moulton T, Mitchell ME, Slavkovich V, Zarate C. Controlled study of meso-2,3-dimercaptosuccinic acid for the management of childhood lead intoxication. J Pediatr 1992; 120(1):133-139.
3. Graziano JH, Lolacono NJ, Meyer P. Dose-response study of oral 2,3-dimercaptosuccinic acid in children with elevated blood lead concentrations. J Pediatr 1988; 113(4):751-757.

SUCRALFATE

Trade: Carafate
Can/Aus/UK: Sulcrate, Novo-Sucralfate, Nu-Sucralfate, Ulcyte, Antepsin
Uses: For peptic ulcers
LRC: L2
AAP: Not reviewed

Sucralfate is a sucrose aluminum complex used for stomach ulcers. When administered orally sucralfate forms a complex that physically covers stomach ulcers.[1]   Less than 5% is absorbed orally. At these plasma levels it is very unlikely to penetrate into breastmilk.

Pregnancy Risk Category: B

Lactation Risk Category: L2

Adult Concerns: Constipation

Pediatric Concerns: None reported via milk. Absorption is very unlikely.

Drug Interactions: The use of aluminum containing antacids and sucralfate may increase the total body burden of aluminum. Sucralfate may reduce the anticoagulant effect of warfarin. Serum digoxin levels may be reduced.   Phenytoin absorption may be decreased. Ketoconazole bioavailability may be decreased. Serum quinidine levels may be reduced. Bioavailability of the fluoroquinolone family may be decreased.

Theoretic Infant Dose:

Relative Infant Dose:

Adult Dose:　　1 g QID

Alternatives:

$T\frac{1}{2}$ =		M/P =		
PHL =		PB =		
T_{max} =		Oral =	< 5%	
MW =	2087	pKa =		
Vd =				

References:
1.　Drug Facts and Comparisons 1995 ed. ed. St. Louis: 1995.

SULCONAZOLE NITRATE
Trade: Exelderm
Can/Aus/UK: Exelderm
Uses: Antifungal cream
LRC: L3
AAP: Not reviewed

Exelderm is a broad spectrum antifungal topical cream.[1]　Although no data exist on transfer into human milk, it is unlikely that the degree of transdermal absorption would be high enough to produce significant milk levels.　Only 8.7% of the topically administered dose is transcutaneously absorbed.

Pregnancy Risk Category:　C

Lactation Risk Category:　L3

Adult Concerns: Rash, skin irritation, burning, stinging

Pediatric Concerns: None reported via milk.

Drug Interactions:

Theoretic Infant Dose:

Relative Infant Dose:

Adult Dose:　　Topical

Alternatives:

References:
1.　Pharmaceutical Manufacturer Prescribing Information. 1996.

SULFAMETHOXAZOLE

Trade: Gantanol
Can/Aus/UK: Apo-Methoxazole, Gantanol, Bactrim, Resprim, Septrin
Uses: Sulfonamide antibiotic
LRC: L3
AAP: Not reviewed

Sulfamethoxazole is a common and popular sulfonamide antimicrobial. It is secreted in breastmilk in small amounts.[1] It has a longer half-life than other sulfonamides. Use with caution in weakened infants and premature infants or neonates with hyperbilirubinemia. Gantrisin (Sulfisoxazole) is considered the best choice of sulfonamides due to reduced transfer to infant. Compatible but exercise caution. PHL= 14.7-36.5 hrs (neonate), 8-9 hrs (older infants).

Pregnancy Risk Category: C

Lactation Risk Category: L3

Adult Concerns: Anemia, blood dyscrasias, allergies

Pediatric Concerns: None reported via milk, but use with caution in hyperbilirubinemic neonates and in infants with G6PD.

Drug Interactions: Decreased effect with paraaminobenzoic acid or PABA metabolites of drugs such as procaine and tetracaine. Increased effect of oral anticoagulants, oral hypoglycemic agents, and methotrexate.

Theoretic Infant Dose:

Relative Infant Dose:

Adult Dose: 1-2 g BID

Alternatives:

$T^{1/2}$ =	10.1 hours	M/P =	0.06
PHL =	14.7-36.5 hours (neonate)	PB =	62%
T_{max} =	1-4 hours	Oral =	Complete
MW =	253	pKa =	
Vd =			

References:

1. Rasmussen F. Mammary excretion of sulphonamides. Acta Pharmacol Toxicol 1958; 15:138-148.

SULFASALAZINE

Trade: Azulfidine
Can/Aus/UK: PMS Sulfasalazine, Salazopyrin, SAS-500
Uses: Anti-inflammatory for ulcerative colitis
LRC: L3
AAP: Drugs associated with significant side effects and should be given with caution

Sulfasalazine is a conjugate of sulfapyridine and 5-Aminosalicylic acid and is used as an anti-inflammatory for ulcerative colitis. Only one-third of the dose is absorbed by the mother. Most stays in the GI tract. Secretion of 5-aminosalicylic acid (active compound) and its inactive metabolite (acetyl -5-ASA) into human milk is very low.

In one study of 12 women receiving 1 to 2 grams/day of sulfasalazine, the amount of sulfasalazine in milk in patients receiving 1 gm/day was far less than 1 mg/L and approximately 0.5 to 2 mg/L in those receiving 2 gm/day.[1] In this study, small milk levels were found in only 2 women. It was estimated by the authors that breastfed infants would receive approximately 0.3 mg/kg/day of sulfapyridine. This very small amount may be regarded as negligible in considering kernicterus because sulfapyridine and sulfadiazine are known to have a poor bilirubin-displacing capacity.

Berlin reported a single case treated with salicylazosulfapyridine (Azulfidine).[2] No 5-amino salicylate compound was found in milk. The sulfapyridine levels were approximately 3 to 6 mg/L. In another study, Jarnerot suggests that while sulfasalazine levels in milk were negligible, sulfapyridine levels were approximately 45% of the maternal serum levels and the infant was likely to receive about 3-4 mg/kg of body weight.[3]

In a study of a patient receiving 1 gm of 5-aminosalicylic acid three times daily, the milk level for 5-ASA and its acetyl derivative (acetyl 5-aminosalicylic acid) was 0.1 ug/mL and 12.3 ug/mL respectively at 5 days postpartum. These results suggest that even with high doses (3gm/d) the amount of 5-ASA transferred is minimal.[4]

Few, if any, adverse effects have been observed in most nursing infants. However, one reported case of toxicity may have been an idiosyncratic allergic response.[5] Use with caution.

Pregnancy Risk Category: B
Lactation Risk Category: L3

Adult Concerns: Watery diarrhea, GI distress, nausea, vomiting, rapid breathing

Pediatric Concerns: Only one reported case of hypersensitivity. Most studies show minimal effects via milk. Observe for diarrhea, GI discomfort.

Drug Interactions: Decreased effect when used with iron, digoxin, and paraaminobenzoic acid containing drugs. Decreased effect of oral anticoagulants, methotrexate, and oral hypoglycemic agents.

Theoretic Infant Dose: 0.3 mg/kg/day

Relative Infant Dose: 1.05%

Adult Dose: 500 mg q 6 hours

Alternatives:

T½ =	7.6 hours	M/P =	0.09-0.17
PHL =		PB =	
T$_{max}$ =	Prolonged	Oral =	Poor
MW =	398	pKa =	
Vd =			

References:
1. Jarnerot G, Into-Malmberg MB. Sulphasalazine treatment during breast feeding. Scand J Gastroenterol 1979; 14(7):869-871.
2. Berlin CM, Jr., Yaffe SJ. Disposition of salicylazosulfapyridine (Azulfidine) and metabolites in human breastmilk. Dev Pharmacol Ther 1980; 1(1):31-39.
3. Janerot G, Into-Malmberg MB. Sulphasalazine treatment during breast feeding. Scand J Gastroenerol 1979; 14(7):869-871.
4. Klotz U, Harings-Kaim A. Negligible excretion of 5-aminosalicylic acid in breastmilk. Lancet 1993; 342(8871):618-619.
5. Branski D, Kerem E, Gross-Kieselstein E, Hurvitz H, Litt R, Abrahamov A. Bloody diarrhea--a possible complication of sulfasalazine transferred through human breastmilk. J Pediatr Gastroenterol Nutr 1986; 5(2):316-317.

SULFISOXAZOLE

Trade: Gantrisin, Azo-Gantrisin
Can/Aus/UK: Novo-Soxazole, Sulfizole
Uses: Sulfonamide antibiotic
LRC: L2
AAP: Maternal Medication Usually Compatible with Breastfeeding

Sulfisoxazole is a popular, sulfonamide antimicrobial. It is secreted in breastmilk in small amounts although the actual levels are somewhat controversial.[1] Kauffman (1980) reports the total amount of sulfisoxazole recovered over 48 hours following a dose of 1 gm every 6 hours (total=4gm) was 0.45% of the total dose.[2] The milk/plasma ratio was quite low for sulfisoxazole, only 0.06, and for n-acetyl sulfisoxazole, 0.22. The infant secreted 1,104 μg total sulfisoxazole in his urine over 24 hours, compared to the 1,142 μg secreted in milk. Less than 1% of the maternal dose is secreted into human milk. This is probably insufficient to produce problems in a normal newborn. Sulfisoxazole appears to be best choice with lowest milk/plasma ratio. Use with caution in weakened infants or those with hyperbilirubinemia.

Pregnancy Risk Category: C

Lactation Risk Category: L2

Adult Concerns: Elevated bilirubin, rash

Pediatric Concerns: None reported via milk. Use with caution in hyperbilirubinemic neonates and in infants with G6PD.

Drug Interactions: The anesthetic effects of thiopental may be enhanced with sulfisoxazole. Cyclosporine concentrations may be decreased by sulfonamides. Serum phenytoin levels may be increased. The risk of methotrexate induced bone marrow suppression may be enhanced. Increased sulfonylurea half-lives and hypoglycemia when used with sulfonamides.

Theoretic Infant Dose:

Relative Infant Dose:

Adult Dose: 1-4 g q 4-6 hours

Alternatives:

T½ =	4.6-7.8 hours	M/P =	0.06
PHL =		PB =	91%
T$_{max}$ =	2-4 hours	Oral =	100%
MW =	267	pKa =	
Vd =			

References:
1. Rasmussen F. Mammary excretion of sulphonamides. Acta Pharmacol Toxicol 1958; 15:138-148.
2. Kauffman RE, O'Brien C, Gilford P. Sulfisoxazole secretion into human milk. J Pediatr 1980; 97(5):839-841.

SULPIRIDE
Trade:
Can/Aus/UK: Dolmatil, Sulparex, Sulpitil
Uses: Antidepressant, antipsychotic
LRC: L2
AAP: Not reviewed

Sulpiride is a selective dopamine antagonist used as an antidepressant and antipsychotic. Sulpiride is a strong neuroleptic antipsychotic drug; however, several studies using smaller doses have found it to significantly increase prolactin levels and breastmilk production in smaller doses that do not produce overt neuroleptic effects on the mother.[1]   In a study with 14 women who received sulpiride (50 mg three times daily), and in a subsequent study with 36 breastfeeding women, Ylikorkala found major increases in prolactin levels and significant but only moderate increases in breastmilk production.[2,3]   In a group of 20 women who received 50 mg twice daily, breastmilk samples were drawn 2 hours after the dose.[4]   The concentration of sulpiride in breastmilk ranged from 0.26 to 1.97 mg/L.   No effects on breastfed infants were noted.   The authors concluded that sulpiride, when administered early in the postpartum period, is useful in promoting initiation of lactation.

In a study by McMurdo, sulpiride was found to be a potent stimulant of maternal plasma prolactin levels.[5]   Interestingly, it appears that the prolactin response to sulpiride is not dose-related and reached a maximum at 3-10 mg and thereafter, further increased doses did not further increase prolactin levels.   Sulpiride is not available in the USA.

Pregnancy Risk Category:

Lactation Risk Category: L2

Adult Concerns: Tardive dyskinesia, extrapyramidal symptoms, sedation, neuroleptic malignant syndrome, cholestatic jaundice

Pediatric Concerns: None reported via milk.

Drug Interactions: Antacids and sucralfate may reduce absorption of sulpiride.   Increased risk of seizure may result from use of tramadol or zotepine with sulpiride.

Theoretic Infant Dose: 0.29 mg/kg/day

Relative Infant Dose: < 20.6%

Adult Dose: 50 mg BID

Alternatives: Metoclopramide, domperidone

T½ =	6-8 hours	M/P =	
PHL =		PB =	
Tmax =	2-6 hours	Oral =	27-34%
MW =	341	pKa =	
Vd =	2.7		

References:
1. Wiesel FA, Alfredsson G, Ehrnebo M, Sedvall G. The pharmacokinetics of intravenous and oral sulpiride in healthy human subjects. Eur J Clin Pharmacol 1980; 17(5):385-391.
2. Ylikorkala O, Kauppila A, Kivinen S, Viinikka L. Sulpiride improves inadequate lactation. Br Med J (Clin Res Ed) 1982; 285(6337):249-251.
3. Ylikorkala O, Kauppila A, Kivinen S, Viinikka L. Treatment of inadequate lactation with oral sulpiride and buccal oxytocin. Obstet Gynecol 1984; 63(1):57-60.

4. Aono T, Shioji T, Aki T, Hirota K, Nomura A, Kurachi K. Augmentation of puerperal lactation by oral administration of sulpiride. J Clin Endocrinol Metab 1979; 48(3):478-482.
5. McMurdo ME, Howie PW, Lewis M, Marnie M, McEwen J, McNeilly AS. Prolactin response to low dose sulpiride. Br J Clin Pharmacol 1987; 24(2):133-137.

SUMATRIPTAN SUCCINATE

Trade: Imitrex
Can/Aus/UK: Imitrex, Imigran
Uses: Anti-migraine medication.
LRC: L3
AAP: Maternal Medication Usually Compatible with Breastfeeding

Sumatriptan is a 5-HT (Serotonin) receptor agonist and a highly effective new drug for the treatment of migraine headache. It is not an analgesic, rather, it produces a rapid vasoconstriction in various regions of the brain, thus temporarily reducing the cause of migraines.

In one study using 5 lactating women, each were given 6 mg subcutaneous injections and samples drawn for analysis over 8 hours.[1] The highest breastmilk levels were 87.2 μg/L at 2.6 hours post-dose and rapidly disappeared over the next 6 hours. The mean total recovery of sumatriptan in milk over the 8 hour duration was only 14.4 μg. On a weight-adjusted basis this concentration in milk corresponded to a mean infant exposure of only 3.5% of the maternal dose. Further, assuming an oral bioavailability of only 14%, the weight-adjusted dose an infant would absorb would be approximately 0.49% of the maternal dose. The authors suggest that continued breastfeeding following sumatriptan use would not pose a significant risk to the sucking infant.

The maternal plasma half-life is 1.3 hours; the milk half-life is 2.22 hours. Although the milk/plasma ratio was 4.9 (indicating significant concentrating mechanisms in milk), the absolute maternal plasma levels were small; hence, the absolute milk concentrations were low.

Pregnancy Risk Category: C

Lactation Risk Category: L3

Adult Concerns: Flushing, hot tingling sensations

Pediatric Concerns: None reported via milk.

Drug Interactions: MAOIs can markedly increase sumatriptan systemic effect and elimination including elevated sumatriptan plasma levels. Ergot containing drugs have caused prolonged vasospastic reactions. There have been rare reports of weakness, hyperreflexia, and incoordination with combined use with SSRIs such as fluoxetine, paroxetine, sertraline and fluvoxamine.

Theoretic Infant Dose: 3 μg/kg/day

Relative Infant Dose: 3.5%

Adult Dose: 25-100 mg BID-TID

Alternatives: Zolmitriptan

T½ =	1.3 hours	M/P =	4.9
PHL =		PB =	14-21%
T$_{max}$ =	12 minutes (IM)	Oral =	10-15%
MW =	413	pKa =	
Vd =			

References:

1. Wojnar-Horton RE, Hackett LP, Yapp P, Dusci LJ, Paech M, Ilett KF. Distribution and excretion of sumatriptan in human milk. Br J Clin Pharmacol 1996; 41(3):217-221.

TACROLIMUS

Trade: Prograf, Protopic
Can/Aus/UK: Protopic
Uses: Immunosuppressant
LRC: L3
AAP: Not reviewed

Tacrolimus is an immunosuppressant formerly known as SK506. It is used to reduce rejection of transplanted organs including liver and kidney.[1] In one report of 21 mothers who received tacrolimus while pregnant, milk concentrations in colostrum averaged 0.79 ng/mL and varied from 0.3 to 1.9 nanograms/mL.[2] Maternal doses (PO) ranged from 9.8 to 10.3 mg/day. Milk/blood ratio averaged 0.54. Using this data and an average daily milk intake of 150 mL/kg, the average dose to the infant per day via milk would be < 0.1 μg/kg/day. Because the oral bioavailability is poor (< 32%), an infant would likely ingest less than 100 ng/kg/day. The usual pediatric dose (PO) for preventing rejection varies from 0.15 to 0.20 mg/kg/day (equivalent to 150,000-200,000 nanograms/kg/day).

In a 32-year-old woman who had taken tacrolimus 0.1 mg/kg/d throughout pregnancy, samples were manually expressed at 0(trough), 1,6, 9, 11, and 12 hours after the morning dose.[3] The C_{max} occurred at 1 hour and was 0.57 μg/L. Using AUC data, the mean milk concentration was calculated to be 0.429 ng/mL. From these measurements, the exclusively breastfed infant would ingest, on average, 0.06 μg/kg/d, which corresponds to 0.06% of the mother's weight-normalized dose. Given the low oral bioavailability of tacrolimus, the maximum amount the baby would receive is 0.02% of the mother's weight-adjusted dose. The milk/blood ratios of tacrolimus at pre-dosing and 1-hour post-dosing concentrations were calculated to be 0.08 and 0.09, respectively. At 2.5 months of age, the infant was developing well both physically and neurologically. The authors suggest that maternal therapy with tacrolimus for liver transplant may be compatible with breastfeeding.

Recently the FDA has approved a topical form of tacrolimus (Protopic) for use in moderate to severe eczema, in those for whom standard eczema therapies are deemed inadvisable because of potential risks, or who are not adequately treated by, or who are intolerant of standard eczema therapies. Absorption via skin is minimal. In a study of 46 adult patients after multiple doses, plasma levels ranged from undetectable to 20 ng/mL, with 45 of the patients having peak blood concentrations less than 5 ng/mL.[1] In another study, the peak blood levels averaged 1.6 ng/mL, which is significantly less than the therapeutic range in kidney transplantation(7-20 ng/mL). While the absolute transcutaneous bioavailability is unknown, it is apparently very low. Combined with the poor oral bioavailability of this product, it is not likely a breastfed infant will receive enough following topical use (maternal) to produce adverse effects.

Pregnancy Risk Category: C

Lactation Risk Category: L3

Adult Concerns: Edema, renal shutdown

Pediatric Concerns: None reported.

Drug Interactions: Drugs that may increase tacrolimus levels include: calcium channel blockers, azole antifungals, macrolide antibiotics (erythromycin, clarithromycin), cisapride, metoclopramide, bromocriptine, cimetidine, cyclosporine, danazol, methylprednisolone, protease inhibitors. Drugs that may decrease tacrolimus blood levels include: carbamazepine, phenobarbital, phenytoin, rifabutin, rifampin.

Theoretic Infant Dose: 0.06 µg/kg/day

Relative Infant Dose: 0.06%

Adult Dose: 0.15-0.3 mg/kg daily

Alternatives:

T½ =	34.2 hours	M/P =	0.54
PHL =	11.5 hours	PB =	99%
T$_{max}$ =	1,6 hours	Oral =	14-32%
MW =	822	pKa =	
Vd =	2.6		

References:
1. Pharmaceutical Manufacturer Prescribing Information.
2. Jain A, Venkataramanan R, Fung JJ, Gartner JC, Lever J, Balan V, Warty V, Starzl TE. Pregnancy after liver transplantation under tacrolimus. Transplantation 1997; 64(4):559-565.
3. French AE, Soldin SJ, Soldin OP, Koren G. Milk transfer and neonatal safety of tacrolimus. Ann Pharmacother 2003; 37(6):815-818.

TAMOXIFEN

Trade: Nolvadex
Can/Aus/UK: Apo-Tamox, Nolvadex, Tamofen, Tamone, Tamoxen, Genox, Eblon, Noltam
Uses: Anti-estrogen, anticancer
LRC: L5
AAP: Not reviewed

Tamoxifen is an nonsteroidal antiestrogen. It attaches to the estrogen receptor and produces only minimal stimulation, thus it prevents estrogen from stimulating the receptor. Aside from this, it also produces a number of other effects within the cytoplasm of the cell and some of its anticancer effects may be mediated by its effects at sites other than the estrogen receptor.

Tamoxifen is metabolized by the liver and has an elimination half-life of greater than 7 days (range 3-21 days).[1] It is well absorbed orally, and the highest tissue concentrations are in the liver (60 fold). It is 99% protein bound and normally reduces plasma prolactin levels significantly (66% after 3 months). At present, there are no data on its transfer into breastmilk; however, it has been shown to inhibit lactation early postpartum in several studies. In one study, doses of 10-30 mg twice daily early postpartum, completely inhibited postpartum engorgement and lactation.[2] In a second study, tamoxifen doses of 10 mg four times daily significantly reduced serum prolactin and inhibited milk production as well.[3] We do not know the effect of tamoxifen on established milk production.

Tamoxifen is potentially teratogenic (category D) and should never be used in pregnant women. Note: it is useful in conjunction with clomiphene to stimulate ovulation...short term use only. It has a pKa of 8.85 which may suggest some trapping in milk compared to the maternal plasma levels.

This product has a very long half-life, and the active metabolite is concentrated in the plasma (2 fold). This drug has all the characteristics that would suggest a concentrating mechanism in breastfed infants over time. Its prominent effect on reducing prolactin levels will inhibit early lactation and may ultimately inhibit established lactation. In this instance, the significant risks to the infant from exposure to tamoxifen probably outweigh the benefits of breastfeeding. Mothers receiving tamoxifen should not breastfeed until we know more about the levels transferred into milk and the plasma/tissue levels found in breastfed infants.

Pregnancy Risk Category: **D**

Lactation Risk Category: **L5**

Adult Concerns: Hot flashes, nausea, vomiting, vaginal bleeding/discharge, menstrual irregularities, amenorrhea

Pediatric Concerns: None reported but caution is urged.

Drug Interactions: Increased anticoagulant effect when used with coumarin-type anticoagulants. Tamoxifen is a potent inhibitor of drug metabolizing enzymes in the liver, observe for elevated levels of many drugs.

Theoretic Infant Dose:

Relative Infant Dose:

Adult Dose: 10-20 mg BID

Alternatives:

T½ =	> 7 days	M/P =	
PHL =		PB =	99%
T$_{max}$ =	2-3 hours	Oral =	Complete
MW =	371	pKa =	8.85
Vd =			

References:
1. Pharmaceutical Manufacturer Prescribing Information. 1997.
2. Shaaban MM. Suppression of lactation by an antiestrogen, tamoxifen. Eur J Obstet Gynecol Reprod Biol 1975; 4(5):167-169.
3. Masala A, Delitala G, Lo DG, Stoppelli I, Alagna S, Devilla L. Inhibition of lactation and inhibition of prolactin release after mechanical breast stimulation in puerperal women given tamoxifen or placebo. Br J Obstet Gynaecol 1978; 85(2):134-137.

TAZAROTENE
Trade: Tazorac
Can/Aus/UK: Zorac
Uses: Anti-psoriatic
LRC: L3
AAP: Not reviewed

Tazarotene is a specialized retinoid for topical use and is used for the topical treatment of stable plaque psoriasis and acne. Following topical application, tazarotene is converted to an active metabolite; transcutaneous absorption is minimal (< 1%).[1] Applied daily, it is indicated for treatment of stable plaque psoriasis of up to 20% of the body surface area. Only 2-3% of the topically applied drug is absorbed transcutaneously. Tazarotene is metabolized to the active ingredient, tazarotenic acid. Tazarotene is used for the topical treatment of stable plaque psoriasis and acne. Following topical application, tazarotene is converted to an active metabolite; transcutaneous absorption is minimal (< 1%). Little compound could be detected in the plasma. At steady state, plasma levels were only 0.09 ng/mL although this value is largely a function of surface area treated. When applied to large surface areas, systemic absorption is increased. Data on transmission to breastmilk are not available. The manufacturer reports some is transferred to rodent milk, but it has not been tested in humans.

Pregnancy Risk Category: X

Lactation Risk Category: L3

Adult Concerns: Hypertriglyceridemia, peripheral edema, pruritus, erythema, burning, contact dermatitis have been reported. This drug is potentially a significant teratogen and should not ever be used in pregnant patients or those not protected with a suitable birth-control measure.

Pediatric Concerns: None via milk. Some caution is recommended if used over large surface areas (20-30%).

Drug Interactions: Do not use concomitantly with drying agents.

Theoretic Infant Dose:

Relative Infant Dose:

Adult Dose: Apply daily

Alternatives:

T½ =	18 hours (met)	M/P =	
PHL =		PB =	99%
T$_{max}$ =	8 hours	Oral =	Complete
MW =	351	pKa =	
Vd =			

References:
1. Pharmaceutical Manufacturer Prescribing Information.

TEA TREE OIL

Trade: Tea Tree Oil
Can/Aus/UK:
Uses: Antibacterial, antifungal
LRC: L3
AAP: Not reviewed

Tee tree oil, as derived from Melaleuca alternifolia, has recently gained popularity for its antiseptic properties. The essential oil, derived by steam distillation of the leaves, contains terpin-4-ol in concentrations of 40% or more.[1] TTO is primarily noted for its antimicrobial effects without irritating sensitive tissues. It is antimicrobial when tested against Candida albicans, E. coli, S. Aureus, Staph. epidermidis, and pseudomonas aeruginosa. In several reports it is suggested to have antifungal properties equivalent to tolnaftate and clotrimazole. Although the use of TTO in adults is mostly nontoxic, the safe use in infants is unknown. Use directly on the nipple should be minimized.

Pregnancy Risk Category:

Lactation Risk Category: L3

Adult Concerns: Toxic effects include allergic eczema. Petechial body rash and leukocytosis in one individual who ingested 1/2 teaspoonful orally. Ataxia and drowsiness following oral ingestion of < 10 cc by a 17 month old infant.

Pediatric Concerns: None reported via milk.

Drug Interactions:

Theoretic Infant Dose:

Relative Infant Dose:

Adult Dose:

Alternatives:

References:
1. Review of Natural Products Ed: Facts and Comparisons 1997.

TECHNETIUM TC 99M SESTAMIBI

Trade: Cardiolite, Sestamibi
Can/Aus/UK:
Uses: Imaging agent
LRC: L4
AAP: Radioactive compound that requires temporary cessation of breastfeeding

Technetium 99M sestamibi is a myocardial imaging agent that is also sometimes used as an oncologic imaging agent. The radioactive technetium-99 ion is chelated to the sestamibi molecule. It is used as an alternative to Thallium-201 imaging.[1] Sestamibi is largely distributed to the myocardium and is a function of myocardial viability.[2] Technetium is a weak gamma emitter with a radioactive half-life of only 6.02 hours. The biological half-life of this product is approximately 6 hours, but the effective half-life (both biological and radioactive) is only about 3 hours. Transfer of significant amounts of sestamibi into human milk is yet unreported but is rather unlikely as sestamibi binds irreversible to myocardial tissue and does not redistribute to other tissues to a significant degree. Other forms of TC-99 have been reported to enter milk, but entry would be largely determined by the chemical form, not the radioactive agent.[3] For current Nuclear Regulatory Commission breastfeeding guidelines consult table in appendix.

Pregnancy Risk Category: C

Lactation Risk Category: L4

Adult Concerns: Dysgeusia, headache, flushing, angina, hypersensitivity, hypertension

Pediatric Concerns: It is not known if the sestamibi chelate is transferred into human milk. But Technetium salts in general do transfer. Pump and dump for 24-30 hours or until all radioactive is gone.

Drug Interactions:

Theoretic Infant Dose:

Relative Infant Dose:

Adult Dose: 10-30 mCi X 1

Alternatives:

T½ =	6 hours	M/P =	
PHL =		PB =	< 1%
T~max~ =		Oral =	Complete
MW =		pKa =	
Vd =			

References:
1. Berman DS. Introduction--Technetium-99m myocardial perfusion imaging agents and their relation to thallium-201. Am J Cardiol 1990; 66(13):1E-4E.
2. Berman DS, Kiat H, Maddahi J. The new Tc-99m myocardial perfusion imaging agents: Tc-99m sestamibi and Tc-99m teboroxime. Circulation 1991; 84((suppl)):7-21.
3. Maisels MJ, Gilcher RO. Excretion of technetium in human milk. Pediatrics 1983; 71(5):841-842.

TECHNETIUM-99M

Trade: Technetium-99m
Can/Aus/UK:
Uses: Radioactive imaging
LRC: L4
AAP: Radioactive compound that requires temporary cessation of breastfeeding

Radioactive technetium-99M (Tc-99m) is present in milk for at least 15 hours to 3 days, and significant quantities have been reported in the thyroid and gastric mucosa of infants ingesting milk from treated mothers. Technetium is one of the halide elements and is handled, biologically, much like iodine. Like iodine, it concentrates in thyroid tissues, the stomach, and breastmilk of nursing mothers. It has a radioactive half-life of 6.02 hours. Following a dose of 15 mCi of Tc-99m for a brain scan, the concentration of Tc-99m in breastmilk at 4, 8.5, 20, and 60 hours was 0.5 uCi, 0.1 uCi, 0.02 uCi, and 0.006 uCi respectively.[1] In another study, following a dose of 10 mCi of NaTcO4, breastmilk levels were 5.7, 1.5, 0.015 uCi/mL at 3.25, 7.5, and 24 hours respectively.[2] The estimated dose to infant was 1,036, 284, and 2.7 uCi/180 mL milk. These authors recommended pumping and discarding milk for 48 hours. Technetium-99m is used in many salt and chemical forms, but the radioactivity and decay are the same although the concentration in milk may be influenced by the salt form.

In another study using Technetium MAG3 in two mothers receiving 150 MBq of radioactivity, the total percent of ingested radioactivity ranged from 0.7 to 1.6% of the total.[3] These authors suggested that the DTPA salt of technetium would produce the least breastmilk levels and would be preferred in breastfeeding mothers. The NRC table in the appendix suggests a duration of interruption of breastfeeding of 12 to 24 hours for 12 and 30 mCi respectively, but this depends on the salt form used.

Pregnancy Risk Category: C

Lactation Risk Category: L4

Adult Concerns:

Pediatric Concerns: None reported, but may be transferred to infant thyroid. Pump and dump for a minimum of 48 hours.

Drug Interactions:

Theoretic Infant Dose:

Relative Infant Dose:

Adult Dose: 15-20 mCi X 1

Alternatives:

T½ =	< 6 hours	M/P =	
PHL =		PB =	
T_{max} =		Oral =	Complete
MW =		pKa =	
Vd =			

References:

1. Rumble WF, Aamodt RL, Jones AE, Henkin RI, Johnston GS. Accidental ingestion of Tc-99m in breastmilk by a 10-week-old child. J Nucl Med 1978; 19(8):913-915.
2. Maisels MJ, Gilcher RO. Excretion of technetium in human milk. Pediatrics 1983; 71(5):841-842.
3. Evans JL, Mountford AN, Herring AN, Richardson MA. Secretion of radioactivity in breastmilk following administration of 99Tcm-MAG3. Nuc Med Comm 1993; 14:108-111.

TEGASEROD MALEATE

Trade: Zelnorm
Can/Aus/UK: Zelnorm
Uses: Treatment of irritable bowel syndrome
LRC: L3
AAP: Not reviewed

Tegaserod is a serotonin agonist (stimulant) used to treat the symptoms of irritable bowel syndrome. Oral absorption is only 10%(fasting) and is reduced 40-65% by food. In patients receiving oral doses of 2, 6, and 12 mg, mean peak plasma concentrations were 0.9, 2.9, and 6.3 µg/L respectively.[2] Studies in rats suggest it transfers with a higher milk/plasma ratio, but this is common for rodent studies and the dose was 320 times that given humans.[2] No data are available on its transfer to human milk. Tegaserod is a lipophilic drug which would assist its transfer into human milk, however, its low plasma levels, poor oral bioavailability (particularly with food), and large volume of distribution suggests that the actual amount transferred into human milk is probably quite low.

Pregnancy Risk Category: B

Lactation Risk Category: L3

Adult Concerns: Adverse events may include abdominal pain, diarrhea, nausea, flatulence, headache, pain, flushing, hypotension, and vertigo.

Pediatric Concerns: None reported via milk, but rat milk levels have been detected.

Drug Interactions: None reported.

Theoretic Infant Dose:

Relative Infant Dose:

Adult Dose: 6 mg twice daily

Alternatives:

T½ =	11 hours	M/P =	
PHL =		PB =	98%
T$_{max}$ =	1 hour	Oral =	10%
MW =	417	pKa =	
Vd =	368		

References:
1. Pharmaceutical Manufacturers prescribing information, 2003.
2. Appel-Dingemanse S. Clinical pharmacokinetics of tegaserod, a serotonin 5 - HT(4) receptor partial agonist with promotile activity. Clin Pharmacokinet 2002; 41(13):1021-1042.

TELMISARTAN

Trade: Micardis, Micardis HCT
Can/Aus/UK: Micardis
Uses: Angiotensin II receptor antagonist
LRC: L3
       L4 if used in neonatal period
AAP: Not reviewed

Telmisartan is a potent antihypertensive that blocks the angiotensin II receptor site. Micardis HCT also contains hydrochlorothiazide 12.5 mg. This agent should never be used in pregnant patients, as fetal demise has been reported with similar agents in this class. No data are available on its use in lactating mothers. However, its use early postpartum in lactating mothers is not recommended due to the sensitivity of newborns to antihypertensives of this family (ACE and AT-1* antagonists).

Pregnancy Risk Category: C during 1 st and 2 nd trimesters
                            D during 3 rd trimester

Lactation Risk Category: L3
          L4 if used in neonatal period

Adult Concerns: UTI infection, back pain, sinusitis and diarrhea have been reported. Flu-like symptoms, myalgia, coughing, hypotension have been reported.

Pediatric Concerns: None reported,   but use caution early postpartum.

Drug Interactions: When coadministered with digoxin, a 50% increase in digoxin peak plasma levels occurred, and a 13-20% increase in trough levels.

Theoretic Infant Dose:

Relative Infant Dose:

Adult Dose: 40 mg daily

Alternatives:

T½ =	24 hours		M/P =	
PHL =			PB =	99.5%
T$_{max}$ =	1 hour		Oral =	42-58%
MW =	514		pKa =	
Vd =	7.14			

References:
1.   Pharmaceutical Manufacturer Prescribing Information.

TEMAZEPAM

Trade: Restoril
Can/Aus/UK: Restoril, PMS-Temazepam, Euhypnos, Noctume, Temaze, Temtabs, Normison
Uses: Short acting benzodiazepine (Valium-like) hypnotic
LRC: L3
AAP: Drugs whose effect on nursing infants is unknown but may be of concern

Temazepam is a short acting benzodiazepine that belongs to the Valium family primarily used as a nighttime sedative.   In one study the milk/plasma ratio varied from < 0.09 to < 0.63 (mean=0.18).[1] Temazepam is relatively water soluble and therefore particians poorly into breastmilk.   Levels of temazepam were undetectable in the infants studied although these studies were carried out 15 hours post-dose. Although the study shows low neonatal exposure to temazepam via breastmilk, the infant should be monitored carefully for sleepiness and poor feeding.

Pregnancy Risk Category: X

Lactation Risk Category: L3

Adult Concerns: Sedation

Pediatric Concerns: None reported via milk, but observe for sedation, poor feeding.

Drug Interactions: Increased effect when used with other CNS depressants.

Theoretic Infant Dose:

Relative Infant Dose:

Adult Dose: 7.5-30 mg daily

Alternatives: Lorazepam, Alprazolam

T½ =	9.5-12.4 hours	M/P =	0.18
PHL =		PB =	96%
T$_{max}$ =	2-4 hours	Oral =	90%
MW =	301	pKa =	1.3
Vd =	0.8-1.0		

References:

1. Lebedevs TH, Wojnar-Horton RE, Yapp P, Roberts MJ, Dusci LJ, Hackett LP, Ilett KF. Excretion of temazepam in breastmilk. Br J Clin Pharmacol 1992; 33(2):204-206.

TERAZOSIN HCL

Trade: Hytrin
Can/Aus/UK: Hytrin
Uses: Antihypertensive
LRC: L4
AAP: Not reviewed

Terazosin is an antihypertensive that belongs to the alpha-1 blocking family. This family is generally very powerful, produces significant orthostatic hypotension and other side effects.[1] As such, for the past 20 years, these drugs have always been used as the STEP II drugs used in hypertension, whereas the beta blockers, ACE inhibitors, calcium channel blockers, and thiazide diuretics have always been used first (STEP I). If the STEP I drugs don't work, then the physician employs a STEP II drug.

Terazosin has rather powerful effects on the prostate and testes producing testicular atrophy in some animal studies (particularly newborn) and is therefore not preferred in pregnant or in lactating women. No data are available on transfer into human milk. Use caution.

Pregnancy Risk Category: C

Lactation Risk Category: **L4**

Adult Concerns: Hypotension, bradycardia, sedation

Pediatric Concerns: None reported, but extreme caution is recommended.

Drug Interactions: Decreased antihypertensive effect when used with NSAIDs. Increased hypotensive effects when used with diuretics and other antihypertensive beta blockers.

Theoretic Infant Dose:

Relative Infant Dose:

Adult Dose: 1-10 mg daily

Alternatives:

T½ =	9-12 hours	M/P =	
PHL =		PB =	94%
T$_{max}$ =	1-2 hours	Oral =	90%
MW =	423	pKa =	
Vd =			

References:
1. Pharmaceutical Manufacturer Prescribing Information. 1995.

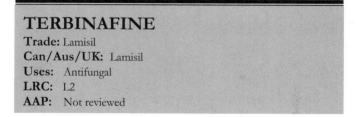

TERBINAFINE

Trade: Lamisil
Can/Aus/UK: Lamisil
Uses: Antifungal
LRC: L2
AAP: Not reviewed

Terbinafine is an antifungal agent primarily used for tinea species such as athlete's foot and ringworm. Systemic absorption following topical therapy is minimal.[1] Following an oral dose of 500 mg in two volunteers, the total dose of terbinafine secreted in breastmilk during the 72 hour post-dosing period was 0.65 mg in one mother and 0.15 mg in another.[2] The total excretion of terbinafine in breastmilk ranged from 0.13% to 0.03 % of the total maternal dose respectively. Topical absorption through the skin is minimal.[3]

Pregnancy Risk Category: **B**

Lactation Risk Category: **L2**

Adult Concerns: Topical: burning, pruritus. Oral: fatigue, headache, GI distress, elevated liver enzymes, alopecia.

Pediatric Concerns: None reported via milk.

Drug Interactions: Terbinafine clearance is decreased 33% by cimetidine, and 16% by terfenadine. Terbinafine increases clearance of cyclosporin(15%). Rifampin increases terbinafine clearance by 100%.

Theoretic Infant Dose:

Relative Infant Dose:

Adult Dose: 250 mg daily

Alternatives: Fluconazole

T½ =	26 hours	M/P =	
PHL =		PB =	99%
Tmax =	1-2 hours	Oral =	80%
MW =	291	pKa =	
Vd =	> 28		

References:
1. Pharmaceutical Manufacturer Prescribing Information. 1996.
2. Drug Facts and Comparisons 1996 ed. ed. St. Louis: 1996.
3. Birnbaum JE. Pharmacology of the allylamines. J Am Acad Dermatol 1990; 23(4 Pt 2):782-785.

TERBUTALINE

Trade: Bricanyl, Brethine
Can/Aus/UK: Bricanyl
Uses: Bronchodilator for asthma
LRC: L2
AAP: Maternal Medication Usually Compatible with Breastfeeding

Terbutaline is a popular Beta-2 adrenergic used for bronchodilation in asthmatics. It is secreted into breastmilk but in low quantities. Following doses of 7.5 to 15 mg/day of terbutaline, milk levels averaged 3.37 µg/L.[1] Assuming a daily intake of 165 mL milk, these levels would suggest a daily intake of less than 0.5 µg/kg/day which corresponds to 0.2 to 0.7% of maternal dose.

In another study of a patient receiving 5 mg three times daily, the mean milk concentrations ranged from 3.2 to 3.7 µg/L.[2] The author calculated the daily dose to infant at 0.4-0.5 µg/kg body weight. Terbutaline was not detectable in the infant's serum. No untoward effects have been reported in breastfeeding infants.

Pregnancy Risk Category: B

Lactation Risk Category: L2

Adult Concerns: Tremors, nervousness, tachycardia

Pediatric Concerns: None reported via milk.

Drug Interactions: Decreased effect when used with beta blockers. May increase toxicity when used with MAOI and TCAs.

Theoretic Infant Dose: 0.5 μg/kg/day

Relative Infant Dose: 0.23%

Adult Dose: 5 mg TID

Alternatives:

$T\frac{1}{2}$ =	14 hours	M/P =	< 2.9
PHL =		PB =	20%
T_{max} =	5-30 minutes	Oral =	33-50%
MW =	225	pKa =	
Vd =	1-2		

References:
1. Lindberg C, Boreus LO, De Chateau P, Lindstrom B, Lonnerholm G, Nyberg L. Transfer of terbutaline into breastmilk. Eur J Respir Dis Suppl 1984; 134:87-91.
2. Lonnerholm G, Lindstrom B. Terbutaline excretion into breastmilk. Br J Clin Pharmacol 1982; 13(5):729-730.

TERCONAZOLE

Trade: Terazol 3, Terazol 7
Can/Aus/UK: Terazol
Uses: Antifungal, vaginal.
LRC: L3
AAP: Not reviewed

Terconazole is an antifungal primarily used for vaginal candidiasis. It is similar to fluconazole and itraconazole. When administered intravaginally, only a limited amount (5 -16%) is absorbed systemically (mean peak plasma level = 6 ng/mL).[1,2] It is well absorbed orally. Even at high doses the drug is not mutagenic, nor fetotoxic. At high doses, terconazole is known to enter breastmilk in rodents although no data are available on human milk. The milk levels are probably too small to be clinically relevant.

Pregnancy Risk Category: C

Lactation Risk Category: L3

Adult Concerns: Vaginal burning, itching, flu-like symptoms

Pediatric Concerns: None reported due to minimal studies.

Drug Interactions:

Theoretic Infant Dose:

Relative Infant Dose:

Adult Dose: 5 g daily

Alternatives: Fluconazole

T½ =	4-11.3 hours	M/P =	
PHL =		PB =	
T$_{max}$ =		Oral =	Complete
MW =	532	pKa =	
Vd =			

References:
1. Pharmaceutical Manufacturer Prescribing Information. 1996.
2. McEvoy GE. (ed):AFHS Drug Information. New York, NY: 2003.

TETRACYCLINE
Trade: Achromycin, Sumycin, Terramycin
Can/Aus/UK: Achromycin, Aureomycin, Tetracyn, Mysteclin, Tetrex, Tetrachel
Uses: Antibiotic
LRC: L2
AAP: Maternal Medication Usually Compatible with Breastfeeding

Tetracycline is a broad spectrum antibiotic with significant side effects in pediatric patients, including dental staining and reduced bone growth. It is secreted into breastmilk in extremely small levels. Because tetracyclines bind to milk calcium they would have reduced oral absorption in the infant.

Posner reports that in a patient receiving 500 mg four times daily, the average concentration of tetracycline in milk was 1.14 mg/L.[1] The maternal plasma level was 1.92 mg/L and the milk/plasma ratio was 0.59. The absolute dose to the infant ranged from 0.17 to 0.39 mg/kg/day. None was detected in the plasma compartment of the infant (limit of detection 0.05 mg/L).

In a mother receiving 275 mg/d, milk levels averaged 1.25 mg/L with a maximum of 2.51 mg/L.[2] None was detected in the infants plasma. In another study of 2-3 patients receiving a single 150 mg/d dose, milk levels ranged from 0.3 to 1.2 mg/L at 4 hours (C$_{max}$). The maximum reported milk level was 1.2 mg/L.[3] A milk/plasma ratio of 0.58 was reported.

From the above studies, the relative infant dose is 0.6%, 4.77% and 8.44%. Thus a high degree of variability exists in these studies. Invariably a mixture of tetracyclines in milk, would greatly limit their oral bioavailability.

The short-term exposure of infants to tetracyclines (via milk) is not contraindicated(< 3 weeks). However, this author does not recommend the long-term exposure of breastfeeding infants to tetracyclines, such as when used daily for acne. The absorption of even small amounts over a prolonged period could result in dental staining.

Pregnancy Risk Category: D

Lactation Risk Category: L2

Adult Concerns: Pediatric: dental staining, decreased bone growth, altered GI flora

Pediatric Concerns: None reported via milk. Poor oral absorption of tetracyclines generally limits effects. Avoid long-term exposure.

Drug Interactions: Absorption may be reduced or delayed when used with dairy products, calcium, magnesium, or aluminum containing antacids, oral contraceptives, iron, zinc, sodium bicarbonate, penicillins, cimetidine. Increased toxicity may result when used with methoxyflurane anesthesia. Use with warfarin anticoagulants may increase anticoagulation

Theoretic Infant Dose: 0.17 mg/kg/day

Relative Infant Dose: 0.6%

Adult Dose: 500 mg QID

Alternatives:

$T\frac{1}{2}$ =	6-12 hours	M/P =	0.58-1.28
PHL =		PB =	25%
T_{max} =	1.5-4 hours	Oral =	75%
MW =	444	pKa =	
Vd =			

References:
1. Posner AC, Prigot A, Konicoff NG. Further observations on the use of tetracycline hydrochloride in prophylaxis and treatment of obstetric infections. New York: Antibiotics Annual 1954-1955. In: Medical Encyclopedia, 1955.
2. Graf von H, Riemann S. Untersuchungen uber die konzentration von pyrrolidino-methyl-tetracyclin in der muttermilch. Dtsch med wochenschr 1959; 84:1694-1696.
3. Matsuda S. Transfer of antibiotics into maternal milk. Biol Res Pregnancy Perinatol 1984; 5(2):57-60.

THALLIUM-201
Trade: Thallium-201
Can/Aus/UK:
Uses: Radioactive tracer
LRC: L4
AAP: Not reviewed

Thallium-201 in the form of thallous chloride is used extensively for myocardial perfusion imaging to delineate ischemic myocardium. Following infusion, almost 85% of the administered dose is extracted into the heart on the first pass. Less than 5% of the dose remains free in the plasma in as little as 5 minutes after administration. Whereas Thallium-201 has a radioactive half-life of only 73 hours, the whole-body half-life of the Thallium ion is about 10 days. Most all radiation will be decayed in 5-6 half-lives (15 days). In a study of one breastfeeding patient who received 111MBq (3 mCi) for a brain scan, the amount of Thallium-201 in breastmilk at 4 hours was 326 Bq/mL and subsequently dropped to 87 Bq/mL after 72 hours.[1] Even without interrupting breastfeeding, the infant would have received less than the NCRP radiation safety guideline dose for infrequent exposure for a 1 year old infant. However, a brief interruption of breastfeeding was nevertheless recommended. The length of interrupted breastfeeding is dependent on age of infant and dose of Thallium. With an interruption time varying from 2, 24, 48, to 96 hours, the respective Thallium dose to the infant would be 0.442, 0.283, 0.197, and 0.101 MBq compared to the maternal dose of 111 MBq.

In another study of a breastfeeding mother who received 111 MBq (3 mCi), the calculated dose an infant (without any interruption of breastfeeding and assuming the consumption of 1000 mL of milk daily) would receive is approximately 0.81 MBq, which is presently less than the maximal allowed radiation dose (NCRP) for an infant.[2] The authors therefore recommend that breastfeeding be discontinued for at least 24-48 hours following the administration of 111 MBq of Thallium-201. The amount of infant exposure from close contact with the mother was also measured and found to be very small in comparison to the orally ingested dose via milk. A brief interruption of breastfeeding for 24-48 hours would dramatically reduce overall exposure of the infant although the Nuclear Regulatory Commission recommends interruption of breastfeeding for 2 weeks (with dose=110 Mbq). See NRC table in appendix.

Pregnancy Risk Category:

Lactation Risk Category: L4

Adult Concerns:

Pediatric Concerns: None reported in one case, but a brief interruption (depending on dose) is advised.

Drug Interactions:

Theoretic Infant Dose:

Relative Infant Dose:

Adult Dose:

Alternatives:

T½ =	73 hours	M/P =
PHL =		PB =
T$_{max}$ =	< 60 minutes	Oral =
MW =		pKa =
Vd =		

References:
1. Johnston RE, Mukherji SK, Perry RJ, Stabin MG. Radiation dose from breastfeeding following administration of thallium-201. J Nucl Med 1996; 37(12):2079-2082.
2. Murphy PH, Beasley CW, Moore WH, Stabin MG. Thallium-201 in human milk: observations and radiological consequences. Health Phys 1989; 56(4):539-541.

THEOPHYLLINE

Trade: Aminophylline, Quibron, Theo-Dur
Can/Aus/UK: Theo-Dur, Pulmophylline, Quibron-T/SR, Austyn, Nuelin
Uses: Bronchodilator
LRC: L3
AAP: Maternal Medication Usually Compatible with Breastfeeding

Theophylline is a methylxanthine bronchodilator. It has a prolonged half-life in neonates which may cause retention. Milk concentrations are approximately equal to the maternal plasma levels. If a mother is maintained at 10-20 µg/mL, the milk concentrations are closely equivalent. Estimates generally indicate that less than 1% of dose is absorbed by infant. Assuming maternal plasma levels of 10-20 µg/mL, the theophylline levels in a neonate would range from 0.9 to 3.6 µg/mL.[1]

In another study of 12 patients receiving 300 mg theophylline, followed 5 hours later by 200 mg, the reported milk concentration was 2.8 mg/L and the milk/plasma ratio ranged from 0.6 to 0.89.[2] The reported maximum concentration was 6.0 mg/L. The relative infant dose would be approximately 5.8% of the weight normalized maternal dose.

One reported case of irritability and fretful sleeping was reported in an infant exposed to breastmilk only on days when the mother reported taking theophylline. The average milk concentration of theophylline in this case was 0.7 mg/L.

Pregnancy Risk Category: C

Lactation Risk Category: L3

Adult Concerns: Irritability, nausea, vomiting, tachycardia, seizures

Pediatric Concerns: None reported via milk. One case of irritability and fretful sleeping.

Drug Interactions: Numerous drug interactions exist. Agents that decrease theophylline levels include barbiturates, phenytoin, ketoconazole, rifampin, cigarette smoking, carbamazepine, isoniazid, loop diuretics, and others. Agents that increase theophylline levels include allopurinol, beta blockers, calcium channel blockers, cimetidine, oral contraceptives, corticosteroids, disulfiram, ephedrine, influenza virus vaccine, interferon, macrolides, mexiletine, quinolones, thiabendazole, thyroid hormones, carbamazepine, isoniazid, and loop diuretics.

Theoretic Infant Dose: 0.42 mg/kg/day

Relative Infant Dose: 5.8%

Adult Dose: 3 mg/kg q 8 hours

Alternatives:

$T\frac{1}{2}$ =	3-12.8 hours	M/P =	0.67
PHL =	30 hours	PB =	56%
T_{max} =	1-2 hours (oral)	Oral =	76%
MW =	180	pKa =	8.6
Vd =	0.3-0.7		

References:

1. Stec GP, Greenberger P, Ruo TI, Henthorn T, Morita Y, Atkinson AJ, Jr., Patterson R. Kinetics of theophylline transfer to breastmilk. Clin Pharmacol Ther 1980; 28(3):404-408.
2. Reinhardt D, Richter O, Brandenburg G. [Pharmacokinetics of drugs from the breast-feeding mother passing into the body of the infant, using theophylline as an example]. Monatsschr Kinderheilkd 1983; 131(2):66-70.
3. Yurchak AM, Jusko WJ. Theophylline secretion into breastmilk. Pediatrics 1976; 57(4):518-520.

THIABENDAZOLE

Trade: Mintezol
Can/Aus/UK: Mintezol
Uses: Anthelmintic, antiparasitic
LRC: L3
AAP: Not reviewed

Thiabendazole is an antiparasitic agent for the treatment of roundworm, pinworm, hookworm, whipworm, and other parasitic infections. After absorption it is completely eliminated from the plasma by 48 hours although most is excreted by 24 hours. Can be used in children. Although it is effective in pinworms, other agents with less side effects are preferred. No reports on its transfer to breastmilk have been found.

Pregnancy Risk Category: C

Lactation Risk Category: L3

Adult Concerns: Hypotension, nausea, vomiting, psychotic reactions (seizures, hallucinations, delirium), rash, pruritus, intrahepatic cholestasis, transient milk hepatitis

Pediatric Concerns: None reported.

Drug Interactions: May increase theophylline and other xanthines levels by 50%.

Theoretic Infant Dose:

Relative Infant Dose:

Adult Dose: 1.5 g BID

Alternatives: Pyrantel

$T\frac{1}{2}$ =		M/P =	
PHL =		PB =	
T_{max} =	1-2 hours	Oral =	Complete
MW =	201	pKa =	
Vd =			

THIOPENTAL SODIUM

Trade: Pentothal
Can/Aus/UK: Pentothal, Intraval
Uses: Barbiturate anesthetic agent
LRC: L3
AAP: Maternal Medication Usually Compatible with Breastfeeding

Thiopental is an ultra short-acting, barbiturate sedative. Used in the induction phase of anesthesia, it rapidly redistributes from the brain to adipose and muscle tissue; hence, the plasma levels are small, and the sedative effects are virtually gone in 20 minutes. Thiopental sodium is secreted into milk in low levels. In a study of two groups of 8 women who received from 5.0 to 5.4 mg/kg thiopental sodium, the maximum concentration in breastmilk 0.9 mg/L in mature milk and in colostrum was 0.34 mg/L.[1] The milk/plasma ratio was 0.3 for colostrum and 0.4 for mature milk. The maximum daily dose to infant would be 0.135 mg/kg or approximately 2.5% of the adult dose.

Pregnancy Risk Category: C

Lactation Risk Category: L3

Adult Concerns: Hemolytic anemia has been reported. Respiratory depression, renal failure, delirium, nausea, vomiting, pruritus.

Pediatric Concerns: None reported in a study of 16 women receiving induction doses.

Drug Interactions: Increased depression when used with CNS depressants (especially opiates and phenothiazines), and with salicylates or sulfisoxazole.

Theoretic Infant Dose: 0.13 mg/kg/day

Relative Infant Dose: 2.5%

Adult Dose: 50-100 mg X 2

Alternatives:

$T\frac{1}{2}$ =	3-8 hours	M/P =	0.3-0.4
PHL =	15 hours	PB =	60-96%
T_{max} =	1-2 minutes	Oral =	Variable
MW =	264	pKa =	
Vd =	1.4		

References:

1. Andersen LW, Qvist T, Hertz J, Mogensen F. Concentrations of thiopentone in mature breastmilk and colostrum following an induction dose. Acta Anaesthesiol Scand 1987; 31(1):30-32.

THIORIDAZINE

Trade: Mellaril
Can/Aus/UK: Apo-Thioridazine, Mellaril, Novo-Ridazine, Aldazine
Uses: Antipsychotic
LRC: L4
AAP: Not reviewed

Thioridazine is a potent phenothiazine tranquilizer. It has a high volume of distribution and long half-life. No data are available on its secretion into human milk, but it should be expected.[1] Pediatric indications (2-12 years of age) are available.

Pregnancy Risk Category: C

Lactation Risk Category: L4

Adult Concerns: Blood dyscrasias, arrhythmias, sedation, gynecomastia, nausea, vomiting, constipation, dry mouth, retinopathy

Pediatric Concerns: None reported due to limited studies.

Drug Interactions: Alcohol may enhance CNS depression. Aluminum salts may reduce GI absorption. Other anticholinergics may reduce the therapeutic actions the phenothiazines. Barbiturates may reduce phenothiazine plasma levels. Bromocriptine effectiveness may be inhibited by phenothiazines. Propranolol and phenothiazines may result in increased plasma levels of both drugs. Tricyclic antidepressant concentrations, serum concentrations may be increased the phenothiazines. Valproic acid clearance may be decreased.

Theoretic Infant Dose:

Relative Infant Dose:

Adult Dose: 100-400 mg daily

Alternatives:

T½ =	21-24 hours	M/P =	
PHL =		PB =	
Tmax =		Oral =	Complete
MW =	371	pKa =	9.5
Vd =	18		

References:
1. O'Brien TE. Excretion of drugs in human milk. Am J Hosp Pharm 1974; 31(9):844-854.

THIOTHIXENE
Trade: Navane
Can/Aus/UK: Navane
Uses: Antipsychotic agent
LRC: L4
AAP: Not reviewed

Thiothixene is an antipsychotic agent similar in action to the phenothiazines, butyrophenones (Haldol), and chlorprothixene. There are no data on its transfer into human milk. Of this family, thiothixene has a rather higher risk of extrapyramidal symptoms and lowered seizure threshold,[1,2] Only two agents in these families have been studied with respect to milk levels: haloperidol and chlorpromazine. Both produced rather low milk levels. However, these agents generally have long half-lives and some concern exists for long-term exposure. Observe infant for sedation, seizures, or jerks.

Pregnancy Risk Category: C

Lactation Risk Category: L4

Adult Concerns: Decreases seizure threshold. Sedation, lethargy, extrapyramidal jerking motion.

Pediatric Concerns: None via milk.

Drug Interactions: Thiothixene may be additive when coadministered with other sedative drugs, alcohol, anticholinergics, and hypotensive agents. Aluminum salts may reduce oral absorption of phenothiazines. Anticholinergics may reduce efficacy of thiothixene. Thiothixene may increase tricyclic antidepressant plasma levels.

Theoretic Infant Dose:

Relative Infant Dose:

Adult Dose: 5-15 mg TID-QID

Alternatives: Haloperidol

$T\frac{1}{2}$ =	34 hours	M/P =	
PHL =		PB =	
T_{max} =	1-2 hours	Oral =	Complete
MW =	443	pKa =	
Vd =			

References:
1. Drug Facts and Comparisons 1999 ed. ed. St. Louis: 1999.
2. McEvoy GE. (ed): AFHS Drug Information. New York, NY: 1999.

THYROID SCAN
Trade: Thyroid Scan
Can/Aus/UK:
Uses: Radiographic scan of thyroid gland
LRC: L4
AAP: Not reviewed

Thyroid scanning with radioiodine (I-131) or technetium 99m is useful in delineating structural abnormalities of the thyroid, eg, to distinguish Grave's disease from multinodular goiter and a single toxic adenoma or to determine the functional state of a single nodule ("hot" vs. "cold").

In one procedure, the radiologist uses radioactive Technetium-99m pertechnate, which has a short half-life of 6.7 hours. At least 97% of the radioactivity would be decayed in 5 half-lives (33.5 hours), after which it would be presumably safe to breastfeed.

In the second procedure (an uptake scan) radioactive Iodine-131 is used. The radioactive half-life of I-131 is 8.1 days. Five half-lives in this situation is 40.5 days. Although the biologic half-life of iodine would be less than the 40.5 days, it is not known with certainty how long is required before breastmilk samples are at background levels. For safety in this case, breastmilk samples should be counted by a gamma counter prior to reinstituting breastfeeding. I-131 is sequestered in high concentrations in breastmilk, and breastmilk levels could be exceedingly high. Excessive exposure of the infants thyroid to I-131 is exceedingly dangerous.[1-6] See NRC table in appendix.

Pregnancy Risk Category:

Lactation Risk Category: L4

Adult Concerns: High milk radioactive levels

Pediatric Concerns: Possible thyroid suppression is possible if high levels of I-131 are used. Count breastmilk samples to determine radiation levels.

Drug Interactions:

Theoretic Infant Dose:

Relative Infant Dose:

Adult Dose:

Alternatives:

References:
1. American Academy of Pediatrics, Committee on Drugs. Transfer of drugs and other chemicals into human milk Pediatrics 1994; 93(1):137-150.
2. Palmer KE. Excretion of 125I in breastmilk following administration of labelled fibrinogen. Br J Radiol 1979; 52(620):672-673.

3. Karjalainen P, Penttila IM, Pystynen P. The amount and form of radioactivity in human milk after lung scanning, renography and placental localization by 131 I labelled tracers. Acta Obstet Gynecol Scand 1971; 50(4):357-361.
4. Hedrick WR, Di Simone RN, Keen RL. Radiation dosimetry from breastmilk excretion of radioiodine and pertechnetate. J Nucl Med 1986; 27(10):1569-1571.
5. Romney B, Nickoloff EL, Esser PD. Excretion of radioiodine in breastmilk. J Nucl Med 1989; 30(1):124-126.
6. Robinson PS, Barker P, Campbell A, Henson P, Surveyor I, Young PR. Iodine-131 in breastmilk following therapy for thyroid carcinoma. J Nucl Med 1994; 35(11):1797-1801.

THYROTROPIN

Trade: Thyrotropin, TSH, Thyrogen
Can/Aus/UK: Thytropar
Uses: Excess TSH, Thyrotropin, hypothyroidism
LRC: L1
AAP: Not reviewed

Thyroid stimulating hormone (Thyrotropin, TSH) is known to be secreted into breastmilk. TSH is extremely elevated in hypothyroid mothers and could presumably cause a hyperthyroid condition in the breastfeeding infant. The level of TSH secreted into milk was determined in a hyperthyroid mother (Plasma TSH=110 mU/L).[1] The breastmilk TSH was low (Milk TSH= 1.4 mU/L) suggesting that human breastmilk does not contain excessive amounts of TSH in the presence of severe maternal hypothyroidism and that breastfeeding is permissible in hypothyroid mothers.

Pregnancy Risk Category: C

Lactation Risk Category: L1

Adult Concerns: Elevated thyroxine levels in breastfeeding infant.

Pediatric Concerns: None reported via milk. Breastfeeding by hyperthyroid mother is permissible.

Drug Interactions:

Theoretic Infant Dose:

Relative Infant Dose:

Adult Dose: 10 units daily

Alternatives:

T½ =		M/P =	
PHL =		PB =	
T$_{max}$ =		Oral =	Poor
MW =		pKa =	
Vd =			

References:
1. Robinson P, Hoad K. Thyrotropin in human breastmilk. Aust N Z J Med 1994; 24(1):68.

TIAGABINE

Trade: Gabitril
Can/Aus/UK: Gabitril
Uses: Anticonvulsant
LRC: L4
AAP: Not reviewed

Tiagabine is a GABA inhibitor useful for the treatment of partial epilepsy.[1] No data are available on its transfer to human milk. It has been used in pediatric patients 3-10 years of age. Use in women who are breastfeeding only if the benefits clearly outweigh the risks.

Pregnancy Risk Category: C

Lactation Risk Category: L4

Adult Concerns: Asthenia, sedation, dizziness, headache, mild memory impairment, and abdominal pain and nausea have been reported.

Pediatric Concerns: None reported via milk.

Drug Interactions: Enhanced clearance of tiagabine has been reported when coadministered with carbamazepine, fosphenytoin, phenytoin, primidone, and phenobarbital. Valproic acid produces a 10% drop in tiagabine plasma levels but with a significant drop in plasma protein binding (may enhance the effect).

Theoretic Infant Dose:

Relative Infant Dose:

Adult Dose: 32-56 mg daily

Alternatives:

$T\frac{1}{2}$ =	7-9 hours	M/P =	
PHL =	3.2-5.7 hours	PB =	95%
T_{max} =	45 minutes	Oral =	90%
MW =		pKa =	
Vd =			

References:
1. Pharmaceutical Manufacturer Prescribing Information. 1999.

TICARCILLIN

Trade: Ticar, Timentin
Can/Aus/UK: Ticar, Tarcil, Ticillin
Uses: Penicillin antibiotic
LRC: L1
AAP: Maternal Medication Usually Compatible with Breastfeeding

Ticarcillin is an extended-spectrum penicillin, used only IM or IV, and is not appreciably absorbed via oral ingestion.[1,2] In a study of 2-3 patients who received 1000 mg IV, only trace amounts were detected in milk and were too low to measure.[3] In a study of 10 patients who received 5 g TID IV, the amount of ticarcillin in milk ranged from 2-2.5 mg/L.[4] Twelve hours after discontinuing ticarcillin, it was undetectable in milk. As with many penicillins, only minimal levels are secreted into milk. Poor oral absorption would limit exposure of breastfeeding infant. May cause changes in GI flora and possibly fungal overgrowth. Timentin is ticarcillin with clavulanate added.

Pregnancy Risk Category: B

Lactation Risk Category: L1

Adult Concerns: Neutropenia, anemia, kidney toxicity. Changes in GI flora, diarrhea, candida overgrowth.

Pediatric Concerns: None reported via milk. Observe for changes in GI flora, diarrhea.

Drug Interactions: Probenecid may increase penicillin levels. Tetracyclines may decrease penicillin effectiveness.

Theoretic Infant Dose: 0.37 mg/kg/day

Relative Infant Dose: 0.18%

Adult Dose: 150-300 mg daily

Alternatives:

$T\frac{1}{2}$ =	0.9-1.3 hours	M/P =		
PHL =	3.5 - 5.6 hours (neonate)	PB =	54%	
T_{max} =	0.5 - 1.25 hours (IM)	Oral =	Poor	
MW =	384	pKa =		
Vd =				

References:

1. Drug Facts and Comparisons 1995 ed. ed. St. Louis: 1995.
2. Pharmaceutical Manufacturer Prescribing Information. 1995.
3. Matsuda S. Transfer of antibiotics into maternal milk. Biol Res Pregnancy Perinatol 1984; 5(2):57-60.
4. von Kobyletzki D, Dalhoff A, Lindemeyer H, Primavesi CA. Ticarcillin serum and tissue concentrations in gynecology and obstetrics. Infection 1983; 11(3):144-149.

TICLOPIDINE

Trade: Ticlid
Can/Aus/UK: Ticlid, Apo-Ticlopidine, Tilodene
Uses: Inhibits platelet aggregation
LRC: L4
AAP: Not reviewed

Ticlopidine is useful in preventing thromboembolic disorders, increased cardiovascular mortality, stroke, infarcts, and other clotting disorders. Ticlopidine is reported to be excreted into rodent milk.[1] No data are available on penetration into human breastmilk. However it is highly protein bound, and the levels of ticlopidine in plasma are quite low. The manufacturer recommends against use in breastfeeding mothers.

Pregnancy Risk Category: B

Lactation Risk Category: L4

Adult Concerns: Bleeding, neutropenia, maculopapular rash

Pediatric Concerns: None reported via milk, but caution is recommended.

Drug Interactions: Antacids may reduce absorption of ticlopidine. Chronic cimetidine administration has reduced the clearance of ticlopidine by 50%. Use of aspirin may alter platelet aggregation. Digoxin plasma levels may be slightly decreased by 15%. Theophylline elimination half-life was significantly increased from 8-10 hours.

Theoretic Infant Dose:

Relative Infant Dose:

Adult Dose: 250 mg BID

Alternatives:

$T\frac{1}{2}$ =	12.6 hours	M/P =		
PHL =		PB =	98%	
T_{max} =	2 hours	Oral =	80%	
MW =	264	pKa =		
Vd =				

References:
1. Pharmaceutical Manufacturer Prescribing Information. 1996.

TIMOLOL

Trade: Blocadren
Can/Aus/UK: Apo-Timol, Blocadren, Timoptic, Novo-Timol, Tenopt, Timpilo, Betim, Timoptol
Uses: Beta blocker for hypertension and glaucoma
LRC: L2
AAP: Maternal Medication Usually Compatible with Breastfeeding

Timolol is a beta blocker used for treating hypertension and glaucoma. It is secreted into milk. Following a dose of 5 mg three times daily, milk levels averaged 15.9 µg/L.[1] Both oral and ophthalmic drops produce modest levels in milk. Breastmilk levels following ophthalmic use of 0.5% timolol drops was 5.6 µg/L at 1.5 hours after the dose.[2] Untoward effects on infant have not been reported. These levels are probably too small to be clinically relevant.

Pregnancy Risk Category: C

Lactation Risk Category: L2

Adult Concerns: Hypotension, bradycardia, depression, sedation

Pediatric Concerns: None reported via milk, but observe for hypotension, weakness, hypoglycemia, sedation, depression.

Drug Interactions: Decreased effect when used with aluminum salts, barbiturates, calcium salts, cholestyramine, NSAIDs, ampicillin, rifampin, and salicylates. Beta blockers may reduce the effect of oral sulfonylureas (hypoglycemic agents). Increased toxicity/effect when used with other antihypertensives, contraceptives, MAO inhibitors, cimetidine, and numerous other products. See drug interaction reference for complete listing.

Theoretic Infant Dose: 2.3 µg/kg/day

Relative Infant Dose: 1.1%

Adult Dose: 10-20 mg BID

Alternatives: Propranolol, Metoprolol

T½ =	4 hours	M/P =	0.8
PHL =		PB =	10%
T$_{max}$ =	1-2 hours	Oral =	50%
MW =	316	pKa =	8.8
Vd =	1-3		

References:
1. Fidler J, Smith V, De Swiet M. Excretion of oxprenolol and timolol in breastmilk. Br J Obstet Gynaecol 1983; 90(10):961-965.
2. Lustgarten JS, Podos SM. Topical timolol and the nursing mother. Arch Ophthalmol 1983; 101(9):1381-1382.

TINZAPARIN SODIUM
Trade: Innohep
Can/Aus/UK: Innohep
Uses: Anticoagulant
LRC: L3
AAP: Not reviewed

Tinzaparin is a low molecular weight heparin with antithrombotic properties used for the treatment of deep vein thrombosis. No data are available on its transfer to milk. However, due to its protein nature and its large molecular weight, breastmilk levels would be expected to be quite low. Some breastfeeding data are available for a similar product, dalteparin. With dalteparin, levels in milk were extraordinarily low.

Pregnancy Risk Category: B

Lactation Risk Category: L3

Adult Concerns: Thrombocytopenia, hypersensitivity, prolonged bleeding times, chest pain, urinary infection, headache

Pediatric Concerns: None reported.

Drug Interactions: Because of increased risk of bleeding, do not use with other anticoagulants, platelet inhibitors, NSAIDs, and thrombolytics.

Theoretic Infant Dose:

Relative Infant Dose:

Adult Dose: 175 IU/kg/d

Alternatives: Dalteparin, enoxaparin

T½ =	3.4 hours	M/P =	
PHL =		PB =	
T_{max} =	3.7 hours S.C.	Oral =	Nil
MW =	7500	pKa =	
Vd =	0.07		

References:
1. Pharmaceutical Manufacturer Prescribing Information.

TINZAPARIN SODIUM

Trade: Innohep
Can/Aus/UK: Innohep, Logiparin
Uses: Anticoagulant low molecular weight heparin
LRC: L3
AAP: Not reviewed

Tinzaparin is a depolymerized heparin (low molecular weight heparin) similar to several others such as dalteparin, enoxaparin, nadroparin or parnaparin. The average molecular weight range of tinzaparin is approximately one-half that of regular (unfractionated) heparin (5500-7500 vs 12,000 daltons). No data are available on the transfer of this anticoagulant into human milk but it is likely low. In studies with dalteparin none was found in milk in one study, and only small amounts in another(see dalteparin). In studies with enoxaparin, no changes in anti-Xa activity were noted in breastfed infants. It is very unlikely any would be orally bioavailable.

Other typical low molecular weight heparins: Dalteparin(Fragmin), enoxaparin(Lovenox), nadroparin(Fraxiparin), parnaparin(Fluxum)

Pregnancy Risk Category: B

Lactation Risk Category: L3

Adult Concerns: Hemorrage, thrombocytopenia, hematoma a site of injection, allergic reaction, and vaginal bleeding

Pediatric Concerns: None reported via milk. Milk levels in other LMWHs are reportedly low, it is likely similar for tinzaparin as well.

Drug Interactions: Do not use with other anticoagulants with includes many NSAIDs, aspirin, herbal remedies, and other agents which inhibit thrombus formation. Check other sources for complete lists.

Theoretic Infant Dose:

Relative Infant Dose:

Adult Dose: 175 IU/kg/day (highly variable)

Alternatives: Dalteparin, enoxaparin

$T\frac{1}{2}$ =	3-4 hours	M/P =	
PHL =		PB =	0%
T_{max} =	4-5 hours (SC)	Oral =	Nil
MW =	< 7500	pKa =	
Vd =	3.1-5.0		

References:
1. Pharmaceutical Manufacturer Prescribing Information.

TIZANIDINE
Trade: Zanaflex
Can/Aus/UK:
Uses: Muscle relaxant
LRC: L4
AAP: Not reviewed

Tizanidine is a centrally acting muscle relaxant. It has demonstrated efficacy in the treatment of tension headache and spasticity associated with multiple sclerosis. It is not known if it is transferred into human milk although the manufacturer states that due to its lipid solubility, it likely penetrates milk.[1] This product has a long half-life, high lipid solubility, and significant CNS penetration, all factors that would increase milk penetration. While the half-life of the conventional formulation is only 4-8 hours, the half-life of the sustained release formulation is 13-22 hours.[2] Further, 48% of patients complain of sedation. Use caution if used in a breastfeeding mother.

Pregnancy Risk Category: C

Lactation Risk Category: L4

Adult Concerns: Hypotension (49%), sedation (48%), dry mouth, asthenia, dizziness, and other symptoms have been reported. Nausea and vomiting have been reported. A high risk of elevated liver enzymes (5%).

Pediatric Concerns: None reported via milk, but caution is recommended.

Drug Interactions: Alcohol may increase plasma levels of tizanidine by 20%. Oral contraceptives may significantly (50%) reduce clearance of tizanidine.

Theoretic Infant Dose:

Relative Infant Dose:

Adult Dose: 8 mg q 6 hours PRN

Alternatives:

$T\frac{1}{2}$ =	13-22 hours	M/P =		
PHL =		PB =	30%	
T_{max} =	1.5 hours	Oral =	40%	
MW =		pKa =		
Vd =	2.4			

References:
1. Pharmaceutical Manufacturer Prescribing Information. 1999.
2. Wagstaff AJ, Bryson HM. Tizanidine. A review of its pharmacology, clinical efficacy and tolerability in the management of spasticity associated with cerebral and spinal disorders. Drugs 1997; 53(3):435-452.

TOBRAMYCIN

Trade: Nebcin, Tobrex
Can/Aus/UK: Nebcin, Tobrex, Tobi, Tobralex
Uses: Ophthalmic antibiotic
LRC: L3
AAP: Not reviewed

Tobramycin is an aminoglycoside antibiotic similar to gentamicin.[1] Although small levels of tobramycin are known to transfer into milk, they probably pose few problems. In one study of 5 patients, following an 80 mg IM dose, tobramycin levels in milk ranged from undetectable to 0.5 mg/L.[2] Tobramycin is poorly absorbed orally and would be unlikely to produce significant levels in an infant.

Pregnancy Risk Category: C

Lactation Risk Category: L3

Adult Concerns: Changes in GI flora

Pediatric Concerns:

Drug Interactions: Increased toxicity when used with certain penicillins, cephalosporins, amphotericin B, loop diuretics, and neuromuscular blocking agents.

Theoretic Infant Dose: 0.075 mg/kg/day

Relative Infant Dose: 6.5%

Adult Dose: 1 mg/kg q 8 hours

Alternatives:

$T\frac{1}{2}$ =	2-3 hours	M/P =	
PHL =	4.6 hours (neonates)	PB =	< 5%
T_{max} =	30-90 minutes (IM)	Oral =	
MW =	468	pKa =	
Vd =	0.22-0.31		

References:
1. Pharmaceutical Manufacturer Prescribing Information. 1996.
2. Takase Z. Laboratory and clinical studies on tobramycin in the field of obstetrics and gynecology. Chemotherapy (Tokyo) 1975; 23:1402.

TOLBUTAMIDE

Trade: Oramide, Orinase
Can/Aus/UK: Apo-Tolbutamide, Mobenol, Novo-Butamide, Orinase, Rastinon, Glyconon
Uses: Antidiabetic
LRC: L3
AAP: Maternal Medication Usually Compatible with Breastfeeding

Tolbutamide is a short-acting sulfonylurea used to stimulate insulin secretion in type II diabetics. Only low levels are secreted into breastmilk. Following a dose of 500 mg twice daily, milk levels in two patients were 3 and 18 μg/L respectively.[1] Maternal serum levels averaged 35 and 45 μg/L. Observe infant closely for jaundice and hypoglycemia.

Pregnancy Risk Category: D

Lactation Risk Category: L3

Adult Concerns: Hypoglycemia, nausea, dyspepsia

Pediatric Concerns: None reported via milk.

Drug Interactions: The hypoglycemic effect may be enhanced by : anticoagulants, chloramphenicol, clofibrate, fenfluramine, fluconazole, H2 antagonists, magnesium salts, methyldopa, MAO inhibitors, probenecid, salicylates, TCAs, sulfonamides. The hypoglycemic effect may be reduced by: beta blockers, cholestyramine, diazoxide, phenytoin, rifampin, thiazide diuretics.

Theoretic Infant Dose: 2.7 μg/kg/day

Relative Infant Dose: 0.018%

Adult Dose: 250-2000 mg daily
Alternatives:

$T\frac{1}{2}$ =	4.5-6.5 hours	M/P =	0.09-0.4
PHL =		PB =	93%
T_{max} =	3.5 hours	Oral =	Complete
MW =	270	pKa =	5.3
Vd =	0.10-0.15		

References:
1. Moiel RH, Ryan JR. Tolbutamide orinase in human breastmilk. Clin Pediatr (Phila) 1967; 6(8):480.

TOLMETIN SODIUM

Trade: Tolectin
Can/Aus/UK: Tolectin
Uses: Non-steroidal analgesic, used for arthritis, etc.
LRC: L3
AAP: Maternal Medication Usually Compatible with Breastfeeding

Tolmetin is a standard non-steroidal analgesic. Tolmetin is known to be distributed into milk but in small amounts. In one patient given 400 mg, the milk level at 0.67 hrs was 0.18 mg/L.[1] The estimate of dose per day an infant would receive is 115 μg/Liter of milk. Tolmetin is sometimes used in pediatric rheumatoid patients (> 2 yrs).

Pregnancy Risk Category: C

Lactation Risk Category: L3

Adult Concerns: GI distress, bleeding, vomiting, nausea, edema

Pediatric Concerns: None reported via milk.

Drug Interactions: May prolong prothrombin time when used with warfarin. Antihypertensive effects of ACEi family may be blunted or completely abolished by NSAIDs. Some NSAIDs may block antihypertensive effect of beta blockers, diuretics. Used with cyclosporin, may dramatically increase renal toxicity. May increase digoxin, phenytoin, lithium levels. May increase toxicity of methotrexate. May increase bioavailability of penicillamine. Probenecid may increase NSAID levels.

Theoretic Infant Dose: 27 μg/kg/day

Relative Infant Dose: 0.47%

Adult Dose: 200-600 mg TID

Alternatives: Ibuprofen

$T^{1/2}$ =	1-1.5 hours	M/P =	0.0055
PHL =		PB =	99%
T_{max} =	0.5-1 hour	Oral =	Complete
MW =	257	pKa =	3.5
Vd =			

References:
1. Sagraves R, Waller ES, Goehrs HR. Tolmetin in breastmilk. Drug Intell Clin Pharm 1985; 19(1):55-56.

TOLTERODINE
Trade: Detrol
Can/Aus/UK: Detrol, Detrusitol
Uses: Urinary incontinence
LRC: L3
AAP: Not reviewed

Tolterodine is a muscarinic anticholinergic agent similar in effect to atropine but is more selective for the urinary bladder.[1] Tolterodine levels in milk have been reported in mice, where offspring exposed to extremely high levels had slightly reduced body weight gain but no other untoward effects. While it is more selective for the urinary bladder, preclinical trials still showed adverse effects including blurred vision, constipation, and dry mouth in adults. While we have no data on human milk, it is unlikely concentrations will be high enough to produce untoward effects in infants. However, the infant should be monitored for classic anticholinergic symptoms including dry mouth, constipation, poor tearing, etc.

Pregnancy Risk Category: C

Lactation Risk Category: L3

Adult Concerns: Blurred vision, constipation, and dry mouth in adults

Pediatric Concerns: None by milk, but observe for anticholinergic symptoms such as dry mouth, constipation, poor tearing, poor urinary output.

Drug Interactions: Fluoxetine reduces metabolism of tolterodine significantly and may increase plasma levels by 4.8 fold.

Theoretic Infant Dose:

Relative Infant Dose:

Adult Dose: 2 mg BID

Alternatives:

T½ =	1.9-3.7 hours	M/P =	
PHL =		PB =	96%
T$_{max}$ =	1-2 hours	Oral =	77%
MW =		pKa =	
Vd =	1.6		

References:
1. Pharmaceutical Manufacturer Prescribing Information.

TOPIRAMATE

Trade: Topamax
Can/Aus/UK: Topamax
Uses: Anticonvulsant
LRC: L3
AAP: Not reviewed

Topiramate is a new anticonvulsant used in controlling refractory partial seizures. In a group of 2 women receiving topiramate (150-200 mg/day) at three weeks postpartum the mean milk/plasma ratio was 0.86 (range=0.67-1.1).[1] The concentration of topiramate in milk averaged 7.9 uM (range= 1.6 to 13.7). The weight normalized relative infant dose (RID), assuming a milk intake of 150 mL/kg/d, was 3-23% of the maternal dose/day. The absolute infant dose was 0.1 to 0.7 mg/kg/day. The plasma concentrations of topiramate in two infants were 1.4 and 1.6 uM, respectively. The plasma level in another infant was undetectable. The plasma concentrations in the two infants were 10-20% of the maternal plasma level. At 4 weeks, the milk/plasma ratio had dropped to 0.69 and plasma levels in the infant were < 0.9 uM and 2.1 uM, respectively.

Topiramate has become increasingly popular due to its fewer adverse side effects.[2-5] Due to the fact that the plasma levels found in breastfeeding infants were significantly less than in maternal plasma, the risk of using this product in breastfeeding mothers is probably acceptable. Close observation for sedation is advised.

Pregnancy Risk Category: C

Lactation Risk Category: L3

Adult Concerns: Topiramate induces a significant Cognitive dysfunction, particularly in older patients. Paresthesias, sedation, weight loss(7%), diarrhea.

Pediatric Concerns: None reported in two cases. Milk levels were moderate and infant plasma levels were 10-20% of maternal levels.

Drug Interactions: A 40% decrease in topiramate concentration has been reported when carbamazepine was added to topiramate therapy. Do not use topiramate with dichlorphenamide due to increased risk of nephrolithiasis. Serum digoxin levels (AUC) are decreased by 12% in patients receiving digoxin and topiramate. Efficacy of combination birth control pills may be reduced when adding topiramate. A 25% decrease in phenytoin levels have been reported when topirmate was added. Phenobarbital may reduce half-life of topirmate by 11%.

Theoretic Infant Dose: 0.69 mg/kg/day

Relative Infant Dose: 24.5%

Adult Dose: 200 mg BID

Alternatives:

T½ =	18-24 hours	M/P =	0.86
PHL =		PB =	15%
T$_{max}$ =	1.5-4 hours	Oral =	75%
MW =	339	pKa =	
Vd =	0.7		

References:
1. Ohman I, Vitols S, Luef G, Soderfeldt B, Tomson T. Topiramate kinetics during delivery, lactation, and in the neonate: preliminary observations. Epilepsia 2002; 43(10):1157-1160.
2. Patsalos PN, Sander JW. Newer antiepileptic drugs. Towards an improved risk-benefit ratio. Drug Saf 1994; 11(1):37-67.
3. Bialer M. Comparative pharmacokinetics of the newer antiepileptic drugs. Clin Pharmacokinet 1993; 24(6):441-452.
4. Britton JW, So EL. New antiepileptic drugs: prospects for the future. J Epilepsy 1995; 8:267-281.
5. Pharmacokinetics of topiramate in pregnancy and lactation-transplacental transfer and excretion in breast-milk. Fifth Eilat Conference on Antiepileptic Drugs, Eilat, Israel. 00 Jun; 2000.

TORSEMIDE
Trade: Demadex
Can/Aus/UK: Demadex, Torem
Uses: Potent Loop diuretic
LRC: L3
AAP: Not reviewed

Torsemide is a potent loop diuretic generally used in congestive heart failure and other conditions which require a strong diuretic.[1]   There are no reports of its transfer into human milk. Its extraordinary high protein binding would likely limit its transfer into human milk. As with many diuretics, reduction of plasma volume and hypotension may adversely reduce milk production although this is rare. See furosemide.

Pregnancy Risk Category: B

Lactation Risk Category: L3

Adult Concerns: Hypotension, hypokalemia, volume depletion, headache, excessive urination, dizziness

Pediatric Concerns: None reported. Renal calcification have been reported with other loop diuretics in premature infants, but not via milk supply.

Drug Interactions: When used with salicylates, elevated plasma salicylate levels may occur. Coadministration with other NSAIDS may increase the risk of renal dysfunction. Cholestyramine administration reduces bioavailability of torsemide. Use caution in using with lithium.

Theoretic Infant Dose:

Relative Infant Dose:

Adult Dose: 5-10 mg daily

Alternatives: Furosemide

$T\frac{1}{2}$ =	3.5 hours	M/P =	
PHL =		PB =	> 99%
T_{max} =	1 hour	Oral =	80%
MW =	348	pKa =	
Vd =	0.21		

References:
1.   Pharmaceutical Manufacturer Prescribing Information. 1997.

TRAMADOL AND ACETAMINOPHEN

Trade: Ultracet
Can/Aus/UK:
Uses: Analgesic
LRC:
AAP: Not reviewed

Ultracet is the combination of 37.5 mg of tramadol(Ultram) and 325 mg acetaminophen. See individual monographs.

TRAMADOL HCL

Trade: Ultram, Ultracet
Can/Aus/UK: Tramal, Nycodol, Tramake, Zydol, Zamadol, Dromadol
Uses: Analgesic
LRC: L3
AAP: Not reviewed

Tramadol is a new class analgesic that most closely resembles the opiates although it is not a controlled substance and appears to have reduced addictive potential.[1]   It appears to be slightly more potent than codeine. After oral use, its onset of analgesia is within 1 hour and reaches a peak in 2-3 hours. Following a single IV 100 mg dose of tramadol, the cumulative excretion in breastmilk within 16 hours was

100 µg of tramadol (0.1% of the maternal dose) and 27 µg of the M1 metabolite.

Pregnancy Risk Category: C

Lactation Risk Category: L3

Adult Concerns: Sedation, respiratory depression, nausea, vomiting, constipation

Pediatric Concerns: None reported via milk. Observe for sedation.

Drug Interactions: Use with carbamazepine dramatically increases tramadol metabolism and reduces plasma levels. Use with MAOI may increase toxicity.

Theoretic Infant Dose:

Relative Infant Dose:

Adult Dose: 50-100 mg q 4-6 hours PRN

Alternatives: Codeine

T½ =	7 hours	M/P =	0.1
PHL =		PB =	20%
Tmax =	2 hours	Oral =	60%
MW =	263	pKa =	
Vd =			

References:
1. Pharmaceutical Manufacturer Prescribing Information. 1996.

TRASTUZUMAB

Trade: Herceptin
Can/Aus/UK:
Uses: Anticancer antibody
LRC: L4
AAP: Not reviewed

Trastuzumab is recombinant DNA-derived humanized monoclonal antibody that selectively binds to receptors common on certain breast cancers. It is indicated in the treatment of patients with metastatic breast cancer whose tumors over express the HER2 protein. It is an IgG1 kappa that contains human framework regions that bind to the HER2 receptors on cancer cells. While IgG transfer minimally into human milk, we do not have data on the transfer of this recombinant product into human milk. Studies on cynomolgus monkeys at doses 25 times the weekly human dose demonstrated that trastuzumab is secreted in milk (levels were not reported). However, it was not associated with any adverse effects on the growth or development of these infant monkeys. It is not likely that this agent at doses used in humans would cause appreciable problems in a breastfeeding human. However, it is not clear that mothers with breast cancer should breastfeed, as we do not yet understand how lactation would affect the mother's response to anticancer agents. Some caution is recommended.

Pregnancy Risk Category: B

Lactation Risk Category: L4

Adult Concerns: Adverse events include pain, asthenia, fever, chills, back and abdominal pain, headache, nausea, diarrhea, vomiting, insomnia, cough, dyspnea, rhinitis, and rash.

Pediatric Concerns: None reported via milk. Studies in monkeys at 25 X doses did not produce toxicity in breastfed offspring.

Drug Interactions: Increased risk of cardiac toxicity when admixed with anthracyclines, and cyclophosphamide. Paclitaxel may increase the plasma levels of trastuzumab by 1.5 times.

Theoretic Infant Dose:

Relative Infant Dose:

Adult Dose: 2 mg/kg/week

Alternatives:

T½ =	1.7-12 days	M/P =	
PHL =		PB =	
T$_{max}$ =		Oral =	Nil
MW =	185,000	pKa =	
Vd =	0.044		

References:
1. Pharmaceutical Manufacturer Prescribing Information. 2003.

TRAZODONE

Trade: Desyrel
Can/Aus/UK: Desyrel, Trazorel, Apo-Trazodone, Novo-Trazodone, Molipaxin
Uses: Antidepressant, serotonin reuptake inhibitor
LRC: L2
AAP: Drugs whose effect on nursing infants is unknown but may be of concern

Trazodone is an antidepressant whose structure is dissimilar to the tricyclics and to the other antidepressants. In six mothers who received a single 50 mg dose, the milk/plasma ratio averaged 0.14.[1] Peak milk concentrations occurred at 2 hours and were approximately 110 µg/L (taken from graph) and declined rapidly thereafter. On a weight basis, an adult would receive 0.77 mg/kg whereas a breastfeeding infant, using this data, would consume only 0.005 mg/kg. The authors estimate that about 0.6 % of the maternal dose was ingested by the infant over 24 hours.

Pregnancy Risk Category: C

Lactation Risk Category: L2

Adult Concerns: Dry mouth, sedation, hypotension, blurred vision

Pediatric Concerns: None reported via milk.

Drug Interactions: May enhance the CNS depressant effect of alcohol, barbiturates, and other CNS depressants. Digoxin serum levels may be increased. Use caution when administering with MAOI. Phenytoin serum levels may be increased. Use with warfarin may increase anticoagulant effect.

Theoretic Infant Dose: 5.0 µg/kg/day

Relative Infant Dose: 0.7%

Adult Dose: 150-400 mg daily

Alternatives:

$T\frac{1}{2}$ =	4-9 hours	M/P =	0.142
PHL =		PB =	85-95%
T_{max} =	1-2 hours	Oral =	65%
MW =	372	pKa =	
Vd =	0.9-1.5		

References:

1. Verbeeck RK, Ross SG, McKenna EA. Excretion of trazodone in breastmilk. Br J Clin Pharmacol 1986; 22(3):367-370.

TRETINOIN

Trade: Retin-A, Renova
Can/Aus/UK: Retin-A, Stieva-A, Vitamin A Acid, Renova, Vesanoid
Uses: Treatment of acne
LRC: L3
AAP: Not reviewed

Tretinoin is a retinoid derivative similar to Vitamin A. It is primarily used topically for acne and wrinkling and sometimes administered orally for leukemias and psoriasis. Used topically, tretinoin stimulates epithelial turnover and reduces cell cohesiveness.[1] Blood concentrations are essentially zero. Absorption of Retin-A via topical sources is reported to be minimal, and breastmilk would likely be minimal to none.[2] However, if it is used orally, transfer into milk is likely and should be used with great caution in a breastfeeding mother.

Pregnancy Risk Category: B for topical Retin-A
                               C for topical Renova
                               D for oral

Lactation Risk Category: L3

Adult Concerns: Leukocytosis, dry skin, skin irritation, blistering, scaling, pigmentary changes, nausea, vomiting.   Side effects of oral use are similar to hypervitaminosis A, and include headache, increased CSF pressure, anorexia, nausea. scaling of skin, fatigue, hepatosplenomegaly.

Pediatric Concerns: None reported via milk.

Drug Interactions: Use other topical medications such as sulfur, resorcinal, benzoyl peroxide or salicylic acid with caution due to accelerated skin irritation.

Theoretic Infant Dose:

Relative Infant Dose:

Adult Dose: Variable

Alternatives:

$T\frac{1}{2}$ =	2 hours		M/P =	
PHL =			PB =	
T_{max} =			Oral =	70%
MW =	300		pKa =	
Vd =	0.44			

References:
1. Zbinden G. Investigation on the toxicity of tretinoin administered systemically to animals. Acta Derm Verereol Suppl(Stockh) 1975; 74:36-40.
2. Lucek RW, Colburn WA. Clinical pharmacokinetics of the retinoids. Clin Pharmacokinet 1985; 10(1):38-62.

TRIAMCINOLONE ACETONIDE

Trade: Nasacort, Azmacort, Tri-Nasal
Can/Aus/UK: Aristocort, Azmacort, Kenalog, Triaderm, Nasacort, Kenalone, Adcortyl
Uses: Corticosteroid
LRC: L3
AAP: Not reviewed

Triamcinolone is a typical corticosteroid (see prednisone) that is available for topical, intranasal, injection, inhalation, and oral use. When applied topically to the nose (Nasacort) or to the lungs (Azmacort), only minimal doses are used and plasma levels are exceedingly low to undetectable.[1]   Although no data are available on triamcinolone secretion into human milk, it is likely that the milk levels would be exceedingly low and not clinically relevant when administered via inhalation or intranasally. While the oral adult dose is 4-48 mg/day, the inhaled dose is 200 μg three times daily, and the intranasal dose is 220 μg/day. See prednisone for more breastfeeding data.

Pregnancy Risk Category: C

Lactation Risk Category: L3

Adult Concerns: Intranasal and inhaled: nasal irritation, dry mucous membranes, sneezing, throat irritation, hoarseness, candida overgrowth.

Pediatric Concerns: None reported via milk. Observe growth rate.

Drug Interactions:

Theoretic Infant Dose:

Relative Infant Dose:

Adult Dose: 200 μg TID-QID

Alternatives:

$T\frac{1}{2}$ =	88 minutes	M/P =	
PHL =		PB =	
T_{max} =		Oral =	Complete
MW =	434	pKa =	
Vd =			

References:
1. Pharmaceutical Manufacturer Prescribing Information. 1996.

TRIAMTERENE

Trade: Dyazide
Can/Aus/UK: Dyrenium, Dyazide, Hydrene
Uses: Diuretic
LRC: L3
AAP: Not reviewed

Triamterene is a potassium-sparing diuretic, commonly used in combination with thiazide diuretics such as hydrochlorothiazide (Dyazide). Plasma levels average 26-30 nanograms/mL.[1] No data are available on the transfer of triamterene into human milk, but it is known to transfer into animal milk. Because of the availability of other less dangerous diuretics, triamterene should be used as a last resort in breastfeeding mothers.

Pregnancy Risk Category: B

Lactation Risk Category: L3

Adult Concerns: Leukopenia, hyperkalemia, diarrhea, nausea, vomiting, hepatitis

Pediatric Concerns: None reported via milk.

Drug Interactions: Hyperkalemia when administered with potassium supplements. Triamterene may reduce clearance of amantadine. May increase plasma potassium levels when administered with amiloride, or ACE inhibitors, cyclosporine. May reduce clearance of lithium. Enhanced bone marrow suppression when administered with methotrexate. Use with spironolactone may result in hyperkalemia.

Theoretic Infant Dose:

Relative Infant Dose:

Adult Dose: 25-100 mg daily

Alternatives: Hydrochlorothiazide

$T^{1/2}$ =	1.5-2.5 hours	M/P =	
PHL =	4.3 hours	PB =	55%
T_{max} =	1.5-3 hours	Oral =	30-70%
MW =	253	pKa =	
Vd =			

References:
1. Mutschler E, Gilfrich HJ, Knauf H, Mohrke W, Volger KD. Pharmacokinetics of triamterene. Clin Exp Hypertens A 1983; 5(2):249-269.

TRIAZOLAM
Trade: Halcion
Can/Aus/UK: Apo-Triazo, Halcion, Novo-Triolam
Uses: Benzodiazepine (Valium-like) hypnotic
LRC: L3
AAP: Not reviewed

Triazolam is a typical benzodiazepine used as a nighttime sedative. Animal studies indicate that triazolam is secreted into milk although levels in human milk have not been reported.[1]   As with all the benzodiazepines, some penetration into breastmilk is likely.

Pregnancy Risk Category: X

Lactation Risk Category: L3

Adult Concerns: Sedation, addiction

Pediatric Concerns: None reported for triazolam, but side effects for benzodiazepines include sedation, depression.

Drug Interactions: See diazepam.

Theoretic Infant Dose:

Relative Infant Dose:

Adult Dose: 0.125-0.25 mg daily

Alternatives: Lorazepam, Alprazolam

T½ =	1.5-5.5 hours	M/P =	
PHL =		PB =	89%
T$_{max}$ =	0.5-2 hours	Oral =	85%
MW =	343	pKa =	
Vd =	1.1-2.7		

References:
1. Drug Facts and Comparisons 1995 ed. ed. St. Louis: 1995.

TRIMEPRAZINE

Trade: Temaril
Can/Aus/UK: Panectyl, Vallergan
Uses: Antihistamine, antipruritic.
LRC: L3
AAP: Not reviewed

Trimeprazine is an antihistamine from the phenothiazine family used for itching. It is secreted into human milk but in very low levels.[1] Exact data are not available.

Pregnancy Risk Category: C

Lactation Risk Category: L3

Adult Concerns: Sedation, hypotension, bradycardia

Pediatric Concerns: None reported, but as with other antihistamines, observe for sedation.

Drug Interactions:

Theoretic Infant Dose:

Relative Infant Dose:

Adult Dose: 5 mg BID

Alternatives:

T½ =	5 hours	M/P =	
PHL =		PB =	
T$_{max}$ =	3.5 hours	Oral =	70%
MW =	298	pKa =	
Vd =			

References:
1. O'Brien TE. Excretion of drugs in human milk. Am J Hosp Pharm 1974; 31(9):844-854.

TRIMETHOBENZAMIDE

Trade: Tigan, Trimazide, Tebamide, T-Gen, Arrestin, Ticon
Can/Aus/UK:
Uses: Antiemetic, antivertigo
LRC: L4
AAP: Not reviewed

Trimethobenzamide is an older generation antiemetics whose use has been supplanted by newer more effective agents. It is most commonly used in suppository form in adults and rarely in infants. Maternal plasma levels following a 500 mg oral dose are 1-2 µg/mL. No data are available on breastmilk levels. But if one were to assume a milk plasma ratio of 1.0(which is probably high), then the theoretical infant dose would only be about 0.3 mg/kg/day, which is far less than the oral dose of 300-400 mg/day used in 15 kg infants. It is unlikely the amount of trimethobenzamide present in breastmilk would produce a clinical effect in an infant.

Pregnancy Risk Category: C

Lactation Risk Category: L4

Adult Concerns: Extrapyramidal symptoms, drowsiness, depression, dizziness, headache, vertigo, blood dyscrasias have been reported following higher oral/IM/rectal doses.

Pediatric Concerns: None reported via milk.

Drug Interactions:

Theoretic Infant Dose:

Relative Infant Dose:

Adult Dose: 250 mg TID-QID

Alternatives: Ondansetron

T½ =	Short	M/P =	
PHL =		PB =	
Tmax =		Oral =	Good
MW =		pKa =	
Vd =			

References:
1.   Drug Facts and Comparisons 1999 ed. ed. St. Louis: 1999.

TRIMETHOPRIM
Trade: Proloprim, Trimpex
Can/Aus/UK: Proloprim, Alprim, Triprim, Ipral, Monotrim, Tiempe
Uses: Antibiotic
LRC: L3
AAP: Maternal Medication Usually Compatible with Breastfeeding

Trimethoprim is an inhibitor of folic acid production in bacteria. In one study of 50 patients, average milk levels were 2.0 mg/L.[1] Milk/plasma ratio was 1.25. In another group of mothers receiving 160 mg 2-4 times daily, concentrations of 1.2 to 5.5 mg/L were reported in milk. Because it may interfere with folate metabolism, use with caution. However, trimethoprim apparently poses few problems in full term or older infants.[2]

Pregnancy Risk Category: C

Lactation Risk Category: L3

Adult Concerns: Rash, pruritus nausea, vomiting, anorexia, altered taste sensation

Pediatric Concerns: None reported via milk.

Drug Interactions: May increase phenytoin plasma levels.

Theoretic Infant Dose: 0.82 mg/kg/day

Relative Infant Dose: 9.02%

Adult Dose: 200 mg daily

Alternatives:

T½ =	8-10 hours	M/P =	1.25
PHL =	14.7-40 hrs (neonate)	PB =	44%
T$_{max}$ =	1-4 hours	Oral =	Complete
MW =	290	pKa =	
Vd =			

References:
1. Miller RD, Salter AJ. The passage of trimethoprim/sulphamethoxazole into breastmilk and its significance. In Daikos GK, ed. Progress in Chemotherapy, Proceedings of the Eight International Congress of Chemotherapy, Athens, 1973. Athens: Hellenic Society for Chemotherapy, 1974.
2. Pagliaro, Levin. Problems in Pediatric Drug Therapy. Hamilton, IL: Drug Intelligence Publications, 1979.

TRIPELENNAMINE

Trade: PBZ, Colrex, Tromide
Can/Aus/UK: Pyrabenzamine
Uses: Antihistamine
LRC: L4
AAP: Not reviewed

Tripelennamine is an older class of antihistamine. This product is generally not recommended in pediatric patients, particularly neonates due to increased sleep apnea.[1] The drug has been shown to be secreted into milk of animals.[2] No human data exist.

Pregnancy Risk Category: B

Lactation Risk Category: L4

Adult Concerns: Sleep apnea in children, peptic ulcer, sedation, dry mouth, GI distress

Pediatric Concerns: None reported, but observe for sedation, sleep apnea.

Drug Interactions: Increased sedation when used with CNS depressants, other antihistamines, alcohol, MAO inhibitors.

Theoretic Infant Dose:

Relative Infant Dose:

Adult Dose: 25-50 mg q 4-6 hours

Alternatives:

$T\frac{1}{2}$ =	2-3 hours	M/P =	
PHL =		PB =	
T_{max} =	2 - 3 hours	Oral =	Complete
MW =	255	pKa =	4.2, 8.7
Vd =	9-12		

References:
1. O'Brien TE. Excretion of drugs in human milk. Am J Hosp Pharm 1974; 31(9):844-854.
2. Pharmaceutical Manufacturer Prescribing Information. 1996.

TRIPROLIDINE

Trade: Actidil, Actacin
Can/Aus/UK: Actifed, Codral, Pro-actidil
Uses: Antihistamine
LRC: L1
AAP: Maternal Medication Usually Compatible with Breastfeeding

Triprolidine is an antihistamine. It is secreted into milk but in very small levels and is marketed with pseudoephedrine as Actifed. In a study of three patients who received 2.5 mg triprolidine, the average concentration in milk ranged from 1.2 to 4.4 μg/L over 24 hours.[1] The relative infant dose is less than 1.8% of the weight-normalized maternal dose. This dose is far too low to be clinically relevant.

Pregnancy Risk Category: C

Lactation Risk Category: L1

Adult Concerns: Sedation, dry mouth, anticholinergic side effects

Pediatric Concerns: None reported. Observe for sedation.

Drug Interactions: Increased sedation when used with CNS depressants, other antihistamines, alcohol, MAO inhibitors.

Theoretic Infant Dose: 0.66 μg/kg/day

Relative Infant Dose: 1.84%

Adult Dose: 2.5 mg q 4-6 hours

Alternatives:

$T\frac{1}{2}$ =	5 hours	M/P =	0.5-1.2
PHL =		PB =	
T_{max} =	2 hours	Oral =	Complete
MW =	278	pKa =	
Vd =			

References:
1. Findlay JW, Butz RF, Sailstad JM, Warren JT, Welch RM. Pseudoephedrine and triprolidine in plasma and breastmilk of nursing mothers. Br J Clin Pharmacol 1984; 18(6):901-906.

TRIPTORELIN PAMOATE

Trade: Trelstar La, Trelstar Depo
Can/Aus/UK:
Uses: Analog of luteinizing hormone releasing hormone
LRC: L3
AAP: Not reviewed

Triptorelin is a potent inhibitor of gonadotropin secretion when given continuously. After chronic administration, a sustained decrease of luteinizing hormone (LH) and follicle stimulating hormone (FSH) secretion and marked reduction of testicular and ovarian steroidogenesis occurs. Continuous use in breastfeeding mothers would ultimately lead to reduced levels of ovulation and sex steroids. In a study in males, prolactin levels were actually increased.[1] Thus it is difficult to discern what, if any, effect this agent would have on milk production in breastfeeding mothers. Some caution is recommended until more is known about this drugs effect on milk production. It is extremely unlikely this agent would penetrate milk due to its high molecular weight. Also, it is not orally bioavailable, so it is very unlikely to harm a breastfeeding infant.

Pregnancy Risk Category: X

Lactation Risk Category: L3

Adult Concerns: Side effects include vaginal dryness, hot flashes, leg pain, headache, breakthrough bleeding, skeletal pain, edema in legs, decreased libido, and dizziness.

Pediatric Concerns: None reported. Unlikely to penetrate milk, or be orally bioavailable.

Drug Interactions:

Theoretic Infant Dose:

Relative Infant Dose:

Adult Dose: 11.25 mg ever 84 days IM

Alternatives:

$T\frac{1}{2}$ =	3 hour IV	M/P =	
PHL =		PB =	0%
T_{max} =	1 week	Oral =	Nil
MW =	1699	pKa =	
Vd =	33		

References:
1. Stoffel-Wagner B, Sommer L, Bidlingmaier F, Klingmuller D. Effects of the gonadotropin-releasing-hormone agonist, D-Trp-6-GnRH, on prolactin secretion in healthy young men. Horm Res. 1995;43:266-272.

TROPISETRON
Trade:
Can/Aus/UK: Navoban
Uses: Antiemetic for chemotherapy
LRC: L3
AAP: Not reviewed

Tropisetron is a serotonergic (5-HT3) receptor antagonist with antiemetic activity similar to ondansetron and many others.[1] No data are available on its transfer to human milk. See ondansetron as alternative in USA.

Pregnancy Risk Category: B3(Australian)

Lactation Risk Category: L3

Adult Concerns: Adverse effects include ocassional extrapyramidal reactions, headache, rash, fever, constipation, fatigue, sedation, dizziness, diarrhea, and hypotension or hypertension.

Pediatric Concerns: None reported via milk.

Drug Interactions: None reported.

Theoretic Infant Dose:

Relative Infant Dose:

Adult Dose: 5 mg orally every 6-24 hours.

Alternatives: Ondansetron

T½	=	5.6-8.6	M/P	=	
PHL	=		PB	=	71%
T$_{max}$	=	2 hours	Oral	=	60%
MW	=		pKa	=	
Vd	=	7.14			

References:
1. Pharmaceutical Manufacturers prescribing information, 2003.

TROVAFLOXACIN MESYLATE
Trade: Trovan, Alatrofloxacin
Can/Aus/UK:
Uses: Antibiotic
LRC: L4
AAP: Not reviewed

Trovafloxacin mesylate is a synthetic broad-spectrum antibiotic for oral use. The IV formula is called alatrofloxacin mesylate which is metabolized to trovafloxacin in vivo. Trovafloxacin is a fluoroquinolone antibiotic similar to ciprofloxacin, norfloxacin, and others. Trovafloxacin was found in measurable but low concentrations in breastmilk of three breastfeeding mothers.[1] Following an IV dose of 300 mg trovafloxacin equivalent and repeated oral 200 mg doses of trovafloxacin mg daily, breastmilk levels averaged 0.8 mg/L and ranged from 0.3 to 2.1 mg per liter of milk. This would average less than 4% of the weight-normalized maternal dose. New data on this antibiotic documents a higher risk of hepatotoxicity and its use is restricted. This agent has been withdrawn from the US market due to risk of acute liver failure.

Pregnancy Risk Category: C

Lactation Risk Category: L4

Adult Concerns: Dizziness, nausea, headache, vomiting, diarrhea have been reported.

Pediatric Concerns: None reported via milk. Only small amounts are secreted in milk.

Drug Interactions: Antacids, Morphine, Sucralfate, and iron significantly reduce oral absorption.

Theoretic Infant Dose: 0.12 mg/kg/day

Relative Infant Dose: 4.2%

Adult Dose: 200-300 mg daily

Alternatives: Norfloxacin, Ofloxacin

T½ =	12.2 hours	M/P =	
PHL =		PB =	76%
Tmax =	1.2 hours	Oral =	88%
MW =	512	pKa =	
Vd =	1.3		

References:
1. Pharmaceutical Manufacturer Prescribing Information.

TUBERCULIN PURIFIED PROTEIN DERIVATIVE
Trade: Tubersol, Aplisol, Sclavo, PPD, Mantoux
Can/Aus/UK:
Uses: Tuberculin skin test
LRC: L2
AAP: Not reviewed

Tuberculin (also called Mantoux, PPD, Tine test) is a skin-test antigen derived from the concentrated, sterile, soluble products of growth of M. Tuberculosis or M. bovis. Small amounts of this purified product when placed intradermally, produce a hypersensitivity reaction at the place of injection in those individuals with antibodies to M. tuberculosis.[1,2] Preliminary studies also indicate that breastfed infants may passively acquire sensitivity to mycobacterial antigens from mothers who are sensitized. There are no contraindications to using PPD tests in breastfeeding mothers as the proteins are sterilized and unlikely to penetrate milk.

Pregnancy Risk Category: C

Lactation Risk Category: L2

Adult Concerns: Local vesiculation, irritation, bruising, and rarely hypersensitivity

Pediatric Concerns: None via milk.

Drug Interactions:

Theoretic Infant Dose:

Relative Infant Dose:

Adult Dose: 5 units X 1

Alternatives:

References:
1. Drug Facts and Comparisons 1999 ed. ed. St. Louis: 1999.
2. McEvoy GE. (ed): AFHS Drug Information. New York, NY: 1999.

TYPHOID VACCINE

Trade: Vivotif Berna, Typhim Vi
Can/Aus/UK: Vivotif Berna
Uses: Vaccination
LRC:
AAP: Maternal Medication Usually Compatible with Breastfeeding

Typhoid vaccine promotes active immunity to typhoid fever. It is available in an oral form (Ty21a) which is a live attenuated vaccine for oral administration.[1] The parenteral (injectable) form is derived from acetone-treated killed and dried bacteria, phenol-inactive bacteria, or a special capsular polysaccharide vaccine extracted from killed S. typhi Ty21a strains. Due to a limited lipopolysaccharide coating, the Ty21a strains are limited in their ability to produce infection.

No data are available on its transfer into human milk. If immunization is required, a killed species would be preferred, as infection of the neonate would be possible.

Pregnancy Risk Category: C

Lactation Risk Category:

Adult Concerns: Following oral administration, nausea, abdominal cramps, vomiting, urticaria. IM preparations may produce soreness at injection site, tenderness, malaise, headache, myalgia, fever.

Pediatric Concerns: None reported, but killed species suggested.

Drug Interactions: Use cautiously in patients receiving anticoagulants. Do not coadminister with plague vaccine. Do not administer the live-attenuated varieties to immunocompromised patients. Phenytoin may reduce antibody response to this product. Do not use with sulfonamides.

Theoretic Infant Dose:

Relative Infant Dose:

Adult Dose: 0.5 mL X 2 over 4 weeks

Alternatives:

References:
1. Pharmaceutical Manufacturer Prescribing Information.

URSODIOL
Trade: Actigall
Can/Aus/UK: Urso, Combidol, Destolit, Lithofalk, Urdox, Ursogal
Uses: Bile acid for dissolving gall stones
LRC: L3
AAP: Not reviewed

Ursodiol (ursodeoxycholic acid) is a bile salt found in small amounts in humans that is used to dissolve cholesterol gallstones. It is almost completely absorbed orally via the portal circulation and is extracted almost completely by the liver. Ursodiol suppresses hepatic synthesis and excretion of cholesterol. Following extraction by the liver, it is conjugated with glycine or taurine and is resecreted into the hepatic bile duct. Only trace amounts are found in the plasma and it is not likely significant amounts would be present in milk.[1] While no breastfeeding data are available, only small amounts of bile salts are known to be present in milk.[2] It is not likely with the low levels of ursodiol in the maternal plasma that clinically relevant amounts would enter milk.

Pregnancy Risk Category: B

Lactation Risk Category: L3

Adult Concerns: Insomnia, headache, abdominal pain, flatulence, cholecystitis, constipation, diarrhea (rare), nausea, vomiting

Pediatric Concerns: None via breastmilk.

Drug Interactions: Cholestyramine, antacids, charcoal and colestipol may interfere with GI absorption.

Theoretic Infant Dose:

Relative Infant Dose:

Adult Dose: 8-10 mg/kg/day in 3 divided doses

Alternatives:

T½ =		M/P =	
PHL =		PB =	
Tmax =		Oral =	90%
MW =	392	pKa =	
Vd =			

References:

1. Bachrach WH, Hofmann AF. Ursodeoxycholic acid in the treatment of cholesterol cholelithiasis. part I. Dig Dis Sci 1982; 27(8):737-761.
2. Forsyth JS, Ross PE, Bouchier IA. Bile salts in breastmilk. Eur J Pediatr 1983; 140(2):126-127.

VALACYCLOVIR

Trade: Valtrex
Can/Aus/UK: Valtrex, Valaciclovir
Uses: Antiviral, for herpes simplex
LRC: L1
AAP: Not reviewed

Valacyclovir is a prodrug that is rapidly metabolized in the plasma to acyclovir. In a study of 5 women who received 500 mg twice daily for 7 days after delivery, the median peak acyclovir concentration in breastmilk was 4.2 mg/L at 4 hours while the average concentration (AUC) was 2.24 mg/L if 12 hour dosing intervals were used.[1] Thus the relative infant dose would be 4.7% of the weight-normalized maternal dose. The ratio of milk/serum ratio was highest 4 hours after the initial dose at 3.4 and reached steady state ratio at 1.85. Valacyclovir is rapidly converted to acyclovir and transfers into breastmilk. However, the amount of acyclovir in breastmilk after valacyclovir administration is considerably less than that used in therapeutic dosing of neonates.

Pregnancy Risk Category: B

Lactation Risk Category: L1

Adult Concerns: Nausea, vomiting, diarrhea, sore throat, edema, and skin rashes

Pediatric Concerns: None reported via milk.

Drug Interactions:

Theoretic Infant Dose: 0.34 mg/kg/day

Relative Infant Dose: 4.7%

Adult Dose: 500-1000 mg BID-TID

Alternatives: Acyclovir

$T^{1/2}$ =	2.5-3 hours	M/P =	0.6-4.1
PHL =	3.2 hours(neonates)	PB =	9-33%
T_{max} =	1.5 hours	Oral =	54%
MW =		pKa =	
Vd =			

References:
1. Sheffield JS, Fish DN, Hollier LM, Cadematori S, Nobles BJ, Wendel GD, Jr. Acyclovir concentrations in human breastmilk after valaciclovir administration. Am J Obstet Gynecol 2002; 186(1):100-102.

VALERIAN OFFICINALIS
Trade: Valerian Root
Can/Aus/UK:
Uses: Herbal sedative
LRC: L3
AAP: Not reviewed

Valerian root is most commonly used as a sedative/hypnotic. Of the numerous chemicals present in the root, the most important chemical group appears to be the valepotriates. This family consists of at least a dozen or more related compounds and is believed responsible for the sedative potential of this plant although it is controversial. The combination of numerous components may inevitability account for the sedative response.   Controlled studies in man have indicated a sedative/hypnotic effect with fewer night awakenings and significant somnolence.[1-3]   The toxicity of valerian root appears to be low, with only minor side effects reported. However, the valepotriates have been found to be cytotoxic, with alkylating activity similar to other nitrogen mustard-like anticancer agents. Should this prove to be so in vivo, it may preclude the use of this product in humans. No data are available on the transfer of valerian root compounds into human milk. However, the use of sedatives in breastfeeding mothers is generally discouraged, due to a possible increased risk of SIDS.

Pregnancy Risk Category:

Lactation Risk Category: L3

Adult Concerns: Ataxia, hypothermia, muscle relaxation. Headaches, excitability, cardiac disturbances.

Pediatric Concerns: None reported via human milk.

Drug Interactions:

Theoretic Infant Dose:

Relative Infant Dose:

Adult Dose:

Alternatives:

References:
1. Leathwood PD, Chauffard F, Heck E, Munoz-Box R. Aqueous extract of valerian root (Valeriana officinalis L.) improves sleep quality in man. Pharmacol Biochem Behav 1982; 17(1):65-71.
2. von Eickstedt KW, Rahman S. [Psychopharmacologic effect of valepotriates]. Arzneimittelforschung 1969; 19(3):316-319.
3. Leathwood PD, Chauffard F. Aqueous extract of valerian reduces latency to fall asleep in man. Planta Med 1985;(2):144-148.

VALGANCICLOVIR
Trade: Valcyte, Cytovene
Can/Aus/UK: Valcyte
Uses: Antiviral
LRC: L3
AAP: Not reviewed

Valganciclovir is a prodrug that is rapidly metabolized to the active antiviral drug ganciclovir.[1] It is used for cytomegalovirus infections particularly in HIV infected patients. The oral bioavailability of valganciclovir is 60% while only 6% with its active metabolite ganciclovir. Further, it is very water soluble and lipophobic, which would suggest milk levels will be low. No data are available on its use in breastfeeding mothers, but its oral absorption in the infant is likely low.

Pregnancy Risk Category: C

Lactation Risk Category: L3

Adult Concerns: Adverse events include diarrhea, neutropenia, nausea, headache, insomnia, abdominal pain, anemia, and catheter-related infections.

Pediatric Concerns: None reported via milk. No studies thus far. Due to its use in HIV infected patients, it is unlikely this agent will be used in breastfeeding mothers. Poor oral bioavailability would limit absorption in an infant.

Drug Interactions: Minimal but check other references.

Theoretic Infant Dose:

Relative Infant Dose:

Adult Dose: 450-900 mg daily

Alternatives:

T½ =	4 hours	M/P =	
PHL =		PB =	1-2%
T$_{max}$ =	1-3 hours	Oral =	61%
MW =	390	pKa =	7.6
Vd =	0.7		

References:
1. Pharmaceutical Manufacturers package insert, 2000.

VALPROIC ACID

Trade: Depakene, Depakote
Can/Aus/UK: Depakene, Novo-Valproic, Deproic, Epilim, Valpro, Convulex
Uses: Anticonvulsant
LRC: L2
AAP: Maternal Medication Usually Compatible with Breastfeeding

Valproic acid is a popular anticonvulsant used in grand mal, petit mal, myoclonic, and temporal lobe seizures. In a study of 16 patients receiving 300-2400 mg/d, valproic acid concentrations ranged from 0.4 to 3.9 mg/L (mean=1.9 mg/L). [1] The milk/plasma ratio averaged 0.05.

In a study of one patient receiving 250 mg twice daily, milk levels ranged from 0.18 to 0.47 mg/L. The milk/plasma ratio ranged from 0.01 to 0.02.[2] Alexander reports milk levels of 5.1 mg/L following a larger dose of up to 1600 mg/d.[3]

In a study of 6 women receiving 9.5 to 31 mg/kg/d valproic acid, milk levels averaged 1.4 mg/L while serum levels averaged 45.1 mg/L.[4] The average milk/serum ratio was 0.027.

Most authors agree that the amount of valproic acid transferring to the infant via milk is low. Breastfeeding would appear safe. However, the infant should be closely monitored for liver and platelet changes.

Pregnancy Risk Category: D

Lactation Risk Category: L2

Adult Concerns: Sedation, thrombocytopenia, tremor, nausea, diarrhea, liver toxicity

Pediatric Concerns: None reported via milk. Observe infant for changes in liver enzymes, clinical status, and platelet levels.

Drug Interactions: Valproic acid levels may be reduced by charcoal, rifampin, carbamazepine, clonazepam, lamotrigine, phenytoin. Valproic acid levels may be increased when used with chlorpromazine, cimetidine, felbamate, salicylates, alcohol. Valproic acid use may increase levels or the effect of barbiturates, warfarin, benzodiazepines, clozapine.

Theoretic Infant Dose: 0.21 mg/kg/day

Relative Infant Dose: 0.68%

Adult Dose: 10-30 mg/kg daily

Alternatives:

T½ =	14 hours	M/P =	0.42
PHL =	10-67 hours (neonate)	PB =	94%
T$_{max}$ =	1-4 hours	Oral =	Complete
MW =	144	pKa =	4.8
Vd =	0.1-0.4		

References:

1. von Unruh GE, Froescher W, Hoffmann F, Niesen M. Valproic acid in breastmilk: how much is really there? Ther Drug Monit 1984; 6(3):272-276.
2. Dickinson RG, Harland RC, Lynn RK, Smith WB, Gerber N. Transmission of valproic acid (Depakene) across the placenta: half-life of the drug in mother and baby. J Pediatr 1979; 94(5):832-835.
3. Alexander FW. Sodium valproate and pregnancy. Arch Dis Child 1979; 54(3):240.
4. Nau H, Rating D, Koch S, Hauser I, Helge H. Valproic acid and its metabolites: placental transfer, neonatal pharmacokinetics, transfer via mother's milk and clinical status in neonates of epileptic mothers. J Pharmacol Exp Ther 1981; 219(3):768-777.

VALSARTAN

Trade: Diovan
Can/Aus/UK: Diovan
Uses: Antihypertensive
LRC: L4
AAP: Not reviewed

Valsartan is a new angiotensin II receptor antagonist used to treat hypertension. While it is believed to enter the milk of rodents, no human data are available.[1,2] Use with caution in breastfeeding mothers.

Pregnancy Risk Category: C during 1st trimester
                                                    D during 2nd and 3rd trimester

Lactation Risk Category: L4

Adult Concerns: Occasional increase in liver enzymes. Small decreases in hemoglobin have been reported. Significant increases (> 20%) in serum potassium levels have been reported. Dizziness, insomnia, viral infection, cough, diarrhea, etc. have been reported.

Pediatric Concerns: None via milk, but caution is recommended.

Drug Interactions: May significantly increase digoxin levels by 49%.

Theoretic Infant Dose:

Relative Infant Dose:

Adult Dose: 80-320 mg daily

Alternatives:

T½ =	9 hours	M/P =		
PHL =		PB =	97%	
T$_{max}$ =	2-4 hours	Oral =	23%	
MW =		pKa =		
Vd =	0.24			

References:
1. Pharmaceutical Manufacturer Prescribing Information. 1999.
2. McEvoy GE. (ed): AFHS Drug Information. New York, NY: 1999.

VANCOMYCIN
Trade: Vancocin
Can/Aus/UK: Vancocin, Vancoled
Uses: Antibiotic
LRC: L1
AAP: Not reviewed

Vancomycin is an antimicrobial agent. Only low levels are secreted into human milk. Milk levels were 12.7 mg/L four hours after infusion in one woman receiving 1 gm every 12 hours for 7 days.[1] Its poor absorption from the infants GI tract would limit its systemic absorption. Low levels in infant could provide alterations of GI flora.

Pregnancy Risk Category: C

Lactation Risk Category: L1

Adult Concerns: Alteration of GI flora, neutropenia, hypotension, kidney and hearing damage

Pediatric Concerns: None reported via milk.

Drug Interactions: When used with aminoglycosides, risk of nephrotoxicity may be increased. Use with anesthetics may produce erythema and histamine-like flushing in children. May increase risk of neuromuscular blockade when used with neuromuscular blocking agents.

Theoretic Infant Dose: 1.9 mg/kg/day

Relative Infant Dose: 6.6%

Adult Dose: 125-500 mg q 6 hours

Alternatives:

T½ =	5.6 hours	M/P =	
PHL =	5.9-9.8 hours (neonates)	PB =	10-30%
T_{max} =		Oral =	Minimal
MW =	1449	pKa =	
Vd =	0.3-0.7		

References:
1. Reyes MP, Ostrea EM, Jr., Cabinian AE, Schmitt C, Rintelmann W. Vancomycin during pregnancy: does it cause hearing loss or nephrotoxicity in the infant? Am J Obstet Gynecol 1989; 161(4):977-981.

VARICELLA VIRUS VACCINE
Trade: Varivax
Can/Aus/UK:
Uses: Vaccination for Varicella (Chickenpox)
LRC: L2
AAP: Not reviewed

A live attenuated varicella vaccine (Varivax - Merck) was recently approved for marketing by the US Food and Drug Administration. Although effective, it does not apparently provide the immunity attained from infection with the parent virus and may not provide life-long immunity. The Oka/Merck strain used in the vaccine is attenuated by passage in human and embryonic guinea pig cell cultures. It is not known if the vaccine-acquired VZV is secreted in human milk, nor its infectiousness to infants. Interestingly, in two women with varicella-zoster infections, the virus was not culturable from milk.[1] Mothers of immunodeficient infants should not breastfeed following use of this vaccine. Recommendations for Use: Varicella vaccine is only recommended for children > 1 year of age up to 12 years of age with no history of varicella infection. Both the AAP[2] and the Center for Disease Control approve the use of varicella-zoster vaccines in breastfeeding mothers, if the risk of infection is high.

Pregnancy Risk Category: C

Lactation Risk Category: L2

Adult Concerns: Tenderness and erythema at the injection site in about 25% of vaccinees and a sparse generalized maculopapular rash occurring within one month after immunization in about 5%. Spread of the vaccine virus to others has been reported. Susceptible, immunodeficient individuals should be protected from exposure.

Pediatric Concerns: None reported via milk, but no studies are available. Immunocompromised infants should not be exposed to this product.

Drug Interactions:

Theoretic Infant Dose:

Relative Infant Dose:

Adult Dose: 0.5 mL X 2 over 4-8 weeks

Alternatives:

References:
1.   Frederick IB, White RJ, Braddock SW. Excretion of varicella-herpes zoster virus in breastmilk. Am J Obstet Gynecol 1986; 154(5):1116-1117.
2.   American Academy of Pediatrics. Committee on Infectious Diseases. Red Book. 1997.

VARICELLA-ZOSTER VIRUS
Trade: Chickenpox
Can/Aus/UK:
Uses: Chickenpox
LRC: L4
AAP: Not reviewed

Chickenpox virus has been reported to be transferred via breastmilk in one 27 year old mother who developed chickenpox postpartum.[1] Her 2 month old son also developed the disease 16 days after mother. Chickenpox virus was detected in the mother's milk and may suggest that transmission can occur via breastmilk. However, in a study of 2 breastfeeding patients who developed varicella-herpes zoster infections, in neither case was the virus isolated and cultured from their milk.[2] According to the American Academy of Pediatrics, neonates born to mothers with active varicella should be placed in isolation at birth and, if still hospitalized, until 21 or 28 days of age, depending on whether they received VZIG (Varicella Zoster Immune Globulin).[3] Candidates for VZIG include: immunocompromised children, pregnant women, and a newborn infant whose mother has onset of VZV within 5 days before or 48 hours after delivery. For an excellent review of VZV and breastfeeding see Merewood and Philipp.[4]

Pregnancy Risk Category:

Lactation Risk Category: L4

Adult Concerns:

Pediatric Concerns: Varicella-zoster virus transfers into human milk. Infants should not breastfeed unless protected with VZIG.

Drug Interactions:

Theoretic Infant Dose:

Relative Infant Dose:

Adult Dose:

Alternatives:

References:

1. Yoshida M, Yamagami N, Tezuka T, Hondo R. Case report: detection of varicella-zoster virus DNA in maternal breastmilk. J Med Virol 1992; 38(2):108-110.
2. Frederick IB, White RJ, Braddock SW. Excretion of varicella-herpes zoster virus in breastmilk. Am J Obstet Gynecol 1986; 154(5):1116-1117.
3. Report of the committee on Infectious Diseases. American Academy of Pediatrics. 1994.
4. Meerwood A, Philipp B. Breastfeeding: Conditions and Diseases. 1st ed. ed. Amarillo, TX: Pharmasoft Publishing L.P., 2001.

VASOPRESSIN

Trade: Pitressin
Can/Aus/UK: Pitressin, Pressyn, Pitresin
Uses: Antidiuretic hormone
LRC: L3
AAP: Not reviewed

Vasopressin, also known as the antidiuretic hormone, is a small peptide (8 amino acids) that is normally secreted by the posterior pituitary.[1] It reduces urine production by the kidney. Although it probably passes to some degree into human milk, it is rapidly destroyed in the GI tract by trypsin and must be administered by injection or intranasally. Hence, oral absorption by a nursing infant is very unlikely. Desmopressin is virtually identical and milk levels have been reported to be very low. See desmopressin.

Pregnancy Risk Category: B

Lactation Risk Category: L3

Adult Concerns: Increased blood pressure, water retention and edema, sweating, tremor, and bradycardia

Pediatric Concerns: None reported via milk.

Drug Interactions:

Theoretic Infant Dose:

Relative Infant Dose:

Adult Dose: 5-10 units BID-QID PRN

Alternatives:

T½ =	10-20 minutes	M/P =	
PHL =		PB =	
T$_{max}$ =	1 hour	Oral =	None
MW =		pKa =	
Vd =			

References:
1. McEvoy GE. (ed):AFHS Drug Information. New York, NY: 2003.

VENLAFAXINE
Trade: Effexor
Can/Aus/UK: Effexor
Uses: Antidepressant, SSRI
LRC: L3
AAP: Not reviewed

Venlafaxine is a new serotonin reuptake inhibitor antidepressant. It inhibits both serotonin reuptake and norepinephrine reuptake. Somewhat similar in mechanism to other antidepressants such as Prozac. Fewer anticholinergic side-effects.

In an excellent study of three mothers (mean age = 34.5 years, 84.5 kg) receiving venlafaxine (225-300 mg/d), the mean milk/plasma ratios for venlafaxine (V) and O-desmethylvenlafaxine (ODV) were 2.5 and 2.7 respectively.[1] The mean maximum concentrations of V and ODV in milk were 1.16 mg/L and 0.796 mg/L. The C_{max} for milk was 2.25 hours. The mean infant exposure was 3.2% for V and 3.2% for ODV of the weight-adjusted maternal dose. V was detected in the plasma of one of seven infants while ODV was detected in four of the seven infants. The infants were healthy and showed no acute adverse effects.

Pregnancy Risk Category: C

Lactation Risk Category: L3

Adult Concerns: Nausea/vomiting, somnolence, dry mouth, dizziness, headache, weakness

Pediatric Concerns: None reported via milk, but no studies are available.

Drug Interactions: Serious, sometimes fatal reactions when used with MAO inhibitors or if used within 7-14 days of their use. Serious organic psychosis has been reported with the co-administration of propafenone(Rythmol). Two recent cases of serotonin-like reactions (agitation, dysarthria, diapyhoresis and extrapyramidal movement disorder) have been reported when metoclopramide was used in patients receiving sertraline or venlafaxine.[2]

Theoretic Infant Dose: 0.29 mg/kg/day

Relative Infant Dose: 6.4%

Adult Dose: 75 mg TID

Alternatives: Sertraline, Paroxetine

T½ =	5 hours(venlafaxine)	M/P =	
PHL =		PB =	27%
T$_{max}$ =	2.25 milk	Oral =	92%
MW =	313	pKa =	9.4
Vd =	4-12		

References:

1. Ilett KF, Kristensen JH, Hackett LP, Paech M, Kohan R, Rampono J. Distribution of venlafaxine and its O-desmethyl metabolite in human milk and their effects in breastfed infants. Br J Clin Pharmacol 2002; 53(1):17-22.
2. Fisher AA, Davis MW. Serotonin syndrome caused by selective serotonin reuptake-inhibitors-metoclopramide interaction. Ann Pharmacother 2002;36(1):67-71.

VERAPAMIL

Trade: Calan, Isoptin, Covera-HS
Can/Aus/UK: Apo-Verap, Isoptin, Novo-Veramil, Anpec, Coridlox, Veracaps SR, Berkatens, Cordilox, Univer
Uses: Calcium channel blocker for hypertension
LRC: L2
AAP: Maternal Medication Usually Compatible with Breastfeeding

Verapamil is a typical calcium channel blocker used as an antihypertensive. It is secreted into milk but in very low levels, which are highly controversial. Anderson reports that in one patient receiving 80 mg three times daily, the average steady-state concentrations of verapamil and norverapamil in milk were 25.8 and 8.8 μg/L respectively.[1] The respective maternal plasma level was 42.9 μg/L. The milk/plasma ratio for verapamil was 0.60. No verapamil was detected in the infant's plasma. Inoue reports that in one patient receiving 80 mg four times daily, the milk level peaked at 300 μg/L at approximately 14 hours.[2] These levels are considerably higher than the aforementioned. In another study of a mother receiving 240 mg daily, the concentrations in milk were never higher than 40 μg/L.[3] See bepridil, diltiazem, nifedipine as alternates. From these three studies, the relative infant dose would vary from 0.15%, 0.98%, and 0.18% respectively. Regardless of the variability, the relative amount transferred to the infant is still quite small.

Pregnancy Risk Category: C

Lactation Risk Category: L2

Adult Concerns: Hypotension, bradycardia, peripheral edema

Pediatric Concerns: None reported via milk. Observe for hypotension, bradycardia, weakness.

Drug Interactions: Barbiturates may reduce bioavailability of calcium channel blockers (CCB). Calcium salts may reduce hypotensive effect. Dantrolene may increase risk of hyperkalemia and myocardial depression. H2 blockers may increase bioavailability of certain CCBs. Hydantoins may reduce plasma levels. Quinidine increases risk of hypotension, bradycardia, tachycardia. Rifampin may reduce effects of CCBs. Vitamin D may reduce efficacy of CCBs. CCBs may increase carbamazepine, cyclosporin, encainide, prazosin levels.

Theoretic Infant Dose: 45 μg/kg/day

Relative Infant Dose: < 0.98%

Adult Dose: 80-100 mg TID

Alternatives: Bepridil, Nifedipine, Nimodipine

$T\frac{1}{2}$ =	3-7 hours	M/P =	0.94
PHL =		PB =	83-92%
T_{max} =	1-2.2	Oral =	90%
MW =	455	pKa =	
Vd =	2.5-6.5		

References:

1. Anderson P, Bondesson U, Mattiasson I, Johansson BW. Verapamil and norverapamil in plasma and breastmilk during breast feeding. Eur J Clin Pharmacol 1987; 31(5):625-627.
2. Inoue H, Unno N, Ou MC, Iwama Y, Sugimoto T. Level of verapamil in human milk. Eur J Clin Pharmacol 1984; 26(5):657-658.
3. Andersen HJ. Excretion of verapamil in human milk. Eur J Clin Pharmacol 1983; 25(2):279-280.

VIGABATRIN

Trade: Sabril
Can/Aus/UK:
Uses: Anticonvulsant
LRC: L3
AAP: Not reviewed

Vigabatrin is a newer anticonvulsant and a synthetic derivative of gamma-aminobutyric acid. It is an effective adjunctive anticonvulsant for the treatment of multi-drug resistant complex partial seizures. It has also shown efficacy in controlling seizures and spasm in infants 3 months and older. No data are available on its transfer into human milk. However, the plasma levels of this drug (dose=1.5 gm) are quite low, 93 μmol/L, which would suggest that the amount in milk would probably be low even if the drug had a milk/plasma ratio of 1 or greater, but this is not known for sure.[1] However, regardless of the kinetics of this drug, it irreversibly inactivates gamma-aminobutyric acid.[2] The effect of this property on neonatal brains is not known. Some caution is recommended in breastfeeding mothers.

Pregnancy Risk Category:

Lactation Risk Category: **L3**

Adult Concerns: Changes in visual field defects have been noted. Drowsiness, fatigue, and acute psychosis (7%) have been described particularly in patients with a history of psychiatric disorders. Psychosis and an increased frequency of seizures have been reported upon abrupt withdrawal of vigabatrin therapy.

Pediatric Concerns: None reported via milk.

Drug Interactions: May decrease phenytoin levels by 30%. Few other interactions are noted which is a plus for this drug.

Theoretic Infant Dose:

Relative Infant Dose:

Adult Dose: 1-4 gm daily

Alternatives:

T½ =	7 hours	M/P =	
PHL =		PB =	0%
T$_{max}$ =	0.5-2 hours	Oral =	50%
MW =	129	pKa =	
Vd =	0.8		

References:

1. Grant SM, Heel RC. Vigabatrin. A review of its pharmacodynamic and pharmacokinetic properties, and therapeutic potential in epilepsy and disorders of motor control. Drugs 1991; 41(6):889-926.
2. Dichter MA, Brodie MJ. New antiepileptic drugs. N Engl J Med 1996; 334(24):1583-1590.

VITAMIN A

Trade: Aquasol A, Del-Vi-A, Vitamin A, Retinol
Can/Aus/UK: Aquasol A, Avoleum
Uses: Vitamin supplement
LRC: L3
AAP: Not reviewed

Vitamin A (retinol) is a typical retinoid. It is a fat soluble vitamin that is secreted into human milk and primarily sequestered in high concentrations in the liver (90%).[1] Retinol is absorbed in the small intestine by a selective carrier-mediated uptake process. Levels in infants are generally unknown. The overdose of Vitamin A is extremely dangerous and adults should never exceed 5000 units/day. Use normal doses. DO NOT use maternal doses > 5000 units /day. Mature human milk is rich in retinol and contains 750 µg/Liter (2800 units). Infants do not generally require vitamin A supplementation.

Pregnancy Risk Category: A

Lactation Risk Category: L3

Adult Concerns: Liver toxicity in overdose

Pediatric Concerns: None reported via milk, but do not use vitamin A in excess of 5000 IU/day.

Drug Interactions:

Theoretic Infant Dose:

Relative Infant Dose:

Adult Dose: < 5000 IU daily

Alternatives:

T½ =		M/P =	
PHL =		PB =	
T$_{max}$ =		Oral =	Complete
MW =	286	pKa =	
Vd =			

References:
1. Lawrence RA. Breastfeeding: A guide for the medical profession. St. Louis: Mosby Publishers, 1994.

VITAMIN B-12

Trade: Cyanocobalamin
Can/Aus/UK: Rubramin, Anacobin, Cytacon
Uses: Vitamin supplement
LRC: L1
AAP: Maternal Medication Usually Compatible with Breastfeeding

Vitamin B-12 is also called cyanocobalamin and is used for the treatment of pernicious anemia. It is an essential vitamin that is secreted in human milk at concentrations of 0.1 µg/100 mL. B-12 deficiency is very dangerous to an infant. Milk levels vary in proportion to maternal serum levels.[1] Vegetarian mothers may have low levels unless supplemented. Supplementation of nursing mothers is generally recommended.

Pregnancy Risk Category: A

Lactation Risk Category: L1

Adult Concerns: Itching, skin rash, mild diarrhea, megaloblastic anemia in vegetarian mothers

Pediatric Concerns: None reported with exception of B-12 deficiency states.

Drug Interactions:

Theoretic Infant Dose: 0.15 μg/kg/day

Relative Infant Dose:

Adult Dose: 25 μg daily

Alternatives:

$T\frac{1}{2}$ =		M/P =	
PHL =		PB =	
T_{max} =	2 hours	Oral =	Variable
MW =	1355	pKa =	
Vd =			

References:
1. Lawrence RA. Breastfeeding: A guide for the medical profession. St. Louis: Mosby Publishers, 1994.

VITAMIN D

Trade: Calciferol, Delta-D, Vitamin D
Can/Aus/UK: Calciferol, Calcijex, Drisdol, Hytakerol, Radiostol
Uses: Vitamin D supplement
LRC: L3
AAP: Maternal Medication Usually Compatible with Breastfeeding

Vitamin D is secreted into milk in limited concentrations and is somewhat proportional to maternal serum levels.[1] Excessive doses can produce elevated calcium levels in the infant;[2] therefore, lower doses are suggested in undernourished mothers (RDA is 200-600 IU/day). There has been some concern that mothers deficient in vitamin D may not provide sufficient vitamin D to the infant and hence impede bone mineralization in their infants. In a study by Greer[3], breastfed infants who received oral vitamin D supplementation had greater bone mineralization than those who were not supplemented. However, a more recent study of Korean women in winter who were not supplemented with vitamin D, and whose infants were either fed with human milk or artificial cow's formula (with vitamin D added), suggested that even though the breastfed groups plasma 25-hydroxyvitamin D concentration was lower, bone mineralization was equivalent in both breastfed and formula-fed infants.[4] The authors speculated that adequate bone mineralization occurs during the breastfeeding period from a predominantly vitamin D independent passive transport mechanism.

Human milk is known to have rather minimal concentrations of vitamin D. On average, breastmilk contains approximately 26 IU/L (range = 5-136).[5] Supplementing a mother with even moderate doses of vitamin D does not substantially increase milk levels. However, supplementing with high therapeutic doses (> 5000 IU/day) for various syndromes can however, significantly elevate milk concentrations of vitamin D leading to potential hypercalcemia in a breastfed infant.[6] Therefore, excessively high therapeutic doses should be used with great caution in a breastfeeding mother.

In 2003 the Academy of Pediatrics, responding to the increased reports of rickets in breastfeeding infants, published a recommendation that all US infants should consume at least 200 IU of vitamin D per day by supplementation if needed.[7] These recommendations are somewhat controversial for at least two reasons. One, we do not know with certainty the minimal but adequate dose of vitamin D required by breastfed infants, and two, they suggest that a mother's milk may in some cases be nutritionally inadequate. Regardless of these concerns, mothers who have limited vitamin D intake due to poor nutrition, or whose bodies have limited exposure to sunlight, probably need supplementation as their milk is likely deficient in vitamin D. In addition, infants of these mothers (who have limited or no exposure to sunlight or inadequate intake) may need supplementation, as these infants (particularly dark skinned) are most at risk for developing rickets.

Pregnancy Risk Category: A

Lactation Risk Category: L3

Adult Concerns: Elevated calcium levels in breastfed infants

Pediatric Concerns: None reported via milk, but do not overdose. Significant renal toxicity can occur in infants.

Drug Interactions:

Theoretic Infant Dose:

Relative Infant Dose:

Adult Dose: 250 µg to 1.5 mg daily

Alternatives:

$T^{1/2}$ =		M/P =	
PHL =		PB =	
T_{max} =		Oral =	Variable
MW =	396	pKa =	
Vd =			

References:
1. Rothberg AD, Pettifor JM, Cohen DF, Sonnendecker EW, Ross FP. Maternal-infant vitamin D relationships during breast-feeding. J Pediatr 1982; 101(4):500-503.
2. Goldberg LD. Transmission of a vitamin-D metabolite in breastmilk. Lancet 1972; 2(7789):1258-1259.

3. Greer FR, Searcy JE, Levin RS, Steichen JJ, Asch PS, Tsang RC. Bone mineral content and serum 25-hydroxyvitamin D concentration in breast-fed infants with and without supplemental vitamin D. J Pediatr 1981; 98(5):696-701.

4. Park MJ, Namgung R, Kim DH, Tsang RC. Bone mineral content is not reduced despite low vitamin D status in breastmilk-fed infants versus cow's milk based formula-fed infants. J Pediatr 1998; 132(4):641-645.

5. Institute of Medicine, Food and Nutrition Board, Standing Committee on the Scientific Evaluation of Dietary Reference Intakes. Vitamin D. In: Dietary Reference Intakes for Calcium, Phosphorus, Magnesium, Vitamin D and Fluoride. Washington, DC: National Academy Press; 1997;250-287.

6. Greer FR, Hollis BW, Napoli JL. High concentrations of vitamin D2 in human milk associated with pharmacologic doses of vitamin D2. J Pediatr 1984;105(1):61-64.

7. Gartner LM, Greer FR. Prevention of rickets and vitamin D deficiency: new guidelines for vitamin D intake. Pediatrics 2003; 111(4 Pt 1):908-910.

VITAMIN E

Trade: Alpha Tocopherol, Aquasol E
Can/Aus/UK: Aquasol E, Bio E
Uses: Vitamin E supplement
LRC: L2
AAP: Not reviewed

Vitamin E (alpha tocopherol) is secreted in milk in higher concentrations than in the maternal serum. Following topical administration to nipples (400 IU/feeding), Vitamin E plasma levels in breastfeeding infants were 40% higher than controls in just 6 days.[1] Studies clearly indicate that high levels of Vitamin E are stored in the liver and tend to accumulate over time. In 1984, over 36 neonates receiving vitamin E in neonatal intensive care units died following the IV administration of just 25-50 IU/day for several weeks.[2] The maternal RDA during lactation is approximately 16 IU/day.[3] Do not overdose. Do not apply to nipples unless concentrations are low (< 50-100 IU) and then, only infrequently. The application of pure vitamin E oil (1000 IU/gm) to nipples should be discouraged.

Pregnancy Risk Category: A

Lactation Risk Category: L2

Adult Concerns:

Pediatric Concerns: None reported via milk, but caution is recommended. Do not use highly concentrated vitamin E oils directly on nipple.

Drug Interactions:

Theoretic Infant Dose:

Relative Infant Dose:

Adult Dose: 16-18 (1 mg d-A-tocopherol) daily

Alternatives:

T½ =	282 hours(IV)	M/P =	
PHL =		PB =	
T$_{max}$ =		Oral =	Variable
MW =	431	pKa =	
Vd =			

References:
1. Marx CM, Izquierdo A, Driscoll JW, Murray MA, Epstein MF. Vitamin E concentrations in serum of newborn infants after topical use of vitamin E by nursing mothers. Am J Obstet Gynecol 1985; 152(6 Pt 1):668-670.
2. Hale TW, Rais-Bahrami K, Montgomery DL, Harkey C, Habersang RW. Vitamin E toxicity in neonatal piglets. J Toxicol Clin Toxicol 1995; 33(2):123-130.
3. Lawrence RA. Breastfeeding: A guide for the medical profession. St. Louis: Mosby Publishers, 1994.

WARFARIN

Trade: Coumadin, Panwarfin
Can/Aus/UK: Coumadin, Warfilone, Marevan
Uses: Anticoagulant
LRC: L2
AAP: Maternal Medication Usually Compatible with Breastfeeding

Warfarin is a potent anticoagulant. Warfarin is highly protein bound in the maternal circulation and therefore very little is secreted into human milk. Very small and insignificant amounts are secreted into milk but it depends to some degree on the dose administered. In one study of two patients who were anticoagulated with warfarin, no warfarin was detected in the infant's serum, nor were changes in coagulation detectable.[1] In another study of 13 mothers, less than 0.08 μmol per liter (25 ng/mL) was detected in milk, and no warfarin was detected in the infants' plasma.[2]

According to these authors, maternal warfarin apparently poses little risk to a nursing infant and thus far has not produced bleeding anomalies in breastfed infants. Other anticoagulants, such as phenindione, should be avoided. Observe infant for bleeding such as excessive bruising or reddish petechia (spots). While the risks in breastfeeding premature infants (which are more susceptible to encranial bleeding) is still low, oral supplementation with vitamin K1 will preclude any chance of hemorrhage. Even modest doses of Vitamin K1 counteract high doses of warfarin.

Pregnancy Risk Category: D

Lactation Risk Category: L2

Adult Concerns: Bleeding, bruising

Pediatric Concerns: None reported via milk, but observe for bleeding, bruising.

Drug Interactions: The drug interactions of warfarin are numerous. Agents that may increase the anticoagulant effect and the risk of bleeding include: acetaminophen, androgens, beta blockers, clofibrate, corticosteroids, disulfiram, erythromycin, fluconazole, hydantoins, ketoconazole, miconazole, sulfonamides, thyroid hormones, and numerous others. Agents that may decrease the anticoagulant effect of warfarin include: ascorbic acid, dicloxacillin, ethanol, griseofulvin, nafcillin, sucralfate, trazodone, amino glutethimide, barbiturates, carbamazepine, etretinate, rifampin. Due to numerous drug interactions, please consult additional references.

Theoretic Infant Dose: 3.75 μg/kg/day

Relative Infant Dose:

Adult Dose: 2-10 mg daily

Alternatives:

T½ =	1-2.5 days	M/P =		
PHL =		PB =	99%	
T$_{max}$ =	0.5-3 days	Oral =	Complete	
MW =	308	pKa =	5.1	
Vd =	0.1-0.2			

References:
1. McKenna R, Cole ER, Vasan U. Is warfarin sodium contraindicated in the lactating mother? J Pediatr 1983; 103(2):325-327.
2. Orme ML, Lewis PJ, De Swiet M, Serlin MJ, Sibeon R, Baty JD, Breckenridge AM. May mothers given warfarin breast-feed their infants? Br Med J 1977; 1(6076):1564-1565.

WEST NILE FEVER
Trade:
Can/Aus/UK:
Uses: Viral febrile infection
LRC:
AAP: Not reviewed

West Nile fever in humans usually is a febrile, influenza-like illness characterized by an abrupt onset (incubation period is 3 to 6 days) of moderate to high fever (3 to 5 days, infrequently biphasic, sometimes with chills), headache (often frontal), sore throat, backache, myalgia, arthralgia, fatigue, conjunctivitis, retrobulbar pain, maculopapular or roseolar rash, lymphadenopathy, anorexia, nausea, abdominal pain, diarrhea, and respiratory symptoms. It is not known whether the virus transfers into human milk, nor if it is communicable if present in milk although its transmission is believed unlikely. Thus far, there has been no documented occurrence of a mother passing the West Nile virus via maternal milk. Infected mosquitoes are the primary vector for West Nile virus although both hard and soft ticks have been found infected with West Nile virus in nature, but their role in the transmission and maintenance of the virus is uncertain. Mosquitoes, largely bird-feeding species, are the principal vectors of West Nile virus. The virus has been isolated from 43 mosquito species, predominantly of the genus Culex.[1-3]

For answers to questions about West Nile virus, please see the CDC web site http://www.cdc.gov/ncidod/dvbid/westnile/q&a.htm and the NYC advisory notice web site http://www.ci.nyc.ny.us/html/doh/html/cd/encalert.html

Pregnancy Risk Category:

Lactation Risk Category:

Adult Concerns: Febrile influenza-like illness, characterized by an abrupt onset of moderate to high fever, headache (often frontal), sore throat, backache, myalgia, arthralgia, fatigue, conjunctivitis, retrobulbar pain, maculopapular or roseolar rash, lymphadenopathy, anorexia, nausea, abdominal pain, diarrhea, and respiratory symptoms.

Pediatric Concerns: No transmission reported via milk but it has not been studied.

Drug Interactions:

Theoretic Infant Dose:

Relative Infant Dose:

Adult Dose:

Alternatives:

References:
1. Hayes C. West Nile Fever. In: Monath TP (ed). The arbovir**Uses:** epidemiology and ecology, Vol 5. Boca Raton, FL: CRC Press, 1989.
2. Shope RE. Other Flavivirus Infections. In: Guerrant RL, Walker DH, and Weller PF (eds). Tropical Infectious Diseases: Principals, Pathogens, and Practice. Philadelphia, PA: Churchill Livingstone, 2004.
3. Hubalek Z, Halouzka J. West Nile fever--a reemerging mosquito-borne viral disease in Europe. Emerg Infect Dis 1999; 5(5):643-650.

XENON-133

Trade: Xenon-133
Can/Aus/UK:
Uses: Evaluation of pulmonary obstruction.
LRC: L3
AAP: Not reviewed

Xenon-133 (T1/2 = 5.3 days) and Xenon-127 (T1/2=36.4 days) are noble gases.[1] As such they are chemically inert and are used often for ventilation and for cerebral blood flow studies. The patient is asked to inhale a gas mixed with either of these isotopes, followed by a brief 5 min wash out period. Obstructions in the lung appear as hot spots. Because these gases are inert, they would not be stored or any length of time in the human and would be rapidly exhaled within minutes. This is a typical case were the biological half-life (time stored in body, minutes in this case) is incredibly short compared to the radioactive half-life (5.3 days). Xenon-133 would not likely be hazardous to a breastfeeding infant as long as a brief wash out period of an hour or more is used.

Pregnancy Risk Category:

Lactation Risk Category: **L3**

Adult Concerns: None

Pediatric Concerns: None if brief wash out period is used.

Drug Interactions:

Theoretic Infant Dose:

Relative Infant Dose:

Adult Dose:

Alternatives:

T½ =	5.3 days	M/P =	
PHL =		PB =	
T$_{max}$ =		Oral =	None
MW =		pKa =	
Vd =			

References:
1. Gopal B, Saha. Fundamentals of Nuclear Pharmacy. 3rd ed. ed. Springer-Verlag Publishers, 1992.

ZAFIRLUKAST
Trade: Accolate
Can/Aus/UK: Accolate
Uses: Leukotriene inhibitor for Asthma
LRC: L3
AAP: Not reviewed

Zafirlukast is a new competitive receptor antagonist of leukotriene D4 and other components of slow-reacting substance of anaphylaxis which are mediators of bronchoconstriction in asthmatic patients. Zafirlukast is not a bronchodilator and should not be used for acute asthma attacks.

Zafirlukast is excreted into milk in low concentrations. Following repeated 40 mg doses twice daily (please note: average adult dose is 20 mg twice daily), the average steady-state concentration in breastmilk was 50 µg/L compared to 255 ng/mL in maternal plasma.[1] Zafirlukast is poorly absorbed when administered with food. It is likely the oral absorption via ingestion of breastmilk would be low. The manufacturer recommends against using in breastfeeding mothers.

Pregnancy Risk Category: B

Lactation Risk Category: L3

Adult Concerns: Pharyngitis, aggravation reaction, headache, nausea, diarrhea have been reported.

Pediatric Concerns: None reported.

Drug Interactions: Erythromycin reduces oral bioavailability of zafirlukast by 40%. Aspirin increase zafirlukast plasma levels by 45%. Theophylline reduces zafirlukast plasma levels by 30%. Zafirlukast increase warfarin anticoagulation by 35%. Terfenadine reduces zafirlukast plasma levels by 54%.

Theoretic Infant Dose: 7.5 µg/kg/day

Relative Infant Dose: 0.65%

Adult Dose: 20 mg BID

Alternatives:

$T\frac{1}{2}$ =	10-13 hours	M/P =	0.15
PHL =		PB =	> 99%
T_{max} =	3 hours	Oral =	Poor
MW =	575	pKa =	
Vd =			

References:
1. Pharmaceutical Manufacturer Prescribing Information. 1997.

ZALEPLON

Trade: Sonata
Can/Aus/UK: Starnoc, Sonata
Uses: Hypnotic agent used for insomnia.
LRC: L2
AAP: Not reviewed

Zaleplon is a nonbenzodiazepine hypnotic sedative that interacts at the GABA receptor. In a study of 5 lactating mothers who received doses of 10 mg orally, the peak milk level occurred at 1.2 hours and averaged 14 μg/L.[1] Milk levels decreased rapidly following a peak at 1.2 hours to less than 3 μg/L four hours following administration. The authors suggest that these levels would be subclinical to the infant.

Pregnancy Risk Category: C

Lactation Risk Category: L2

Adult Concerns: Headache, drowsiness, peripheral edema, dizziness have been reported. Avoid alcohol and other depressants.

Pediatric Concerns: None reported via milk. Milk levels were reported to be subclinical.

Drug Interactions: Zaleplon potentiates the CNS effects of alcohol, imipramine, thioridazine. Rifampin decreases the plasma levels of zaleplon. Cimetidine produces a significant increase in plasma levels of zaleplon.

Theoretic Infant Dose: 2.1 μg/kg/day

Relative Infant Dose: 1.4%

Adult Dose: 10 mg nightly

Alternatives:

$T\frac{1}{2}$ =	1.2 hours	M/P =	0.5
PHL =		PB =	
T_{max} =	1.2 hours	Oral =	Complete
MW =		pKa =	
Vd =			

References:

1. Darwish M, Martin PT, Cevallos WH, Tse S, Wheeler S, Troy SM. Rapid disappearance of zaleplon from breastmilk after oral administration to lactating women. J Clin Pharmacol 1999; 39(7):670-674.

ZANAMIVIR

Trade: Relenza
Can/Aus/UK: Relenza
Uses: Treatment of Influenza viral infections
LRC: L3
AAP: Not reviewed

Zanamivir is a viral neuraminidase inhibitor that blocks or prevents viral seeding or release from infected cells and prevents viral aggregation.[1] It is only moderately effective and is believed to reduce symptoms by only 30% or several days, and only if treatment is instituted within 2 days of infection.

It is administered via inhalation using a Diskhaler device. Only 4-17% of the inhaled drug is systemically absorbed. Peak plasma concentrations are only 17-142 ng/mL within 2 hours of administration and then rapidly decline. The manufacturer reports that it is present in the milk of rodents; although, no human data are available.[2] Due to the poor oral or inhaled absorption and the incredibly low plasma levels, it is unlikely to produce untoward effects in breastfed infants. However, due to its limited efficacy (reduces length of illness by 1 to 1.5 days), its use in breastfeeding mothers is probably not warranted, unless in high-risk patients with other severe medical conditions.

Pregnancy Risk Category: B

Lactation Risk Category: L3

Adult Concerns: Bronchospasm may occur in patients with asthma or obstructive pulmonary disease.

Pediatric Concerns: None reported via milk but not studies exist.

Drug Interactions: None yet reported.

Theoretic Infant Dose:

Relative Infant Dose:

Adult Dose: 10 mg twice daily

Alternatives:

T½ =	2.5-5.1 hours	M/P =	
PHL =		PB =	< 10%
T$_{max}$ =	1-2 hours	Oral =	4-17%
MW =	332	pKa =	
Vd =			

References:

1. Pharmaceutical Manufacturer Package Insert, 2000.
2. Drug Facts and Comparisons. 1999 ed. Facts and Comparison, St. Louis.

ZINC SALTS
Trade: Zinc
Can/Aus/UK:
Uses: Zinc supplements
LRC: L2
AAP: Not reviewed

Zinc is an essential element that is required for enzymatic function within the cell. Zinc deficiencies have been documented in newborns and premature infants with symptoms such as anorexia nervosa, arthritis, diarrheas, eczema, recurrent infections, and recalcitrant skin problems.

The Recommended Daily Allowance for adults is 12-15 mg/day. The average oral dose of supplements is 25-50 mg/day; higher doses may lead to gastritis. Doses used for treatment of cold symptoms averaged 13.3 mg (lozenges) every 2 hours while awake for the duration of cold symptoms. The acetate or gluconate salts are preferred due to reduced gastric irritation and higher absorption. Zinc sulfate should not be used. Excessive intake is detrimental. Eleven healthy males who ingested 150 mg twice daily for 6 weeks showed significant impairment of lymphocyte and polymorphonuclear leukocyte function and a significant reduction of HDL cholesterol.

Interestingly, absorption of dietary zinc is nearly twice as high during lactation as before conception. In 13 women studied, zinc absorption at preconception averaged 14% and during lactation, 25%.[1] There was no difference in serum zinc values between women who took iron supplements and those who did not although iron supplementation may reduce oral zinc absorption. Zinc absorption by the infant from human milk is high, averaging 41%, which is significantly higher than from soy or cow formulas (14% and 31% respectively). Minimum daily requirements of zinc in full term infants vary from 0.3 to 0.5 mg/kg/day.[2] Daily ingestion of zinc from breastmilk has been estimated to be 0.35 mg/kg/day and declines over the first 17 weeks of life as older neonates require less zinc due to slower growth rate. Supplementation with 25-50 mg/day is probably safe, but excessive doses are discouraged. Another author has shown that zinc levels in breastmilk are independent of maternal plasma zinc concentrations or dietary zinc intake.[3] Other body pools of zinc (ie, liver and bone) are perhaps the source of zinc in breastmilk. Therefore, higher levels of oral zinc intake probably have minimal effect on zinc concentrations in milk but excessive doses are not recommended.

Pregnancy Risk Category:

Lactation Risk Category: L2

Adult Concerns: Oral Zinc salts may cause gastritis, GI upset. Gluconate salts, and lower doses are preferred.

Pediatric Concerns: None reported via milk.

Drug Interactions: Zinc may reduce absorption of ciprofloxacin, tetracyclines, norfloxacin, ofloxacin. Iron salts may reduce absorption of zinc. Foods containing high concentrations of phosphorus, calcium (dairy foods), or phytates (bran, brown bread) may reduce oral zinc absorption. Coffee reduces zinc absorption by 50%.

Theoretic Infant Dose: 0.35 μg/kg/day

Relative Infant Dose:

Adult Dose: 15 mg daily

Alternatives:

T½ =		M/P =	
PHL =		PB =	
T$_{max}$ =		Oral =	41%
MW =		pKa =	
Vd =			

References:
1. Fung EB, Ritchie LD, Woodhouse LR, Roehl R, King JC. Zinc absorption in women during pregnancy and lactation: a longitudinal study. Am J Clin Nutr 1997; 66(1):80-88.
2. Drug Facts and Comparisons 1997 ed. ed. St. Louis: 1997.
3. Krebs NF, Reidinger CJ, Hartley S, Robertson AD, Hambidge KM. Zinc supplementation during lactation: effects on maternal status and milk zinc concentrations. Am J Clin Nutr 1995; 61(5):1030-1036.

ZIPRASIDONE

Trade: Geodon
Can/Aus/UK:
Uses: Antipsychotic
LRC: L4
AAP: Not reviewed

Ziprasidone is an atypical antipsychotic agent chemically unrelated to phenothiazines or butyrophenones.[1] No data are available on its transfer into human milk. Until data are available, risperidone or olanzapine should be suggested.

Pregnancy Risk Category: C

Lactation Risk Category: L4

Adult Concerns: Side effects include somnolence, prolonged QT/QTc intervals, nausea, dyspepsia, headache, skin rash, elevated liver enzymes. Relative incidence of extrapyramidal symptoms is low. Elevation of serum prolactin levels is common with this family and should be expected, although it appears minimal with this agent. Prolonged QT intervals are potentially quite hazardous so should be used with caution in individuals with bradycardia, hypokalemia, and/or hypomagnesemia.

Pediatric Concerns: None reported via milk, but it is not studied.

Drug Interactions: None reported as yet.

Theoretic Infant Dose:

Relative Infant Dose:

Adult Dose: 20 mg BID

Alternatives: Risperidone, Olanzapine

T½ =	7 hours	M/P =	
PHL =		PB =	99%
T$_{max}$ =	4-5 hours	Oral =	60%
MW =	419	pKa =	
Vd =	1.5		

References:
1. Pharmaceutical Manufacturers prescribing information, 2003.

ZOLMITRIPTAN

Trade: Zomig, Zomig-ZMT
Can/Aus/UK: Zomig, Rapimelt
Uses: Migraine analgesic
LRC: L3
AAP: Not reviewed

Zolmitriptan is a selective serotonin-1D receptor antagonist that is specifically indicated for treating acute migraine headaches. Peak plasma levels of zolmitriptan during migraine attacks are generally 8-14 ng/mL and occur before 4 hours.[1,2] Zolmitriptan is structurally similar to sumatriptan but has better oral bioavailability, higher penetration into the CNS, and may have dual mechanisms of action. No data are available on its penetration into human milk. See sumatriptan as preferred alternate.

Pregnancy Risk Category: C

Lactation Risk Category: L3

Adult Concerns: Asthenia, dizziness, paresthesias, drowsiness, nausea, throat tightness, tight chest. Tachycardia and palpitations have been reported.

Pediatric Concerns: None reported via milk. See sumatriptan as alternative.

Drug Interactions:

Theoretic Infant Dose:

Relative Infant Dose:

Adult Dose: 2.5 mg q 2 hours PRN

Alternatives: Sumatriptan

T½ =	3 hours	M/P =	
PHL =		PB =	
T$_{max}$ =	2-4 hours	Oral =	48%
MW =		pKa =	
Vd =			

References:

1. Seaber E, On N, Dixon RM, Gibbens M, Leavens WJ, Liptrot J, Chittick G, Posner J, Rolan PE, Pack RW. The absolute bioavailability and metabolic disposition of the novel antimigraine compound zolmitriptan (311C90). Br J Clin Pharmacol 1997; 43(6):579-587.
2. Palmer KJ, Spencer CM. Zolmitriptan (Adis new drug profile). CNS Drugs Jun 1997; 7(6):468-478.

ZOLPIDEM TARTRATE

Trade: Ambien
Can/Aus/UK:
Uses: Sedative, sleep aid
LRC: L3
AAP: Maternal Medication Usually Compatible with Breastfeeding

Zolpidem, although not a benzodiazepine, interacts with the same GABA-BZ receptor site and shares some of the same pharmacologic effects of the benzodiazepine (Valium) family.[1] In a study of 5 lactating mothers receiving 20 mg daily, the maximum plasma concentration occurred between 1.75 and 3.75 hours and ranged from 90 to 364 µg/L.[2] The authors suggest that the amount of zolpidem recovered in breastmilk 3 hours after administration ranged between 0.76 and 3.88 µg or 0.004 to 0.019% of the total dose administered. Breastmilk clearance of zolpidem is very rapid and none was detectable (below 0.5 ng/mL) by 4-5 hours postdose.

One case of infant sedation and poor appetite related to zolpidem use has been reported following the nightly use of sertraline(100mg) and 10 mg Zolpidem.[3] Upon discontinuation of zolpidem, the infant regained appetite and became more alert.

Pregnancy Risk Category: B

Lactation Risk Category: L3

Adult Concerns: Sedation, anxiety, fatigue, irritability

Pediatric Concerns: One case of infant drowsiness and poor feeding.

Drug Interactions: Use with food may significantly decrease plasma levels by 25%.

Theoretic Infant Dose:

Relative Infant Dose:

Adult Dose: 5-10 mg daily

Alternatives:

T½ =	2.5-5 hours	M/P =	0.13-0.18
PHL =		PB =	92.5%
T$_{max}$ =	1.6 hours	Oral =	70%
MW =	307	pKa =	
Vd =			

References:
1. Pharmaceutical Manufacturer Prescribing Information. 1996.
2. Pons G, Francoual C, Guillet P, Moran C, Hermann P, Bianchetti G, Thiercelin JF, Thenot JP, Olive G. Zolpidem excretion in breastmilk. Eur J Clin Pharmacol 1989; 37(3):245-248.
3. A.K. Personnal communication. 1999.

ZONISAMIDE

Trade: Zonegran
Can/Aus/UK:
Uses: Anti-convulsant
LRC: L5
AAP: Not reviewed

Zonisamide is a broad-spectrum anti-seizure drug chemically classified as a sulfonamide. It has a long half-life and high pKa which from the data below leads to high maternal milk and plasma concentrations. In a study of one patient receiving 100 mg three times daily of zonisamide on postpartum day 0, 3, 6, 14, and 30, the reported milk levels were drawn at 1.5 to 2.5 hours following administration of the medication.[1] The reported milk levels ranged from 8.25 to 10.5 mg/L (mean=9.5) while the maternal plasma levels ranged from 9.52 to 10.6 mg/L (mean=10.13). The milk/plasma ratio averaged 0.93. Using the highest reported milk level, the relative infant dose would be 33% of the maternal dose. This is quite high. Significant caution is recommended with this medication as a number of pediatric adverse effects have been noted in older children.

Pregnancy Risk Category: C

Lactation Risk Category: L5

Adult Concerns: Adverse reactions include somnolence, dizziness, headache, nausea, anorexia, agitation, irritability, speech abnormalities, diplopia, chest pain, paresthesias, psychosis, leukopenia, weight loss, SJ syndrome, oligohidrosis and hyperthermia in pediatric patients. Seizures on withdrawal have been reported. Nephrolithiasis is reported in 4% of patients.

Pediatric Concerns: None via breastmilk, but levels are extremely high.

Drug Interactions: Carbamazepine may increase the plasma clearance of zonisamide. Do not use with Evening primrose oil or Ginko as seizure thresholds may be lowered. Phenobarbital reduces plasma half-life of zonisamide signficantly.

Theoretic Infant Dose: 1.4 mg/kg/day

Relative Infant Dose: 33.2%

Adult Dose: 100-200 mg/day

Alternatives:

$T\frac{1}{2}$ =	63 hours	M/P =	0.93
PHL =		PB =	40%
T_{max} =	2-6 hours	Oral =	
MW =	212	pKa =	10.2
Vd =	1.45		

References:

1. Shimoyama R, Ohkubo T, Sugawara K. Monitoring of zonisamide in human breastmilk and maternal plasma by solid-phase extraction HPLC method. Biomed Chromatogr 1999; 13(5):370-372.

ZOPICLONE

Trade:
Can/Aus/UK: Apo-Zopiclone, Dom-Zopiclone, PMS-Zopiclone, Rhovan, Alti-Zopiclone, Ratio-Zopiclone, Imovane, Zileze
Uses: Hypnotic sedative.
LRC: L2
AAP: Not reviewed

Zopiclone is a sedative/hypnotic which, although structurally dissimilar to the benzodiazepines, shares their pharmacologic profile.[1] In a group of 12 women who received 7.5 mg of Zopiclone, the average peak milk concentration at 2.4 hours was 34 μg/L[2], but the average milk concentration was 10.92 μg/L. The milk half-life was 5.3 hours compared to the maternal plasma half-life of 4.9 hours. The milk/plasma AUC ratio was 0.51 and ranged from 0.4 to 0.7. The authors report that the average infant dose of Zopiclone via milk would be 1.4% of the weight adjusted dose ingested by the mother.

Pregnancy Risk Category:

Lactation Risk Category: L2

Adult Concerns: Sedation

Pediatric Concerns: None reported via milk.

Drug Interactions:

Theoretic Infant Dose: 1.6 µg/kg/day

Relative Infant Dose: 1.5%

Adult Dose: 7.5 mg orally

Alternatives:

$T\frac{1}{2}$ =	4-5 hours	M/P =	0.51	
PHL =		PB =	45%	
T_{max} =	1.6 hours	Oral =	75%	
MW =	388	pKa =		
Vd =	1.51			

References:
1. Gaillot J, Heusse D, Hougton GW, Marc AJ, Dreyfus JF. Pharmacokinetics and metabolism of zopiclone. Pharmacology 1983; 27 Suppl 2:76-91.
2. Matheson I, Sande HA, Gaillot J. The excretion of zopiclone into breastmilk. Br J Clin Pharmacol 1990; 30(2):267-271.

Appendix

Glossary

adipose	the fat tissue in the body
analgesic	drugs used to treat pain
androgen	drug that mimics the action of the male hormone testosterone
antiangina	drug used to treat the pain associated with reduced coronary flow in the heart
antidepressant	drugs that elevate or treat mental depression
antiemetic	compound used to treat nausea and vomiting.
antihypertensive	drug used to treat high blood pressure
antimetabolite	drug generally used to inhibit the immune response, such as in arthritis or cancer
antineoplastic	drug used to treat neoplasms, or cancers
antivertigo	compound used to treat dizziness bradycardia slow heart rate
anxiolytic	reduces anxiety. sedative drug
arthropathy	painful inflammation of joints
bronchodilator	drug that dilates the bronchi in the lungs
CCB	calcium channel blocker
candidiasis	fungal infection, candida, yeast, thrush
cholinergic	nerve transmitter, acetylcholine
diuretic	drug that induces excretion of water by kidneys
dL	deciliter, 100ml
DNA	deoxyribonucleic acid, chromosome, genetic components of human cells
estrogen	drugs that mimic the action of estrogens, or female hormones.
flora	bacteria normally residing within the intestine.
GI	gastrointestinal
half-life	the time required for the concentration of a drug to diminish by one-half in the specified compartment (blood).
hepatoxic	drug that produces liver damage
hyperglycemia	elevated blood sugar (dextrose)
hypoglycemia	low blood sugar (dextrose)
hypotension	low blood pressure
immune	antibody system which fights infection, foreign protein, etc.
immunosuppressive	drugs that diminish or reduce the immune (antibody) response.
L	liter, 1000 ml, 1000 cc, approximately 1 quart
lipid	fat
maternal	mother
mg	milligram, one thousandth of gram
mg/L	milligram per Liter
milk-plasma ratio	ratio of drug in milk to plasma. Higher ratios indicate more drug penetration into milk. A ratio of 1 means that the amount of drug in milk is identical to that in plasma.

ng	nanogram, 1×10^{-9} gm
NICU	Neonatal intensive care unit
NSAID	Nonsteroidal anti-inflammatory
perineal	area between the anus and scrotum.
progestational	drug that mimics the action of progesterone, a female hormone.
prolactin	hormone that promotes breast milk production.
pseudomembranous colitis	severe, sometimes bloody diarrhea caused by overgrowth of offending colonic bacteria.
RNA	ribonucleic acid, genetic component of human cell.
tachycardia	rapid heart rate
teratogenic	drugs or conditions that produce birth defects in pregnant women.
µg	microgram, one millionth of a gram
µg/L	microgram per liter

Normal Growth During Development

BOYS	Weight (lb).	Length (in.)	Head Circumference (in.)
Birth	7.5	19.9	13.9
3 months	12.6	23.8	16.1
6 months	16.7	26.1	17.3
9 months	20.0	28	18.1
12 months	22.2	29.6	18.6
15 months	23.7	30.9	18.9
18 months	25.2	32.2	19.2
24 months	27.7	34.4	19.6

Please note, these data were not derived from exclusively breastfed infants.

Normal Growth During Development

GIRLS	Weight (lb).	Length (in.)	Head Circumference (in.)
Birth	7.2	19.7	13.5
3 months	11.8	23.5	15.6
6 months	15.9	25.8	16.7
9 months	18.8	27.7	17.4
12 months	21.0	29.3	17.9
15 months	22.5	30.6	18.4
18 months	23.9	31.9	18.6
24 months	26.3	34.0	18.8

Please note, these data were not derived from exclusively breastfed infants.

Radiocontrast agents and their reported milk concentrations*

Drug	Dose	Milk (C_{max})	Clinical Significance	Bio-availability	References
Gadopentetate	6.5 g	3.09 μmol/L	Only 0.023% of maternal dose; total dose = 0.013 μmol/24h;safe	0.8%	See Mono-graph
Iohexol	0.75 g/kg	35 mg/L	Mean milk level was only 11.4 mg/L; virtually unabsorbed; safe	<0.1%	See Mono-graph
Iopanoic Acid	2.77 g	20.8 mg/19-29 h	Only 0.08% of maternal dose; virtually unabsorbed; safe	Nil	See Mono-graph
Metrizamide	5.06 g	32.9 mg/L	Only 0.02% maternal dose recovered over 44.3 h; poor oral absorption; safe	0.4%	See Mono-graph
Metrizoate	580 mg	14 mg/L	Mean milk level 11.4 mg/24h; only 0.3% of maternal dose; safe	Nil	See Mono-graph

* Adapted from Hale TW, Ilett KF. Drug Therapy and Breastfeeding: From Theory to Clinical Practice, First Edition ed. London: Parthenon Publishing; 2002

Activities of Radiopharmaceuticals That Require Instructions and Records When Administered to Patients Who Are Breast-Feeding an Infant or Child.*

Radiopharmaceutical	COLUMN 1 Activity Above Which Instructions Are Required		COLUMN 3 Examples of Recommended Duration of Interruption of Breast-Feeding*
	MBq	mCi	
I-131 NaI	0.01	0.0004	Complete cessation (for this infant or child)
I-123 NaI	20	0.5	
I-123 OIH	100	4	
I-123 mIBG	70	2	24 hr for 370 MBq (10mCi) 12 hr for 150 MBq (4 mCi)
I-125 OIH	3	0.08	
I-131 OIH	10	0.30	
Tc-99m DTPA	1,000	30	
Tc-99m MAA	50	1.3	12.6 hr for 150 Mbq (4mCi)
Tc-99m Pertechnetate	100	3	24 hr for 1,100 Mbq (30mCi) 12 hr for 440 Mbq (12 mCi)
Tc-99m DISIDA	1,000	30	
Tc-99m Glucoheptonate	1,000	30	
Tc-99m HAM	400	10	
Tc-99m MIBI	1,000	30	
Tc-99m MDP	1,000	30	
Tc-99m PYP	900	25	
Tc-99m Red Blood Cell In Vivo Labeling	400	10	6 hr for 740 Mbq (20 mCi)

Radiopharma ceutical	COLUMN 1 Activity Above Which Instructions Are Required		COLUMN 3 Examples of Recommended Duration of Interruption of Breast-Feeding*
Tc-99m Red Blood Cell In Vitro Labeling	1,000	30	
Tc-99m Sulphur Colloid	300	7	6 hr for 440 Mbq (12 mCi)
Tc-99m DTPA Aerosol	1,000	30	
Tc-99m MAG3	1,000	30	
Tc-99m White Blood Cells	100	4	24 hr for 1,100 Mbq (5 mCi) 12 hr for 440 Mbq (2 mCi)
Ga-67 Citrate	1	0.04	1 month for 150 Mbq (4 mCi) 2 weeks for 50 Mbq (1.3 mCi) 1 week for 7 Mbq (0.2 mCi)
Cr-51 EDTA	60	1.6	
In-111 White Blood Cells	10	0.2	1 week for 20 Mbq (0.5 mCi)
Tl-201 Chloride	40	1	2 weeks for 110 Mbq (3 mCi)

* The duration of interruption of breast-feeding is selected to reduce the maximum dose to a newborn infant to less than 1 millisievert (0.1 rem), although the regulatory limit is 5 millisieverts (0.5 rem). The actual doses that would be received by most infants would be far below 1 millisievert (0.1 rem). Of course, the physician may use discretion in the recommendation, increasing or decreasing the duration of the interruption.

If there is no recommendation in Column 3 of this table, the maximum activity normally administered is below the activities that require instructions on interruption or discontinuation of breast-feeding.

*Source: Nuclear Regulatory Commission. For a more complete table see : http://neonatal.ama.ttuhsc.edu/lact/radioactive.html

Thyroid Function Tests

T_4(thyroxine)	1-7 days	10.1-20.9 μg/dL
	8-14 days	9.8-16.6 μg/dL
	1 month-1year	5.5-16 μg/dL
	>1 year	4-12 μg/dL
FTI	1-3 days	9.3-26.6
	1-4 weeks	7.6-20.8
	1-4 months	7.4-17.9
	4-12 months	5.1-14.5
	1-6 years	5.7-13.3
	>6 years	4.8-14
T_3 by RIA	Newborns	100-470 ng/dL
	1-5 years	100-260 ng/dL
	5-10 years	90-240 ng/dL
	10 years-adult	70-210 ng/dL
T_3 uptake		35-45%
TSH	Cord	3-22 μIU/mL
	1-3 days	<40 μIU/mL
	3-7 days	<25 μIU/mL
	>7 days	0-10 μIU/mL

Therapeutic Drug Levels

Reference (Normal) Values

Drug	Therapeutic Range	
Acetaminophen	10-20	µg/ml
Theophylline	0-20	µg/ml
Carbamazepine	4-10	µg/ml
Ethosuximide	40-100	µg/ml
Phenobarbital	15-40	µg/ml
Phenytoin		
Neonates	6-14	µg/ml
Children, adults	10-20	µg/ml
Primidone	5-15	µg/ml
Valproic Acid	5-15	µg/ml
Gentamicin		
Peak	5-12	µg/ml
Trough	< 2.0	µg/ml
Vancomycin		
Peak	20-40	µg/ml
Trough	5-10	µg/ml
Digoxin	0.9-2.2	µg/ml
Lithium	0.3-1.3	mmol/L
Salicylates	20-25	mg/dL

From Therapeutic Drug Monitoring Guide, WE Evan, Editor, Abbott Laboratories, 1988.

864

Pediatric Laboratory Values

Test	Age	Range	Units
pH	< 1 mo.	7.3-7.46	
pCO_2	2-5d	4.1-6.3	kPa(mmHg)
pCO_2	2-5d	5.6-7.7	kPa(mmHg)
Total CO_2	< 1 yr.	15-35	mmol/L
Albumin, Serum	< 1 yr.	3-4.9	gm/dL
Phenylalamine	Newborn	0.7-3.5	umol/L
Ammonia	< 1 yr.	68	umol/L
Total Bilirubin	< 2 w	< 11.7	mg/dL
	< 10 yr.	< 0.9	mg/dL
Calcium	< 1 yr.	7.8-11.2	mg/dL
Chloride	< 2 yr.	100-110	mmol/dL
Cholesteral Total	< 1 yr.	93-260	mg/dL
Copper, Serum	1-5 yr.	80-150	µg/dL
Copper, Wiring	< 6 yr.	8-17	µg/dL
Creatine Kinose	1-3 yr.	50-305	IU/L
Creatine, Serum	< 10 yr.	0.2-1.02	mg/dL
Ferritin	1-4 yr.	6-24	µg/L
Fructosamine	5-17 yr.	1.4-2.2	mmol/L
Glucose	1-6 yr.	74-127	mg/dL
Hemoglobin A_{1C}	2-12 yr.	5.1	%HbA_{1C}
Cholesterol (HDL)	1-9 yr.	35-82	mg/dL
Iron	< 2 yr.	11-150	µg/dL
Magnesium	< 1 yr.	1.6-2.6	mg/dL
Osmolality	28d	274-305	mmol/dL
Phosphatose, alkaline	2-9 yr.	100-400	IU/L
Phosphorus, Serum	< 2 yr.	2.5-7.1	mg/dL
Potassium	< 2 mo.	3-7.0	mmol/dL
Prolactin	0-18 yr.	20 or less	ng/mL
Protein, Total	< 1 yr.	5-7.5	mg/dL
Protein, Urine	< 1 yr.	130-145	mmol/dL
Sodium, Urinary	1-6 mo.		
breast-fed		6.1	mmol/L
formula-fed		13.2	mmol/L

Typical Radioactive Half-Lives

Radioactive Element	Half-Life
Mo-99	2.75 Days
TI-201	3.05 Days
TI-201	73.1 Hours
Ga-67	3.26 Days
Ga-67	78.3 Hours
I-131	8.02 Days
Xe-133	5.24 Days
In-111	2.80 Days
Cr-51	27.7 Days
I-125	60.1 Days
Sr-89	50.5 Days
Tc-99m	6.02 Hours
I-123	13.2 Hours
Sm-153	47.0 Hours

Common Radiopaque Agents

Generic Name (Iodine Content)	Trade Name
Iocetamic Acid (62% Iodine)	Cholebrine
Iopanoic Acid (66.68% Iodine)	Telepaque
Ipodate Calcium (61.7% Iodine)	Oragrafin Calcium
Ipodate Sodium (61.4% Iodine)	Bilivist,Oragrafin Sodium
Tyropanoate Sodium (57.4% Iodine)	Bilopaque
Diatrizoate Sodium 41.66% (24.9% Iodine)	Hypaque Sodium
Diatrizoate Meglumine 66% and Diatrizoate Sodium 10% (37% Iodine)	Gastrografin, MD-Gastroview
Diatrizoate Meglumine 30% (14.1% Iodine)	Hypaque Meglumine 30%, Reno-M-Dip, Urovist Meglumine DIU/CT
Gadopentetate Dimeglumine 46.9%	Magnevist
Iodamide Meglumine 24% (11.1% Iodine)	Renovue-Dip
Iohexol (46.36% Iodine)	Omnipaque
Iopamidol 26% (12.8% Iodine)	Isovue-128
Iothalamate Meglumine 30% (14.1 % Iodine)	Conray 30
Ioversol 34% (16% Iodine)	Optiray 160
Metrizamide (48.25% Iodine)	Amipaque
Diatrizoate Meglumine 28.5% and Diatrizoate Sodium 29.1% (31% Iodine)	Renovist II
Diatrizoate Meglumine 50% and Diatrizoate Sodium 25% (38.5% Iodine)	Hypaque-M, 75%
Diatrizoate Meglumine 52% and Diatrizoate Sodium 8% (29.3% Iodine)	Angiovist 292, MD-60, Renografin-60
Diatrizoate Meglumine 60% and Diatrizoate Sodium 30% (46.2% Iodine)	Hypaque-M, 90%

Generic Name (Iodine Content)	Trade Name
Diatrizoate Meglumine 66% and Diatrizoate Sodium 10% (37% Iodine)	Angiovist 370, Hypaque-76, MD-76, Renografin-76
Iothalamate Meglumine 52% and Iothalamate Sodium 26% (40% Iodine)	Vascoray
Ioxaglate Meglumine 39.3% and Ioxaglate Sodium 19.6% (32% Iodine)	Hexabrix
Diatrizoate Meglumine 18% (8.5% Iodine)	Cystografin Dilute
Diatrizoate Meglumine 30% (14.1% Iodine)	Cystografin, Hypaque-Cysto, Reno-M-30, Urovist Cysto
Diatrizoate Sodium 20% (12% Iodine)	Hypaque Sodium 20%
Iothalamate Meglumine 17.2% (8.1% Iodine)	Cysto-Conray II

Oxytocin Intranasal Spray

Oxytocin intranasal spray is no longer available on the US market, but oxytocin powder is available through several vendors. Below is one.

Hawkins Chemical   800-328-5460

Drugs that are usually contraindicated in lactating women*

Drug	Nature of possible infant risk
Amiodarone	Relative infant dose 4-6% of maternal dose; may accumulate because of very long half-life; adverse cardiovascular and thyroid effects possible
Antineoplastic agents	Overtly toxic; avoid exposure; bone marrow suppression, damage to intestinal epithelial cells possible.
Chloramphenicol	Relative infant dose 2% of maternal dose. Blood dyscrasias, aplastic anemia, etc. possible
Ergotamine	Symptoms of ergotism (vomiting and diarrhea) reported; potential to inhibit prolactin secretion
Gold salts	Relative infant dose varies from 1-7%. Long half-life in adults suggests potential for accumulation. Possibility of diarrhea, dermatitis, nephrotoxicity and blood dyscrasias
Lithium	Not recommended as relative infant dose is around 18-23% of maternal dose, and severe rash also reported. Caution if use.
Phenindione	Relative infant dose calculated at around 18% of maternal dose and abnormal blood coagulation in an infant has been reported

Drugs that are usually contraindicated in lactating women

Drug	Nature of possible infant risk
Radiopharmaceuticals	Temporary discontinuation of breastfeeding may be necessary. See NRC table.
Retinoids	Secretion into milk is unknown, but is likely to be significant as these drugs are usually very lipid soluble (e.g. isotretinoin). Contraindicated because if the wide range of adverse effects in adults and mutagenic and carcinogenic actions in animals
Tetracyclines (Chronic)	While the short-term use of tetracyclines for up to 3 weeks is OK, chronic use over many months may lead to staining of immature teeth, or changes in epiphyseal bone growth
Pseudoephedrine	Recently published data by the authors indicate that pseudoephedrine may inhibit milk production significantly

* Adapted from Hale TW, Ilett KF. Drug Therapy and Breastfeeding: From Theory to Clinical Practice, First Edition ed. London: Parthenon Publishing; 2002

Is It a Cold or the Flu?

Symptoms	Cold	Flu
fever	rare	characteristic, high (102-104F); lasts 3-4 days
headache	rare	prominent
general aches, pains	slight	usual; often severe
fatigue, weakness	quite mild	can last up to 2-3 weeks
extreme exhaustion	never	early and prominent
stuffy nose	common	sometimes
sneezing	usual	sometimes
sore throat	common	sometimes
chest discomfort, cough	mild to moderate; hacking cough	common; can become severe

(Source: National Institute of Allergy and Infectious Diseases)

Publication No. (FDA) 99-1264
http://www.fda.gov/fdac/features/896_flu.html

Neuromuscular Blocking Agents				
Agent (BRANDNAME)	Pharmac- ological Properties	Time of Onset (min.)	Clinical Duration (min.)	Half- Life (min.)
Succinylcholine (ANECTINE)	ultrashort duration	1 – 1.5	5 – 8	< 1 min
d-Tubocurarine	long duration	4 – 6	80 – 120	173 min
Atracurium (TRACRIUM)	intermediate duration	2 – 4	30 – 60	16 – 20 min
Doxacurium (NUROMAX)	long duration	4 – 6	90 – 120	120 min
Mivacurium (MIVACRON)	Short duration	2 – 4	12 – 18	1.8 – 2 min
Pancuronium (PAVULON)	long duration	4 – 6	120 – 180	89 – 140 min
Pipecuronium (ARDUAN)	long duration	2 – 4	80 – 100	137 – 161 min
Rapacuronium (RAPLON)	intermediate duration	1 – 2	15 – 30	72 – 175 min
Rocuronium (ZEMURON)	intermediate duration	1 – 2	30 – 60	84 – 131 min
Vecuronium (NORCURON)	intermediate duration	2 – 4	60 – 90	80 min

Cold Remedies

Trade Name	Ingredients	Comments
666 cold preparation, maximum strength liquid	Acetaminophen, Dexchlorpheniramine, Pseudoephedrine, Dextromethorphan	Probably safe but may suppress milk supply.
Actifed cold & allergy tablets	Triprolidine, Pseudoephedrine	Probably safe; observe for sedation and may suppress milk supply.
Actifed cold & sinus maximum strength tablets	Acetaminophen, Chlorpheniramine, Pseudoephedrine	Probably safe; observe for sedation and may suppress milk supply.
Advil cold & sinus tablets	Ibuprofen, Pseudoephedrine	Probably safe but may suppress milk supply.
Advil flu & body ache tablets	Ibuprofen, Pseudoephedrine	Probably safe but may suppress milk supply.
Alavert	Loratadine	Safe
Alavert D-12	Loratadine, Pseudoephedrine	Probably safe but may suppress milk supply.
Aleve cold & sinus tablets	Naproxen, Pseudoephedrine	Probably safe but may suppress milk supply.
Aleve sinus & headache tablets	Naproxen, Pseudoephedrine	Probably safe but may suppress milk supply.
Alka-Seltzer plus cold & cough medicine effervescent tablets	Chlorpheniramine, Phenylephrine, Dextromethorphan	Probably safe; observe for sedation.
Alka-Seltzer plus cold & cough liquid-gels	Acetaminophen, Chlorpheniramine, Dextromethorphan	Probably safe; observe for sedation.
Alka-Seltzer plus cold & flu liqui-gels	Acetaminophen, Pseudoephedrine, Dextromethorphan	Probably safe but may suppress milk supply.
Alka-Seltzer plus cold & sinus liqui gels	Acetaminophen, Pseudoephedrine	Probably safe but may suppress milk supply.
Alka-Seltzer plus cold & sinus tablets	Acetaminophen Phenylephrine	Probably safe
Alka-Seltzer plus cold medicine effervescent tablets	Acetaminophen, Chlorpheniramine, Phenylephrine	Probably safe; observe for sedation.
Alka-Seltzer plus cold medicine liquid-gels	Acetaminophen, Chlorpheniramine, Pseudoephedrine	Probably safe; observe for sedation and may suppress milk supply.
Alka-Seltzer plus flu medicine effervescent tablets	Aspirin, Chlorpheniramine, Dextromethorphan	Probably safe; observe for sedation.

Cold Remedies

Trade Name	Ingredients	Comments
Alka-Seltzer plus liquid-gels flu medicine	Acetaminophen, Pseudoephedrine, Dextromethorphan	Probably safe but may suppress milk supply.
Alka-Seltzer plus nightTime cold liquid-gels	Acetaminophen, Dexchlorpheniramine, Pseudoephedrine, Dextromethorphan	Probably safe; observe for sedation and may suppress milk supply.
Alka-Seltzer plus night-time cold medicine effervescent	Dexchlorpheniramine, Phenylephrine, Dextromethorphan	Probably safe; observe for sedation.
Allegra-D tablets	Fexofenadine, Pseudoephedrine	Probably safe but may suppress milk supply.
Allerest maximum strength tablets	Chlorpheniramine, Pseudoephedrine	Probably safe; observe for sedation and may suppress milk supply.
Aprodine tablets	Triprolidine, Pseudoephedrine	Probably safe; observe for sedation and may suppress milk supply.
Benadryl allergy & cold tablets	Acetaminophen, Diphenhydramine, Pseudoephedrine	Probably safe; observe for sedation and may suppress milk supply.
Benadryl allergy & sinus fastmelt dissolving tablets	Diphenhydramine Pseudoephedrine	Probably safe; observe for sedation and may suppress milk supply.
Benadryl allergy & sinus headache tablets	Acetaminophen, Diphenhydramine, Pseudoephedrine	Probably safe; observe for sedation and may suppress milk supply.
Benadryl allergy & sinus liquid	Diphenhydramine, Pseudoephedrine	Probably safe; observe for sedation and may suppress milk supply.
Benadryl allergy & sinus tablets	Diphenhydramine, Pseudoephedrine	Probably safe; observe for sedation and may suppress milk supply.
Benadryl maximum strength severe allergy & sinus headache tablets	Acetaminophen, Diphenhydramine, Pseudoephedrine	Probably safe; observe for sedation and may suppress milk supply.
Benylin expectorant liquid	Guaifenesin, Dextromethorphan	Probably safe
Bromfed capsules	Brompheniramine, Pseudoephedrine	Probably safe; observe for sedation and may suppress milk supply.
Bromfed syrup	Brompheniramine, Pseudoephedrine	Probably safe; observe for sedation and may suppress milk supply.
Bromfed tablets	Brompheniramine, Pseudoephedrine	Probably safe; observe for sedation and may

Cold Remedies

Trade Name	Ingredients	Comments
		suppress milk supply.
Cardec DM syrup	Carbinoxamine, Pseudoephedrine, Dextromethorphan	Probably safe; observe for sedation and may suppress milk supply.
Cepacol sore throat liquid	Acetaminophen, Pseudoephedrine	Probably safe but may suppress milk supply.
Cheracol cough syrup	Guaifenesin, Codeine	Probably safe; observe for sedation.
Cheracol D cough formula syrup	Guaifenesin, Dextromethorphan	Probably safe
Cheracol plus liquid	Guaifenesin, Dextromethorphan	Probably safe
Chlor-Trimeton allergy-D 12 hour tablets	Chlorpheniramine, Pseudoephedrine	Probably safe; observe for sedation and may suppress milk supply.
Chlor-Trimeton allergy-D 4 hour tablets	Chlorpheniramine, Pseudoephedrine	Probably safe; observe for sedation and may suppress milk supply.
Claritin-D 12 hour tablets	Loratadine, Pseudoephedrine	Probably safe but may suppress milk supply.
Claritin-D 24 hour tablets	Loratadine, Pseudoephedrine	Probably safe but may suppress milk supply.
Codiclear DH syrup	Guaifenesin, Hydrocodone	Probably safe; observe for sedation.
Codimal DH syrup	Pyrilamine, Phenylephrine, Hydrocodone	Probably safe; observe for sedation.
Codimal DM syrup	Pyrilamine, Phenylephrine, Dextromethorphan	Probably safe; observe for sedation.
Coldec D tablets	Carbinoxamine, Pseudoephedrine	Probably safe; observe for sedation and may suppress milk supply.
Coldmist LA tablets	Guaifenesin, Pseudoephedrine	Probably safe but may suppress milk supply.
Comtrex allergy-sinus treatment, maximum strength tablets	Acetaminophen, Chlorpheniramine, Pseudoephedrine	Probably safe; observe for sedation and may suppress milk supply.
Comtrex cough and cold relief, multi-symptom maximum strength tablets	Acetaminophen, Chlorpheniramine, Pseudoephedrine, Dextromethorphan	Probably safe; observe for sedation and may suppress milk supply.
Comtrex day & night cold & cough relief, multi-symptom maximum strength	Acetaminophen, Chlorpheniramine, Pseudoephedrine, Dextromethorphan	Probably safe; observe for sedation and may suppress milk supply.

Cold Remedies		
Trade Name	**Ingredients**	**Comments**
tablets		
Comtrex flu therapy & fever relief day & night, multi-symptom maximum strength tablets	Acetaminophen, Chlorpheniramine, Pseudoephedrine	Probably safe; observe for sedation and may suppress milk supply.
Comtrex multi-symptom deep chest cold & congestion relief softgels	Acetaminophen, Guaifenesin, Pseudoephedrine, Dextromethorphan	Probably safe but may suppress milk supply.
Comtrex multi-symptom maximum strength non-drowsy cold & cough relief tablets	Acetaminophen, Pseudoephedrine, Dextromethorphan	Probably safe but may suppress milk supply.
Contac day & night allergy/sinus	Acetaminophen, Diphenhydramine, Pseudoephedrine	Probably safe; observe for sedation and may suppress milk supply.
Contac day & night cold & flu tablets	Acetaminophen, Diphenhydramine, Pseudoephedrine, Dextromethorphan	Probably safe; observe for sedation and may suppress milk supply.
Contac severe cold & flu maximum strength tablets	Acetaminophen, Chlorpheniramine, Pseudoephedrine, Dextromethorphan	Probably safe; observe for sedation and may suppress milk supply.
Coricidin 'D' cold, flu & sinus tablets	Acetaminophen, Chlorpheniramine, Pseudoephedrine	Probably safe; observe for sedation and may suppress milk supply.
Coricidin HBP cold & flu tablets	Acetaminophen, Chlorpheniramine	Probably safe; observe for sedation.
Coricidin HBP cough & cold tablets	Chlorpheniramine, Dextromethorphan	Probably safe; observe for sedation.
Coricidin HBP maximum strength flu tablets	Acetaminophen, Chlorpheniramine, Dextromethorphan	Probably safe; observe for sedation.
Deconamine SR capsules	Chlorpheniramine, Pseudoephedrine	Probably safe; observe for sedation and may suppress milk supply.
Deconamine syrup	Chlorpheniramine, Pseudoephedrine	Probably safe; observe for sedation and may suppress milk supply.
Deconamine tablets	Chlorpheniramine, Pseudoephedrine	Probably safe; observe for sedation and may suppress milk supply.

Cold Remedies

Trade Name	Ingredients	Comments
Dihistine DH elixir	Chlorpheniramine, Pseudoephedrine, Codeine	Probably safe; observe for sedation and may suppress milk supply.
Dimetane-DX cough	Brompheniramine, Pseudoephedrine, Dextromethorphan	Probably safe; observe for sedation and may suppress milk supply.
Dimetapp cold & allergy elixir	Brompheniramine, Pseudoephedrine	Probably safe; observe for sedation and may suppress milk supply.
Dristan cold multi-symptom formula tablets	Acetaminophen, Chlorpheniramine, Phenylephrine	Probably safe; observe for sedation.
Dristan cold non-drowsy maximum strength tablets	Acetaminophen, Pseudoephedrine	Probably safe but may suppress milk supply.
Dristan sinus tablets	Ibuprofen, Pseudoephedrine	Probably safe but may suppress milk supply.
Drixoral allergy sinus tablets	Acetaminophen, Dexbrompheniramine, Pseudoephedrine	Probably safe; observe for sedation and may suppress milk supply.
Drixoral cold & allergy tablets	Dexbrompheniramine, Pseudoephedrine	Probably safe; observe for sedation and may suppress milk supply.
Duratuss GP tablets	Guaifenesin, Pseudoephedrine	Probably safe but may suppress milk supply.
Duratuss HD elixir	Guaifenesin, Pseudoephedrine, Hydrocodone	Probably safe; observe for sedation and may suppress milk supply.
Duratuss tablets	Guaifenesin, Pseudoephedrine	Probably safe but may suppress milk supply.
Dura-Vent/DA tablets	Chlorpheniramine, Phenylephrine, Methscopolamine	Probably safe; observe for sedation.
Dynex tablets	Guaifenesin, Pseudoephedrine	Probably safe but may suppress milk supply.
Endal tablets	Guaifenesin, Pseudoephedrine	Probably safe but may suppress milk supply.
Entex HC liquid	Guaifenesin, Phenylephrine, Hydrocodone	Probably safe; observe for sedation.
Entex LA tablets	Guaifenesin, Phenylephrine	Probably safe
Entex liquid	Guaifenesin, Phenylephrine	Probably safe
Entex PSE tablets	Guaifenesin, Pseudoephedrine	Probably safe but may suppress milk supply.
Genac tablets	Triprolidine, Pseudoephedrine	Probably safe; observe for sedation and may suppress milk supply.

Cold Remedies

Trade Name	Ingredients	Comments
Guaifed capsules	Guaifenesin, Pseudoephedrine	Probably safe but may suppress milk supply.
Guaifed-PD capsules	Guaifenesin, Pseudoephedrine	Probably safe but may suppress milk supply.
Guaifenex PSE 120 tablets	Guaifenesin, Pseudoephedrine	Probably safe but may suppress milk supply.
Guaifenex-Rx tablets	Guaifenesin, Pseudoephedrine	Probably safe but may suppress milk supply.
Guiatuss PE liquid	Guaifenesin, Pseudoephedrine	Probably safe but may suppress milk supply.
Histex liquid	Chlorpheniramine, Pseudoephedrine	Probably safe; observe for sedation and may suppress milk supply.
Histex SR capsules	Brompheniramine, Pseudoephedrine	Probably safe; observe for sedation and may suppress milk supply.
Histussin HC syrup	Chlorpheniramine, Phenylephrine, Hydrocodone	Probably safe; observe for sedation and may suppress milk supply.
Hycodan syrup	Hydrocodone, Homatropine	Probably safe; observe for sedation.
Hycodan tablets	Hydrocodone, Homatropine	Probably safe; observe for sedation.
Levall 5.0 liquid	Guaifenesin, Phenylephrine, Hydrocodone	Probably safe; observe for sedation.
Levall liquid	Carbetapentane, Guaifenesin, Phenylephrine	Probably safe; observe for sedation.
Lodrane liquid	Brompheniramine, Pseudoephedrine	Probably safe; observe for sedation and may suppress milk supply.
Motrin sinus headache tablets	Ibuprofen, Pseudoephedrine	Probably safe but may suppress milk supply.
Naldecon senior DX liquid	Guaifenesin, Dextromethorphan	Probably safe
Nucofed expectorant syrup	Guaifenesin, Pseudoephedrine, Codeine	Probably safe; observe for sedation and may suppress milk supply.
Nucotuss expectorant syrup	Guaifenesin, Pseudoephedrine, Codeine	Probably safe; observe for sedation and may suppress milk supply.
OMNIhist LA tablets	Chlorpheniramine, Phenylephrine, Methscopolamine	Probably safe; observe for sedation.
PanMist JR tablets	Guaifenesin, Pseudoephedrine	Probably safe but may suppress milk supply.
PanMist LA tablets	Guaifenesin, Pseudoephedrine	Probably safe but may suppress milk supply.

Cold Remedies

Trade Name	Ingredients	Comments
PanMist-DM syrup	Guaifenesin, Pseudoephedrine, Dextromethorphan	Probably safe but may suppress milk supply.
PanMist-S syrup	Guaifenesin, Pseudoephedrine	Probably safe but may suppress milk supply.
Percogesic extra strength tablets	Acetaminophen, Diphenhydramine	Probably safe; observe for sedation.
Percogesic tablets	Acetaminophen, Phenyltoloxamine	Probably safe; observe for sedation.
Phenergan VC syrup	Promethazine, Phenylephrine	Caution; observe for sedation
Polaramine expectorant liquid	Dexchlorpheniramine, Guaifenesin, Pseudoephedrine	Probably safe; observe for sedation and may suppress milk supply.
Primatene tablets	Guaifenesin, Ephedrine	Unsafe
Prolex DH liquid	Hydrocodone, K Guaicolsulfonate	Probably safe; observe for sedation.
Prometh VC w/codeine cough syrup	Promethazine, Phenylephrine, Codeine	Unsafe
Promethazine HCL with codeine cough syrup	Promethazine, Codeine	Unsafe
Rescon-GG liquid	Guaifenesin, Phenylephrine	Probably safe
Robitussin allergy & cough liquid	Brompheniramine, Pseudoephedrine, Dextromethorphan	Probably safe; observe for sedation and may suppress milk supply.
Robitussin CF syrup	Guaifenesin, Pseudoephedrine, Dextromethorphan	Probably safe but may suppress milk supply.
Robitussin cold sinus & congestion tablets	Acetaminophen, Guaifenesin, Pseudoephedrine	Probably safe but may suppress milk supply.
Robitussin cold, cold & congestion softgels & tablets	Guaifenesin, Pseudoephedrine, Dextromethorphan	Probably safe but may suppress milk supply.
Robitussin cold, cold & cough softgels	Guaifenesin, Pseudoephedrine, Dextromethorphan	Probably safe but may suppress milk supply.
Robitussin cold, multi-symptom cold & flu softgels	Acetaminophen, Guaifenesin, Pseudoephedrine, Dextromethorphan	Probably safe but may suppress milk supply.
Robitussin cold, multi-symptom cold & flu tablets	Acetaminophen, Guaifenesin, Pseudoephedrine, Dextromethorphan	Probably safe but may suppress milk supply.
Robitussin cough	Guaifenesin,	Probably safe

Cold Remedies		
Trade Name	**Ingredients**	**Comments**
& congestion formula liquid	Dextromethorphan	
Robitussin flu liquid	Acetaminophen, Chlorpheniramine, Pseudoephedrine, Dextromethorphan	Probably safe; observe for sedation and may suppress milk supply.
Robitussin honey cough & cold liquid	Pseudoephedrine, Dextromethorphan	Probably safe but may suppress milk supply.
Robitussin Honey Flu Multisymptom liquid	Acetaminophen, Pseudoephedrine, Dextromethorphan	Probably safe but may suppress milk supply.
Robitussin honey flu nighttime syrup	Acetaminophen, Chlorpheniramine, Pseudoephedrine, Dextromethorphan	Probably safe; observe for sedation and may suppress milk supply.
Robitussin honey flu non-drowsy syrup	Acetaminophen, Pseudoephedrine, Dextromethorphan	Probably safe but may suppress milk supply.
Robitussin maximum strength cough & cold syrup	Pseudoephedrine, Dextromethorphan	Probably safe but may suppress milk supply.
Robitussin night relief liquid	Acetaminophen, Pyrilamine, Pseudoephedrine, Dextromethorphan	Probably safe; observe for sedation and may suppress milk supply.
Robitussin PE liquid	Guaifenesin, Pseudoephedrine	Probably safe but may suppress milk supply.
Robitussin severe congestion liquid-gels	Guaifenesin, Pseudoephedrine	Probably safe but may suppress milk supply.
Robitussin sugar free cough liquid	Guaifenesin, Dextromethorphan	Probably safe
Robitussin-DM liquid	Guaifenesin, Dextromethorphan	Probably safe
Rondec syrup	Brompheniramine, Pseudoephedrine	Probably safe; observe for sedation and may suppress milk supply.
Rondec tablets	Carbinoxamine, Pseudoephedrine	Probably safe; observe for sedation and may suppress milk supply.
Rondec-DM syrup	Brompheniramine, Pseudoephedrine, Dextromethorphan	Probably safe; observe for sedation and may suppress milk supply.
Rondec-TR tablets	Carbinoxamine, Pseudoephedrine	Probably safe; observe for sedation and may suppress milk supply.
Ryna liquid	Chlorpheniramine,	Probably safe; observe

Cold Remedies

Trade Name	Ingredients	Comments
	Pseudoephedrine	for sedation and may suppress milk supply.
Ryna-12 S suspension	Pyrilamine, Phenylephrine	Probably safe; observe for sedation.
Ryna-C liquid	Chlorpheniramine, Pseudoephedrine, Codeine	Probably safe; observe for sedation and may suppress milk supply.
Rynatan pediatric suspension	Chlorpheniramine, Phenylephrine	Probably safe; observe for sedation.
Rynatan tablets	Chlorpheniramine, Phenylephrine	Probably safe; observe for sedation.
Rynatuss tablets	Chlorpheniramine, Carbetapentane, Ephedrine	Unsafe
Singlet for adults tablets	Acetaminophen, Chlorpheniramine, Pseudoephedrine	Probably safe; observe for sedation and may suppress milk supply.
Sinutab non-drying liquid caps	Guaifenesin, Pseudoephedrine	Probably safe but may suppress milk supply.
Sinutab sinus allergy, maximum strength tablets	Acetaminophen, Chlorpheniramine, Pseudoephedrine	Probably safe; observe for sedation and may suppress milk supply.
Sinutab sinus without drowsiness maximum strength tablets	Acetaminophen, Pseudoephedrine	Probably safe but may suppress milk supply.
Sinutab sinus without drowsiness regular strength tablets	Acetaminophen, Pseudoephedrine	Probably safe but may suppress milk supply.
Sudafed cold & allergy maximum strength tablets	Chlorpheniramine, Pseudoephedrine	Probably safe; observe for sedation and may suppress milk supply.
Sudafed cold & sinus non-drowsy liqui-caps	Acetaminophen, Pseudoephedrine	Probably safe but may suppress milk supply.
Sudafed maximum strength sinus nighttime plus pain relief tablets	Acetaminophen, Diphenhydramine, Pseudoephedrine	Probably safe; observe for sedation and may suppress milk supply.
Sudafed multi-symptom cold & cough liquid caps	Acetaminophen, Guaifenesin, Pseudoephedrine, Dextromethorphan	Probably safe but may suppress milk supply.
Sudafed non-drowsy non-drying sinus liquid caps	Guaifenesin, Pseudoephedrine	Probably safe but may suppress milk supply.
Sudafed non-	Acetaminophen,	Probably safe but may

Cold Remedies

Trade Name	Ingredients	Comments
drowsy severe cold formula maximum strength tablets	Pseudoephedrine, Dextromethorphan	suppress milk supply.
Sudafed sinus headache non-drowsy tablets	Acetaminophen, Pseudoephedrine	Probably safe but may suppress milk supply.
Sudafed sinus nighttime maximum strength tablets	Triprolidine, Pseudoephedrine	Probably safe; observe for sedation and may suppress milk supply.
Tanafed suspension	Chlorpheniramine, Pseudoephedrine	Probably safe; observe for sedation and may suppress milk supply.
Tavist allergy/sinus/head ache tablets	Acetaminophen, Clemastine, Pseudoephedrine	Unsafe
Tavist sinus maximum strength tablets	Acetaminophen, Pseudoephedrine	Probably safe but may suppress milk supply.
TheraFlu cold & cough nightTime powder	Acetaminophen, Chlorpheniramine, Pseudoephedrine, Dextromethorphan	Probably safe; observe for sedation and may suppress milk supply.
TheraFlu flu & cold medicine for sore throat, maximum strength powder	Acetaminophen, Chlorpheniramine, Pseudoephedrine	Probably safe; observe for sedation and may suppress milk supply.
TheraFlu flu & cold medicine original	Acetaminophen, Chlorpheniramine, Pseudoephedrine	Probably safe; observe for sedation and may suppress milk supply.
TheraFlu flu & cough nightTime maximum strength powder	Acetaminophen, Chlorpheniramine, Pseudoephedrine, Dextromethorphan	Probably safe; observe for sedation and may suppress milk supply.
TheraFlu flu & sore throat night time, maximum strength powder	Acetaminophen, Chlorpheniramine, Pseudoephedrine	Probably safe; observe for sedation and may suppress milk supply.
TheraFlu flu & sore throat, maximum strength powder	Acetaminophen, Chlorpheniramine, Pseudoephedrine	Probably safe; observe for sedation and may suppress milk supply.
TheraFlu flu, cold & cough and sore throat maximum strength powder	Acetaminophen, Chlorpheniramine, Pseudoephedrine, Dextromethorphan	Probably safe; observe for sedation and may suppress milk supply.
TheraFlu flu, cold	Acetaminophen,	Probably safe; observe

Cold Remedies

Trade Name	Ingredients	Comments
& cough nightTime maximum strength powder	Chlorpheniramine, Pseudoephedrine, Dextromethorphan	for sedation and may suppress milk supply.
TheraFlu flu, cold & cough powder	Acetaminophen, Chlorpheniramine, Pseudoephedrine, Dextromethorphan	Probably safe; observe for sedation and may suppress milk supply.
TheraFlu maximum strength flu & congestion non-drowsy powder	Acetaminophen, Guaifenesin, Pseudoephedrine, Dextromethorphan	Probably safe but may suppress milk supply.
TheraFlu maximum strength flu, cold & congestion powder	Acetaminophen, Guaifenesin, Pseudoephedrine, Dextromethorphan	Probably safe but may suppress milk supply.
TheraFlu maximum strength nightTime formula flu, cold & cough medicine	Acetaminophen, Chlorpheniramine, Pseudoephedrine, Dextromethorphan	Probably safe; observe for sedation and may suppress milk supply.
TheraFlu non-drowsy flu, cold & cough maximum strength powder	Acetaminophen, Pseudoephedrine, Dextromethorphan	Probably safe but may suppress milk supply.
TheraFlu non-drowsy formula maximum strength tablets	Acetaminophen, Pseudoephedrine, Dextromethorphan	Probably safe but may suppress milk supply.
TheraFlu severe cold & congestion nightTime maximum strength powder	Acetaminophen, Chlorpheniramine, Pseudoephedrine, Dextromethorphan	Probably safe; observe for sedation and may suppress milk supply.
TheraFlu severe cold & congestion non-drowsy maximum strength powder	Acetaminophen, Pseudoephedrine, Dextromethorphan	Probably safe but may suppress milk supply.
Triaminicin cold, allergy, sinus medicine tablets	Acetaminophen, Chlorpheniramine, Pseudoephedrine	Probably safe; observe for sedation and may suppress milk supply.
Triotann pediatric suspension	Chlorpheniramine, Pyrilamine, Phenylephrine	Probably safe; observe for sedation.
Tussend syrup	Chlorpheniramine, Pseudoephedrine, Hydrocodone	Probably safe; observe for sedation and may suppress milk supply.

Cold Remedies

Trade Name	Ingredients	Comments
Tussend tablets	Chlorpheniramine, Pseudoephedrine, Hydrocodone	Probably safe; observe for sedation and may suppress milk supply.
Tussi-12 tablets	Carbetapentane, Chlorpheniramine	Probably safe; observe for sedation.
Tussionex pennkinetic suspension	Chlorpheniramine, Hydrocodone	Probably safe; observe for sedation.
Tussi-Organidin-DM NR liquid	Guaifenesin, Dextromethorphan	Probably safe
Tylenol allergy sinus nightTime, maximum strength tablets	Acetaminophen, Diphenhydramine, Pseudoephedrine	Probably safe; observe for sedation and may suppress milk supply.
Tylenol allergy sinus, maximum strength tablets, gelcaps and geltabs	Acetaminophen, Chlorpheniramine, Pseudoephedrine	Probably safe; observe for sedation and may suppress milk supply.
Tylenol cold complete formula tablets	Acetaminophen, Chlorpheniramine, Pseudoephedrine, Dextromethorphan	Probably safe; observe for sedation and may suppress milk supply.
Tylenol cold non-drowsy formula gel-caps and tablets	Acetaminophen, Pseudoephedrine, Dextromethorphan	Probably safe but may suppress milk supply.
Tylenol flu maximum strentgh non-drowsy gelcaps	Acetaminophen, Pseudoephedrine, Dextromethorphan	Probably safe but may suppress milk supply.
Tylenol flu nightTime maximum strength liquid	Acetaminophen, Doxylamine, Pseudoephedrine, Dextromethorphan	Probably safe; observe for sedation and may suppress milk supply.
Tylenol flu nightTime, maximum strength gelcaps	Acetaminophen, Diphenhydramine, Pseudoephedrine	Probably safe; observe for sedation and may suppress milk supply.
Tylenol multi-symptom cold severe congestion tablets	Acetaminophen, Guaifenesin, Pseudoephedrine, Dextromethorphan	Probably safe but may suppress milk supply.
Tylenol PM extra strength tablets, gelcaps and geltabs	Acetaminophen, Diphenhydramine	Probably safe; observe for sedation.
Tylenol severe allergy tablets	Acetaminophen, Diphenhydramine	Probably safe; observe for sedation.

Cold Remedies

Trade Name	Ingredients	Comments
Tylenol sinus nightTime, maximum strength tablets	Acetaminophen, Doxylamine, Pseudoephedrine	Probably safe; observe for sedation and may suppress milk supply.
Tylenol sinus non-drowsy maximum strength geltabs, tablets and gelcaps	Acetaminophen, Pseudoephedrine	Probably safe but may suppress milk supply.
Vicks 44D cough & head congestion relief liquid	Pseudoephedrine, Dextromethorphan	Probably safe but may suppress milk supply.
Vicks 44E cough & chest congestion relief	Guaifenesin, Dextromethorphan	Probably safe
Vicks 44M cough, cold & flu relief liquid	Acetaminophen, Chlorpheniramine, Pseudoephedrine, Dextromethorphan	Probably safe; observe for sedation and may suppress milk supply.
Vicks DayQuil Liqui Caps Multisymptom Cold/Flu Relief Capsules	Acetaminophen, 0, Pseudoephedrine, Dextromethorphan	Probably safe but may suppress milk supply.
Vicks DayQuil multi-symptom cold/flu relief liquid	Acetaminophen, Pseudoephedrine, Dextromethorphan	Probably safe but may suppress milk supply.
Vicks NyQuil cough syrup	Doxylamine, Dextromethorphan	Probably safe; observe for sedation.
Vicks NyQuil multi-symptom cold & flu relief liquiCaps capsules	Acetaminophen, Doxylamine, Pseudoephedrine, Dextromethorphan	Probably safe; observe for sedation and may suppress milk supply.
Vicks NyQuil multi-symptom cold/flu relief liquid	Acetaminophen, Doxylamine, Pseudoephedrine, Dextromethorphan	Probably safe; observe for sedation and may suppress milk supply.
Vicodin Tuss syrup	Guaifenesin, Hydrocodone	Probably safe; observe for sedation.
Z-Cof DM syrup	Guaifenesin, Pseudoephedrine, Dextromethorphan	Probably safe but may suppress milk supply.
Zyrtec-D 12 hour tablets	Cetirizine, Pseudoephedrine	Probably safe but may suppress milk supply.

Nasal Products

Product Name	Ingredients	Safety
Nasal Spray	Sodium chloride 0.9%	Safe
Pretz Moisturizing		Safe
Afrin Saline, Extra Moisturizing		Safe
Simply Saline		Safe
Pretz Irrigation		Safe
SalineX	0.4% sodium chloride	Safe
Ayr Saline	0.65% sodium chloride	Safe
Breathe Free		Safe
HuMist Moisturizing Mist		Safe
NaSal		Safe
Nasal Moist		Safe
Ocean		Safe
Mycinaire Saline Mist		Safe
Rhinaris Lubricating Mist Solution	15% polyethylene glycol, 5% propylene glycol	Safe
Rhinaris Lubricating Mist Gel	15% polyethylene glycol, 20% propylene glycol	Safe
Nasalcrom Nasal Spray	Cromolyn sodium	Safe
Nasal-Ease with Zinc	Zinc Acetate	Safe
Nasal-Ease with Zinc Gluconate	Zinc Gluconate	Safe

Nasal Decongestants

Oxymetazoline HCl	Oxymetazoline 0.05%	Safe: observe for nervousness, insomnia, excitation.*
12 Hour Nasal		Safe: see above
Twice-A-Day 12 Hour Nasal		Safe: see above
Neo-Synephrine 12 Hour Extra Moisturizing		Safe: see above
Neo-Synephrine 12 Hour		Safe: see above

Nasal Decongestants

Duration	Oxymetazoline 0.05%	Safe: see above
Afrin 12 Hour Original Pump Mist		Safe: see above
Afrin 12 Hour Original		Safe: see above
Afrin Severe Congestion w/ Menthol		Safe: see above
Afrin Sinus with Vapornase		Safe: see above
Afrin No-Drip 12 Hour		Safe: see above
Afrin No-Drip 12 Hour Extra Moisturing		Safe: see above
Afrin No-Drip 12 Hour Severe Congestion w/ Menthol		Safe: see above
Afrin No-Drip Sinus w/ Vapornase		Safe: see above
Dristan 12 Hr. Nasal		Safe: see above
Duramist Plus 12 Hr. Decongestant		Safe: see above
Genasal		Safe: see above
Nasal Decongestant, Maximum Strength		Safe: see above
Nasal Relief		Safe: see above
Nostrilla 12 Hour		Safe: see above
Vicks Sinex 12 Hour Long-Acting		Safe: see above
Vicks Sinex 12 Hour Ultra Fine Mist for Sinus Relief		Safe: see above
Tyzine Pediatric	Tetrahydrozoline HCl 0.05%	Safe: see above
Tyzine	Tetrahydrozoline HCl 0.1%	Safe: see above
Otrivin Pediatric Nasal	Xylometazoline HCl 0.05%	Safe: see above
Natru-Vent		Safe: see above
Otrivin	Xylometazoline HCl 0.1%	Safe: see above
Natru-Vent		Safe: see above

Nasal Decongestants		
Dristan Fast Acting Formula	0.5% phenylephrine HCl and 0.2% pheniramine maleate	Safe: see above
Benzedrex	250 mg propylhexedrine	Unsafe
Vicks Vapor Inhaler	50 mg I-desoxyephedrine	Unsafe
Little Noses Gentle Formula, Infants & Children	Phenylephrine HCl 0.125%	Safe
Afrin Children's Pump Mist	Phenylephrine HCl 0.25%	Safe
Little Colds For Infants and Children		Safe
Neo-Synephrine 4-Hour Mild Formula		Safe
Rhinall		Safe
Neo Synephrine 4-Hour Regular Strength	Phenylephrine HCl 0.5%	Safe
Vicks Sinex Ultra Fine Mist		Safe
Phenylephrine HCl	Phenylephrine HCl 1%	Safe
4-Way Fast Acting		Safe
Neo-Synephrine 4-Hour Extra Strength		Safe
Adrenaline Chloride	Epinephrine HCl 1 mg/ml	Caution
Pretz-D	Ephedrine Sulfate 0.25%	Unsafe
Privine	Naphazoline HCl 0.05%	Safe

*Products with Oxymetazoline, Tetrahydrozoline, and Naphazoline should only be used briefly in breastfeeding mothers, if at all. If overdosed, breastfed infants could potentially be agitated and tremulous. Do not use in infants with hypertension or cardiac syndromes.

Radiologic Procedures and Dosing Ranges*

Procedure Name	Radiopharmaceutical	Dosing Range
Adrenocortical Scan	^{131}I-Iodomethyinorcholesterol	2 mCi
Bone scan	^{99}mTc-MDP, -HDP	<30 mCi
Bone marrow scan	^{99}mTc-SC	<20 mCi
Brain scan	^{99}mTc-D$_4$-, -DTPA, -GH	<20-30 mCi
Brain scan-SPECT	^{99}mTc-Ceretec^R or Neurolite^R	20-30 mCi
Cardiac first pass	^{99}mTc, Cardiolite^R or Myoview^R	7-30 mCi
Cardiac Studies	^{99}mTc, Cardiolite^R or Myoview^R	7- 30 mCi
Cardiac stress test	^{201}Tl	2.5-3.5 mCi
Cardiac dual-Isotope: Rest Stress Perfusion	^{201}Tl ^{99}mTc, Cardiolite^R or Myoview^R ^{99}mTc, Cardiotec^R	2-3 mCi 20 mCi
CEA-Scan^R	^{99}mTc-arcitumomab	20-30 mCi
Cisternogram	^{111}Indium-DTPA	0.5-1.5 mCi
Cystogram (voiding)	^{99}mTc-SC, ^{99}mTc-O$_4$-	0.5-1 mCi
Gallium scan for infections	^{67}Ga	5-10 mCi
Gallium scan (tumor)	^{67}Ga	5-10 mCi
Gastric emptying	^{99}mTc-SC	0.5-1 mCi
GI bleed	^{99}mTc-pyp-RBCs	20-30 mCi
HIDA (cholescintigraphy)	^{99}mTc-Choletec, Hepatolite,	3-5 mCi
Liver/spleen scan	^{99}mTc-SC (sulfur colloid)	2-4 mCi

Procedure Name	Radiopharmaceutical	Dosing Range
Liver SPECT (hemangioma)	^{99m}Tc-pyp-RBCs	20-30 mCi
Lung perfusion imaging	^{99m}Tc-MAA (microaggregated albumin)	2-4 mCi
Lung ventilation imaging	^{133}Xe	10-15 mCi
Lung ventilation imaging	^{99m}Tc-DTPA (labeled aerosol)	30 mCi
Lymphoscintigraphy	^{99m}Tc-SC	100-800 μCi
Meckel's diverticulum	^{99m}Tc-O$_4$-	10-15 mCi
MIBG (adrenal medulla)	^{131}I-MIBG	0.5 mCi
MUGA scan	^{99m}Tc-labeled-RBCs	20-30 mCi
Myocardial (MI) scan	^{99m}Tc-pyp	20-30 mCi
OctreoScan^R	^{111}In-pentetriotide	6 mCi
OncoScint^R	^{111}In-satumomab pendetide	4-6 mCi
Parathyroid scan Subtraction:	^{99m}Tc-Cardiolite^R ^{201}Tl ^{99m}Tc-D$_4$-	16-30 mCi 2-3 mCi 5-12 mCi
Pheochromocytoma scan	^{123}I and ^{131}I-mIBG ^{123}I ^{131}I	3-10 mCi 0.5-1 mCi
ProstaScint^R	^{111}In-CYT-356	5-17 mCi
Renal scan	^{99m}Tc-DTPA	10-15 mCi
Renal scan	^{99m}Tc-DMSA	3-10 mCi
Renal scan	^{99m}Tc-MAG3	3-10 mCi
Renogram	^{131}I-OIH	150-300 μCi
Schilling	B$_{12}$-^{57}Co	0.3-0.5 μCi
Scintimammography	^{99m}Tc-Cardiolite^R	20 mCi
Testicular scan	^{99m}TcO$_4$	0-25 mCi

Procedure Name	Radiopharmaceutical	Dosing Range
Thyroid ablation	^{131}I Sodium	30-300 mCi
Thyroid hyperthyroid therapy	^{131}I Sodium diffuse nodular	1-10 mCi <30 mCi
Thyroid uptake and scan	^{123}I ^{131}I	< 350 μCi < 100 μCi
Thyroid scan (substernal)	^{131}I	< 100 μCi
Thyroid scan	^{99}mTcO$_4$	1-2 mCi
WBC scan	^{99}mTc-WBC ^{99}mTc-Ceretec^R ^{111}In-WBC	10-15 mCi 10-24 mCi 500 μCi
Whole-body ^{131}I carcinoma work-up	^{131}I	1-5 mCi

* Please note that doses vary significantly from one source to another. These were partially derived from: Saha, GB. Fundamentals of Nuclear Pharmacy. Springer-Verlag, 1998.

Radioactive Diagnostic Procedures

Diagnostic Procedure	Isotope	Tracer	Dose (mCi)	Comments*
Cardiac perfusion and stress tests	^{201}Tl	Chloride	3+1	2 week interruption for 3 mCi
Infections	^{67}Ga	Citrate	5	1 month interruption for 4 mCi
			5	2 weeks interruption for 1.3 mCi
Tumors imaging				1 weeks interruption for 0.2 mCi
Lung ventilation	^{133}Xe	Gas	10-30	1 hour interruption for washout
Thyroid Diagnostic imaging – (post thyroidectomy	^{131}I	Sodium	5	Complete cessation of breast-feeding or count
Tumor Imaging	^{131}I	MIBG	1.5	
Renal Blood flow and clearance	^{131}I	Hippuran	0.25	

* Check Table 3. Activities of Radiopharmaceuticals from NRC for exact recommendations.

Radioactive Diagnostic Procedures				
Diagnostic Procedure	**Isotope**	**Tracer**	**Dose (mCi)**	**Comments***
Gastroesophageal emptying time-liquids	99mTc	Sulfur Colloid	1	6 hours for 12 mCi
Gastroesophageal emptying time for solids			0.5	6 hours for 12 mCi
SPECT Analysis – Liver			5	6 hours for 12 mCi
Biliary Atresia - Cholecystitis	99mTc	IDA derivative	5	
Perfusion studies of Lung	99mTc	MAA	3	12.6 hours for 4 mCi
CNS Perfusion Renal perfusion/filtration	99mTc	DTPA	30 10 or 20	No interruption for 30 mCi or less
Kidney parenchyma imaging kidney DTPA + DMSA	99mTc	DMSA glucoheptonate	5 10	

Radioactive Diagnostic Procedures				
Diagnostic Procedure	**Isotope**	**Tracer**	**Dose (mCi)**	**Comments***
Renal Blood Flow, Clearance	^{99m}Tc	MAG3	10	No interruption for 30 mCi or less
Bone – osteomyelitis	^{99m}Tc	MDP	20	No interruption for 30 mCi or less
Infections – labeled with HMPAO		WBC	3-10	24 hour interruption for 5 mCi 12 hour interruption for 2 mCi
Thyroid Imaging Scans	^{123}I	Sodium	0.4	Complete cessation of breast-feeding or until counts are baseline.
CSF – cisternogram, shunt patency **CSF** – shunt patency	^{111}In	DTPA	0.5 0.5	1 week interruption for 0.5 mCi
Infections	^{99m}Tc	WBC	0.5	1 week interruption for 0.5 mCi

B

C

D

E

F

G

I

J

K

L

M

O

P

R

Q

S

T

U

V

Ordering Information

Pharmasoft Publishing

1712 N. Forest

Amarillo, Texas, USA 79106-7017

8:00 AM to 5:00 PM CST

Call......	806-376-9900
Sales.....	800-378-1317
FAX......	806-376-9901

http://www.iBreastfeeding.com